Passport for the Orthop
Examination

Cyril Mauffrey • David J. Hak
Editors

Passport for the Orthopedic Boards and FRCS Examination

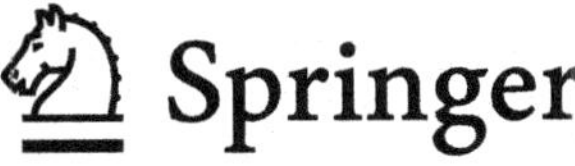

Editors
Cyril Mauffrey, MD, FACS, FRCS
Director of Orthopaedic Trauma
Denver Health Medical Center
Associate Professor of Orthopaedics
University of Colorado School of Medicine
Denver
USA

David J. Hak, MD, FACS, MBA
Department of Orthopaedic Surgery
Denver Health Medical Center
Professor of Orthopaedics
University of Colorado School of Medicine
Denver
USA

ISBN 978-2-8178-0563-4 ISBN 978-2-8178-0475-0 (eBook)
DOI 10.1007/978-2-8178-0475-0
Springer Paris Heidelberg New York Dordrecht London

Printed on acid-free paper

Springer is part of Springer Science+Business Media (www.springer.com)

'Success is the ability to go from one failure to another with no loss of enthusiasm'

Winston Churchill

We collectively dedicate this book to our hardworking residents from the University of Colorado School of Medicine.

This book is dedicated to my wife Marzia and daughters Oceane, Manon and Chiara. Their love and support is my engine. To my parents for leading the way by example.

Cyril Mauffrey

For Kimberly and Hailey, whose love and support make all things possible

David Hak

Contents

Part I
Anatomy and Surgical Approaches

David Seligson and Jason M. McKean

Upper Limb Anatomy and Surgical Approaches

Jason M. McKean and David Seligson

1 Shoulder

- Anterior (deltopectoral) Approach
  - Indications
    - Access to anterior glenohumeral joint, anterior glenoid, and proximal humerus
  - Superficial dissection
    - Internervous plane.
      - Deltoid (axillary nerve) and pectoralis major (medial and lateral pectoral nerves).
      - The cephalic vein can serve as a guide to delineate where the deltoid and pectoralis major meet.
    - Dangers
      - Cephalic vein is found in deltopectoral groove.
      - Multiple branches are found medially and laterally and need to be ligated or cauterized for hemostasis.

J.M. McKean, MD (✉)
Department of Orthopaedics, Lincoln Medical Center, Bronx, USA
e-mail: jasonmckean@gmail.com

D. Seligson, MD
Department of Orthopaedics, University of Louisville Hospital, Louisville, KY, USA
e-mail: seligson@louisville.edu

C. Mauffrey, D.J. Hak (eds.), *Passport for the Orthopedic Boards and FRCS Examination*, DOI 10.1007/978-2-8178-0475-0_1

- Deep dissection
  - Short head of biceps and coracobrachialis are retracted medially.
    - Both supplied by musculocutaneous nerve.
    - Both attach to the coracoid process as the conjoint tendon.
  - The subscapularis tendon is exposed deep to the deltoid (laterally) and the conjoint tendon (medially).
  - The subscapularis tendon can be elevated after incision through the lateral aspect of the tendon or an osteotomy of the lesser tuberosity of the proximal humerus.
  - The joint capsule is located just deep to the subscapularis.
  - Dangers
    - Musculocutaneous nerve.
      - Inserts into coracobrachialis and short head of biceps medially to each muscle.
      - Over-retraction of the conjoint tendon can put the nerve on stretch and cause injury.
    - Axillary nerve
      - Passes just below the subscapularis and wraps around the posterior proximal humerus, innervating the deltoid and teres minor.
      - Adducting the shoulder will help prevent injury to nerve by decreasing tension on nerve and keeping it more inferior to subscapularis.
      - Axillary sheath
        - Contains brachial plexus and axillary vessels.
        - Travels under the clavicle, medial to coracoid, deep to pectoralis minor, the short head of the biceps, and the coracobrachialis.
        - Extensive medial dissection or retraction can cause injury.

- <u>Lateral Approach</u>
  - Indications
    - Access to greater tuberosity and proximal humerus
    - Access to subacromial pathology
    - Repair of lateral rotator cuff tears
  - Superficial dissection
    - Internervous plane
      - No true internervous plane
      - Split the fibers of the deltoid longitudinally at the junction of the anterior 1/3 and posterior 2/3 of the muscle

- Deep dissection
  - Subacromial bursa is directly under the deltoid proximally.
    - Can be excised for better visualization of proximal humerus.
  - Insertion of supraspinatus to the greater tuberosity can be visualized.
    - Access to the supraspinatus tendon can be difficult as the tendon is significantly retracted medially.
  - Dangers
    - Axillary nerve
      - The nerve travels through the quadrilateral space (medial, long head of triceps; lateral, humerus; superior, teres minor; inferior, teres major) and then wraps around humerus with posterior circumflex arteries.
      - The axillary nerve enters the deltoid slightly posteriorly, approximately 7 cm inferior to the acromion.
      - Placing a stay suture at the inferior apex of the deltoid split to prevent unintentional distal dissection and axillary nerve damage.

- <u>Posterior (Judet) Approach</u>
  - Indications
    - Access to posterior glenohumeral joint
    - Access to scapula
  - Superficial dissection
    - Internervous plane
      - Deltoid (axillary nerve) and the infraspinatus (suprascapular nerve)
    - Detach origin of deltoid off the scapular spine
      - The plane between the deltoid and the infraspinatus is easier to appreciate more laterally.
  - Deep dissection
    - Internervous plane
      - Infraspinatus (suprascapular nerve) and the teres minor (axillary nerve).
      - The infraspinatus should be retracted superiorly and the teres minor should be retracted inferiorly.
    - The posteroinferior aspect of the glenohumeral joint capsule is then exposed.
    - Joint capsule should be incised longitudinally.
    - Dangers

- Axillary nerve
  - The nerve courses through the quadrilateral space under the teres minor, so it is important to stay superior to teres minor and exploit the interval between the infraspinatus and teres minor.
- Suprascapular nerve
  - The nerve courses under the suprascapular ligament as it passes through the suprascapular notch, then around the base of the scapular spine as it descends from the supraspinatus fossa to the infraspinatus fossa.
  - Innervates both the supraspinatus and the infraspinatus.
  - Aggressive medial retraction should be avoided to prevent stretching of the nerve.

2 Arm

- Anterior Approach
  - Indications
    - Access to humerus and anterior structures of the arm
  - Superficial dissection
    - Essentially this is a distal extension of the deltopectoral approach.
    - Internervous plane
      - Proximally
        - Deltoid (axillary nerve) and pectoralis major (medial and lateral pectoral nerves)
      - Distally
        - Lateral fibers of brachialis muscle (radial nerve) and medial fibers of brachialis muscle (musculocutaneous nerve)
    - The deltoid inserts into the deltoid tuberosity distally and laterally to the insertion of the pectoralis major.
    - The belly of the brachialis is distal and medial to the insertion of the deltoid.
    - The brachialis is exposed by developing the interval between it and the biceps brachii, then retracting the biceps medially.
  - Deep dissection
    - The pectoralis major tendon covers the bicipital groove and inserts into the humerus lateral to groove.
      - This insertion may need to be partially elevated subperiosteally to gain access to proximal third of humeral shaft.

- The brachialis fibers should be split longitudinally along the midline to preserve the innervation medially and laterally.
  - Flexing the elbow will relieve some tension of the fibers to assist with retraction and exposure of the anterior humerus.
- Dangers
  - Anterior circumflex humeral vessels
    - Encountered deep between the deltoid and pectoralis major in the proximal humerus.
    - Vessels need to be either ligated or cauterized.
  - Radial nerve
    - Proximally
      - Primarily a posterior structure in the proximal two thirds of the humerus.
      - Courses along the spiral groove and exits the groove 10–14 cm proximal to the lateral epicondyle
      - Despite being located posteriorly, the nerve can be damaged during an anterior approach by retractors, drill bits, and depth gauges.
      - To minimize risk, stay subperiosteal during dissection and retractor placement.
    - Distally
      - The nerve courses anterior as it pierces the lateral intermuscular septum between the triceps and the brachialis.
      - It enters the anterior compartment of the arm between the brachioradialis and the brachialis muscles (approximately 7.5–10 cm proximal to distal articular surface of humerus).
      - If the brachialis is split along the midline, the lateral portion will protect the radial nerve during retraction.
  - Axillary nerve
    - Courses deep to deltoid and wraps around posterior and lateral to proximal humerus
    - At risk during vigorous retraction of deltoid

- <u>Anterolateral Approach</u>
  - Indications
    - Provides better exposure to distal humerus than direct anterior approach
  - Superficial dissection
    - Internervous plane
      - No true internervous plane.
      - The brachioradialis and the lateral half of the brachialis are both innervated by the radial nerve.

    - Retracting the biceps medially will expose the brachialis medially and the brachioradialis laterally.
    - The radial nerve is found between the brachialis and the brachioradialis.
      - Bluntly dissect this interval.
      - Identify and protect the radial nerve.
      - The nerve can be traced proximally to where it pierces the lateral intermuscular septum.
    - Deep dissection
      - Internervous plane
        - There is no internervous plane at this level.
      - Carry out dissection medial to radial nerve.
      - The lateral aspect of the brachialis is incised, and bony anatomy of the distal anterior humeral shaft is revealed.
  - Dangers
    - Superficially
      - Lateral cutaneous nerve of the forearm
        - Branches off the musculocutaneous nerve and surfaces from between the brachialis and the biceps brachii
        - Strictly sensory in function and innervates the radial aspect of the forearm
    - Deep
      - The radial nerve must be identified and protected in the lateral aspect of the dissection.
- <u>Lateral Approach</u>
  - Indications
    - Access to lateral condyle of distal humerus
  - Superficial
    - Internervous plane
      - There is no true internervous plane.
      - Both the triceps brachii and the brachioradialis muscle are innervated by the radial nerve.
    - Dissection can be carried down straight to bone after identifying the plane between the brachioradialis and the triceps.
  - Deep dissection
    - Internervous plane

  - Proximally there is no internervous plane as described above.
  - If the exposure needs to extend distally to reveal the radiocapitellar joint, then the anconeus (radial nerve) can be retracted posteriorly, while the extensor carpi ulnaris (posterior interosseous nerve) can be retracted anteriorly.
    - This is essentially extending the lateral humerus approach into the posterolateral elbow approach.
 - The brachioradialis is retracted anteriorly and the triceps posteriorly.
 - The common extensor origin is found on the lateral epicondyle and can be taken down as needed for exposure.
- Dangers
 - The distal exposure is free of significant neurovascular structures.
 - The radial nerve must be identified and protected if proximal extension of this approach is to be performed.

- <u>Posterior Approach</u>
  - Indications
    - Provides access to the distal three fourths of the humerus
    - Ideal approach for exploring radial nerve in spiral groove
  - Superficial dissection
    - Internervous plane
      - There is no internervous plane.
        - The dissection goes directly through the triceps brachii.
        - Innervation of the triceps is by the radial nerve, and the nerve enters the muscle proximally at its origin.
        - The medial head of the triceps receives contributing innervation from the ulnar nerve as well.
        - Splitting the muscle longitudinally does not cause denervation from either source.
      - The triceps brachii has two layers.
        - The outer layer has two heads.
          - Lateral head originates from lateral lip of spiral groove.
          - Long head originates off the infraglenoid tubercle of the scapula.
        - The inner layer
          - Medial (deep) head originates over the entire width of the posterior humerus distal to the spiral groove.

  - Dissection of the outer layer is best done starting proximal to where they form a confluent tendon.
    - Interval can be developed with blunt dissection.
    - Several smaller vessels cross the muscle more distally and need to cauterized.
- Deep dissection
  - The deep (medial) head of the triceps lies deep to the outer two heads.
  - The radial nerve passes around the posterolateral aspect of the humerus just proximal to the origin of the deep head.
  - Dissection through the medial head should be midline and down to the periosteum, and any further dissection medial or lateral should be done subperiosteal to prevent injury of the radial nerve proximally and the ulnar nerve medially.
    - The ulnar nerve pierces the medial intermuscular septum as it passes from anterior to posterior.
- Dangers
  - Radial nerve
    - Dissection to bone in the proximal two thirds of the humerus should not be performed until the nerve has been identified and protected.
  - Ulnar nerve
    - Courses deep to the medial head of the triceps in distal third of arm.
    - Dissection must be done subperiosteally in this region to prevent injury.

3 Elbow

- Posterolateral (Kocher) Approach
  - Indications
    - Access to the radiocapitellar joint
  - Superficial dissection
    - Internervous plane
      - Anconeus (radial nerve) and the extensor carpi ulnaris (posterior interosseous nerve).

    - The interval between the anconeus and the extensor carpi ulnaris is easier to appreciate more distally as the two muscles share a common aponeurosis proximally.
      - A fat stripe sometimes helps define the interval.
    - Releasing the proximal aspect of the anconeus where it attaches to the lateral epicondyle of the humerus will aid in exposure.
  - Deep dissection
    - There is no internervous plane in the deep dissection.
      - The supinator (posterior interosseous nerve) is traversed to gain access to the joint.
    - The posterolateral aspect of the supinator is incised to expose the joint capsule.
      - The arm should be pronated during the deep dissection to protect the posterior interosseous nerve and move it further from the operative field.
    - The joint capsule is incised longitudinally to expose the radial head, capitellum, and annular ligament.
      - This should be done about 1 cm above the supinator crest which will keep the incision at the anterior border of the lateral ulnar collateral ligament.
  - Dangers
    - Posterior interosseous nerve
      - Staying proximal to the annular ligament and pronation of the forearm will help to protect the nerve.
      - Keep retractors subperiosteal in this region.
    - Radial nerve
      - Close in proximity to operative field (anterior to elbow joint).
      - Open capsule laterally and not anteriorly to prevent injury.
    - Lateral collateral ligament complex
      - Lies below the equator of the capitellum.
      - Preservation of this complex will prevent instability of the elbow.
- <u>Lateral (Kaplan) Approach</u>
  - Indications
    - Access to radiocapitellar joint
      - Avoids the lateral ulnar collateral ligament complex

- Superficial dissection
  - Internervous plane
    - No true internervous plane as there is dual innervation in both interval muscles
      - Extensor digitorum communis (posterior interosseous nerve with some contribution from radial nerve) and extensor carpi radialis brevis (posterior interosseous nerve with some contribution from radial nerve)
  - The interval is easier to define distally.
  - The extensor carpi radialis brevis is retracted anteriorly and the extensor digitorum communis is retracted posteriorly.
- Deep dissection
  - Internervous plane
    - There is no internervous plane.
  - The supinator can be released to gain better exposure.
  - Often the annular ligament is split, but the lateral ulnar collateral ligament remains intact so there is not instability of the elbow.
- Dangers
  - Posterior interosseous nerve
    - The lateral approach puts the posterior interosseous nerve at more of a risk than the posterolateral approach as it puts the surgical field more anterior.
    - The forearm should be pronated to protect the nerve as much as possible.
    - Aberrant retractor placement can cause nerve injury in this approach.

- <u>Medial Approach</u>
  - Indications
    - Provides access to the ulnohumeral joint, the coronoid, and the medial humeral condyle/epicondyle.
  - Superficial dissection
    - Internervous plane
      - Proximally the plane is between the brachialis muscle (musculocutaneous nerve) and the triceps muscle (radial nerve).
      - Distally the plane is between the brachialis muscle (musculocutaneous nerve) and the pronator teres (medial nerve).

        - The medial antebrachial cutaneous nerve is found superficially in the fascia anterior to the medial intermuscular septum.
          - Protect to prevent postoperative a neuroma.
        - The superficial dissection should start with identifying and isolating the ulnar nerve.
          - The nerve courses posterior to the medial intermuscular septum just proximal to the elbow joint then wraps around the posterior aspect of the medial epicondyle.
          - Without significant swelling, the nerve can be palpated subcutaneously before an incision is made.
        - Proximally define the plane between the brachialis and the triceps.
          - The medial intermuscular septum is a stout structure that helps delineate this plane.
        - Distally develop the interval between the pronator teres and the brachialis muscles.
          - The median nerve enters the pronator teres near the midline of the anterior proximal forearm.
        - The medial epicondyle can be osteotomized for maximum exposure.
        - The pronator teres is retracted medially.
      - Medial (Hotchkiss) Approach
        - Similar to interval described above
          - Primary difference is that the medial epicondyle is not osteotomized.
          - The deep interval is between the pronator teres and the flexor carpi ulnaris along with the remainder of the flexor pronator group.
          - The pronator teres is elevated from its origin leaving a cuff of tissue for later repair.
          - Pronator is retracted laterally exposing the anterior elbow.
      - Deep dissection
        - Incise the capsule and expose the joint.
      - Dangers
        - Medial antebrachial cutaneous nerve
          - Encountered early in the dissection before reaching the muscular anatomy
        - Ulnar nerve
          - Must be identified at the start of the dissection and protected throughout the case

- Median nerve
  - Vulnerable to traction injury due to its multiple branches to the pronator teres.
  - The anterior interosseous nerve is its major branch and can also be injured during over-aggressive retraction.

- Posterior Approach
  - Indications
    - Excellent exposure to entire elbow joint.
    - Depending on the objectives of the surgery and surgeon's comfort level, there are different methods of exposure of the posterior elbow.
      - Olecranon osteotomy
        - Exposes 57 % of joint
        - Potential for nonunion at site of osteotomy
      - Triceps reflecting
        - Exposes 46 % of joint
      - Triceps splitting
        - Exposes 35 % of joint
  - Superficial dissection
    - Internervous plane
      - There is no internervous plane.
    - The first structure to identify and protect is the ulnar nerve on the medial aspect of the elbow joint as it courses posterior to the medial epicondyle.
  - Olecranon osteotomy
    - Score the olecranon longitudinally with an osteotome to have a reference point for anatomic rotational reduction when repairing osteotomy.
    - Make a chevron osteotomy at midpoint of the olecranon fossa with an oscillating saw approximately 2 cm distal the tip with the apex pointing distally.
    - Use osteotome to complete cut in order to create slight irregularity that can be fit together at the end of the procedure when reducing the osteotomy.
    - Release the soft tissue attached to the olecranon tip to allow reflection and exposure of the joint.
    - Elevate the deep head of the triceps from the posterior humerus.
      - Proximally beyond the distal fourth of the humerus, the radial nerve will be encountered.

- Triceps reflecting
  - After isolating the ulnar nerve, a periosteal elevator is used to remove the triceps muscle off the distal humerus medial to lateral.
  - The triceps tendon, olecranon periosteum, and forearm fascia are retracted medial to lateral.
    - The triceps tendon is sharply dissected off the olecranon.
    - A wafer of bone can be lifted off the olecranon to facilitate bone-to-bone healing instead of tendon-to-bone healing.
    - The extensor mechanism and the posterior capsule are reflected as a single unit.
    - The elbow is flexed to expose the joint.
    - Extensor mechanism repair
      - Two transosseous drill holes in a crossed fashion and one in a transverse fashion.
      - The tendon is held down with nonabsorbable suture.
- Triceps splitting
  - After isolating and protecting the ulnar nerve, a longitudinal incision is made in the proximal triceps tendon and extended to the olecranon.
  - The anconeus is reflected subperiosteally and laterally off the proximal ulna, and the flexor carpi ulnaris is reflected medially off the proximal ulna.
  - Alternatively the musculotendinous junction can be incised in an inverted V shape so it can later be repaired in a V to Y fashion if lengthening is needed (capsular release in stiff elbow).
    - The tendon is then repaired with nonabsorbable suture.
- Dangers
  - Ulnar nerve
    - Isolate and protect throughout the surgery to prevent traction or compression injury during manipulation of elbow.
  - Median nerve
    - Lies anterior to distal humerus.
    - Staying subperiosteal in the anterior dissection will prevent injury.
  - Radial nerve
    - At risk if dissection is performed more proximally than the distal third of the humerus.

- <u>Anterior Approach</u>
  - Indications
    - Access to

    – Distal biceps tendon
    – Radial nerve
    – Median nerve
    – Brachial artery
    – Anterior elbow joint

– Superficial dissection

  • Internervous plane

    – Proximally

      • Brachioradialis (radial nerve) and brachialis (musculocutaneous nerve)

    – Distally

      • Brachioradialis (radial nerve) and pronator teres (median nerve)

  • Numerous veins lie superficially and need to be ligated.
  • Lateral cutaneous nerve of the forearm (branch of the musculocutaneous nerve) emerges from between the biceps tendon and the brachialis.
  • Incise the bicipital aponeurosis close to its biceps tendon origin and reflect it laterally.

    – The bicipital aponeurosis, also referred to as the lacertus fibrosus, connects the biceps tendon to the medial fascia covering the flexor wad.

  • The radial artery is deep to the bicipital aponeurosis and superficial to the biceps tendon.

    – Trace radial artery up to the brachial artery proximally.

  • The median nerve lies medial to the radial artery.
  • The radial nerve courses between the brachialis and the brachioradialis.

    – Radial nerve branches into posterior interosseous nerve and superficial radial nerve just proximal to elbow joint.

– Deep dissection

  • This approach is primarily used for access to the neurovascular structures.
  • Retracting the biceps and brachialis muscles medially and the brachioradialis muscle laterally will expose the supinator.
  • Fully supinating the forearm will place the posterior interosseous nerve in a relatively protected position under the supinator.
  • Elevating the supinator subperiosteally laterally will expose the anterior capsule and the biceps tubercle (insertion of distal biceps tendon).

– Dangers

  • Lateral cutaneous nerve of the forearm

- At risk during incision of the deep fascia
- Found emerging from between the biceps tendon and the brachialis

- Radial artery
  - Found just deep to bicipital aponeurosis.
  - Avoid injury while incising bicipital aponeurosis.
- Posterior interosseous nerve
  - Branches off the radial nerve and wraps around neck of radius within the muscle of the supinator.
  - Keep forearm in supination while detaching insertion of supinator.

4 Forearm

- Volar (Henry) Approach to Radial Shaft
  - Indications
    - Utilitarian approach to radius
  - Superficial dissection
    - Internervous plane
      - Proximally brachioradialis (radial nerve) and pronator teres (median nerve)
      - Distally brachioradialis (radial nerve) and flexor carpi radialis (median nerve)
    - The interval is easier to appreciate distally; therefore dissection should start distally and progress proximally.
    - The superficial radial nerve branches off the radial nerve just proximal to the elbow joint and runs distally under the brachioradialis.
      - Preserve this sensory nerve to prevent postoperative numbness and neuroma.
    - Proximally the brachioradialis receives arterial branches from the radial artery (recurrent radial artery) just distal to the elbow.
      - Ligate this recurrent vessel so the brachioradialis is free to move laterally.
    - The radial artery is beneath the brachioradialis in the mid forearm.
  - Deep dissection
    - Distal third

    - The flexor pollicis longus and the pronator quadratus originate on the anterior aspect of the radius.
    - Sharply dissect the periosteum at the distal anterior radius and elevate the pronator quadratus along with the flexor pollicis longus from the radial side and retract them ulnarly.
  - Middle third
    - Pronator teres and flexor digitorum superficialis muscles cover the anterior radius in the middle third of the forearm.
    - Pronating the forearm takes some tension off the pronator teres, and the insertion can be better appreciated on the lateral aspect of the radius.
    - Sharply elevate the muscle subperiosteally and retract ulnarly to access the bone surface.
  - Proximal third
    - Incision of a small bursa just lateral to the distal biceps insertion to the bicipital tuberosity will give access to the proximal radius.
    - The radial artery is superficial and medial to the biceps tendon.
    - The supinator covers the proximal radius with the posterior interosseous nerve coursing through the muscle.
    - Fully supinating the forearm will bring the nerve lateral and away from the surgical field, as well as expose the insertion of the supinator on the anterior aspect of the proximal radius.
    - To expose the proximal radius, incise the supinator at its origin ulnarly and elevate subperiosteally and retract laterally.
      - Refrain from placing retractors on the posterior aspect of the radial neck to prevent iatrogenic nerve palsy.
- Dangers
  - Radial artery
    - Most vulnerable structure during aspects of the approach
      - Mobilizing the brachioradialis puts the artery at risk due to the recurrent radial branches and the small gauge of the vessel after exsanguination and tourniquet use.
      - The artery lies just medial to the distal biceps tendon, so it is important to stay lateral to biceps tendon during the proximal dissection.
  - Recurrent radial arteries
    - Feed into the brachioradialis in the proximal forearm.
    - There are two groups, one anterior to the superficial radial nerve and one posterior to the nerve.
      - Both must be ligated for immobilization of the nerve, radial artery, and brachioradialis.

- Posterior interosseous nerve
  - In order to adequately protect the nerve, the supinator must be elevated subperiosteally at its origin when the arm is fully supinated.
- Superficial radial nerve
  - Courses distally along the forearm just deep to the brachioradialis.
  - Nerve is at risk for a stretch or crush injury during lateral retraction of the "mobile wad" (brachioradialis, extensor carpi radialis brevis, extensor carpi radialis longus).

- <u>Dorsal (Thompson) Approach to Radial Shaft</u>
- Indications
  - Access to dorsal aspect of entire radius.
    - Radius is more superficial dorsally.
- Superficial dissection
  - Internervous plane
    - Proximally
      - Extensor carpi radialis brevis (radial nerve) and extensor digitorum communis (posterior interosseous nerve)
    - Distally
      - Extensor carpi radialis brevis (radial nerve) and extensor pollicis longus (posterior interosseous nerve)
  - Develop plane between extensor carpi radialis brevis and extensor digitorum communis
    - Plane is more obvious distally where the abductor pollicis longus and the extensor pollicis brevis emerge from between the two muscles.
    - Proximally the two muscles come together into a common aponeurosis.
  - Continue the dissection proximally to expose the supinator lying deep in this interval
- Deep dissection
  - Proximal third
    - The supinator covers the dorsal aspect of the proximal radius
      - The posterior interosseous nerve runs within the muscle proximally and then emerges about 1 cm proximal to the distal edge of the muscle.
      - The nerve then divides and enters the extensors of the wrist, fingers, and thumb.

        - After identification of the nerve, fully supinate the forearm and release the insertion of the supinator from the radius subperiosteally to expose the proximal radial shaft.

    - Middle third

        - The abductor pollicis longus and the extensor pollicis brevis cover the radius in this region.
        - Elevate subperiosteally under the muscle bellies proximally and distally along the mid shaft, and these muscles can then be mobilized for access to bony anatomy.

    - Distal third

        - Separating the extensor carpi radialis brevis from the extensor pollicis longus gives direct access to the radius.

- Dangers

    - Posterior interosseous nerve

        - Identification of the nerve can be difficult due to the variable branching and small caliber of the branches at the distal edge of the supinator.
        - During initial approach going from superficial to deep dissection the arm should be pronated to keep the nerve distally and more radial.

- <u>Ulnar Shaft Approach</u>

    - Indications

        - Utilitarian access to the ulnar shaft

    - Superficial dissection

        - Internervous plane

            - Distal

                - Extensor carpi ulnaris (posterior interosseous nerve) and flexor carpi ulnaris (ulnar nerve)

            - Proximal

                - Anconeus (radial nerve) and flexor carpi ulnaris (ulnar nerve)

        - Begin distally where the bone is nearly subcutaneous.
        - In the middle third, some fibers of the flexor carpi ulnaris need to be divided to reach the bone.

    - Deep dissection

        - Incise periosteum longitudinally and elevate dorsally or volarly.
        - Very proximally the broad insertion of the triceps will need to be elevated for exposure as needed.

- Dangers
  - Ulnar nerve
    - Courses between the flexor carpi ulnar and the flexor digitorum profundus.
    - Nerve is safe if dissection remains subperiosteal.
    - Most at risk during proximal dissection.

5 Wrist

- Dorsal Approach
  - Indications
    - Access to extensor tendons
    - Access to dorsal distal radius
    - Access to dorsal wrist joints
  - Superficial dissection
    - Internervous plane
      - No true internervous plane.
      - The interval used at this level is primarily between tendons and musculotendinous junctions.
        - Innervations of these muscles are proximal, so exploiting these intervals is safe.
    - Different intervals can be used depending on the intent of the surgery.
  - Deep dissection
    - A common interval is between the third compartment (extensor pollicis longus) and the fourth compartment (extensor digitorum communis and extensor indicis).
      - The third compartment is released, and the extensor pollicis longus is retracted radially.
      - The fourth compartment is elevated subperiosteally.
        - More compartments can be elevated as needed.
  - Dangers
    - Superficial radial nerve
      - Emerges from the beneath the tendon of the brachioradialis just proximal to the wrist joint.
      - Taking the incision down to retinaculum before dissecting radially and ulnarly usually protects the nerve as is dwells within the subcutaneous fat.

- Posterior interosseous nerve
  - Found deep to fourth extensor compartment

- Volar approach to distal radius
  - Indications
    - Access to volar distal radius
  - Superficial dissection
    - Internervous plane
      - No internervous plane
  - Deep dissection
    - Anterior forearm approach
      - The interval is between the flexor carpi radialis and the radial artery.
      - Complicated by branches of radial artery crossing the field.
    - Flexor Carpi Radialis Approach
      - The flexor carpi radialis sheath is opened, and the tendon is retracted radially.
      - The floor of the tendon sheath is incised longitudinally on the radial aspect (to avoid the palmar cutaneous branch of the median nerve).
      - The flexor pollicis longus is found deep to the sheath.
      - Sharply dissect the periosteum at the distal anterior radial border of the radius and elevate the pronator quadratus along with the flexor pollicis longus and retract them ulnarly.
    - Dangers
      - Palmar cutaneous branch of median nerve
        - Injury to this cutaneous branch can cause a painful neuroma or complex regional pain syndrome.
        - Emerges from the median nerve 5 cm proximal to the palmar flexion crease.
        - The branch travels along the ulnar border of the flexor carpi radialis sheath for 3 cm before approaching the dermis for innervation.

6 Hand and Wrist

6.1 Carpal Approaches

- Carpal tunnel
  - Indications
    - Open carpal tunnel release
    - Perilunate dislocations

- Superficial dissection
  - Location of incision varies.
  - Divide volar fascia longitudinally to expose transverse carpal ligament.
- Deep dissection
  - Longitudinally incise the transverse carpal ligament and the antebrachial fascia found distally to enter the carpal tunnel.
    - A volar fat pad distal to the transverse carpal ligament acts as a landmark to signify where the carpal tunnel release should stop.
- Dangers
  - Median nerve
    - Staying ulnar while incising the transverse carpal ligament will protect palmar cutaneous branch of the nerve.
  - Preservation of crossing nerves during superficial dissection above the transverse carpal ligament has not shown to improve postoperative scar pain.

- <u>Guyon Canal Approach</u>
  - Indications
    - Access to ulnar nerve and ulnar artery at the level of the wrist
    - Access to pisotriquetral joint, pisiform, and hook of hamate
  - Superficial
    - Preserve superficial branches of the ulnar nerve subcutaneously.
    - Divide palmaris brevis muscle and volar carpal ligament longitudinally in distal aspect of wound.
      - This exposes the ulnar nerve.
    - Divide the antebrachial fascia proximally.
    - The pisiform is located in the tendon of the flexor carpi ulnaris and can be shelled out subperiosteally as needed.
  - Deep dissection
    - Divide the fibrous arch at the origin of the hypothenar muscles.
      - This provides access to the motor branch of the ulnar nerve.
      - The main motor branch courses adjacent to the distal aspect of the hook of hamate as it travels laterally to innervate the interossei.

- Dangers
    - Motor branch of abductor digiti quinti
        - Runs distal and medial around the pisiform
    - Motor branch of ulnar nerve

- Dorsal Midline Approach
    - Indications
        - Utilitarian approach to carpus
    - Superficial dissection
        - Dissection is performed down to retinaculum before raising flaps.
        - Identify extensor pollicis longus ulnar to the Lister tubercle in the third dorsal compartment and released.
        - Elevate the fourth dorsal compartment subperiosteally.
        - The third and second dorsal compartments can be elevated radially.
    - Deep dissection
        - After elevating the dorsal compartments away from the midline, the following structures are revealed:
            - Dorsal radiocarpal joint capsule
            - Dorsal intercarpal ligament
            - Dorsal radiocarpal ligament
        - Use an inverted T capsule incision to further expose carpus by incising along the dorsal radial cuff and dorsal radioulnar ligament.
            - This provides access to the radial styloid, triangular fibrocartilage complex, and both carpal rows.
            - The pisiform and trapezium are not accessible from this approach.
    - Dangers
        - Superficial dorsal radial nerve
            - Branches cross at distal incision
        - Superficial dorsal ulnar nerve
            - Branches cross at distal incision

- Dorsolunar Approach
    - Indications
        - Access to ulnar-sided proximal carpal row and triangular fibrocartilage complex

- Superficial dissection
  - Dissect down over the distal radioulnar joint.
  - Divide the extensor retinaculum.
    - Either open the fifth dorsal compartment or divide between the fifth and sixth dorsal compartments.
  - Perform a capsulotomy to expose the joint.
- Dangers
  - Dorsal sensory branch of the ulnar nerve
    - Found subcutaneously during approach
  - Dorsal radioulnar ligament
    - Preserve this structure to prevent distal radioulnar joint instability.

- Scaphoid Approach (Volar)
  - Indications
    - Scaphoid waist fractures and nonunions
      - Able to correct humpback deformity easier than dorsal approach.
      - Preserve dorsal blood supply.
  - Superficial dissection
    - Open sheath of flexor carpi radialis and retract tendon ulnarly.
    - Longitudinally incise floor of sheath and capsule.
  - Deep dissection
    - Incise radioscaphocapitate and long radiolunate ligaments for exposure of the scaphoid waist and proximal pole.
    - To expose the distal pole of the scaphoid, perform a volar radial transverse capsulotomy in the scaphotrapezial joint.
    - Repair volar ligaments at the end of the case.
  - Dangers
    - Superficial branch of the radial nerve

6.2 Metacarpals

- Dorsal Approach
  - Indications
    - Utilitarian approach

- Superficial dissection
  - Dissection occurs either radial or ulnar to extensor tendons.
  - If two adjacent metacarpals need to be exposed, then a single incision can be used for both.
  - The metacarpals are subcutaneous dorsally.
- Dangers
  - Superficial branch of the radial nerve or dorsal sensory branch of ulnar nerve
    - Depends on which metacarpal is being exposed.
    - Retract during approach to protect.

6.3 Phalanges

- Dorsal Approach
  - Indications
    - Utilitarian approach
  - Superficial dissection
    - Middle and proximal phalanges
      - Dissection of the extensor mechanism is performed for exposure of bony anatomy.
        - Extensor mechanism can be split longitudinally over the proximal or middle phalanges.
        - The extensor mechanism can also be elevated by incising the transverse retinacular ligaments at the proximal interphalangeal joint and retracting the extensor mechanism radially or ulnarly.
  - Distal phalanges and distal interphalangeal joint
    - The distal phalanx is essentially subcutaneous.
    - Perform capsulotomy in the interval between the collateral ligament and the terminal tendon.
  - Dangers
    - Germinal matrix
      - Distal extension of incisions must avoid the germinal matrix and eponychial fold.
      - The average distance from terminal extensor insertion to the proximal edge of the germinal matrix is about 1.2 mm.
    - Terminal tendon insertion
      - Preserve insertion to prevent postoperative deformity.

Bibliography

1. Catalano LW, Zlotolow DA, Hitchcock PB, Shah SN, Barron OA. Surgical exposures of the radius and ulna. J Am Acad Orthop Surg. 2011;19:430–8.
2. Cheung EV, Steinmann SP. Surgical approaches to the elbow. J Am Acad Orthop Surg. 2009;17:325–33.
3. Hoppenfeld S, deBoer P, Buckley R. Surgical exposures in orthopaedics. The anatomic approach. 4th ed. Philadelphia: Lippincott Williams & Wilkins; 2009.
4. Zlotolow DA, Catalano LW, Barron OA, Glickel SZ. Surgical exposures of the humerus. J Am Acad Orthop Surg. 2006;14:754–65.

Lower Limb Anatomy and Surgical Approaches

Jason M. McKean, John Riehl, and David Seligson

1 Pelvis

- Approach to the anterior pelvic ring
  - Indications
    - Access to pubic symphysis and superior pubic ramus
  - Superficial dissection
    - Internervous plane
      - No internervous plane
      - Rectus abdominis muscles receive segmental innervation so they are not denervated
    - Incise through subcutaneous fat down to rectus sheath
    - Ligate superficial epigastric arteries and veins
    - Split the rectus muscles vertically along the midline raphe
  - Deep dissection
    - Develop the space of Retzius with blunt dissection

J.M. McKean, MD (✉)
Department of Orthopaedics, Lincoln Medical Center, Bronx, USA
e-mail: jasonmckean@gmail.com

J. Riehl, MD
Department of Orthopaedics, Andrews Institute for Orthopaedics, Pensacola, USA
e-mail: jtriehl@hotmail.com

D. Seligson, MD
Department of Orthopaedics, University of Louisville Hospital, Louisville, KY, USA
e-mail: seligson@louisville.edu

C. Mauffrey, D.J. Hak (eds.), *Passport for the Orthopedic Boards and FRCS Examination*, DOI 10.1007/978-2-8178-0475-0_2

        - Subperiosteally dissect superior pubic ramus to reveal the symphysis and pubic crest
    - Dangers
        - Bladder
            - Mobilization of space of Retzius (anterior to bladder and posterior to pubic symphysis) may be dangerous if there are adhesions present
        - Corona mortis
            - Anastomosis between external iliac and obturator vessels
            - These vessels vary in size but are fairly consistently present
            - Ligate as they course over the lateral third of the superior pubic ramus
- <u>Anterior approach to sacroiliac (SI) joint</u>
    - Indications
        - Access to anterior sacroiliac joint
    - Superficial dissection
        - Internervous plane
            - No internervous plane
        - Incision in line with iliac crest and continues anteromedially beyond anterior superior iliac spine
        - Incise through subcutaneous fat down to iliac crest
        - The deep fascia can be elevated off the crest with subperiosteal elevation along the inner table of the pelvis, or an osteotomy of the iliac crest can be performed for bony healing after closure
    - Deep dissection
        - Raise the iliacus muscle subperiosteally off the inner wall of the ilium heading medially until the sacroiliac joint is exposed
            - Hip flexion can aid in this dissection
    - Dangers
        - Lateral cutaneous nerve of the thigh
            - If osteotomy is used, then nerve may have to be sacrificed for exposure which will result in numbness of the lateral thigh
        - Sacral nerve roots
            - At risk where they emerge from the sacral foramina
            - Dissection should stop at approximately 1 cm from the anterior edge of the SI joint
            - Care must be taken with retractor positioning and positioning plates medially

2 Hip and Acetabulum

- Anterior (Smith-Petersen) approach to the hip
  - Indications
    - Access to anterior hip joint
  - Superficial dissection
    - Internervous plane
      - Sartorius (femoral nerve) and tensor fasciae latae (superior gluteal nerve)
    - Identify the plane between the sartorius and the tensor fasciae latae 2–3 cm below the anterior superior iliac spine
    - Dissect through subcutaneous fat along the interval (alternatively can dissect through fascia of tensor fasciae latae to avoid lateral femoral cutaneous nerve)
      - Take care to preserve the lateral femoral cutaneous nerve of the thigh
      - The nerve runs over the fascia of the sartorius
    - Incise deep fascia on medial aspect of tensor fasciae latae
    - Retract the tensor fasciae latae posteriorly and inferiorly and the sartorius superiorly and medially
      - Release the tensor fasciae latae from its origin (lateral anterior iliac crest) as needed to gain exposure
    - Ligate or cauterize the large ascending branch of the lateral femoral circumflex artery that crosses inferior to the anterior superior iliac spine
  - Deep dissection
    - Internervous plane
      - Rectus femoris (femoral nerve) and gluteus medius (superior gluteal nerve)
    - The rectus femoris has two heads
      - One originates from anterior inferior iliac spine, and the other originates from the superior lip of the acetabulum/anterior capsule of hip joint
    - Detach the rectus femoris from its origins and retract medially to expose the hip capsule
    - The iliopsoas is found in the inferomedial aspect of the wound and inserts into the lesser trochanter of the femur
      - Retract medially

  - Adduct and externally rotate the hip to put the capsule on stretch
  - Incise the capsule to expose the hip joint

- Dangers

  - Lateral cutaneous nerve of the thigh

    - Passes the sartorius muscle approximately 2.5 cm distal to the anterior superior iliac spine
    - Cutting the nerve can cause a painful neuroma

  - Femoral nerve

    - Courses directly anterior to the hip joint within the femoral triangle (superiorly, inguinal ligament; laterally, sartorius; medially, adductor magnus)
    - Nerve is medial to rectus and not in field
    - If anatomy becomes unclear, feel for the femoral pulse which is medial to the nerve and well medial to dissection plane

  - Ascending branch of lateral femoral circumflex artery

    - Ligate as it crosses operative field proximally between tensor fasciae latae and sartorius muscles

- <u>Anterolateral (Watson-Jones) approach to the hip</u>
  - Indications

    - Access to anterolateral hip joint

  - Superficial dissection

    - Internervous plane

      - No true internervous plane
      - Gluteus medius and the tensor fasciae latae are both innervated by the superior gluteal nerve

        - Avoid extremely proximal dissection between these two muscles, and the nerve will remain intact

    - Incise subcutaneous fat until reaching deep fascia of the thigh over the greater trochanter
    - Incise the fascia lata and the bursa over the greater trochanter
    - Incise the fascia lata in line with its fibers heading toward the anterior superior iliac spine
    - Extend fascial incision distally to expose the vastus lateralis
    - Reflect the fascial flap anteriorly to better expose the interval between the tensor fasciae latae and the gluteus medius

      - Branches of the superior gluteal artery are found in this interval and must be ligated or cauterized

- Deep dissection
  - The abductor mechanism needs to be retracted to gain better exposure of the hip joint
    - The greater trochanter can be osteotomized and reflected superiorly and repaired
    - The anterior one third of the tendinous insertion of the gluteus medius can be partially released from its insertion on the greater trochanter
  - Retract the gluteus medius and minimus laterally and superiorly
  - To put the capsule on stretch, fully externally rotate and adduct the hip
  - Elevate the vastus lateralis off the vastus lateralis ridge to expose the anterior aspect of the joint capsule
  - Bluntly clear the anterior aspect of the hip capsule and detach the reflected head of the rectus femoris off the anterior lip of the acetabulum
    - Partially flexing the hip will make this easier
  - Incise the capsule and the hip joint is exposed
- Dangers
  - Femoral nerve
    - Courses directly anterior to the hip joint within the femoral triangle (superiorly, inguinal ligament; laterally, sartorius; medially, adductor magnus)
    - The most common problem is compression neuropraxia secondary to overzealous medial retracting
    - If anatomy becomes unclear, feel for the femoral pulse which is medial to the nerve and well medial to dissection plane
  - Femoral artery and vein
    - At risk with aberrant retractor placement

- <u>Lateral (Hardinge) approach to the hip</u>
  - Indications
    - Access to anterior hip joint
  - Superficial dissection
    - Internervous plane
      - There is no internervous plane
    - Dissect through subcutaneous fat down to fascia over the greater trochanter of the proximal femur
    - Incise the deep fascia in line with the incision and retract the edges of the fascia to pull the tensor fasciae latae anteriorly and the gluteus maximus posteriorly

        - The gluteus medius and the vastus lateralis are now exposed, and both attach to the greater trochanter

    - Deep dissection

        - Split the fibers of the gluteus medius longitudinally starting at the middle third of the greater trochanter

            - Put a stay suture in the muscle fibers to prevent dissection of greater than 3 cm proximal to the greater trochanter so there is no denervation of the superior gluteal nerve

        - Split fibers of the vastus lateralis in the same line as the gluteus medius
        - Form an anterior flap consisting of the gluteus medius (with some underlying gluteus minimus) and the vastus lateralis
        - The proximal and distal muscle units will be connected by the tendinous region that is elevated off the greater trochanter
        - As this anterior flap is elevated and retracted medially to expose the hip capsule, the gluteus minimus insertion to the greater trochanter will need to be released
        - The capsule is now exposed and a capsulotomy can be performed

    - Dangers

        - Superior gluteal nerve

            - Courses between the gluteus medius and minimus 3–5 cm proximal to the greater trochanter
            - A stay suture can help prevent unintended proximal dissection and potential nerve injury

        - Femoral nerve

            - Courses directly anterior to the hip joint within the femoral triangle (superiorly, inguinal ligament; laterally, sartorius; medially, adductor magnus)
            - At risk for inappropriately placed retractors

        - Femoral artery and vein

            - At risk with aberrant retractor placement

        - Transverse branch of the lateral femoral circumflex artery

            - Must be cauterized during approach to allow mobilization of vastus lateralis

- <u>Ilioinguinal approach to the acetabulum</u>

    - Indications

        - Access to anterior column of acetabulum

- Superficial dissection
  - Internervous plane
    - There is no internervous plane
  - Dissect down to aponeurosis of external oblique muscle along the iliac crest
  - The lateral cutaneous nerve of the thigh will be exposed in the lateral aspect of this dissection, and often it needs to be transected
  - Incise the aponeurosis of the external oblique from the superficial inguinal ring to the anterior superior iliac spine
    - This exposes the spermatic cord in the male and the round ligament in the female
    - Tag these structures when identified
  - Divide the anterior rectus sheath medially to expose the underlying rectus abdominis muscle
  - Dissect the iliacus muscle off the iliac fossa exposing the anterior iliosacral joint and pelvic brim
- Deep dissection
  - Release the rectus abdominis muscle off the insertion of the pubic symphysis, leaving a cuff for later repair
  - Bluntly open the space of Retzius between the bladder and pubic symphysis
  - Divide the internal oblique muscle and the transverse abdominis muscles both medially and laterally to the deep inguinal ring
    - Together these two muscles form the posterior wall of the inguinal canal
    - Ligate the inferior epigastric vessels that arise near the deep inguinal ring
  - The extraperitoneal fat is now exposed and should be bluntly swept superiorly to reveal the femoral vessels, the femoral nerve, and the tendon of the iliopsoas
    - The iliopectineal fascia separates the iliopsoas and femoral nerve from the femoral artery and vein
  - Identify the anterior aspect of the femoral vessels and the lymphatics in the midportion of the incision
  - Place one sling around the femoral sheath and another around the iliopsoas with the femoral nerve lying superficial to it
  - This creates three "windows"

    - Lateral window: lateral aspect of wound to iliopsoas (iliopectineal fascia)
        - Provides access to the iliac wing, the quadrilateral plate, and anterior sacroiliac joint
    - Middle window: between the external iliac vessels and the iliopsoas (iliopectineal fascia)
        - Provides access to the pelvic brim, the quadrilateral plate, and the lateral aspect of the superior pubic ramus
    - Medial window: medial aspect of wound to external iliac vessels
        - Provides direct access to pubic rami
  - Dangers
    - Femoral nerve
      - Courses beneath the inguinal canal on the iliopsoas
        - Stretching the nerve with aggressive retraction can lead to postoperative quadriceps weakening
    - Lateral cutaneous nerve of the thigh
      - Often need to be sacrificed
    - Femoral artery and vein
      - These should be kept together in the femoral sheath as opposed to dissecting them out separately
    - Inferior epigastric vessels
      - Should be ligated to provide access to deeper structures
    - Spermatic cord
      - The vas deferens and the testicular artery are found within the cord
      - Avoid overtightening around the cord during closure to prevent ischemic damage to testicle

- <u>Modified Stoppa approach to the acetabulum</u>
  - Indications
    - Access to
      - Quadrilateral plate
      - Superior pubic ramus
      - Ilium
      - Medial aspect of posterior column
      - Sciatic buttress
      - Anterior sacroiliac joint

- Superficial dissection
  - Internervous plane
    - There is no internervous plane
  - Dissect through subcutaneous fascia down to rectus fascia and incise vertically in midline
  - Incise transversalis fascia superior to pubic symphysis
  - Bluntly open the space of Retzius and pack with sponges to protect the bladder
- Deep dissection
  - Using subperiosteal elevation, expose the superior pubic ramus, posterior surface of the ramus, pelvic brim, and internal iliac fossa
    - Protect the external iliac vessels during this dissection
  - The corona mortis (anastomosis between the external iliac vessels and the obturator vessels) will be encountered as the artery and vein course over the superior pubic ramus toward the obturator foramen
    - Ligate these vessels to gain exposure along the pelvic brim and quadrilateral surface
  - Detach the iliopectineal fascia over the anterior column to gain additional exposure along the pelvic brim
  - Continue dissection toward anterior sacroiliac joint to expose entire pelvic brim
  - Expose the quadrilateral surface and posterior column while protecting the obturator neurovascular bundle
- Dangers
  - Corona mortis
    - These vessels vary in size but are consistently present
    - Ligate as they course over the lateral third of the superior pubic ramus
  - External iliac vessels
    - Must be mobilized and protected to provide adequate exposure to iliac fossa
  - Obturator vessels
    - Must be retracted and protected during exposure of the quadrilateral plate and posterior column
  - Bladder
    - Protect throughout case by using a Foley catheter to deflate the bladder and placing sponges and/or a malleable retractor anterior to bladder

- Spermatic cord/round ligament
  - Avoid far lateral dissection to prevent injury; it exits the deep inguinal ring

- Posterior (Kocher-Langenbeck) approach to the hip and acetabulum
  - Indications
    - Access to
      - Posterior hip joint
      - Posterior wall of acetabulum
      - Posterior column of acetabulum
      - Medial aspect of posterior column
  - Superficial dissection
    - Internervous plane
      - There is no internervous plane
    - Dissect through subcutaneous fascia down to fascia lata on the lateral aspect of the femur and incise longitudinally and distally
    - Continue fascial incision proximally toward the gluteus maximus and bluntly split the muscle in line with its fibers
  - Deep dissection
    - Retract split gluteus maximus anteriorly and posteriorly to expose the deep tissues
    - The short external rotators insert into the posterior aspect of the greater trochanter
      - From superior to inferior, these external rotators include
        - Piriformis muscle (largest and comes in at a more inferior angle than the others
        - Superior gemellus muscle
        - Obturator internus muscle (only muscle in the pelvis that makes a 90° turn)
        - Inferior gemellus
      - The sciatic nerve most commonly courses
        - Anterior to the piriformis
        - Posterior to the gemelli, obturator internus, and quadratus femoris
        - Anterior to gluteal sling insertion to femur
      - Internally rotate hip to put external rotators on stretch and incise the tendinous insertions 1.5 cm medial to the insertion on the greater trochanter (to preserve blood supply to the femoral head) or at the trochanter for arthroplasty procedures

    - Reflect the external rotators medially to expose the capsule of the hip joint
    - Perform capsulotomy to expose joint
    - To expose more of the posterior wall of the acetabulum, elevate the gluteus minimus subperiosteally and retract anteriorly

- Dangers
  - Sciatic nerve
    - Retractors should be placed on the muscle bellies of the short external rotators as they are reflected medially to protect the sciatic nerve
  - Inferior gluteal artery
    - Exits pelvis inferior to the piriformis
    - If the artery is torn at its trunk, control of bleeding can be difficult
      - Interventional radiology may be an option depending on facility

- <u>Medial approach to the hip</u>
  - Indications
    - Soft tissue releases
    - Biopsy
    - Open reduction of congenital hip dislocation
  - Superficial dissection
    - Internervous plane
      - There is no internervous plane
      - Adductor longus and gracilis are both innervated by the anterior division of the obturator nerve
    - With a finger bluntly develop a plane between the gracilis and adductor longus
  - Deep dissection
    - Continue dissection between adductor brevis and adductor magnus in the direction of the lesser trochanter of the femur
  - Dangers
    - Anterior division of the obturator nerve
      - Courses superficially to the obturator externus and continues down the medial side of the thigh between the adductor longus and adductor brevis
      - Provides innervation to adductor longus, adductor brevis, and gracilis
      - Preserve unless object of surgery is to divide in order to relieve muscular spasticity

- Posterior division of the obturator nerve
  - Innervates and is found within the substance of the obturator externus
  - Supplies the adductor magnus
  - Preserve unless object of surgery is to divide in order to relieve muscular spasticity
- Medial femoral circumflex artery
  - Passes around the medial side of the distal aspect of the psoas tendon

3 Femur

- Lateral approach
  - Indications
    - Utilitarian approach to the femur
  - Superficial dissection
    - Internervous plane
      - There is no internervous or intermuscular plane
      - Vastus lateralis (femoral nerve) is split
    - Incise fascia lata in line with skin incision
  - Deep dissection
    - Split directly through the vastus lateralis to expose the lateral femur
  - Dangers
    - Perforating branches of the profunda femoris artery
      - Traverse vastus lateralis
      - They should be cauterized or ligated
- Posterolateral approach
  - Indications
    - Utilitarian approach to the femur
  - Superficial dissection
    - Internervous plane
      - Vastus lateralis (femoral nerve) and hamstring muscles (sciatic nerve)

    - Incise fascia lata in line with skin incision which exposes the vastus lateralis

  - Deep dissection

    - Follow the vastus lateralis posteriorly to find the intermuscular septum and retract the vastus lateralis anteriorly
    - Continue to free the vastus lateralis from the intermuscular septum until the femur is reached along the linea aspera
    - Use sharp dissection to release the vastus lateralis off the linea aspera and then continue to elevate off the femur subperiosteally

  - Dangers

    - Perforating branches of the profunda femoris artery

      - Pierce the lateral intermuscular septum to supply the vastus lateralis
      - They should be cauterized or ligated

- <u>Anteromedial approach</u>

  - Indications

    - Access to distal two thirds of femur

  - Superficial dissection

    - Internervous plane

      - There is no internervous plane
      - The approach exploits the interval between the rectus femoris and the vastus medialis muscles which are both innervated by the femoral nerve proximal in the thigh

    - Incise deep fascia in line with skin incision and identify the interval between the rectus femoris and the vastus medialis

  - Deep dissection

    - Begin the dissection distally by opening the knee joint capsule cutting through the medial patellar retinaculum
    - Extend the dissection proximally incising the quadriceps tendon

      - Leaving a cuff of quadriceps tendon allows easier closure

    - As the vastus intermedius is encountered proximally, split the muscle in line with its fibers
    - The femur is now exposed and further exposure should be done subperiosteally

- Dangers
    - Medial superior genicular artery
        - Crosses operative field just superior to knee joint
        - Ligate to prevent postoperative hematoma
    - Medial patellofemoral ligament
        - Can be disrupted during approach
        - Meticulous closure is essential

- Posterior approach
    - Indications
        - Access to posterior femur
        - Access to sciatic nerve
    - Superficial dissection
        - Internervous plane
            - Vastus lateralis (femoral nerve) and hamstring muscles (sciatic nerve)
                - Plane is between the lateral intermuscular septum (which covers the vastus lateralis) and the biceps femoris
        - Incise deep fascia in line with skin incision and avoid the posterior femoral cutaneous nerve (runs longitudinally under the deep fascia)
        - In the proximal wound, bluntly dissect the plane between the lateral border of the biceps femoris and vastus lateralis
    - Deep dissection
        - Begin the dissection proximally by retracting the biceps femoris medially and the vastus lateralis laterally
        - The short head of the biceps femoris is located along the linea aspera of the femur and sharply dissected off to expose the posterior aspect of the femur
        - To gain distal exposure, retract the long head of the biceps laterally to expose the sciatic nerve
        - Identify the sciatic nerve and gently retract laterally
        - Elevate the musculature deep to the sciatic nerve subperiosteally to expose the femur
    - Dangers
        - Sciatic nerve
            - Courses distally through the posterior compartment in the thigh
                - In proximal wound, the nerve is located medial to the biceps
                - Distally the nerve is in the operative field
            - Avoid aggressive retraction

4 Knee

- Medial parapatellar approach
  - Indications
    - Utilitarian approach to knee joint
  - Superficial dissection
    - Internervous plane
      - No internervous plane
    - Incise down to deep fascia and expose the quadriceps tendon, medial border of the patella, and the patellar tendon
    - Sharply incise the capsule starting on the medial side of the patella, making sure to leave a cuff of fascia for repair
    - Proximally divide the quadriceps tendon medial to the midline to allow repair, and distally finish capsulotomy medial to the patellar tendon
    - Excise or retract the anterior infrapatellar fat pad depending on intent of surgery
  - Deep dissection
    - Extend the knee, dislocate the patella laterally and flip it 180° so the articular surface is facing anterior, and then flex the knee
      - If there is difficulty adequately dislocating the patella, extend the incision proximally and release further up the quadriceps
      - As a last resort, the patellar tendon can be removed from the tibia with a block of bone to be repaired later
    - The knee joint is now exposed
  - Dangers
    - Infrapatellar branch of the saphenous nerve
      - Often sacrificed during the approach
      - The patient can have postoperative painful neuroma or numbness inferior and lateral to the patella
- Medial approach
  - Indications
    - Access to medial structures about the knee
  - Superficial dissection
    - Internervous plane
      - No internervous plane

  - Incise down to fascia and raise skin flaps
  - From the incision, exposure can include from the midline anteriorly to the posteromedial corner
  - Sacrifice the infrapatellar branch of the saphenous nerve

- Deep dissection
  - Anterior to medial collateral ligament
    - Access to
      - Superficial medial collateral ligament
      - Anteromedial meniscus
      - And the anterior cruciate ligament
    - Incise fascia along the anterior border of the sartorius from its insertion in the tibia and extend proximally 5 cm about the joint line
    - Flex up the knee to allow the sartorius muscle to retract posteriorly, revealing the rest of the pes anserinus (sartorius semitendinosus and gracilis muscles)
    - Retracting the three muscles of the pes anserinus exposes the tibial insertion of the superficial medial collateral ligament, which lies deep to the anterior edge of the sartorius
      - The ligament inserts 6–7 cm below the joint line
    - If access to the joint is desired, incise along the medial aspect of the patella to enter the anterior aspect of the joint
  - Posterior to the superficial medial collateral ligament
    - Access to
      - Posterior third of medial meniscus
      - Posteromedial corner of the knee
    - Incise the fascia anterior to the sartorius muscle as described above for the anterior approach
    - Retract the sartorius, semitendinosus, and gracilis muscles posteriorly
    - If there is no posteromedial corner injury and the capsule is intact, then expose the posteromedial corner of the joint by separating the medial head of the gastrocnemius muscle from the semimembranosus muscle
      - Both muscles are supplied by the tibial nerve, but the semimembranosus muscle receives the innervation well proximal, and the gastrocnemius receives its innervation well distal so the interval is safe
    - With blunt dissection, separate the gastrocnemius from the posterior capsule almost to the midline

- Dangers
  - Infrapatellar branch of the saphenous nerve
    - Sacrificed during the approach
    - Burry the cut end in fat to prevent painful neuroma
  - Saphenous nerve
    - Courses out from between the gracilis and sartorius muscles
    - Should be preserved as it provides sensation for part of the foot
  - Saphenous vein
    - Found in posterior corner of superficial dissection
    - Can be used for vascular procedures so should be preserved
  - Medial inferior genicular artery
    - Curves around the proximal tibia near the medial belly of the gastrocnemius
    - Can be damaged during retraction and cause a postoperative hematoma
  - Popliteal artery
    - Courses distally along the posterior joint capsule in the midline
    - Adjacent to the medial head of the gastrocnemius

- Lateral approach
  - Indications
    - Access to supporting structures found on the lateral aspect of the knee
  - Superficial dissection
    - Internervous plane
      - Dissection is between the iliotibial band (fascial aponeurosis formed proximally by fascia from tensor fasciae latae and gluteus maximus muscles supplied by the superior gluteal nerve and the inferior gluteal nerve, respectively) and the biceps femoris muscle (sciatic nerve)
    - Incise down to deep fascia and create skin flaps
    - Locate the iliotibial band (attaches to anterolateral tibia at Gerdy's tubercle) and the biceps femoris posterior to it (attaches to the fibular head)
    - Exploit the interval between the iliotibial band and the biceps femoris while avoiding the common peroneal nerve coursing along the posterior aspect of the biceps tendon

    - Retracting the iliotibial band anteriorly and the biceps femoris posteriorly reveals the fibular collateral ligament (runs from lateral epicondyle of femur to the fibular head)

  - Deep dissection

    - Anterior to fibular collateral ligament

      - Incise capsule inferior to ligament to access the anterior meniscus

    - Posterior arthrotomy

      - To access the posterolateral meniscus, locate the lateral head of the gastrocnemius at its origin at the posterior aspect of the lateral femoral condyle
      - Dissect between it and the capsule

        - Ligate the superior geniculate arteries in this area

      - Of note, in this region, the popliteus muscle inserts onto the femur inside the joint
      - Excision of the capsule in this region should be done superior to joint line to prevent damage to the meniscus and the popliteus tendon

  - Dangers

    - Common peroneal nerve

      - Most at risk during this approach
      - Isolate and protect early in dissection

    - Lateral superior genicular artery

      - Found between the lateral head of the gastrocnemius and the posterolateral capsule
      - Must be ligated for access to that region of the knee

- <u>Posterior approach</u>

  - Indications

    - Primarily for access to neurovascular structures

  - Superficial dissection

    - Internervous plane

      - No true internervous plane

    - Create skin flaps with subcutaneous fat
    - Do not fully exsanguinate leg before elevating tourniquet in order to make identification of the venous structures easier

    - Identifying the saphenous vein helps locate the medial sural cutaneous nerve running lateral to it, which acts as a guide to the tibial nerve deeper in the fossa
    - Incise the fascia medial to the small saphenous vein and follow the medial sural cutaneous nerve up to the tibial nerve
    - Continue superiorly in the popliteal fossa following the tibial nerve
      - The superior apex of the fossa is formed by the semimembranosus muscle on the medial side and the biceps femoris muscle on the lateral side
    - The proximal tibial nerve dissection will lead to the common peroneal nerve branch which can then be followed distally
    - The popliteal artery has five branches about the knee
      - Two superior genicular arteries
      - Two inferior genicular arteries
      - One middle genicular artery
    - Ligate at least one branch to mobilize artery
  - Deep dissection
    - Posteromedial joint capsule access
      - Detaching the tendinous origin of the medial head of the gastrocnemius from the posterior femur and retracting the head inferiorly and laterally will provide exposure to the posteromedial corner of the joint
    - Posterolateral joint capsule access
      - Detach the tendinous origin of the lateral head of the gastrocnemius from the lateral posterior femur
      - Develop the interval between it and the biceps femoris and the posterolateral corner of the joint is accessible
  - Dangers
    - Common peroneal nerve
      - Injury at this level causes paralysis of extensors and evertors of the foot
    - Tibial nerve
      - Injury at this level causes paralysis of the flexors of the toes and feet
    - Medial sural cutaneous nerve
      - At risk early in dissection
      - Injury to nerve can cause painful neuroma or anesthesia

5 Tibia and Fibula

- Anterior approach to tibia
  - Indications
    - Utilitarian approach to access anterior tibia
  - Superficial dissection
    - Internervous plane
      - No internervous plane
    - Incise through skin and subcutaneous fat 1 cm lateral to tibial crest
  - Deep dissection
    - Elevate full thickness skin flap to tibial crest, and then incise deep fascia and periosteum longitudinally next to tibial crest.
    - Retract anterior compartment musculature laterally to expose lateral face of the tibia
    - Alternatively, tibia can be approached directly medially where the bone lies directly subcutaneously
  - Dangers
    - Long saphenous vein
      - Runs along the medial side of the calf
- Anterolateral approach to tibia
  - Indications
    - Provides access to tibia with good soft tissue coverage
  - Superficial dissection
    - Internervous plane
      - Peroneus brevis muscle (superficial peroneal nerve) and extensor digitorum longus muscle (deep peroneal nerve)
      - Tibialis posterior muscle (tibial nerve) and extensor muscles of ankle and foot (deep peroneal nerve)
    - Incise through skin and subcutaneous fat to expose fascia
      - Avoid short saphenous vein
    - Incise fascia to expose the peroneal muscles and bluntly develop plane between peroneus brevis and extensor digitorum longus
      - This plane with lead to the anterolateral aspect of the fibula

    - The superficial peroneal nerve courses along the peroneus brevis muscle
  - Deep dissection
    - Bluntly release the extensor musculature from the anterior surface of the interosseous membrane
      - Following this membrane medially will lead to the lateral border of the tibia
      - Stay close to membrane as the anterior neurovascular bundle is just anterior to membrane and at risk for injury
    - Elevate the tibialis anterior subperiosteally as needed at the posterolateral aspect of the tibia
  - Dangers
    - Superficial peroneal nerve
      - Course down the leg in the lateral compartment
      - Branches for muscular innervation are proximal to this approach so injury will cause only anesthesia in this region
    - Anterior tibial artery with deep peroneal nerve
      - Course distally in the anterior compartment just anterior to interosseous membrane
      - Stay close to membrane while dissecting lateral to medial
- <u>Posterolateral approach to tibia</u>
  - Indications
    - Access to posterior tibia
  - Superficial dissection
    - Internervous plane
      - Dissection is between the posterior and lateral compartments
        - Gastrocnemius, soleus, and flexor hallucis longus muscles (tibial nerve) and peroneal muscles (superficial peroneal nerve)
    - Incise down to fascia creating flaps and avoiding short saphenous vein
    - Enter the fascia and develop plane between the anterior edge of the gastrocnemius/soleus complex and the posterior aspect of the peroneal muscles
    - Retract the lateral border of the soleus and gastrocnemius medially and posteriorly exposing the flexor hallucis longus
  - Deep dissection
    - Release the origins of the soleus and flexor hallucis longus from the fibula and retract both posteriorly to gain adequate exposure

- Continue medially elevating the tibialis posterior off the interosseous membrane
    - The posterior tibial artery and the tibial nerve are between the soleus and the tibialis posterior
    - Stay against fibula then interosseous membrane going from lateral to medial to prevent injury to these structures
- Follow the interosseous membrane to the posterolateral border of the tibia and elevate as needed

– Dangers

- Branches of the peroneal artery
    - Cross plane between gastrocnemius and peroneus brevis muscles
    - Ligate or cauterize to maintain hemostasis
- Posterior tibial artery and tibial nerve
    - Structures are protected by keeping dissection plane along the interosseous membrane

- <u>Approach to proximal fibula</u>
  - Indications
    - Utilitarian approach to the fibula
  - Superficial dissection
    - Internervous plane
      - Peroneal muscles (superficial peroneal nerve) and flexor muscles (tibial nerve)
    - Incise deep fascia and identify the common peroneal nerve as it courses posterior to the biceps femoris tendon and wraps around the fibular neck
    - Define the border between the peroneals and soleus along the fibula
  - Deep dissection
    - Strip the muscle off the fibula as needed from distal to proximal with a sharp elevator
  - Dangers
    - Common peroneal nerve
      - Most vulnerable as it wraps around neck of fibula
        - Identify it early and protect throughout case

6 Ankle and Foot

- Anterior approach to ankle joint
  - Indications
    - Utilitarian approach to anterior ankle joint
  - Superficial dissection
    - Internervous plane
      - No true internervous plane
      - Plane is between extensor hallucis longus and extensor digitorum longus (both innervated by deep peroneal nerve)
    - Incise down to fascia and incise through extensor retinaculum between the extensor hallucis longus tendon and the extensor digitorum longus tendons a few centimeters above the ankle joint
    - Identify the neurovascular bundle just medial to the extensor hallucis longus which includes the anterior tibial artery and the deep peroneal nerve
    - Retract the tendon of the extensor hallucis longus medially with the neurovascular bundle and the tendons of the extensor digitorum longus laterally
  - Deep dissection
    - With the tendons retracted, the anterior capsule of the tibiotalar joint will be exposed
    - Expose entire ankle joint as needed by detaching the anterior capsule from the ankle joint by sharp dissection
  - Dangers
    - Superficial peroneal nerve
      - Courses close to incision
      - Use caution to preserve nerve
    - Anterior neurovascular bundle (deep peroneal nerve and anterior tibial artery
      - Identify and protect early in dissection
        - Superior to ankle joint, the bundle courses between the extensor hallucis longus and the tibialis anterior
        - At the level of the joint, the extensor hallucis longus crosses the bundle toward the medial direction
- Medial approach to the ankle (with osteotomy)
  - Indications
    - Utilitarian approach to medial ankle

- Superficial dissection
  - Internervous plane
    - No true internervous plane
  - Develop skin flaps posterior to medial malleolus avoiding the long saphenous vein and saphenous nerve, both found anterior to the medial malleolus
- Deep dissection
  - Make a small incision in the capsule in the anterior aspect of the medial malleolus to establish where the medial malleolus attaches to the tibial shaft
  - Incise the flexor retinaculum posterior to the medial malleolus and expose the posterior tibialis tendon
    - Retract tendon posteriorly
  - Score the junction of the medial malleolus and the shaft of the tibia longitudinally to assist in repair at the end of the case
    - Drill holes before the osteotomy to establish alignment of medial malleolus during repair
  - Use an oscillating saw or osteotome to osteotomize the medial malleolus
    - Can be angled or step cut
    - Exits intra-articular at the superomedial corner of the joint
  - Retract the medial malleolus inferior hinging on the deltoid ligament to expose the tibiotalar joint
    - Evert the foot for better exposure
- Dangers
  - Saphenous nerve
    - Preserve to prevent painful neuroma
  - Tendon of posterior tibialis
    - Protect during osteotomy

- Posteromedial approach to the ankle
  - Indications
    - Frequently used for access to soft tissue structures of posteromedial ankle
  - Superficial dissection
    - Internervous plane
      - No true internervous plane

    - Dissect down to plane of fat between Achilles tendon and deep fascia of posterior ankle
        - Incise fascia to expose flexor hallucis longus and tibial nerve
- Deep dissection
    - Locate the lateral aspect of the flexor hallucis longus and tract medially to expose the posterior ankle joint
    - The structures in the posteromedial ankle from anterior to posterior are *t*ibialis posterior, flexor *d*igitorum longus, posterior tibial *a*rtery, tibial *n*erve, and flexor *h*allucis longus
        - *T*om, *D*ick, *a*nd *n*ervous *H*arry
- Dangers
    - Posterior tibial artery and tibial nerve
        - Identify and protect during this approach

- Posterolateral approach to the ankle
    - Indications
        - Access to soft tissue and bony structures of posterolateral ankle
    - Superficial dissection
        - Internervous plane
            - Peroneus brevis muscle (superficial peroneal nerve) and flexor hallucis longus (tibial nerve)
        - Mobilize skin flaps while preserving the short saphenous vein and the sural nerve which run posterior to the lateral malleolus
        - Incise deep fascia and expose the peroneal tendons as they run posterior to the lateral malleolus
            - The peroneus brevis tendon is anterior to the peroneus longus at the level of the ankle joint, and its muscle belly extends more distal
        - Release the peroneal retinaculum to release the tendons and retract them anteriorly if access to the posterior fibula is necessary
        - The flexor hallucis longus muscle is medial to the peroneal tendons
            - It is the only structure at this level that has a significant muscle belly as opposed to pure tendon
    - Deep dissection
        - Release the fibers of the flexor hallucis longus that adhere to the medial fibula and retract the muscle medially
        - The posterior tibia and posterior ankle joint are now exposed

- Dangers
  - Saphenous nerve
    - Preserve along with short saphenous vein to prevent neuroma formation
- <u>Lateral approach to the hindfoot</u>
  - Indications
    - Access to talocalcaneonavicular, posterior talocalcaneal, and calcaneocuboid joints
  - Superficial dissection
    - Internervous plane
      - Peroneus tertius tendon (deep peroneal nerve) and peroneal tendons (superficial peroneal nerve)
    - Refrain from creating large skin flaps to prevent devascularization of skin
    - Open the deep fascia at the lateral aspect of the hind foot transversely to extensor tendons and curving posteriorly under fibula
    - Retract peroneus tertius and extensor digitorum longus tendons medially
  - Deep dissection
    - Sharply partially detach the fat pad in the sinus tarsi
      - Leave attached to skin flap
    - Sharply detach the origin of the extensor digitorum brevis under the fat pad and retract distally
      - This will expose the talocalcaneonavicular joint and the calcaneocuboid joint laterally
    - Releasing the peroneal tendons will prove access to the posterior talocalcaneal joint
  - Dangers
    - Skin flap necrosis
      - Keep skin flaps thick and avoid aggressive retracting to prevent breakdown
- <u>Dorsal approach to the midfoot</u>
  - Indications
    - Access to midfoot joints and insertion of foot inverters and evertors
      - Tibialis anterior
        - Inserts into medial and undersurface of medial cuneiform, base of first metatarsal

    - Peroneus longus
        - Inserts into lateral side of the medial cuneiform
    - Peroneus brevis
        - Inserts into base of lateral fifth metatarsal
    - Tibialis posterior
        - Broad insertion into the tuberosity of the navicular, inferior surface of the medial cuneiform; the middle cuneiform; and the base of the second, third, and fourth metatarsals
  - Superficial dissection
    - Internervous plane
      - No internervous plane
    - Make incision directly over structure or joint of interest
    - Keep skin flaps thick
    - Spare superficial nerves if possible
- <u>Dorsal approach to metatarsophalangeal joint of great toe</u>
  - Indications
    - Utilitarian approach to metatarsophalangeal joint
  - Superficial dissection
    - Internervous plane
      - No internervous plane
      - Bone is subcutaneous
    - Dorsomedial incision
      - Incise down to dorsomedial aspect of the metatarsophalangeal joint
      - Laterally retract the dorsal digital branch of the medial cutaneous nerve
      - Create a U-shaped capsulotomy with the capsule attached to the proximal aspect of the first proximal phalanx
    - Dorsal incision
      - Incise fascia over extensor hallucis longus and retract tendon laterally
      - Incise dorsal aspect of capsule longitudinally
  - Deep dissection
    - Longitudinally incise the periosteum of the proximal phalanx and first metatarsal and elevate the periosteum as needed for procedure

- Dangers
  - Tendon of extensor hallucis longus
    - Preserve tendon to maintain function of great toe
  - Tendon of flexor hallucis longus
    - Preserve tendon to maintain function of great toe
  - Dorsal sensory nerve of great toe

Bibliography

1. Archdeacon MT, Kazemi N, Guy P, Sagi HC. The modified stoppa approach for the acetabulum. J Am Acad Orthop Surg. 2011;19:170–5.
2. Hoppenfeld S, deBoer P, Buckley R. Surgical exposures in orthopaedics. The anatomic approach. 4th ed. Philadelphia: Lippincott Williams & Wilkins; 2009.

Spine Anatomy and Surgical Approaches

Jason M. McKean and David Seligson

1 Cervical Spine

- Posterior approach
  - Indications
    - Fusion
    - Biopsy
    - Discectomy
    - Utilitarian access to posterior cervical spine
  - Superficial dissection
    - Internervous plane
      - No internervous plane
      - Midline between paracervical muscles (segmental innervation by cervical rami)
    - Incise down to posterior aspect of cervical spinous processes
    - Elevate the paraspinal muscles off the cervical vertebra subperiosteally off the levels and side (for herniated disc) or sides (for fusion) as needed
      - Elevate as far lateral exposing lamina, facets, and transverse processes as needed

J.M. McKean, MD (✉)
Department of Orthopaedics, Lincoln Medical Center, Bronx, USA
e-mail: jasonmckean@gmail.com

D. Seligson, MD
Department of Orthopaedics, University of Louisville Hospital, Louisville, KY, USA
e-mail: seligson@louisville.edu

C. Mauffrey, D.J. Hak (eds.), *Passport for the Orthopedic Boards and FRCS Examination*, DOI 10.1007/978-2-8178-0475-0_3

- Deep dissection
  - Sharply dissect the ligamentum flavum from the leading edge of the inferior lamina
  - Protect the dura underneath the ligamentum flavum and remove as much as needed to provide access to the dura, nerve roots, or lamina for a laminectomy
  - Retracting the spinal cord medially will provide access to the cervical disc and vertebral body
- Dangers
  - Spinal cord and nerve roots
    - Avoid aggressive spinal cord and nerve root retraction
  - Venous plexus surrounding cord
    - Venous plexus in the spinal canal is vulnerable to tearing with retraction
      - Bipolar cautery is recommending in this proximity to the spinal cord

- <u>Anterior approach</u>
  - Indications
    - Discectomy
    - Fusion
    - Biopsy
  - Superficial dissection
    - Internervous plane
      - No internervous plane superficially through the platysma (innervated by branches of the facial nerve)
      - Deeper dissection is between the sternocleidomastoid muscle (spinal accessory nerve) and the strap muscles of the neck (segmental innervation from C1, C2, and C3)
      - Deepest muscle dissection is between the left and right longus colli muscles (segmental innervation from C2 to C7)
    - Incise the fascia over the platysma and split the muscle in line with the fibers
    - Incise the fascia anterior to the sternocleidomastoid and retract it laterally
    - Retract the sternohyoid and sternothyroid strap muscles medially and anteriorly
      - The trachea and esophagus are just deep to these structures
    - Open the pretracheal sheath and develop a plane between the carotid sheath laterally and the thyroid, trachea, and esophagus medially

- Retract the carotid sheath with its vessels laterally with the sternocleidomastoid muscle
  - If the superior and inferior thyroid arteries coming from the carotid sheath prevent adequate exposure, then ligate these vessels as needed
- The prevertebral fascia and the longus colli muscles lie just anterior to the cervical vertebra

– Deep dissection
  - Dissect through the midline of the longus colli muscle longitudinally over the vertebra
    - Elevate subperiosteally along with the anterior longitudinal ligament and retract to expose vertebra
  - Localize the cervical level by placing a needle in the vertebral disc and obtaining a lateral radiograph

– Dangers
  - Recurrent laryngeal nerve
    - At the greatest risk during deep dissection
    - Keeping the retractors under the medial edge of the longus muscles will help protect the nerve
  - Sympathetic nerves and stellate ganglion
    - Injury to nerves can cause Horner's syndrome
    - Protect the nerves by retracting subperiosteally in the deep dissection
  - Carotid sheath contents (the carotid artery, carotid vein, and vagus nerve)
    - Courses deep to and along the anterior border of the sternocleidomastoid
    - Do not place retractors directly against the carotid sheath

2 Thoracic Spine

- Posterior approach
  - Indications
    - Fusion
    - Biopsy
    - Utilitarian access to the posterior thoracic spine
  - Superficial dissection
    - Internervous plane

    - The paraspinal muscles are innervated segmentally from the posterior primary rami of the thoracic nerve roots

  - Dissect down directly over the posterior spinous process

    - Staying within the plane between the paraspinal muscles superficially will avoid major bleeding

- Deep dissection

  - Dissect along the spinous process and laminae, elevating the paraspinal muscles subperiosteally
  - Using a Cobb elevator, continue dissection laterally and strip the muscles off the laminae and transverse processes

- Dangers

  - Segmental vessels

    - Arise between the transverse processes to supply the paraspinal muscles
    - Branch directly off the aorta
    - Use cautery to obtain hemostasis

  - Posterior primary rami

    - Arise from between the transverse processes near the facet joints
    - There is significant overlap in paraspinal innervation so individual injury to rami is not damaging overall

- <u>Anterior (transthoracic) approach</u>

  - Indications

    - Access to the anterior thoracic spine from T2 to T12
    - Should be done with the assistance of a thoracic surgeon or in a facility with expedited access to one

  - Superficial dissection

    - Internervous plane

      - There is no internervous plane

    - Entering the chest from the right side avoids the aorta
    - Divide through the latissimus dorsi and serratus anterior muscles in line with the skin incision to expose the ribs
    - Perform a partial rib resection to gain better exposure or exploit the intercostal space for access

      - The section of removed rib can be used as bone graft
      - It is safe to resect the posterior three fourths of the ribs

    - For exposure to thoracic levels above T10, use the fifth intercostal space

      - The scapula covers the healing site

        - For access to levels T10 and below, use the sixth intercostal space
            - The scapula does not fully cover this area, and there may be clicking as it slides over the callus
        - Using cautery, dissect over the superior aspect of the rib to avoid the neurovascular bundle found inferior to each rib
        - Insert a rib spreader to hold the ribs apart
    - Deep dissection
        - After entering the thoracic cavity, have the anesthesiologist deflate the lung
        - Locate the esophagus medially and incise the overlaying pleura
        - Expose and mobilize the esophagus with blunt dissection and retract it from the anterior surface of the spine
        - Intercostal vessels cross the operative field
            - Ligate vessels sparingly to prevent ischemia of the spinal cord
            - Contributions to the spinal cord from these vessels vary
        - Expose vertebral bodies as needed
    - Dangers
        - Lungs
            - Have anesthesia expand the lungs every 30 min to prevent microatelectasis
        - Intercostal vessels
            - At risk during superficial dissection under the ribs and during the deep dissection where they course over the anterior aspect of the thoracic vertebrae

3 Lumbar Spine

- Posterior approach
    - Indications
        - Herniated disc removal
        - Nerve root exploration
        - Fusion
        - Access to tumors
    - Superficial dissection
        - Internervous plane

    - No internervous plane
    - Between erector spinae muscles (innervation by segmental primary rami of lumbar nerves)

  - Incise through the skin, fat, and fascia down to the posterior tip of the spinous process
  - Release the paraspinal muscles subperiosteally from the spinous process and lamina
  - Follow the lamina laterally continuing subperiosteal dissection to reach the facet joint

    - Only expose facet as needed to prevent joint instability

  - Continue laterally over the descending facet and over the joint to the mammillary process of the ascending facet to reach the transverse process

- Deep dissection

  - Release the attachment of the ligamentum flavum from the leading edge of the inferior lamina with a curet or sharp instrument

    - This will expose the underlying epidural fat and the dura

  - Retracting the dura and the nerve root will provide access to the posterior aspect of the intervertebral disc

- Dangers

  - Superficial dissection

    - Segmental vessels supplying the paraspinal muscles close to the facet joints can cause excessive bleeding

      - Vigorous cauterization is often necessary

    - Primary rami of the lumbar nerves innervate the paraspinal muscles but obliteration of these nerves do not denervate the muscle

  - Deep dissection

    - Nerve roots

      - Lateral dissection will make it easier to locate and protect the nerve root, but dissecting too far lateral will expose and destabilize the facet joint

    - Venous plexus

      - Surround nerves and floor of the vertebra

        - May cause extensive bleeding during blunt dissection accessing the disc
        - Bipolar cautery, Gelfoam, and thrombin-soaked cotton patties all can be used to control bleeding

- Anterior (transperitoneal) approach
  - Indications
    - Anterior access to the lumbar spine
  - Superficial dissection
    - Internervous plane
      - No internervous plane
      - Midline plane is between the abdominal muscle (segmentally supplied by branches from the seventh to the twelfth intercostal nerves)
    - Dissect down to the midline of the fibrous rectus sheath
    - Incise the linea alba longitudinally starting inferiorly
    - Bluntly separate the rectus abdominus with a finger
      - The peritoneum covered by the transversalis fascia is just deep to this
    - Sharply dissect through the transversalis fascia to expose the peritoneum
    - Carefully open remainder of the wound while protecting the viscera below
  - Deep dissection
    - Retract the bladder distally and the abdominis muscles laterally
    - Place the table in Trendelenburg's position at 30° and pack bowels superiorly
    - Incise the posterior peritoneum draping the anterior lumbar vertebra
    - The sacral artery must be ligated as it courses the anterior surface of the sacrum
    - The ureters are lateral to dissection
    - The L5–S1 disc space is below the bifurcation of the aorta
      - The space can be localized using an 18 gauge needle and a radiograph
    - Accessing the L4–L5 disc space requires more exposure
      - Mobilize the colon superiorly by incising the peritoneum at the base of the sigmoid colon
      - The bifurcation of the aorta will become exposed
      - Gently mobilize the aorta along the left side
        - Ligate the fourth and fifth lumbar vessels
      - Gently retract the aorta, vena cava, and left common iliac vessels to the right in order to expose the L4–L5 disc space
        - The ureter is more at risk in this region
  - Dangers
    - Presacral plexus of parasympathetic nerves

- Important for sexual function
  - Injury can cause retroejaculation and impotence in men
- Injecting saline into presacral tissue helps identify and preserve the plexus

- Aorta and inferior vena cava
  - The lumbar vessels tether the vessels to the anterior lumbar vertebra
  - Ligate these smaller vessels to allow mobilization of great vessels
    - If vessels are torn of the base of the aorta or vena cava, then hemostasis will be extremely difficult to achieve
- Ureter
  - When exposing L4–L5 the ureter must be mobilized laterally
  - Ensure identification by gently pinching ureter with smooth forces to cause peristalsis

- <u>Anteriolateral (retroperitoneal) approach</u>
  - Indications
    - Anterior access to the lumbar spine (easier access to L1–L4 compared to transperitoneal approach)
  - Superficial dissection
    - Internervous plane
      - No internervous plane
      - External oblique, internal oblique, and transverse abdominis muscles are all innervated segmentally
    - Exposure is often performed on the left side because the aorta (much tougher than the vena cava) is on the left
    - Dissect down to external oblique aponeurosis under the 12th rib and dissect in line with fibers
    - Dissect across internal oblique perpendicular to its fibers and in line with external oblique fibers
    - Dissect across the third layer of the muscle (transversus abdominis) in the same line as previous two layers
      - The retroperitoneal space is deep to this layer
    - Bluntly form a plane between the retroperitoneal fat and the psoas muscle
  - Deep dissection
    - Follow the plane anterior to the psoas heading medially, and the aorta will be encountered

    - The aorta is fixed to the vertebral bodies through the segmental lumbar vessels
    - Ligate these vessels to mobilize the aorta and vena cava
  - Place a radiopaque maker into the desired disc space and take a radiograph to confirm the level
- Dangers
  - Genitofemoral nerve
    - Courses along the anterior aspect of the psoas
    - Must preserve the nerve
  - Sympathetic chain
    - Found on the lateral aspect of the vertebral body and medial to the psoas
    - Preserve during dissection
  - Aorta and inferior vena cava
    - The largest vessels encountered
    - Must ligate segmental lumbar vessels to free up the aorta and vena cava
  - Ureter
    - Will be medial to approach
    - Usually move with the peritoneum when it is retracted forward
      - If there is a question of whether or not a structure is a ureter, a gentle stroke will induce peristalsis and confirm its identification

Bibliography

1. Hoppenfeld S, deBoer P, Buckley R. Surgical exposures in orthopaedics. The anatomic approach. 4th ed. Philadelphia: Lippincott Williams & Wilkins; 2009.

Part II
Basic Sciences

Gregory J. Della Rocca

Tissues

Sharath S. Bellary, Wellington K. Hsu, Phuc Dang, Ranjan Gupta, Bastián Uribe-Echevarría, Brian R. Wolf, Matthew T. Provencher, Daniel J. Gross, Amun Makani, and Petar Golijanin

1 Bone

Sharath S. Bellary and Wellington K. Hsu

Take-Home Message

- Bone regeneration depends on an osteoinductive stimulus, osteoconductive matrix, source of responding cells, and sufficient vascular supply.
- The mechanical environment will influence bone grown in accordance with Wolff's Law.
- If one or more of these factors is lacking, new bone formation is significantly decreased.

S.S. Bellary, MD (✉) • W.K. Hsu, MD
Department of Orthopaedic Surgery, Northwestern University Feinberg School of Medicine, Chicago, Illinois, USA

P. Dang, MD • R. Gupta, MD
Department of Orthopaedic Surgery, University of California – Irvine, Orange, California, USA

B. Uribe-Echevarría, MD • B.R. Wolf, MD
Department of Orthopaedics and Rehabilitation, University of Iowa, Iowa City, Iowa, USA

M.T. Provencher, MD
Sports Medicine and Surgery, Harvard Medical School, Massachusetts General Hospital, 175 Cambridge St. Suite 400, Boston, MA 02114, USA
e-mail: mtprovencher@partners.org

D.J. Gross, MD • A. Makani, MD • P. Golijanin, BA
Sports Medicine and Surgery, Massachusetts General Hospital, 175 Cambridge St. Suite 400, Boston, MA 02114, USA
e-mail: danielgross23@gmail.com; amakani@partners.org; pgolijanin@partners.org

C. Mauffrey, D.J. Hak (eds.), *Passport for the Orthopedic Boards and FRCS Examination*, DOI 10.1007/978-2-8178-0475-0_4

Osteoinduction

- Characterized by the process of recruitment of immature pluripotent cells.
- Subsequent stimulation causes differentiation into pre-osteoblasts.
- Several growth factors have been identified as critical components in osteoinduction (Table 1 and Figure 1).
- The most widely studied are those in the bone morphogenetic protein (BMP) family, of which over 20 have been identified.
- BMPs are members of the TGF-β [beta] superfamily of growth hormones with BMP-2 and BMP-7 having the most development for therapeutic applications.
- BMP supplementation is FDA-approved to augment spinal arthrodesis and to treat nonunion or open fractures of long bones.
- Absorbable collagen sponges have been commercialized as a method of local delivery of BMP to surgical sites; endogenous BMP molecules are also naturally released during trauma to bone and during bone remodeling.
- Inflammatory cytokines and damage to the bone ECM can liberate matrix-bound growth factors which induce differentiation and proliferation of osteoprogenitor cells.

Table 1 Mediators of bone formation

Type	Source	Action
Bone morphogenetic protein –2, –7 (TGF-β[beta] superfamily)	MSCs, ECM, vascular endothelium	Recruitment and osteoblastic differentiation of mesenchymal cells, ossification of ECM
Fibroblast growth factor – 18	Vascular endothelium basement membrane	Bone development
Insulin-like growth factor	Liver	Activation of osteocytes, anabolic for bone tissue
Platelet-derived growth factor	Platelets, smooth muscle cells, activated macrophages, vascular endothelium	Mitogen for mesenchymal cells, angiogenesis
Vascular endothelium growth factor	Vascular endothelium, smooth muscle	Angiogenesis
Hydroxyapatite	Osteocytes, major component of bone ECM	Contributes to density and strength of bone, initiation of osteoblastic differentiation from MSCs
Osteoprotegerin (TNF-α [alpha] superfamily)	Vascular endothelium and smooth muscle, osteocytes	Blocks RANK ligand interaction with RANK receptor
RANK ligand	Vascular endothelium and smooth muscle, osteocytes	Osteoclastic differentiation and activation

Sources: Refs. [2, 3, 7, 10–18, 23]

TGF transforming growth factor, *MSC* mesenchymal stem (stromal) cell, *ECM* extracellular matrix, *TNF* tumor necrosis factor

- Under the influence of an osteoinductive environment, these cells terminally differentiate into osteoblasts and begin to deposit calcified extracellular matrix (ECM).

Osteoconduction

- The process of bone growth on a surface or scaffold, the initial deposit of osteoid and its conversion to woven and lamellar bone, is an example of this process.
- Implantation of bone grafts and scaffolds are other examples of osteoconduction.
- There are many characteristics of a scaffold that optimize its ability to aid bone regeneration such as compressive strength, biocompatibility, adhesive properties, and pore size.
- It has been previously reported that osteoconduction does not occur on some materials such as copper and silver, with increasing success on materials of higher biocompatibility such as titanium.
- Due to stress shielding, bone growth around and within a scaffold is optimized when the Young's modulus (stiffness) of the scaffold closely correlates to that of bone; pore size of the scaffold can be adjusted to meet this requirement in non-absorbable scaffolds.
- Increased porosity allows for a greater surface area upon which recruited cells may grow, too much of which makes the matrix unstable.
- Scaffolds are also often coated with or made from biologic agents to encourage cell recruitment and adhesion or provide extended release of osteoinductive compounds.
- Materials such as chitin, Gelfoam, hydroxyapatite, polyethylene glycol, or collagen have been investigated.
- With rapidly absorbable scaffolds, the rate of degradation should correlate with the rate of new bone growth, presenting a challenge in the design of novel material implants.

Responding Cells

- There are four primary cell types in bone tissue: osteocytes, osteoblasts, osteoclasts, and osteoprogenitor cells.
- A source of responding cells is required to provide a renewable source of primary osteoblasts and osteoclasts that will aid in the continuous formation and remodeling of bone.
- Cells can either be delivered through a cell-based strategy or endogenously confined through binding epitopes. Each strategy is designed to offer a long-term source of osteogenic activity.
- Cell-based therapies often require concomitant regeneration of vasculature in addition to bone and therefore osteogenic and vasculogenic cell types have been grown in coculture to promote heterotypic interactions.
- During an acute fracture, bone marrow is the main source of stem cells for bone repair. Mesenchymal cells under the influence of chemotactic agents are recruited

to the site of injury, where local osteoinductive effects encourage differentiation of these cells into pre-osteoblasts.

- These osteoprogenitor cells further differentiate into osteoblasts and after a period of months may terminally differentiate into osteocytes.
- Osteoblasts are responsible for bone formation by depositing osteoid and mineralizing it. The absolute number of osteoblasts tends to decrease with age.
- Osteocytes are long-lived stellate cells that are trapped within the matrix they secrete.
- Osteoclastic cells are derived from hematopoietic progenitor cells which differentiate under influence from mesenchymal stromal cells. The balance between osteoblast and osteoclast activity is responsible for the continuous remodeling of bone tissue.

Vascular Supply

- Bone is a highly vascular tissue, receiving 10–20 % of the resting cardiac output.
- Fracture healing is a delicate physiological process dependent on adequate vascular supply to damaged tissue.
- Preservation of tissue planes during surgical exposure is an important tenet to avoid disrupting the existing blood supply to the area.
- Osteocytes receive nutrition via cell–cell communication through bone canaliculi, while Volkmann and Haversian canals allow routes for blood vessels to penetrate through bone tissue.
- The ultimate strength of bony repair hinges on the vascular supply to the anatomic area. For example, fractures which occur in a rich vascular environment (distal radius metaphysis) have a much higher healing rate than those with poor circulation (scaphoid).
- Avascular necrosis (AVN) of bone tissue has been well described (femoral head AVN, Kienbock's disease). It is also well known that poor vascular supply is associated with unfavorable outcomes following surgery.
- VEGF has been shown to be the most important growth factor for angiogenesis and bone healing at a fracture site. Hypoxia has been shown to enhance angiogenic response and levels of VEGF in rodent bone marrow cells.
- Local delivery of these factors may lead to enhanced angiogenesis which may affect outcomes. Vascular tissue is an important source not only for nutrition and a route for responding cells, but also for osteoinductive stimuli.

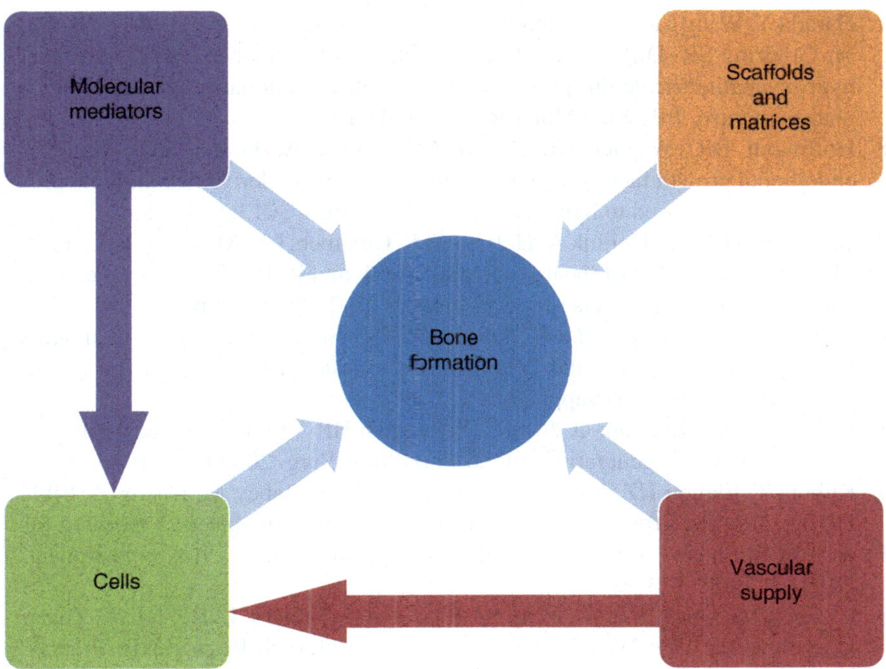

Fig. 1 Factors influencing bone formation

Bibliography

1. Albrektsson T. The healing of autologous bone grafts after varying degrees of surgical trauma. A microscopic and histochemical study in the rabbit. J Bone Joint Surg Br. 1980;62:403–10.
2. Albrektsson T, Johansson C. Osteoinduction, osteoconduction and osseointegration. Eur Spine J. 2001;10(Suppl 2):S96–101.
3. Beenken A, Mohammadi M. The FGF family: biology, pathophysiology and therapy. Nat Rev Drug Discov. 2009;8:235–53.
4. Caplan AI. Mesenchymal stem cells. J Orthop Res. 1991;9:641–50.
5. Chan O, Coathup MJ, Nesbitt A, Ho CY, Hing KA, Buckland T, Campion C, Blunn GW. The effects of microporosity on osteoinduction of calcium phosphate bone graft substitute biomaterials. Acta Biomater. 2012;8:2788–94.
6. Cui Q, Botchwey EA. Emerging ideas: treatment of precollapse osteonecrosis using stem cells and growth factors. Clin Orthop Relat Res. 2011;469:2665–9.

7. Harada Y, Wang JT, Doppalapudi VA, Willis AA, Jasty M, Harris WH, Nagase M, Goldring SR. Differential effects of different forms of hydroxyapatite and hydroxyapatite/tricalcium phosphate particulates on human monocyte/macrophages in vitro. J Biomed Mater Res. 1996;31:19–26.
8. Hoffmann BR, Wagner JR, Prisco AR, Janiak A, Greene AS. Vascular endothelial growth factor-A signaling in bone marrow-derived endothelial progenitor cells exposed to hypoxia. Physiol Genomics. 2013;45:1021–34.
9. Kempen DH, Lu L, Heijink A, Hefferan TE, Creemers LB, Maran A, Yaszemski MJ, Dhert WJ. Effect of local sequential VEGF and BMP-2 delivery on ectopic and orthotopic bone regeneration. Biomaterials. 2009;30:2816–25.
10. Keramaris NC, Calori GM, Nikolaou VS, Schemitsch EH, Giannoudis PV. Fracture vascularity and bone healing: a systematic review of the role of VEGF. Injury. 2008;39(Suppl 2):S45–57.
11. Kleinheinz J, Stratmann U, Joos U, Wiesmann HP. VEGF-activated angiogenesis during bone regeneration. J Oral Maxillofac Surg. 2005;63:1310–6.
12. Kubota T, Elalieh HZ, Saless N, Fong C, Wang Y, Babey M, Cheng Z, Bikle DD. Insulin-like growth factor-1 receptor in mature osteoblasts is required for periosteal bone formation induced by reloading. Acta Astronaut. 2013;92:73–8.
13. Lamplot JD, Qin J, Nan G, Wang J, Liu X, Yin L, Tomal J, Li R, Shui W, Zhang H, Kim SH, Zhang W, Zhang J, Kong Y, Denduluri S, Rogers MR, Pratt A, Haydon RC, Luu HH, Angeles J, Shi LL, He TC. BMP9 signaling in stem cell differentiation and osteogenesis. Am J Stem Cells. 2013;2:1–21.
14. Lounev VY, Ramachandran R, Wosczyna MN, Yamamoto M, Maidment AD, Shore EM, Glaser DL, Goldhamer DJ, Kaplan FS. Identification of progenitor cells that contribute to heterotopic skeletogenesis. J Bone Joint Surg Am. 2009;91:652–63.
15. Luginbuehl V, Zoidis E, Meinel L, von Rechenberg B, Gander B, Merkle HP. Impact of IGF-I release kinetics on bone healing: a preliminary study in sheep. Eur J Pharm Biopharm. 2013;85:99–106.
16. Matsubara H, Hogan DE, Morgan EF, Mortlock DP, Einhorn TA, Gerstenfeld LC. Vascular tissues are a primary source of BMP2 expression during bone formation induced by distraction osteogenesis. Bone. 2012;51:168–80.
17. Nagayama T, Okuhara S, Ota MS, Tachikawa N, Kasugai S, Iseki S. FGF18 accelerates osteoblast differentiation by upregulating Bmp2 expression. Congenit Anom (Kyoto). 53:83–8.
18. Rao RR, Stegemann JP. Cell-based approaches to the engineering of vascularized bone tissue. Cytotherapy. 2013;15:1309–22.
19. Ross M. Bone In: Pawlina W, editor. Histology: a text and atlas. Philadelphia: Lippincott Williams & Wilkins; 2010. p. 218–53.
20. Sanghani A, Chimutengwende-Gordon M, Adesida A, Khan W. Applications of stem cell therapy for physeal injuries. Curr Stem Cell Res Ther. 2013;8:451–5.
21. Stevenson S, Emery SE, Goldberg VM. Factors affecting bone graft incorporation. Clin Orthop Relat Res. 1996;(324):66–74.

22. Szpalski C, Nguyen PD, Cretiu Vasiliu CE, Chesnoiu-Matei I, Ricci JL, Clark E, Smay JE, Warren SM. Bony engineering using time-release porous scaffolds to provide sustained growth factor delivery. J Craniofac Surg. 2012;23:638–44.
23. Tsiridis E, Upadhyay N, Giannoudis P. Molecular aspects of fracture healing: which are the important molecules? Injury. 2007;38(Suppl 1):S11–25.
24. Wang X, Wang Y, Gou W, Lu Q, Peng J, Lu S. Role of mesenchymal stem cells in bone regeneration and fracture repair: a review. Int Orthop. 2013;37:2491–8.
25. Wang H, Zhi W, Lu X, Li X, Duan K, Duan R, Mu Y, Weng J. Comparative studies on ectopic bone formation in porous hydroxyapatite scaffolds with complementary pore structures. Acta Biomater. 2013;9:8413–21.
26. Yang F, Wang J, Hou J, Guo H, Liu C. Bone regeneration using cell-mediated responsive degradable PEG-based scaffolds incorporating with rhBMP-2. Biomaterials. 2013;34:1514–28.
27. Yang J, Wang J, Yuan T, Zhu XD, Xiang Z, Fan YJ, Zhang XD. The enhanced effect of surface microstructured porous titanium on adhesion and osteoblastic differentiation of mesenchymal stem cells. J Mater Sci Mater Med. 2013;24(9):2235–46.

2 Peripheral Nervous System

Phuc Dang and Ranjan Gupta

Take-Home Message

- Axons are surrounded by three layers of connective tissue including the endoneurium, the perineurium (blood–nerve barrier), and the epineurium.
- Seddon's classification of nerve injury: neurapraxia, axonotmesis, neurotmesis.
- Early tension-free nerve repair in young patients results in best chances for functional recovery.

Definitions The primary cellular components of peripheral nerves are axons from neurons and glial cells. Neurons are polarized cells with dendrites and axons that process and transmit information through electrochemical signals.

In the peripheral nervous system (PNS), the primary glial cell is the Schwann cell which serves to ensheathe axons in myelin and provides trophic support through release of important neurotrophic factors.

Peripheral nerves are part of the PNS that convey signals between the spinal cord to the limbs and organs. Nerves are composed of cellular processes from multiple different neurons including motor, sensory, and autonomic. The efferent neurons (motor and autonomic) receive signals from the central nervous systems (CNS) and transmit messages to their target end organs. Afferent nerves receive signals from specialized cell types, such as Pacinian corpuscles for fine sensation, and relay this information to the CNS.

Embryology The PNS are primarily derived from neural crest cells. Neural crest cells are groups of ectodermal cells that delaminate from the dorsal neural tube in early development. These cells then migrate throughout the body and develop into neurons, glia, and neurosecretory cells of the PNS.

Histology/Physiology A neuron usually ranges from 5 to 150 μm in diameter and contains a cell body and at least two cellular processes, the dendrite and the axon (Fig. 2). Impulses from the dendrites are directed toward the cell body, which in turn generate an action potential which is directed down the axon toward the synapse, or a target end organ such as a neuromuscular junction (NMJ). Axons can be myelinated (large fibers such as motor) or unmyelinated (small fibers such as type C pain fibers) (Table 2). Myelin, produced by the Schwann cells, acts as insulation surrounding the axon and serves to reduce the dissipation of action potential into the surrounding environment. Within myelinated axons, there are gaps without myelin called nodes of Ranvier, which allows propagation of action potential via saltatory conduction so as to increase nerve conduction velocity without increasing the diameter of an axon.

Cross-Sectional Anatomy The peripheral nerve is surrounded by three layers of connective tissue (Fig. 3). The innermost layer is the endoneurium and consists of loose collagenous matrix that nourishes and protects each axon. The middle layer is

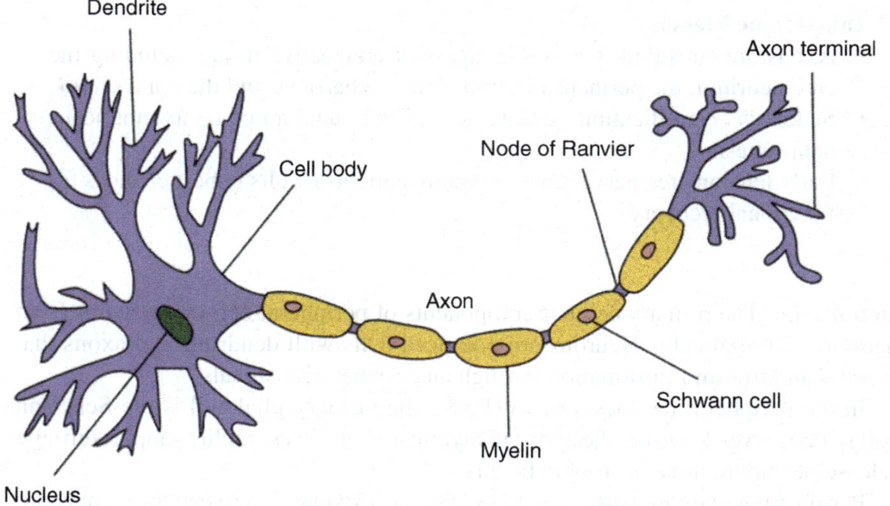

Fig. 2 Neuron morphology

Table 2 Nerve fiber types and function

Nerve fiber types		Function	Myelination	CV (m/s)
A	alpha	Motor – skeletal muscle	Yes	100
	beta	Touch, pressure		30–70
	delta	Muscle spindle, proprioception		15–30
	gamma	Fast pain (cold/touch)		12–30
B		Preganglionic autonomic	Yes	3–15
C		Pain (thermal), mechanoreceptor	No	0.5–2
		Postganglionic autonomic		0.7–2.3

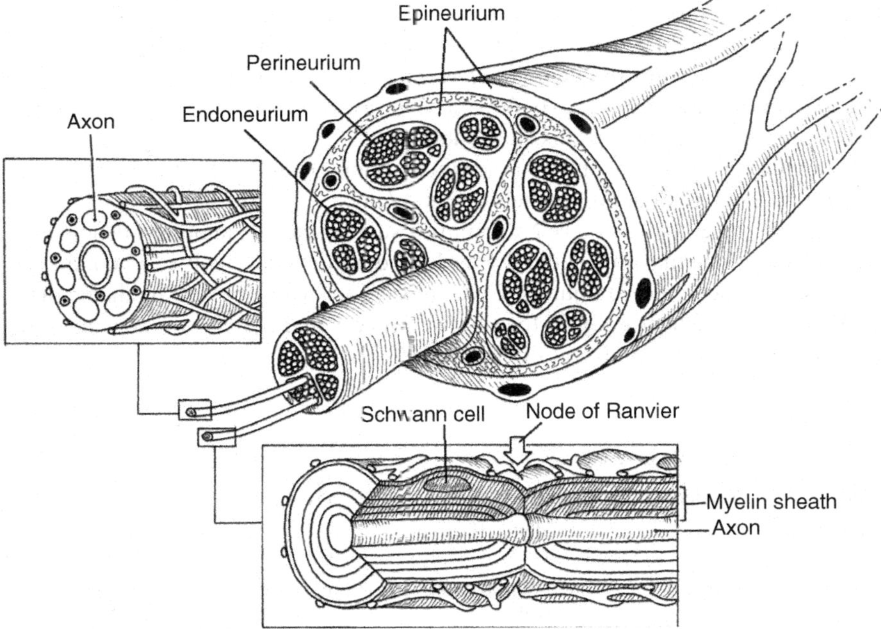

Fig. 3 Cross-sectional anatomy of the peripheral nerve (Adapted with permission from Lundborg G. Nerve injury and repair. New York: Churchill Livingstone; 1988. p. 33.)

the perineurium and consists of flattened fibroblasts that surround a fascicle of axons so as to act as a blood–nerve barrier via tight and gap junctions. The perineural layer is the major contributor to nerve tensile strength and has high resistance to compression and longitudinal traction. The outermost connective tissue layer is the epineurium and consists of an inner and outer layer. The outer layer surrounds and protects the nerve from external stresses while the inner layer pads the nerve's multiple fascicles and perineurium.

Neural blood supply is derived from a complex network of blood vessels. There are two major arterial systems and one minor longitudinal system that are linked together by anastomoses. The major systems consist of vessels that lie superficially on the nerve and within the interfascicular epineurium while the minor blood vessel system consists of blood vessels located in the endoneurium and perineurium.

Injury Injury to peripheral nerve can be acute or chronic.

Acute peripheral nerve injuries were initially described by Seddon and later refined by Sunderland. Seddon classified nerve injuries into three groups: neurapraxia, axonotmesis, and neurotmesis. A neurapraxia is characterized by myelin damage without neuronal injury so that distal neural degeneration does not occur. Axonotmesis is characterized by loss of axonal continuity with the preservation of connective tissue elements so as to provide a framework for healing. Importantly, the distal axon does undergo a series of cellular and molecular changes known as Wallerian degeneration to prepare for neural regeneration. Neurotmesis is the physiologic disruption of entire nerve with the ensuing distal axon undergoing degeneration without a framework for healing unless surgical repair is performed.

Sunderland further divided axonotmetic injuries into three types depending on severity of injury to connective tissues (Table 3).

After injury, axonal growth from proximal stump occurs with the growth cone regenerating at a rate of approximately 1–3 mm/day.

Chronic nerve compression (CNC) injuries such as carpal tunnel syndrome are common conditions that are acquired over long duration and involve ischemia and fibrosis. Unlike acute nerve injuries, CNC injuries are Schwann cell-mediated and lack axonal involvement early in the disease process and thereby do not undergo Wallerian degeneration or changes in the NMJ.

Table 3 Classification of nerve injuries

Seddon	Sunderland	Injury	Prognosis
Neurapraxia	Grade I	Focal demyelination	Complete recovery in hours to months
Axonotmesis	Grade II	Disruption of axon and myelin	Functional recover months to years
		Intact epi-, peri-, and endoneurium	May not be complete
	Grade III	Disruption of axon, myelin, and endoneurium	Recovery range from poor to complete Depends on degree of intrafascicular fibrosis
		Intact epineurium and perineurium	
	Grade IV	Disruption of axon, myelin, endo- and perineurium	Spontaneous recovery nearly impossible
		Intact epineurium	Recovery depends on surgery
			Complete recovery unlikely
Neurotmesis	Grade V	Complete physiologic nerve disruption	Spontaneous recovery impossible
			Recovery depends on surgery
			Complete recovery unlikely

Treatment Acute nerve injury can result in motor and sensory deficits with life-altering outcomes for patients. Reconstruction of nerve after transection or segmental loss is essential to achieve functional reinnervation. Prerequisites for nerve repair are clean wound, good vascular supply, and adequate tissue coverage. Microscope, capable surgeons and team, and patient participation are essential for success. Early surgical repairs tend to have better functional recovery as there is diminished neural retraction and reduced requirement for grafting. If tension-free repair cannot be achieved, nerve grafting must be performed with an autograft (same donor), an allograft (donor from same species), or a nerve conduit. The current gold standard for grafting remains the autograft.

Nerve repair can be performed via suturing the epineurium or group of fascicles (Fig. 4). Epineural repair establishes continuity of the nerve without tension and properly aligns the fascicles.

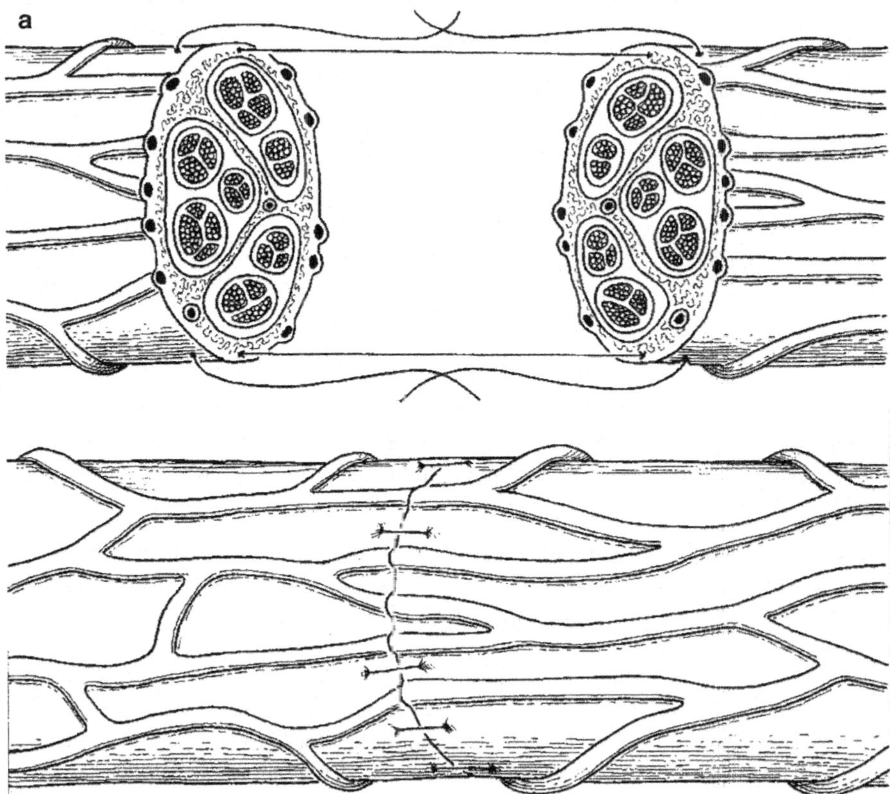

Fig. 4 (**a**) Group fascicular repair (Adapted with permission from Lundborg G. Nerve injury and repair. New York: Churchill Livingstone; 1988. p. 199). (**b**) Group fascicular repair (Adapted with permission from Lundborg G. Nerve injury and repair. New York: Churchill Livingstone; 1988. p. 200)

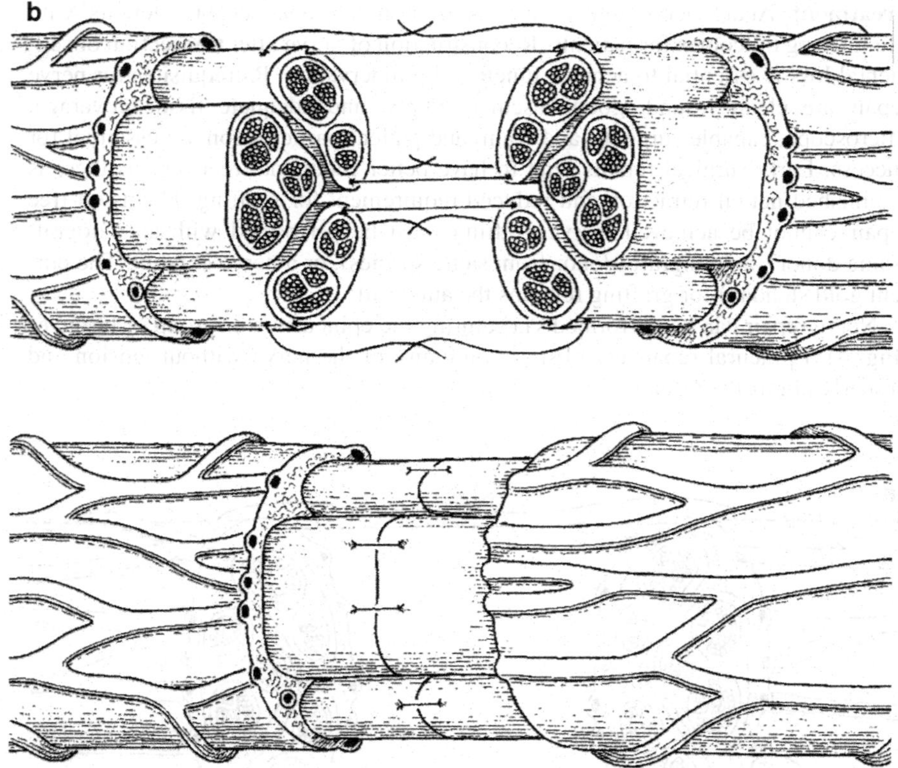

Fig. 4 (continued)

Group fascicle repair aligns proper fascicles (sensory–sensory, motor–motor) and allows proper reinnervation. In theory, group fascicular repair should produce a better clinical outcome; however, multiple studies have not shown improved functional outcomes.

Prognosis Meaningful functional recovery (M3-against gravity, S3-pain and touch with >15 mm 2-point discrimination) can be achieved in approximately 60 % of patients with best results achieved with median nerve repair and worst outcomes with ulnar nerve repair.

Young patient, early repair, single function nerve, distal repairs, and short or no nerve graft are important prognostic factors for improving results. Future directions for improving functional neural recovery include developing strategies to improve the rate of regeneration, to improve the specificity of regeneration, to create novel allografts, and to prevent target end-organ degeneration of the neuromuscular junction.

Bibliography

1. Chao T, Frump D, Lin M, Caiozzo VJ, Mozaffar T, Steward O, Gupta R. Matrix metalloproteinase 3 deletion preserves denervated motor endplates after traumatic nerve injury. Ann Neuro. 2013;73(2):210–23.
2. Chemnitz A, Bjorkman A, Dahlin LB, Rosen B. Functional outcome thirty years after median and ulnar nerve repair in childhood and adolescence. J Bone Joint Surg Am. 2013;95(4):329–37.
3. Gupta R, Steward O. Chronic nerve compression induces concurrent apoptosis and proliferation of Schwann cells. J Comp Neuro. 2003;461(2):174–86.
4. Gupta R, Nassiri N, Hazel A, Bathen M, Mozaffar T. Chronic nerve compression alters Schwann cell myelin architecture in a murine model. Muscle Nerve. 2012;45(2):231–41.
5. Hammert CW, Chung CK. Peripheral nerve conditions: using evidence to guide treatment. Hand Clin. 2013:29; 317–458.
6. Khuong TH, Midha R. Advances in nerve repair. Curr Neuro Neurosci Rep. 2013;13:332.
7. Kim HD, Kam CA, Chandika P, Tiel LR, Kline D. Surgical management and outcomes in patients with medial nerve lesions. J Neurosurg. 2001;95: 584–94.
8. Kim HD, Han K, Tiel LR, Murovic AJ, Kline GD. Surgical outcomes of 654 ulnar nerve lesions. J Neurosurg. 2003;98:993–1004.
9. Lee KS, Wolfe WS. Peripheral nerve injury and repair. J Am Acad Orthop Surg. 2000;8:243–52.
10. Li R, Liu Z, Pan Y, Chen L, Zhang Z, Lu L. Peripheral nerve injuries treatment: a systematic review. Cell Biochem Biophys. 2014;68:449–54.
11. Menorca MGR, Fussell TS, Elfar JC. Nerve physiology: mechanisms of injury and recovery. Hand Clin. 2013:29;317–30.
12. Murovic JA. Upper-extremity peripheral nerve injuries: a Louisiana State University Health Sciences Center literature review with comparison of the operative outcomes of 1837 Louisiana State University Health Sciences Center median, radial, and ulnar nerve lesions. Neurosurgery. 2009;65(4 Suppl): A11–7.
13. Purves D, Augustine JG, Fitzpatrick D, Hall CW, LaMantia A-S, McNamara OJ, William MS. Neuroscience 3rd ed. Sinauer Associates: Massachusetts; 2004.
14. Seddon HJ. Surgical disorders of the peripheral nerves. Baltimore: Williams & Wilkins; 1972. pp. 68–88.
15. Sunderland S. Nerve injuries and their repair: a critical appraisal. New York: Churchill Livingstone; 1991.

3 Skeletal Muscle

Bastián Uribe-Echevarría and Brian R. Wolf

Take-Home Message

- Muscle>fascicle>muscle fiber (single cell)>myofibril>myofilament> sarcomere
- Actin-binding site for myosin are blocked by tropomyosin.
- Contraction: sliding of actin and myosin.
- Bands: A, I, H, M, and Z. Bands H and I shorten during contraction.
- Maximal force is proportional to physiologic cross-sectional area (PCSA). Maximal excursion and velocity are proportional to length.
- Eccentric contraction generates highest tension and risk of injury.

Muscle Morphology Muscle fiber: single multinucleated cell.

Muscle fibers are made from myofibrils that are divisible into myofilaments (functional units composed of sarcomeres arranged in series) (Fig. 5).

Myofibrils are surrounded by sarcoplasmic reticulum (SR) and its transverse tubules (T tubules). The SR is an endoplasmic reticulum specialized in storing and pumping Ca^{2+} ions. T tubules are continuous with the sarcolemma (cell membrane), extending the extracellular space into the muscle fiber.

No syncytial bridges as opposed to cardiac muscle.

Endomysium: connective tissue (CT) surrounding individual fibers.

Perimysium: CT surrounding collections of fibers.

Epimysium: CT covering entire muscle.

Cross-striations are identified by letters. A sarcomere is the area between two Z lines in a myofibril. Contraction results in H- and I-band shortening. A-band remains the same.

Contractile proteins

- *Thick filaments*

  Myosin-II: long tail and two globular heads that contain an actin-binding site and a catalytic site that hydrolyzes ATP.

- *Thin filaments*

  Actin: long double helix
  Tropomyosin: filaments located in the groove between chains of actin
  Troponin: located along tropomyosin molecules. Three subunits:

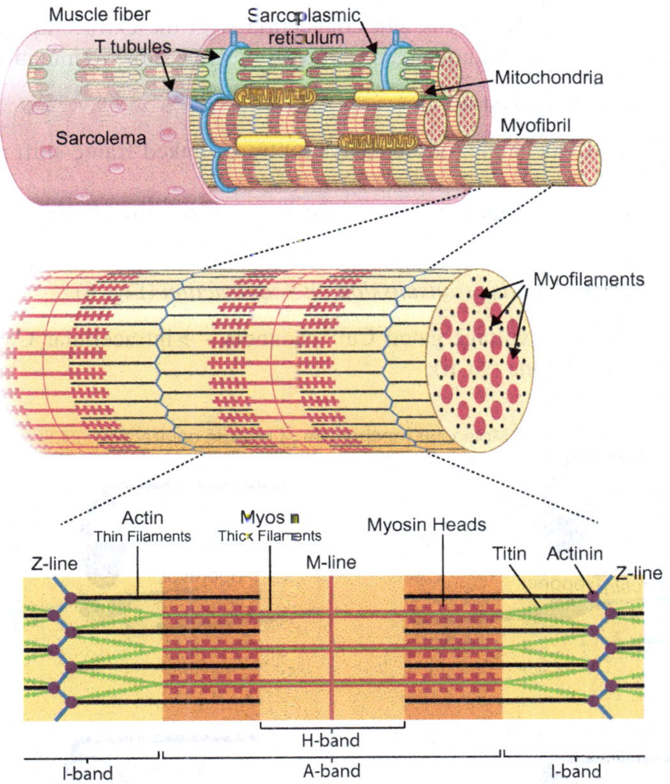

Fig. 5 Morphology (Adapted. Permission license BAS59347 McGraw-Hill Education)

T binds to tropomyosin.
C binds to Ca^{2+} producing a conformational change affecting subunit I.
I inhibits the interaction of myosin with actin.

Structural proteins

Actinin binds actin to Z lines.
Titin connects Z lines to M lines and provides scaffolding and passive elasticity of the muscle. Largest known protein (3,800,000 Da). When stretched (unfolding

of folded domains), quickly increases resistance protecting sarcomere structure.

Desmin binds Z lines to plasma membrane.

Dystrophin: scaffolding for fibrils and connection with the extracellular environment. One of the longest known genes, therefore susceptible to mutation.

Pathologies affecting dystrophin:

If absent, produces Duchenne muscular dystrophy, X-linked frame-shift mutation, fatal by 30.

If altered or reduced, produces Becker muscular dystrophy, X-linked mutated gene.

Muscle Physiology *Impulse transmission and contraction* (Fig. 6)

- Action potential – >voltage-gated Ca^{2+} channels – >intracellular Ca^{2+} causes release of acetylcholine (ACh).

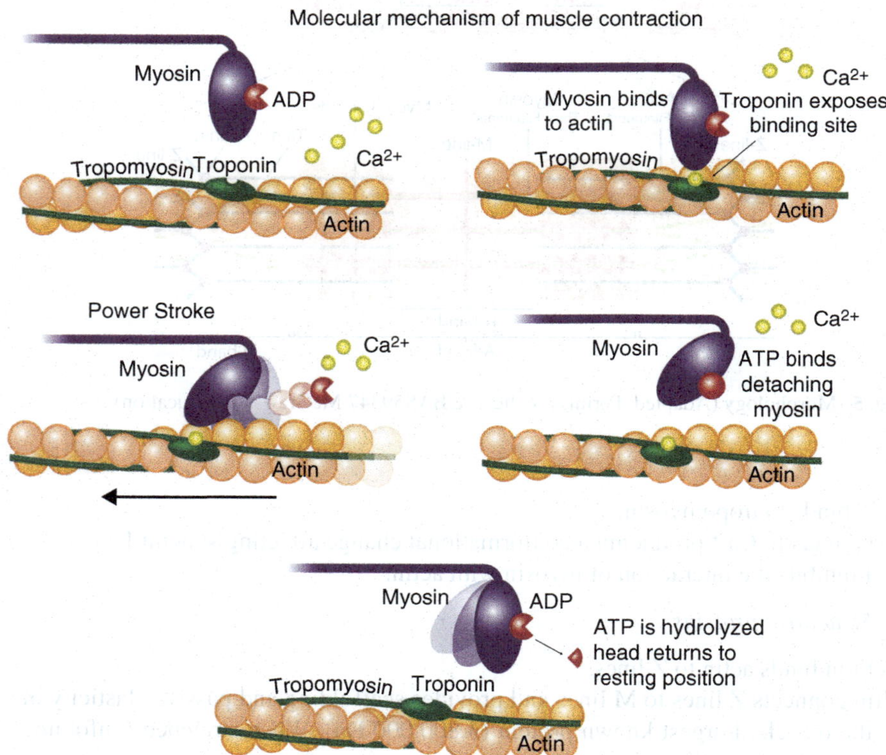

Fig. 6 Muscle contraction (Adapted from Muskel-molekular.png. Wikimedia Commons. Hank van Helvete. 2006 licensed with Cc-by-sa-2.5)

- Activation of nicotinic ACh receptor (nAChR) leads to depolarization of the motor end plate (muscle cell).
- Depolarization spreads along muscle cell and T tubules.
- Voltage-sensitive dihydropyridine receptor on the T tubules couples with ryanodine receptor (also Ca^{2+} sensitive) on SR, inducing Ca^{2+} release. Effect amplified by calcium-induced Ca^{2+} release.
- Ca^{2+} binds to troponin C, causing conformational change, exposing binding site on actin, allowing myosin–actin crossbridges.
- Myosin releases bound adenosine diphosphate (ADP) and bends at the junction of the head and neck, sliding actin over myosin, shortening the sarcomere (power stroke).
- ATP binds to now-exposed site on myosin, detaching it from actin.
- ATP is hydrolyzed into ADP. Myosin head returns to resting position.

Each power stroke shortens the sarcomere by 1 % (10 nm). Muscles shorten 35–50 %. Myosin crossbridge action *repeats several times* during contraction, if ATP available and Ca^{2+} present.

Electronic response of the muscle fiber is similar to that of the nerve (5 ms). Contraction and relaxation are slower (100 ms), making temporal summation of contractions possible. Repeated stimulations before relaxation produce a response added to the contraction already present. When frequency is high enough to produce a continuous contraction without relaxation, it is called tetanic contraction.

Types of muscle fibers: a continuum. Classifications are made for research (Table 4).

Table 4 Types of muscle fibers

	Type 1	Type 2A	Type 2B
Morphology	Red	White	White
	Small muscle fiber	Medium muscle fiber	Large muscle fiber
	High concentration of mitochondria	Intermediate	Low concentration of mitochondria
	High capillary density	High capillary density	Low capillary density
Physiology	Slow twitch	Fast twitch	Fast twitch
	Low strength	High strength	High strength
Metabolism	Slow oxidative (SO)	Fast oxidative/glycolytic (FOG)	Fast glycolytic (FG)
	High aerobic capacity	Medium aerobic capacity	Low aerobic capacity
	Fatigue resistant	Intermediate resistance to fatigue	Least resistant to fatigue
Training needed		Endurance	Strength

3.1 Contraction Types

- Isometric: muscle remains the same length, muscular strength matches load.
- Isotonic: muscle contracts, maintaining constant tension.
- Isovelocity (isokinetic): contraction velocity remains constant; force may vary. Rare in natural state. Primarily an analysis method.
- Concentric: muscle force overcomes resistance, muscle shortens.
- Eccentric: resistance overcomes muscle force, muscle lengthens. Higher risk of injury.

3.2 Contraction Physiology

Excursion and velocity are proportional to muscle fiber length, yielded by sarcomeres arranged in series (Fig. 7).

Maximum tetanic tension is proportional to the physiologic cross-sectional area (PCSA) (Fig. 7). PCSA is dependent on anatomic cross-sectional area, pennation (angle of fibers), muscle density, and fiber length.

Force–length relationship, also called length–tension curve (Fig. 8). Muscles operate with greatest active force when close to an ideal length (often resting length). Based on the amount of overlapping molecules of myosin and actin that can interact at a specific length. Due to the presence of elastic proteins within a muscle (such as titin), when muscle is stretched beyond a given length, entirely passive forces oppose lengthening.

Force–velocity relationship (Fig. 9): Under experimental conditions, contraction speed (regulated by load) affects force. Force is inversely proportional in a hyperbolic fashion to velocity.

Max velocity: zero force

Zero velocity: isometric max force

Negative velocity (eccentric contraction): force above isometric maximum (absolute maximum)

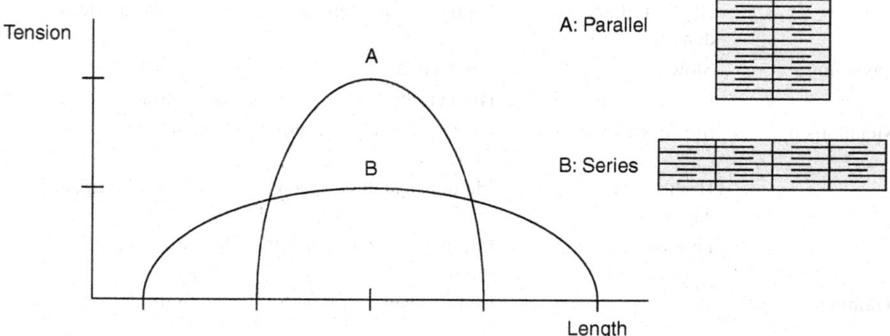

Fig. 7 Sarcomeres arrangement tension, excursion and velocity

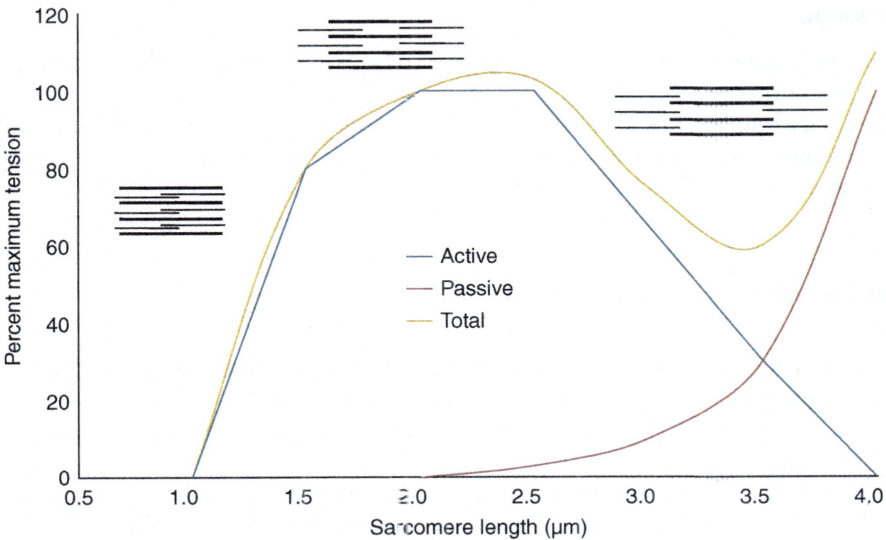

Fig. 8 Force-length relationship curve

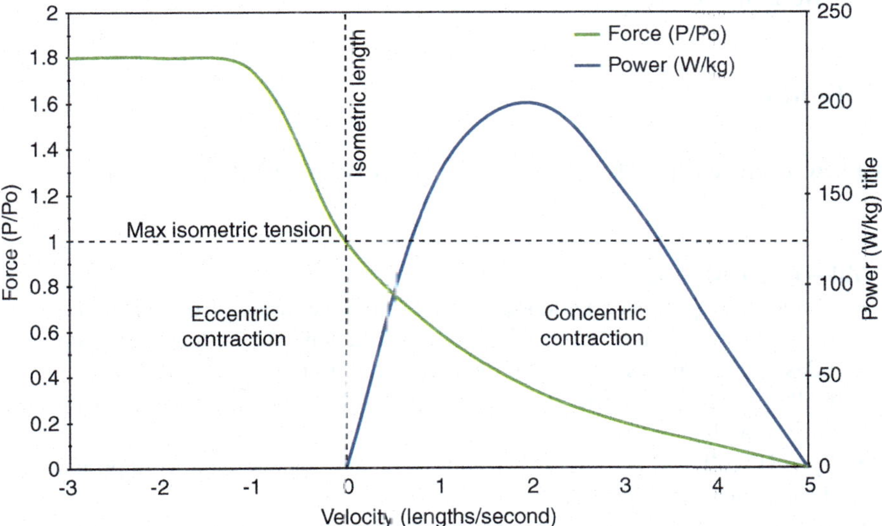

Fig. 9 Force-velocity relationship

Power: Product of force and velocity. The muscle does not generate power at isometric force (due to zero velocity) nor maximal velocity (due to zero force). Optimal shortening velocity for power generation is approximately one-third of maximum shortening velocity (Fig. 9).

Training

Strength training: high load, low repetition. Produces hypertrophy of all fiber types, especially type 2B

Endurance training: low load, high repetition. Muscle increases efficiency. Increase in capillarity, mitochondrial size, number, and density. Increase in oxidative capacity in all fiber types, especially type 2A

Bibliography

1. Barrett KE, Boitano S, Barman SM, Brooks HL, editors. Ganong's review of medical physiology. 24 ed. New York: McGraw-Hill; 2010.
2. Herzog W, editor. Skeletal muscle mechanics. From mechanisms to function. West Sussex: Wiley; 2000.
3. Lieber RL. Skeletal muscle, structure, function, and plasticity. The physiological basis of rehabilitation. 2nd ed. Philadelphia: Lippincott Williams & Wilkins; 2002.
4. Lieberman JR, editor. AAOS comprehensive orthopaedic review. Rosemont: AAOS; 2009.
5. Nigg BM, Herzog W, editors. Biomechanics of the musculo-skeletal system. 3rd ed. West Sussex: Wiley; 2007.

4 Tendon

Matthew T. Provencher, Daniel J. Gross, Amun Makani, and Petar Golijanin

Take-Home Message

- Tendons are produced by tenocytes and primarily formed from water. The dry weight is primarily formed of type I collagen. The collagen polypeptides form a triple helix, which then cross-link to form fibrils.
- Collagen's parallel fibril arrangement with cross-linking contributes to tensile strength.
- Type III collagen is found in the endotenon and epitenon and is important during early healing and remodeling.
- Nutrition is derived from synovial fluid for intrasynovial tendons, where as extrasynovial tendons are able to remain metabolically active regardless of environment.
- The transition zone for tendon insertion consists of four layers: tendon, unmineralized fibrocartilage, mineralized fibrocartilage (Sharpey's fibers), and bone.

- Tendons follow a stress–strain relationship, and its characteristics can be illustrated on a load–elongation curve.
- Tendon healing follows four stages of repair: inflammation, proliferation, matrix formation, and remodeling.
- Tendons are weakest at 7–10 days during inflammation stage and generally reach maximum strength at 6 months.

Anatomy

- Composition:
  - Primarily composed of collagen (approximately 85 % of dry weight) with a high concentration of proteoglycans (and elastin)
- Collagen:
  - Basic structural unit of tendon
    - Type I collagen is predominant.
    - Type III collagen is found in the endotenon and epitenon and increases during the early phase of healing and remodeling.
  - Collagen polypeptides form a triple helix which then combines to form fibrils with cross-linking.
    - This parallel fibril arrangement with cross-linking contributes to the tensile strength of tendon.
  - Produced by tenocytes.
- Proteoglycans:
  - Interact with the collagen fibrils, helping to form a matrix that disperses load between fibrils.
  - Composed of subunits known as glycosaminoglycans (GAGs).
  - Negatively charged, hydrophilic molecules resist compressive force.
  - Responsible for viscoelasticity
- Viscoelasticity:
  - Describes a rate-dependent response to load.
  - Is a function of the internal friction of the material.
  - Tendons are less viscoelastic than ligaments.
- Histology and Microanatomy:
  - Fibroblasts (tenocytes) are the predominant cell type.
  - Tendons are composed of bundles of collagen called fascicles (See Fig. 10).

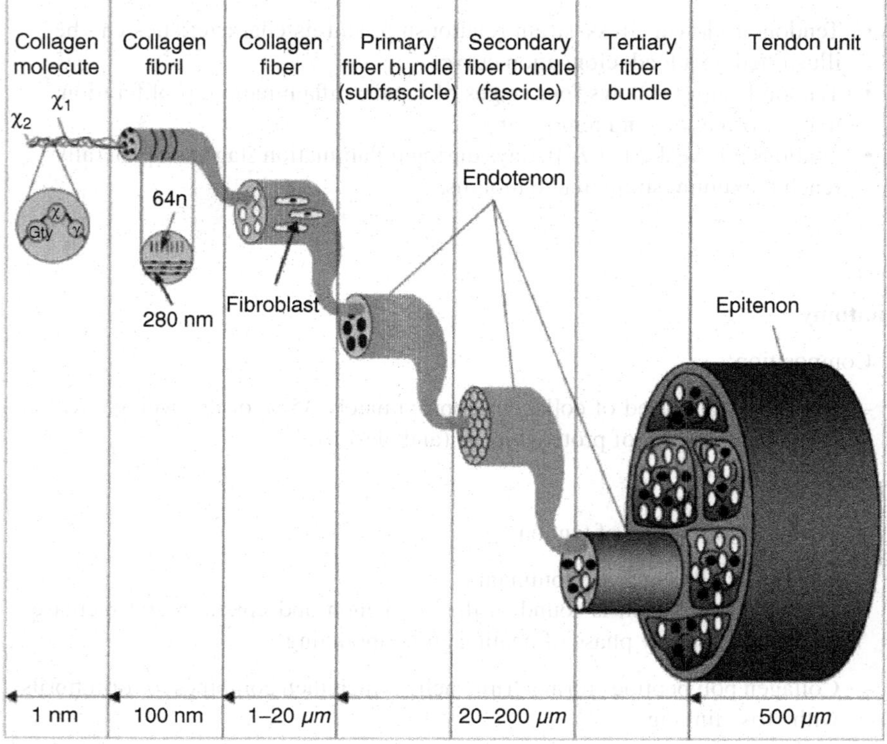

Fig. 10 Architecture of tendon

- Fascicles are groups of collagen fibrils running in parallel to the long axis of the tendon.
- Resist tensile force.
- Grouped into individual fascicles that are surrounded by endotenon.
- Groups of fascicles are surrounded by epitenon.
- Epitenon is a synovial-like outer membrane containing blood vessels, nerves, and lymphatics.

- Blood supplies two types of tendons:
  - Paratenon-covered (vascular): patellar tendon, Achilles tendon
    - Vascular tendons with capillary system contained within paratenon
    - Greater healing potential than avascular tendons
  - Sheathed (avascular) tendon: hand flexor tendons
    - Vincula (vascular mesotenons) carry a vessel that supplies only one tendon segment.
    - Avascular areas receive nutrition via diffusion from vascularized segments including musculotendinous and tendon–bone junction.

- Nutrition:
  - Intrasynovial: tendons are dependent on the synovial fluid for nutrition.
    - Regenerative ability is decreased when removed from this environment.
  - Extrasynovial: able to remain metabolically active regardless of environment.
    - Nutrition is derived from several sources including perimysium, periosteal attachments, and surrounding tissues.
- Insertion:
  - Two types of insertion: direct and indirect
  - Fibrocartilaginous (Direct): transition zone consisting of four layers:
    - Tendon
    - Unmineralized fibrocartilage
    - Mineralized fibrocartilage (Sharpey's fibers)
    - Bone
      - Transition zone allows gradual dissipation of force.
      - "Direct" refers to the absence of periosteum.
      - Present in distal insertion of medial collateral ligament (MCL) on proximal tibia.
  - Fibrous (Indirect): collagen fibers of the tendon enter bone via perforating collagen fibers (periosteum).
    - Present in proximal insertion of MCL on distal femur

Biomechanics

- Tendons are oriented along lines of stress.
- Load transmission:
  - Stress-strain relationship: Time-dependent, nonlinear viscoelastic properties with stress being force per unit area and strain being the change in length.
  - Stress-relaxation:
    - Stress (or deformation) decreases with time if the strain is held constant.
  - Creep:
    - Strain increases with time if the stress is held constant (increased deformation under a constant load).
- Load–elongation curve: Four distinct regions (See Fig. 11):

- Toe region: greatest amount of deformation for given load
  - Relaxed (crimped) fibers of a tendon are straightened and oriented to take up load.

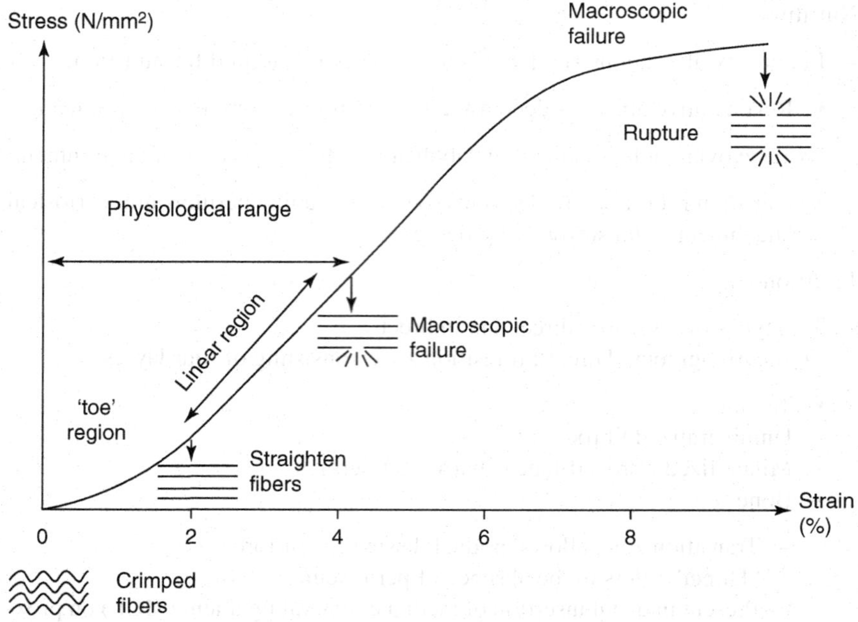

Fig. 11 Tendon stress–strain curve (load–elongation curve)

- Linear region: constant load-elongation behavior
  - Tendon fibers are oriented parallel to the direction of the load, and tissue stiffness is represented by the slope.
- Yield Point: tendon transitions from elastic (reversible) to plastic (irreversible).
- Failure: curve beings to decline

- Hysteresis: energy dissipation
  - Loading and unloading curves differ due to energy dissipated during loading of tendon.

Injury and Repair Tendon–bone healing (Fig. 12):

- Bony avulsion of tendon insertions heals more rapidly than midsubstance tears.

- Tendon healing follows four stages of repair:
  - Inflammation: 0–5 days
    - Primary cells: neutrophils and macrophages.
    - Initial production of type III collagen.
    - Tendon is at its weakest during this stage of healing (weakest at 7–10 days).

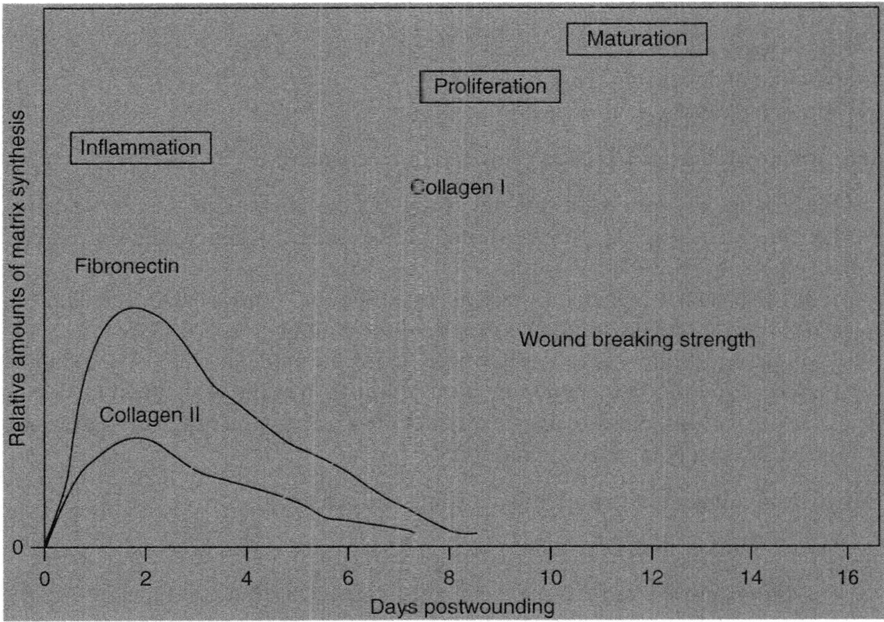

Fig. 12 Phases of healing

- Proliferation: 4–14 days
  - Five growth factors shown to be significantly upregulated during healing (TGF-β[beta], BMPs (−12, −13, −14), PDGF, IGF-1, VEGF, bFGF) promote differentiation and proliferation of fibroblasts.
- Matrix formation: >14 days
  - Increased angiogenesis
  - Deposition of large amounts of disorganized collagen
- Remodeling: up to 18 months
  - Fibrosis
  - Tissue may continue to remodel for approximately 1 year, but it generally reaches maximum strength by 12 months.
  - Type I collagen begins replacing type III collagen.
  - In bone–tendon healing, bone grows into the fibrovascular scar tissue over time. While this coincides with significant increase in strength, this scar tissue at the site of repair will limit the ultimate strength.

- Known factors that impede healing:
  - NSAIDs
  - Smoking

- EtOH
- Diabetes
- Vitamin D deficiency
- Stress overload

Current Knowledge and Trends Post-injury mechanics:

- Early range of motion (ROM) and cyclic loading after surgical tendon repair have been shown to help avoid postoperative stiffness, reduce adhesions, and regain maximal ROM.
- It has also been shown to increase the inflammatory response at the repair site, which may affect the terminal strength of the tendon–bone interface.
- Postoperative immobilization has been shown to modulate the early inflammatory response, but its end effect on terminal strength of the tendon–bone interface is inconclusive, and potential complications include postoperative stiffness as well as reduced final ROM.

• Biological augmentation for tendon healing and repair:

  - Growth factors and stem cells:

    • Various growth factors and stem cells have been shown to be effective at augmenting tendon–bone healing, but delivery to the site continues to be the limiting factor to their effectiveness.
    • Investigators continue to look toward bioscaffolds and gene therapy to improve delivery, as well as optimal combinations of both growth factors and stem cells to improve effectiveness.

Bibliography

1. Brophy RH, Kovacevic D, Imhauser CW, Stasiak M, Bedi A, Fox AJS, et al. Effect of short-duration low-magnitude cyclic loading versus immobilization on tendon-bone healing after ACL reconstruction in a rat model. J Bone Joint Surg Am. 2011;93(4):381–93.
2. Isaac C, Gharaibeh B, Witt M, Wright VJ, Huard J. Biologic approaches to enhance rotator cuff healing after injury. J Shoulder Elbow Surg. 2012;21(2): 181–90.
3. Lui PP, Wong OT. Tendon stem cells: experimental and clinical perspectives in tendon and tendon-bone junction repair. Muscles Ligaments Tendons J. 2012;2(3):163–8. Print 2012 Jul.

Bibliography

1. American Academy of Orthopaedic Surgeons. Symposium (1987: Savannah Ga.), Woo SLY, Buckwalter JA, American Academy of Orthopaedic Surgeons, National Institute of Arthritis and Musculoskeletal and Skin Diseases (U.S.). Injury and repair of the musculoskeletal soft tissues: workshop, Savannah, Georgia, June 1987. Park Ridge: American Academy of Orthopaedic Surgeons; 1988. p. 548.
2. Benjamin M, Evans EJ, Copp L. The histology of tendon attachments to bone in man. J Anat. 1986;149:89–100.
3. Benjamin M, Toumi H, Ralphs JR, Bydder G, Best TM, Milz S. Where tendons and ligaments meet bone: attachment sites ('entheses') in relation to exercise and/or mechanical load. J Anat. 2006;208(4):471–90.
4. Brophy RH, Kovacevic D, Imhauser CW, Stasiak M, Bedi A, Fox AJS, et al. Effect of short-duration low-magnitude cyclic loading versus immobilization on tendon-bone healing after ACL reconstruction in a rat model. J Bone Joint Surg Am. 2011;93(4):381–93.
5. Bruns J, Kampen J, Kahrs J, Plitz W. Achilles tendon rupture: experimental results on spontaneous repair in a sheep-model. Knee Surg Sports Traumatol Arthrosc. 2000;8(6):364–9.
6. Burger S. Influence of intermittent compressive force on proteoglycan content in calcifying growth plate cartilage in vitro. J Biochemistry, 1987;262 (32):15490–15495.
7. Butler DL, Grood ES, Noyes FR, Zernicke RF. Biomechanics of ligaments and tendons. Exerc Sport Sci Rev. 1978;6:125–81.
8. Chang C-H, Chen C-H, Su C-Y, Liu H-T, Yu C-M. Rotator cuff repair with periosteum for enhancing tendon-bone healing: a biomechanical and histological study in rabbits. Knee Surg Sports Traumatol Arthrosc. 2009;17(12):1447–53.
9. Dagher E, Hays PL, Kawamura S, Godin J, Deng X-H, Rodeo SA. Immobilization modulates macrophage accumulation in tendon-bone healing. Clin Orthop Relat Res. 2009;467(1):281–7.
10. Einhorn TA, Simon SR, American Academy of Orthopaedic Surgeons. Orthopaedic basic science: biology and biomechanics of the musculoskeletal system. 2nd ed. Rosemont: American Academy of Orthopaedic Surgeons; 2000. p. 873, xix
11. Eliasson P, Andersson T, Aspenberg P. Achilles tendon healing in rats is improved by intermittent mechanical loading during the inflammatory phase. J Orthop Res. 2012;30(2):274–9.
12. Fallon J, Blevins FT, Vogel K, Trotter J. Functional morphology of the supraspinatus tendon. J Orthop Res. 2002;20(5):920–6.
13. Fenwick SA, Hazleman BL, Riley GP. The vasculature and its role in the damaged and healing tendon. Arthritis Res. 2002;4(4):252–60.

14. Ginsburg JH, Whiteside LA, Piper TL. Nutrient pathways in transferred patellar tendon used for anterior cruciate ligament reconstruction. Am J Sports Med. 1980;8(1):15–8.
15. Hashimoto Y, Naka Y, Fukunaga K, Nakamura H, Takaoka K. ACL reconstruction using bone-tendon-bone graft engineered from the semitendinosus tendon by injection of recombinant BMP-2 in a rabbit model. J Orthop Res. 2011;29(12):1923–30.
16. Hays PL. The role of macrophages in early healing of a tendon graft in a bone tunnel. J Bone Joint Surg Am. 2008;90(3):565.
17. Hettrich CM, Gasinu S, Beamer BS, Fox A, Ying O, Deng XH, et al. The effect of immobilization on the native and repaired tendon-to-bone interface. J Bone Joint Surg Am. 2013;95(10):925–30.
18. Hoppe S, Alini M, Benneker LM, Milz S, Boileau P, Zumstein MA. Tenocytes of chronic rotator cuff tendon tears can be stimulated by platelet-released growth factors. J Shoulder Elbow Surg. 2013;22(3):340–9.
19. Isaac C, Gharaibeh B, Witt M, Wright VJ, Huard J. Biologic approaches to enhance rotator cuff healing after injury. J Shoulder Elbow Surg. 2012;21(2): 181–90.
20. Kaeding C, Best TM. Tendinosis: pathophysiology and nonoperative treatment. Sports Health. 2009;1(4):284–92.
21. Kastelic J, Galeski A, Baer E. The multicomposite structure of tendon. Connect Tissue Res. 1978;6(1):11–23.
22. Katzel EB, Wolenski M, Loiselle AE, Basile P, Flick LM, Langstein HN, et al. Impact of Smad3 loss of function on scarring and adhesion formation during tendon healing. J Orthop Res. 2011;29(5):684–93.
23. Kim HM, Galatz LM, Das R, Havlioglu N, Rothermich SY, Thomopoulos S. The role of transforming growth factor beta isoforms in tendon-to-bone healing. Connect Tissue Res. 2011;52(2):87–98.
24. Kondo E, Yasuda K, Katsura T, Hayashi R, Kotani Y, Tohyama H. Biomechanical and histological evaluations of the doubled semitendinosus tendon autograft after anterior cruciate ligament reconstruction in sheep. Am J Sports Med. 2012;40(2):315–24.
25. Lundborg G, Myrhage R, Rydevik B. The vascularization of human flexor tendons within the digital synovial sheath regio--tructural and functional aspects. J Hand Surg Am. 1977;2(6):417–27.
26. Lundborg G, Holm S, Myrhage R. The role of the synovial fluid and tendon sheath for flexor tendon nutrition. An experimental tracer study on diffusional pathways in dogs. Scand J Plast Reconstr Surg. 1980;14(1):99–107.
27. Manske PR. Flexor tendon healing. J Hand Surg Br. 1988;13(3):237–45.
28. Manske PR, Lesker PA. Flexor tendon nutrition. Hand Clin. 1985;1(1): 13–24.
29. Martinek V, Latterman C, Usas A, Abramowitch S, Woo SLY, Fu FH, et al. Enhancement of tendon-bone integration of anterior cruciate ligament grafts with bone morphogenetic protein-2 gene transfer: a histological and biomechanical study. J Bone Joint Surg Am. 2002;84-A(7):1123–31.

30. Molloy T, Wang Y, Murrell G. The roles of growth factors in tendon and ligament healing. Sports Med. 2003;33(5):381–94.
31. Oshiro W, Lou J, Xing X, Tu Y, Manske PR. Flexor tendon healing in the rat: a histologic and gene expression study. J Hand Surg. 2003;28(5):814–23.
32. Ota S, Uehara K, Nozaki M, Kobayashi T, Terada S, Tobita K, et al. Intramuscular transplantation of muscle-derived stem cells accelerates skeletal muscle healing after contusion injury via enhancement of angiogenesis. Am J Sports Med. 2011;39(9):1912–22.
33. Prisk V, Huard J. Muscle injuries and repair: the role of prostaglandins and inflammation. Histol Histopathol. 2003;18:1243–56.
34. Rodeo SA. Biologic augmentation of rotator cuff tendon-healing with use of a mixture of osteoinductive growth factors. J Bone Joint Surg Am. 2007;89(11):2485.
35. Rodeo SA, Suzuki K, Deng XH, Wozney J, Warren RF. Use of recombinant human bone morphogenetic protein-2 to enhance tendon healing in a bone tunnel. Am J Sports Med. 1999;27(4):476–88.
36. Rodeo SA, Kawamura S, Kim HJ, Dynybil C, Ying L. Tendon healing in a bone tunnel differs at the tunnel entrance versus the tunnel exit: an effect of graft-tunnel motion? Am J Sports Med. 2006;34(11):1790–800.
37. Rodeo SA, Delos D, Williams RJ, Adler RS, Pearle A, Warren RF. The effect of platelet-rich fibrin matrix on rotator cuff tendon healing: a prospective, randomized clinical study. Am J Sports Med. 2012;40(6):1234–41.
38. September AV, Schwellnus MP, Collins M. Tendon and ligament injuries: the genetic component. Br J Sports Med. 2007;41(4):241–6; discussion 6.
39. Sharma P. Tendon injury and tendinopathy: healing and repair. J Bone Joint Surg Am. 2005;87(1):187.
40. Sharma P, Maffulli N. Basic biology of tendon injury and healing. Surgeon. 2005;3(5):309–16.
41. Sharma P, Maffulli N. Biology of tendon injury: healing, modeling and remodeling. J Musculoskelet Neuronal Interact. 2006;6(2):181–90.
42. Sharma P, Maffulli N. Tendinopathy and tendon injury: the future. Disabil Rehabil. 2008;30(20–22):1733–45.
43. Su B, O'Connor JP. NSAID therapy effects on healing of bone, tendon, and the enthesis. J Appl Physiol. 2013;115:892–9.
44. Tanaka E, Aoyama J, Tanaka M, van Eijden T, Sugiyama M, Hanaoka K, et al. The proteoglycan contents of the temporomandibular joint disc influence its dynamic viscoelastic properties. J Biomed Mater Res. 2003;65A(3): 386–92.
45. Thomopoulos S, Genin GM, Galatz LM. The development and morphogenesis of the tendon-to-bone insertion – what development can teach us about healing. J Musculoskelet Neuronal Interact. 2010;10(1):35–45.
46. Viidik. Tendon tensile strength. Acta Orthop Scand. 2007:1–12.
47. Wang JH, Guo Q, Li B. Tendon biomechanics and mechanobiology-a minireview of basic concepts and recent advancements. J Hand Ther. 2012; 25(2):133–41.
48. Wang JHC. Mechanobiology of tendon. J Biomech. 2006;39(9):1563–82.

Orthopaedic Diseases

Susan V. Bukata, Katherine Edwards, Amanda Marshall, Brian A. Mosier, Daniel T. Altman, Joyce M. Wilson, Michael Pensak, and Jennifer Moriatis Wolf

1 Genetics

Susan V. Bukata

> **Take-Home Message**
> - Genetic anomalies can result in significant musculoskeletal issues and perioperative complications and risks.

1.1 Modes of Inheritance

Autosomal Dominant A single copy of the mutated gene is sufficient to create the disorder; if the gene is present, the disorder will occur.

S.V. Bukata, MD
Division Chief Oncology, UCLA Health System, Los Angeles, CA, USA

K. Edwards, MD
University of Missouri Department of Physical Medicine and Rehabilitation, Columbia, Missouri, USA

J.M. Wilson, MD
Orthopedic Surgery, Jefferson City Medical Group, Jefferson City, Missouri, USA

M. Pensak, MD • J.M. Wolf, MD
Department of Orthopaedic Surgery, University of Connecticut, Farmington, Connecticut, USA

A. Marshall, MD
University of Texas Health Science Center at San Antonio, San Antonio, TX, USA

B.A. Mosier, MD
Department of Orthopaedic Surgery, Allegheny General Hospital, Pittsburgh, PA USA

D.T. Altman, MD
Orthopaedic Surgery, Allegheny General Hospital, 1307 Federal St, 2nd Floor, Pittsburgh, PA 15212, USA
e-mail: daltman@wpahs.org

C. Mauffrey, D.J. Hak (eds.), *Passport for the Orthopedic Boards and FRCS Examination*, DOI 10.1007/978-2-8178-0475-0_5

Autosomal Recessive Two copies of the mutated gene are for this person to be affected with the disease; single copy of the gene creates a gene carrier but that will not have the disease

X-Linked Dominant A disorder of a gene on the X chromosome causes a disorder to be expressed in all individuals (both males and females)

Females more frequently affected; no male-to-male transmission.

X-Linked Recessive Disorder in a gene on the X chromosome, but the disorder will only occur in males and females with two mutated copies of the gene; no male-to-male transmission

Variable Inheritance (Penetrance) Spectrum of disease severity from a genetic mutation known to cause disease, ranging from no obvious disease to mild to severe. Even within the same family with the same gene mutation, significant variation in disease severity can occur.

Chromosomal Abnormalities A structural anomaly in the chromosomes resulting in missing, abnormal, or excess DNA compared to normal chromosomes; can occur in all cells in the body or only in select cells (mosaicism)

1.2 Down Syndrome

Definition Chromosomal anomaly associated with cognitive delay, muscle hypotonia, and other birth defects

Etiology Trisomy 21 (extra copy of chromosome 21 from one parent), more common from egg but can be from sperm

Rate: 1 per 691 births in the USA.

Can also occur from unbalanced translocation of chromosome 21 and another chromosome. One or both parents may not be affected due to a balanced translocation, but this translocation can become unbalanced in their child(ren), leading to disease.

Pathophysiology Distinctive facial appearance, 50 % have heart defect, joint instability (hip, patella, neck, and foot), muscle hypotonia in infants, and cataracts

Treatment Supportive treatment for symptomatic defects, physical therapy, and surveillance

1.3 Turner Syndrome

Definition Chromosomal anomaly in females that affects development

Etiology Single X chromosome (50 % of cases) or severely dysfunctional second X chromosome in females

Rate: 1 per 2,500 in females, can present as mosaicism with only some cells affected

SHOX gene on X chromosome most associated with musculoskeletal anomalies in the syndrome

Pathophysiology Normal intelligence, early ovarian failure (most do not undergo puberty and are infertile), webbed neck (30 %), low hairline, lymphedema of limbs (70 %), skeletal anomalies, renal defects, heart defects (30–50 %), and hypothyroid (10–30 %)

Increased risk of congenital hip dislocation, scoliosis (10 %), delayed skeletal maturation (85 %), short 4th metacarpal, and osteoporosis

Treatment Hormone therapy to induce puberty, supportive care, physical therapy, and surveillance

1.4 Von Willebrand Disease

Definition Bleeding disorder with slowed clotting process resulting in easy bruising and prolonged bleeding after injury

Etiology Most common genetic bleeding disorder

Estimated incidence: 1 per 100 to 1 per 10,000 people

Diagnosis Bleeding time, tests for von Willebrand factor (quantity and quality)

Pathophysiology Mutations in the VWF gene reducing the amount of von Willebrand factor produced.

Von Willebrand factor essential for platelet adhesion and stabilizes other clotting proteins preventing their breakdown.

Impaired function prevents clots from forming normally.

Clinical Manifestations Easy bruising, heavy or prolonged menstrual bleeding, prolonged bleeding after injury, nosebleeds, and excessive bleeding after dental work

Classification

Type I: decreased von Willebrand factor levels, most common type (75 % of patients), mildest form, variable quantities of von Willebrand factor in bloodstream, and autosomal dominant inheritance.

Type II: abnormally functioning von Willebrand factor, intermediate in severity, and autosomal recessive inheritance.

Type III: most severe form with no von Willebrand factor produced, extremely rare (1 per 500,000), autosomal recessive inheritance; mutation creates short nonfunctional protein.

Treatment Desmopressin nasal spray stimulates release of von Willebrand factor from vascular endothelium.

For severe cases: von Willebrand factor and factor VIII transfusions

For surgery/procedures: may need to have blood products including von Willebrand factor available

1.5 Hemophilia

Definition Factor deficiency that slows blood clotting process; its classic form is factor VIII deficiency.

Etiology X-linked recessive mutation in F8 gene; rate: 1 in 5000 males
Produces abnormal version of coagulation protein
Leads to prolonged prothrombin time (PTT)

Pathophysiology Continuous bleeding after injury, surgery, or dental work, sometimes spontaneous bleeding (joints, muscles, brain)

Treatment IV replacements with recombinant factor VIII preoperatively, continue 5 days postoperatively, 21 days for bone procedures

Hemophilic Arthropathy Synovitis and cartilage destruction in a joint due to repeated bleeds

Treatment Factor replacement, physical therapy, bracing, arthroscopic synovectomy, or total knee replacement for more severe cases

1.6 Christmas Disease

Definition Clotting disorder deficiencies in factor IX

Etiology X-linked defect in F9 gene liposomal protein production, second most common form of hemophilia; rate: 1 per 20,000 in males

Pathophysiology Form of hemophilia, similar effects and treatments as common hemophilia

Treatment IV infusion factor IX (plasma or recombinant), desmopressin applied directly small wounds

1.7 Gaucher's Disease

Definition Cell storage disorder that affects beta-glucocerebrosidase enzyme activity and allows accumulation of glucocerebroside within cells to toxic levels.

Etiology Autosomal recessive mutations in GBA gene; rate: 1 per 50,000–100,000
In people of Ashkenazi Jewish descent; rate: 1 per 500–1000

Pathophysiology Hepatosplenomegaly, anemia, thrombocytopenia, bone pain and pathologic fractures, abnormal bone remodeling, delayed healing, arthritis, and lung disease
Increased perioperative bleeding and infection risk

Classification

Type I: most common form, non-neuropathic, more frequent with Ashkenazi Jewish descent
Type II: added effect on the central nervous system and brain, begins in infancy, with brain damage, seizures, and abnormal eye movements
Type III: also affect the central nervous system, slower progression than type II

Treatment IV enzyme replacement for types 1 and 3

1.8 Sickle Cell Anemia

Definition Disorder that affects hemoglobin protein and causes red blood cells to distort into crescent/sickle shape

Etiology Autosomal recessive mutations in HBB gene affect beta-globin subunit of hemoglobin (hemoglobin S form)

Hemoglobin has four subunit: two alpha-globins and two beta-globins

Most common in those of African descent; rate: one for 70,000 in the USA, one in 500 African-Americans, and one in 1,000 Hispanic Americans

Classification

Sickle cell trait: at least one beta-globin subunit replaced by hemoglobin S
Sickle cell disease: globulin subunit replaced I hemoglobin S

Pathophysiology Symptoms of sickle cell disease seen in early childhood

Anemia, pain episodes, repeated infection, shortness of breath, fatigue, delayed growth and development, osteonecrosis, and pulmonary hypertension

Pain episodes occur when cells undergoes cyclic and have trouble passing through blood vessels.

Treatment Decitabine or hydroxyurea (induces production of fetal hemoglobin), pain medications, fluids, rest, oxygen if levels are low, and blood transfusion for severe anemia or perioperatively

1.9 Thalassemias

Definition Disorder that reduces hemoglobin production resulting in difficulties carrying oxygen to cells of the body

Etiology Defect in quantity in either the alpha or beta subunit of hemoglobin production resulting in low hemoglobin levels

Can occur as major form (both genes for the subunit effected, got one from each parent) or minor form (one gene for the subunit effected, other is normal)

Classification

Alpha thalassemia: involves the alpha subunit of hemoglobin, losses from two genes involved (HBA 1/HBA 2); two forms: HbBart (severe, with loss of all 4 alleles of HBA genes) and HbH (milder, loss of 3 of the 4 alleles; more common in Southeast Asia and Mediterranean countries; complex inheritance because it involves gene copy number

Beta thalassemia: involves the beta subunit of hemoglobin, common globally but most frequent with Mediterranean decent, involves mutations in the HBB gene that range from complete loss of beta-globin production to decreased quantity, generally autosomal recessive inheritance/rare autosomal dominance

Pathophysiology Decrease oxygen delivery to tissues. Anemia, weakness, fatigue, increased risk of blood clots, jaundice, hepatosplenomegaly, osteoporosis and fragility fractures, and growth retardation

Treatment Blood transfusions, folate supplementation, iron chelation, and perioperative caution with increased clotting risk

2 Calcium and Phosphate Metabolism

Kate Edwards

Take-Home Message

- Calcium is an important mineral in the body that is tightly regulated by intact parathyroid hormone, vitamin D, and calcitonin. It is involved in many physiologic processes. Both too much and too little calcium can be pathologic.
- Rickets – failure of osteoid to calcify in children resulting in bony abnormalities
- Osteomalacia – incomplete mineralization of osteoid following growth plate closure

2.1 Calcium

Calcium is the most abundant mineral in the body with 98–99 % housed in the bone and teeth as hydroxyapatite. In the plasma, 50 % is ionized and active, while 45 % is protein bound (albumin) and 5 % is bound to phosphate and citrate. The total amount of calcium in the extracellular fluid is approximately 1 g. In contrast, the bone contains 1 kg of calcium!

Serum calcium concentration is 8.5–10.2 mg/dL.

To correct for a low albumin, use the following equation: ([4-plasma albumin in g/dL] × 0.8 + serum calcium).

Calcium is required for many physiologic processes including: muscle contraction, enzyme cofactor for hormonal secretion, vascular contraction and dilation, membrane stability, intracellular signaling, bone structure and mineralization, and nerve conduction.

Recommended amount of dietary calcium per the Institute of Medicine is 700–1,300 mg/day based on age with an upper limit of 1,000–3,000 mg/day.

The gut absorbs only 30–40 % of ingested calcium. In contrast, the kidneys are quite efficient and absorb 97–98 % of circulating calcium. Approximately 500 mg of calcium is exchanged daily in the bone with remodeling.

pH is important in calcium regulation. In states of acidemia, there is decreased calcium binding to albumin which increases ionized calcium, while the reverse is true for alkalemia.

Calcium is closely regulated by parathyroid hormone (PTH), vitamin D, and calcitonin. Calcium levels are also affected by magnesium and phosphorous.

2.2 PTH

- Stimulates bone resorption
- Stimulates calcium reabsorption at the distal tubule of the kidney
- Stimulates phosphate excretion
- Stimulates conversion of 25 hydroxyvitamin D2 to 1,25 dihydroxyvitamin D3
- Indirectly increases gut absorption due to the increased vitamin D

PTH has a very short half-life of 5 min.

PTH receptors are found on osteoblasts. It is thought that PTH inhibits osteoblast function and increases osteoclastic activity via cell-to-cell communication.

The parathyroid gland is extremely sensitive to changes in ionized calcium as detected by calcium-sensing receptors (CaSR) which ultimately regulates the release of PTH.

2.3 Calcitonin

Is a hormone released by the thyroid parafollicular cells in response to elevated calcium levels.

In the bone, it inhibits resorption of calcium, and in the kidney, it inhibits reabsorption of both calcium and phosphate.

2.4 Vitamin D

- Stimulates calcium absorption in the gut
- Stimulates bone resorption
- Stimulates renal reabsorption of calcium
- Regulates PTH release

Check serum 25(OH) level, desired level is >30 ng/dL

25(OH) has a longer half-life than the active form, 1,25 dihydroxyvitamin D3 (15 days vs. 4 h), and its concentration is 1,000-fold greater.

As far as oral supplementation, D2(ergocalciferol) and D3(cholecalciferol) are traditionally regarded as equivalents.

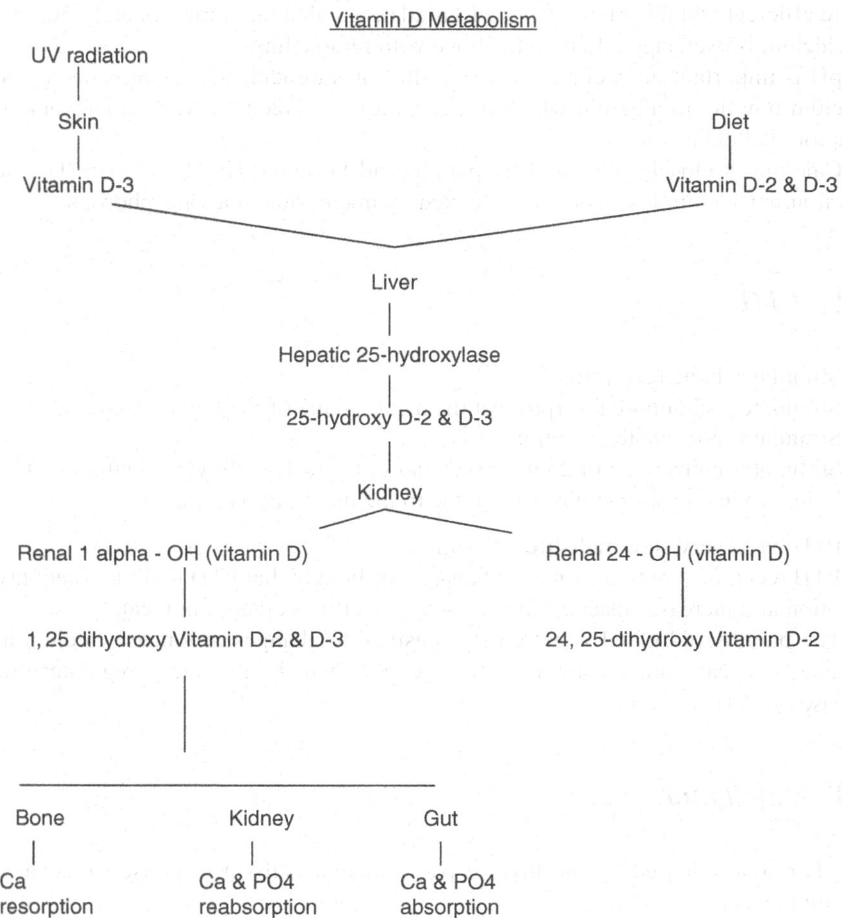

2.5 *Phosphorous*

Most phosphorous in the body is present as phosphate.

80–90 % of ingested phosphorous is absorbed by the gut.

Serum levels are primarily maintained by the rate of kidney excretion.

Serum concentration is 3–4 mg/dL.

Helps maintain physiologic pH.
Deficiency is uncommon except in genetic disorders of phosphate metabolism.
Calcium and phosphate are both deposited and resorbed from bone together.

2.6 *Hypocalcemia*

Definition Serum calcium <10.5 mg/dL or ionized calcium <1.0 mmol/L

Causes Renal failure, vitamin D deficiency, magnesium deficiency, acute pancreatitis, hypoparathyroidism, hyperphosphatemia, and medication effect
Very common in hospitalized patients

Symptoms

Acute – syncope, perioral numbness, fatigue, muscle cramps, and congestive heart failure
Chronic – psoriasis, dry skin, coarse hair, brittle nails, poor dentition, and cataracts

Severe hypocalcemia can but rarely causes tetany, arrhythmias, hypotension, and seizures as well as other signs/symptoms of neuromuscular irritability.

Diagnosis Ionized calcium level
Check liver function test, albumin, iPTH, magnesium, BUN, and creatinine to assess for secondary causes.
Treatment is with oral versus IV supplementation.

2.7 *Hypercalcemia*

Definition Serum calcium >10.5 mg/dL or ionized calcium >2.5 mmol/L

Causes

90 % caused by malignancy or hyperparathyroidism
10 % caused by increased vitamin D levels, thiazide diuretics, renal failure, rapid bone turnover, and familial causes

Symptoms Anxiety, depression, coma, somnolence, arrhythmia, nephrolithiasis, hypertension, nausea, vomiting, anorexia, and osteoporosis (“stones, bones, abdominal groans, psychiatric moans”)

Treatment IV fluids, loop diuretics, IV bisphosphonates, calcitonin, dialysis, and glucocorticoids

2.8 *Rickets*

Definition Disease of growing bone affecting children

Causes Failure of osteoid to calcify typically from prolonged vitamin D deficiency.

Vitamin D deficiency → decreased serum calcium → +PTH → increased renal phosphorous loss → decreased deposition of calcium in the bone

Demographics More common in exclusively breastfed babies and those with little sunlight exposure. Also present in conditions that cause malabsorption such as celiac disease and seen in severe renal disease.

Physical Exam Skeletal deformity (bow leg, knock knee, rachitic rosary), short stature, dental defects, kyphoscoliosis, and delay in closure of fontanels

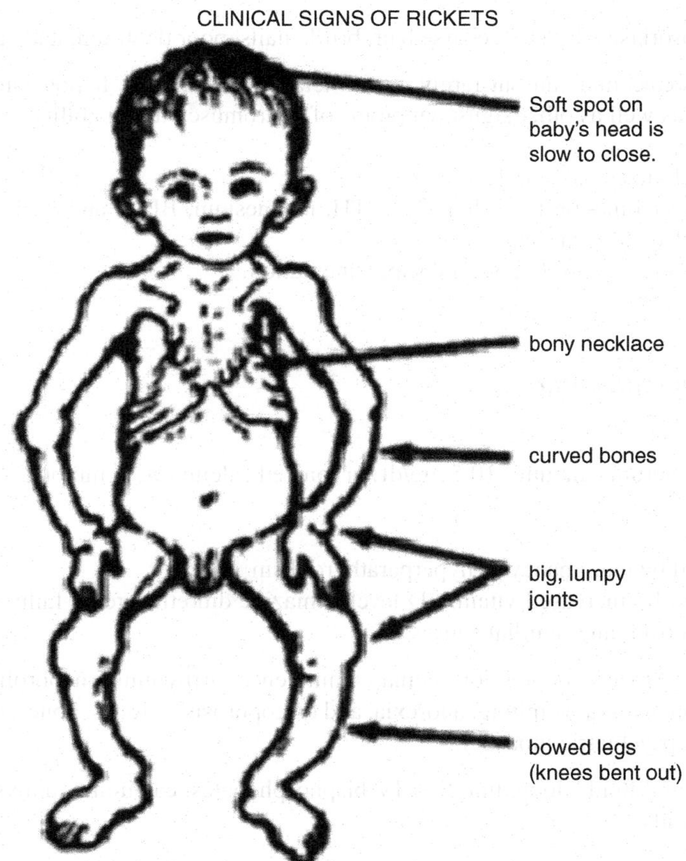

Laboratory

Low calcium, phosphorous, and vitamin D levels
Elevated alkaline phosphate and PTH

Radiography Anterior view of the knee will show cupping and widening of the metaphyses

Treatment Vitamin D and calcium supplementation, may need surgical intervention for skeletal deformities

2.9 Osteomalacia

Similar to rickets but occurs in adults

Definition Incomplete mineralization of osteoid following growth plate closure. Normal amount of collagen, too little calcium.

Not to be confused with osteoporosis, which is a decrease in bone mass with NORMAL mineralization

Causes Most commonly from vitamin D deficiency.

Can also be caused by celiac disease, anticonvulsants, kidney and liver disease, surgeries that remove part of the stomach or small intestine, low phosphorous intake, and cancer

Symptoms Bone pain, muscle weakness, and fractures

Physical Exam Patients may exhibit a waddling gait.

Workup Low levels of serum calcium, vitamin D, and phosphorous

Radiology Radiography may show Looser's transformation zones (pseudofractures)

Diagnosis Bone biopsy can definitively make the diagnosis, usually blood work, and radiography is sufficient for diagnosis.

Treatment Vitamin D and calcium supplementation, braces, and surgical intervention in severe cases

3 Joint Arthridites: Osteoarthritis and Inflammatory Arthritis

Amanda Marshall

Osteoarthritis Degenerative joint disease affecting the articular cartilage of synovial joints; inflammation is not the major component of the disorder.

Primary (most common) – develops in the absence of a known cause, aka idiopathic
Secondary – results from hereditary, developmental, metabolic, traumatic, infectious, or neurologic condition

Inflammatory Arthritis Inflammatory process from various triggers mediating synovial proliferation and inflammation ultimately resulting in soft tissue and bone destruction. The most common type is rheumatoid arthritis (affecting 0.5–1 % of US adults), but other conditions include systemic lupus erythematosus (SLE), ankylosing spondylitis, and psoriatic arthritis.

Pathophysiology

Osteoarthritis: sequence of changes within the matrix affecting the structure and function of the articular cartilage.

Stage I, matrix alteration – increased water content, decreased proteoglycan aggregation, and decrease in glycosaminoglycan chain length, but no change in type II collagen concentration.

Stage II, chondrocyte response – increase in matrix synthesis, turnover, and chondrocyte proliferation. Matrix metalloproteinases (MMPs) destroy aggrecan and activate collagenase.

Stage III, decline in chondrocyte response – accumulation of molecules within the matrix.

The bone responds to the degeneration of articular cartilage by increasing subchondral bone density, formation of cysts, and development of bony and cartilaginous outgrowths later forming osteophytes. End-stage disease represented by complete loss of cartilage and resultant denuded bone.

Inflammatory arthritis: migration of mononuclear cells via induction of IL-8, and IL-1β incites inflammatory response directed at periarticular tissues. Midkine (heparin-binding growth factor) upregulates osteoclast differentiation.

Diagnostic Criteria

Characteristic	Rheumatoid arthritis	Osteoarthritis
Patient age	Varies: begin any time in life.	>55 years of age
Speed of onset	Relatively rapid, over weeks to months	Slow, over years
Joint symptoms	Pain, swelling, and stiffness	Achiness, pain, minimal swelling
	Synovitis, joint destruction	Reduced ROM, crepitus
Pattern of joints that are affected	Symmetrical, involving both small and large joints	Usually asymmetric: DIPs, large weight-bearing joints (hips, knees), or the spine
Duration/timing of stiffness	Morning stiffness lasts >30 min	Morning stiffness <1 h; returns at the end of the day or after periods of activity
Radiologic findings	Erosions, narrowing of joint space	Joint space narrowing, osteophytes, sclerosis, subchondral cysts
Serology	ANA, RF, Anti-CCP, ESR, CRP	Normal
Synovial fluid analysis	>50,000 WBCs	<50,000 WBCs
Systemic symptoms	Frequent fatigue and anorexia	None

Ankylosing Spondylitis Manifests frequently during second decade of life. It usually presents as back pain characterized as insidious in onset, present for greater than 3 months; morning stiffness improves with exercise, worsens with rest. Extraspinal features include enthesitis, dactylitis, and uveitis. Radiographic changes include early squaring of the vertebral bodies progressing to bamboo spine chronically. MRI most sensitive for sacroiliac involvement. +HLA-B27

Psoriatic Arthritis Occurs in 15–20 % of patients with psoriasis. Skin lesions (scaly erythematous plaques) appear prior to onset of arthritic symptoms in 80 % of patients. Most common presentation is asymmetrical oligoarthritis (50 %). Spondylitis present in up to 40 % of patients. Synovial fluid analysis WBC 5,000–15,000. Radiographic features include mild erosive disease. Arthritis mutilans = "pencil in cup" deformity of hands.

Biochemical Markers

Osteoarthritis: Several biochemical markers have been investigated, but none have proven sufficiently discriminatory in the diagnosis and/or prognosis of OA. Recent studies show promise for serum, urine, and synovial fluid biomarkers such as uCTX-II (urinary cross-linked C-telopeptide of collagen), sCOMP (serum cartilage oligomeric matrix protein) fragment, sfNT (synovial fluid nitrotyrosine), and CXCL12 (serum and synovial fluid stromal cell-derived factor).

Rheumatoid arthritis: The serum biochemical markers associated with RA are "inflammation"-based and include IL-6, leptin, resistin, CRP, MMP-1 and MMP-3, and YKL-40 (chitinase-3-like protein 1 aka CH13L1). A commercially available kit is available for use in clinical practice.

Treatment Physical therapy

NSAIDS

Disease-modifying antirheumatic drugs (DMARDS)

Biologic agents: Apremilast, Phosphodiesterase-4 inhibitor, ustekinumab

Surgery:

Arthroscopic synovectomy

Joint replacement

Arthrodesis

Bibliography

1. Lafeber FPJG, Van Spil WE. Osteoarthritis year 2013 in review: biomarkers; reflecting before moving forward, one step at a time. Osteoarthritis Cartilage. 2013;21:1452–64.

4 Infection, Septic Arthritis, and Osteomyelitis

Brian A. Mosier, Daniel T. Altman

Take-Home Message

- *S. aureus* is the most common species involved in bone infections.
- Intravenous drug users have a predilection for *Pseudomonas aeruginosa* and gram-negative infections.
- Definitive diagnosis is based on cultures from bone and soft tissue specimens.
- Biofilms can exist on orthopedic devices in a sessile state and contribute to chronic bacterial infections.

Definitions

- Biofilm: Communities of microorganisms encased within an extracellular polymeric slime matrix.
- Osteomyelitis
  - Sequestra: Dead infected bone seen in acute osteomyelitis. Serves as a substrate for biofilm formation
  - Involucrum: New periosteal bone that forms in chronic osteomyelitis encasing and supporting the weakened area of dead infected bone

Etiology *Septic Arthritis*

- Adult Septic Arthritis
  - Mechanisms of inoculation are hematogenous seeding, direct inoculation, and contiguous spread.
  - Most frequently involved joints: Knee, hip, elbow, and ankle.
  - Two major patient groups:
    - <40: the most common organism is *N. gonorrhoeae*.
    - Elderly: the most common organism is *S. aureus*.
- Pediatric Septic Arthritis
  - Source is dependent on age and blood vessel flow patterns.
    - Neonates: adjacent osteomyelitis due to vessels crossing the physis
    - Infants/children: hematogenous spread most common. May have spread from adjacent portions of intracapsular metaphyseal areas such as in the wrist, hip, and knee and humerus.

Osteomyelitis

- Adult Osteomyelitis
  - Most common mechanisms are contiguous spread and direct inoculation.
  - Staphylococcus is the most common organism involved due to its inherent adherence mechanisms.
- Pediatric Osteomyelitis
  - Most common organism is *S. Aureus*.
    - In neonates, suspect group A streptococci.
  - Mechanism usually via hematogenous spread.
  - Due to robust blood supply in the metaphyseal region of children, acute osteomyelitis may prelude septic arthritis.

Pathophysiology

Septic Arthritis

Proteolytic enzymes produced by PMNs cause irreversible destruction of articular cartilage.

Osteomyelitis

Acute suppurative infection can disrupt the vascular supply to the bone leading to areas of necrosis. The sequestra serve as a medium for biofilm formation with chronic infection ensuing unless an intervention occurs.

Biofilms

- Can develop on implanted orthopedic devices or dead bone and may mature over months or years with few signs of inflammation.
- Imparts resistance to host immunity, responds poorly to antibiotics, is chronic in nature, and is often culture negative.
- Detection and management are difficult and evolving.

Radiology

Septic Arthritis

Radiographs:

- Useful for assessing bony involvement or presence of hardware

MRI:

- Convenient to rule out periarticular soft tissue infection or abscess

Ultrasound

- Preferred method for determining deep joint distension/effusion in pediatric septic arthritis

Osteomyelitis

Radiographs:

- Early osteomyelitis: adjacent soft tissue swelling and joint effusions. Most useful for ruling out presence of fractures, implant loosening.
- Late osteomyelitis: bone destruction and necrosis within the sequestrum signified by periosteal reactions, bone cysts, and focal areas of resorption. Demonstrates mixed destructive-sclerotic lesions.

MRI:

- Findings are seen 2–3 weeks before any changes are observed on plain radiographs.
- Low signal on T1 study, edema on T2 study, and enhancement on post-gadolinium study.

Radionuclide Imaging

Technetium Bone Scan

- Sensitive to tumor, infection, arthritis, or trauma
- Combination of indium (^{111}In) and technetium (^{99}Tn) labeling provides the most sensitive and specific imaging in acute bone infections.

PET Scan

- Expensive
- PET scans with FDG (fluorodeoxyglucose) labeling are valuable and have increased utility in diagnosing periprosthetic joint infections.

Diagnosis

Septic Arthritis

Serum Blood Tests:

- CBC: leukocyte count usually elevated.
- ESR/CRP: CRP always elevated; ESR is sometimes normal.
- Blood cultures required.

Joint Fluid Aspirate:

- Mandatory for diagnosis and identification of the inciting organism
- Send for cell count with differential, gram stain, glucose level, crystal analysis, and culture (aerobic/anaerobic, fungal, mycobacterial).
- Characteristics of a likely infected aspirate:
  - Cloudy or purulent
  - Glucose <60 % serum level
  - >75 % PMNs
  - 50,000 cells/mm^3

Osteomyelitis

- CBC: leukocyte count elevated or normal in acute osteomyelitis. Most often normal in chronic osteomyelitis
- ESR/CRP: Elevated in both acute and chronic osteomyelitis
  - Monitor CRP level to determine effectiveness of treatment.
  - CRP dissipates after 1 week of effective treatment.
  - ESR is elevated in 90 % of cases and peaks after 3–5 days.

Definitive diagnosis is based on cultures obtained from bone biopsies.

Classification Osteomyelitis: Cierny-Mader Staging System for Osteomyelitis (Fig. 1)

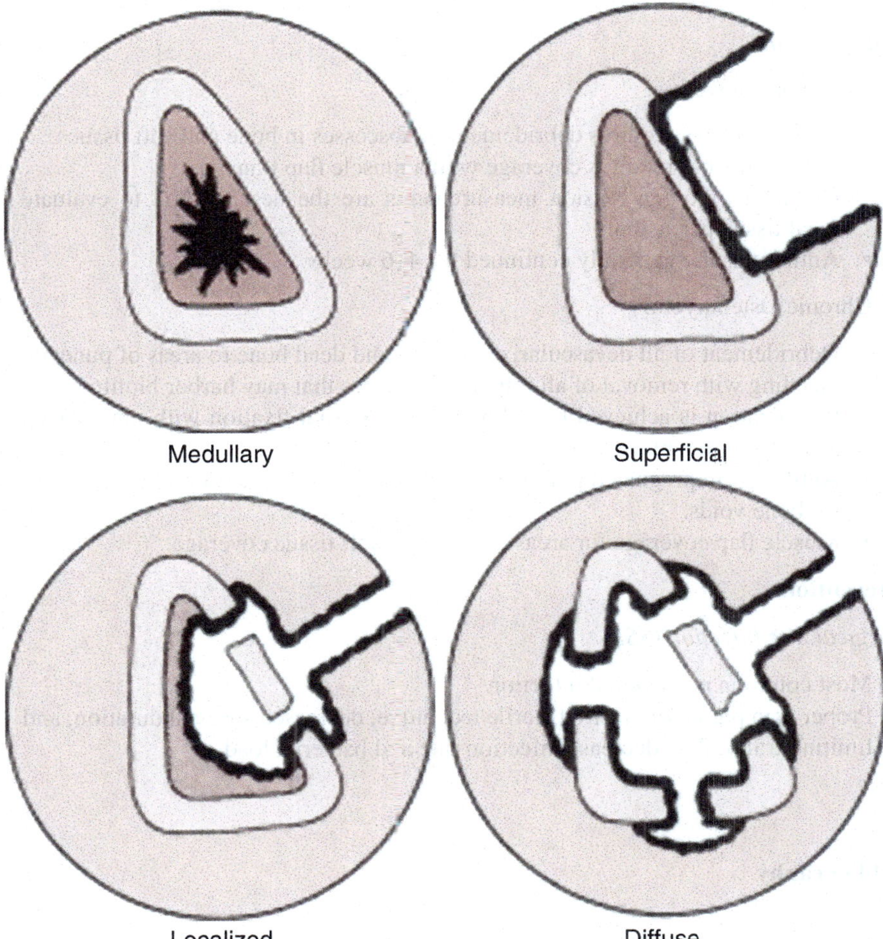

Fig. 1 Cierny anatomic classification of adult osteomyelitis (Cierny III G, Mader JT, Pennink JJ. A clinical staging system for adult osteomyelitis. Contemo Orthop. 1985;10:17–37)

- Based on anatomic site of infection and physiologic class of the host including systemic and local factors.
- Relates medical context of the host to their ability to respond to an infection.
- Weak hosts require more aggressive treatment.

Treatment

Septic Arthritis

Main goal of treatment is the preservation of articular cartilage by eliminating proteolytic enzymes that rapidly destroy the articular cartilage.

- Serial aspirations: monitor joint fluid polymorphonuclear cell count to assess adequacy of treatment.
- Open debridement: Highest chance of clearing offending agents.

Osteomyelitis

Acute Osteomyelitis:

- Almost always requires debridement of abscesses in bone and soft tissues.
- Soft tissue loss requires coverage with a muscle flap transfer.
- Cutaneous oxygen tension measurements are the best method to evaluate local tissue perfusion.
- Antibiotics are generally continued for 4–6 weeks.

Chronic Osteomyelitis

- Debridement of all devascularized tissues and dead bone to areas of punctate bleeding with removal of all implanted devices that may harbor biofilms.
- Stabilization is achieved by splint/cast or external fixation with pins placed away from the infection site.
- Antibiotic-impregnated polymethylmethacrylate may be used to temporarily fill bone voids.
- Muscle flap coverage for areas deficient of soft tissue coverage.

Prevention

Surgical Site Infection (SSI)

- Most common nosocomial infection
- Proper skin preparation, strict sterile technique, decreased surgical duration, and limiting traffic flow decrease infection rate and bacterial load.

Bibliography

1. Harrop JS, Radcliff KE, Styliaras JC, et al. Contributing factors to surgical site infections. J Am Acad Orthop Surg. 2012;20(2):94–101.
2. McPherson EJ, Peters CL. Musculoskeletal infection. In: Flynn JM, editor. OKU 10. Rosemont: American Academy of Orthopaedic Surgeons; 2011. p. 239–58.

3. Miller M, Thompson S, Hart J. Review of orthopaedics. 6th ed. Philadelphia: Elsevier Saunders. 2012.
4. Stoodley P, Ehrlich GD, Altman DT, et al. Orthopaedic biofilm infections. Curr Orthop Pract. 2011;22(6):558–63.

5 Complex Regional Pain Syndrome

Joyce M. Wilson

Take-Home Message

- Symptom complex of pain, allodynia, vasomotor instability, swelling, and dystrophic skin changes and motor dysfunction.
- Peripheral and central nervous system is involved.
- Treatment is multidisciplinary and should start as early as possible.
- Treatment is directed toward improving limb function and pain symptoms.

Definition Regional pain with autonomic dysfunction, atrophy, and functional impairment affecting musculoskeletal, neural, and vascular structures.

Diagnostic criteria include hyperalgesia (often non-anatomic), allodynia, vasomotor instability, motor dysfunction, and trophic symptoms.

Etiology Common cause is trauma to an extremity.

Peripheral and central nervous system sensitization.

Causative mechanisms may differ across patients and within a patient over time.

Risk factors include prolonged immobilization, smoking, substance abuse, genetic, and psychological factors (anxiety, depression).

Pathophysiology

Unknown, multifactorial; begins with initial trauma

- Upregulation of alpha 1-adenoreceptor in the peripheral nervous system and in the spinal cord.
- Primary afferent nociceptive mechanisms demonstrate abnormally heightened sensation, including spontaneous pain and hyperalgesia.
- Inflammatory response increases in interleukin (IL) – 1β [beta], 2, 6; tumor necrosis factor (TNF) – α [alpha]; calcitonin gene-related peptide (CGRP); bradykinin; and substance P. Decrease in IL-10.
- Brain plasticity causes decreased representation of the affected limb in the in somatosensory cortex causing greater pain intensity and hyperalgesia, impaired tactile discrimination, and perception of sensations outside of the nerve distribution.

Imaging X-rays: show regional osteopenia in 80 % of patients

Triple phase bone scan: diffusely increased periarticular uptake involving multiple joints in the affected extremity; imaging modality with greatest sensitivity and negative predictive value for ruling out CRPS type 1

MRI: may show bone marrow edema, skin edema, uptake of the skin, joint effusion, and intra-articular uptake

Total digital microvascular flow: analyzed by digital temperature measurements, laser Doppler fluxmetry, and vital capillaroscopy

Classification

Type 1: initiated by minor trauma to an extremity compounded by external forces (tight cast, dependant positioning, excessive swelling). "Classic RSD"
Type 2: associated with an identifiable peripheral nerve injury or "causalgia"
Type 3: nontraumatic cause producing extremity pain such as myofascial syndrome

Warm vs. cold CRPS describes temperature changes of limb.
Cold – more chronic state, poorer prognosis.
Historical stages – times and stages are not absolute.

Stage 1 (lasts 1–3 months):

- Changes in skin temperature, switching between warm and cold
- Faster growth of nails and hair
- Muscle spasms and joint pain
- Severe burning, aching pain that worsens with slight touch or breeze
- Skin becomes blotchy, purple, pale, or red; thin and shiny; swollen; sweatier

Stage 2 (lasts 3–6 months):

- Continued changes in the skin
- Nails that are cracked and break more easily
- Pain that is becoming worse
- Slower hair growth
- Stiff joints and weak muscles

Stage 3 (irreversible changes can be seen)

- Limited movement – contracted muscles and tendons
- Muscle atrophy
- Pain in the entire limb

Treatment Multidisciplinary treatment is key (PCP, therapy, pain management, support groups, psychotherapy, etc.).

Identify reversible causes (injured nerve), and correct if possible, especially in CRPS type 2.

Start physical and occupational therapy as early as possible – improve mobility and strength.

Medications

- Antidepressants – relieve post-traumatic depression; provide analgesia and modulate sympathetic hyperactivity in the peripheral nervous system and CNS

(tricyclic antidepressants, tetracyclic antidepressants, atypical antidepressants, and selective serotonin reuptake inhibitors)

- Anticonvulsants – treat hyperpathic pain; thought to stabilize excitable nerve membranes, limit neuronal hyperexcitability, and inhibit trans-synaptic neuronal impulses in the CNS
- Local and oral anesthetic agents – only used in severe, refractory cases due to significant side effects
- Adrenergic medications – peripheral vasodilation, increases nutritional blood flow, and affects α[alpha]1 and α[alpha]2 receptors
- Calcium channel blockers decrease sympathetic tone
- Bisphosphonates – provide analgesia by preventing bone resorption; some act on inflammatory mediators, including IL-1, IL-6, lactic acid, and TNF-α[alpha].

Parenteral Medications

- Intravenous regional infusions – pain management specialists may use; bretylium tosylate (only FDA-approved medication) and corticosteroids most common
- Percutaneous neural or ganglionic blockade
- Sympathetic blockade – continuous infusion of a local anesthetic around stellate ganglion or paravertebral ganglia, along the brachial plexus, or within the epidural space

Implantable Devices

- Peripheral nerve stimulator – for gray matter, the dorsal column, the spinal cord, and peripheral nerves; improve pain relief, improve sleep, decrease the use of addictive pain medication, and improve health-related quality of life
- Spinal cord stimulator – invasive, high complication rate, results diminish with time, but can help in carefully selected patients

Central nervous system ablative techniques – sympathectomy; only short-term palliation; may make some patients worse

Biofeedback/acupuncture – useful in properly selected patients

Complications

- Cognitive impairment
- Depression
- Loss of muscle size or strength in the affected limb
- Worsening of the affected limb
- Complications from surgical procedures

Prognosis Varies

Children and teenagers – good recovery

Early intervention and rehabilitation can limit severity and duration on symptoms.

Some patients will develop unremitting pain and crippling, irreversible changes despite treatment.

Prevention

- Vitamin C following wrist fracture. 500 mg daily for 45–50 days
- Early mobilization and ambulation following a stroke or other extremity trauma

Bibliography

1. Bruehl S. An update on the pathophysiology of complex regional pain syndrome. Anesthesiology. 2010;113:713–25.
2. Cappello ZJ, Kasdan ML, Louis DS. Meta-analysis of imaging techniques for the diagnosis of complex regional pain syndrome type I. J Hand Surg Am. 2012;37A:288–96.
3. Marinus J, Moseley GL, Birklein F, Baron R, Maihöfner C, Kingery WS, van Hilten JJ. Clinical features and pathophysiology of complex regional pain syndrome. Lancet Neurol. 2011;10(7):637–48.

6 Connective Tissue Disorders

Michael Pensak, Jennifer Moriatis Wolf

Take-Home Message

- Ehlers-Danlos is a connective tissue disorder of collagen metabolism characterized by skin elasticity, fragility, and hypermobile joints.
- Marfan's syndrome is a connective tissue disorder resulting from autosomal dominant mutation in fibrillin-1 gene – aortic root dilation/dissection, joint laxity, and scoliosis.
- Neurofibromatosis-1 is an autosomal dominant disorder characterized by neurofibroma masses, congenital pseudarthrosis, café au lait spots, and axillary/groin freckling.
- Homocystinuria is an inborn error of methionine metabolism, with typical laxity, and scoliosis; diagnosed by urine sulfur amino acid and treated with pyridoxine.

6.1 Ehlers-Danlos

Definition

- Connective tissue disorder characterized by skin elasticity, fragility, and joint hypermobility due to abnormal collagen metabolism resulting from a variety of mutations.

Etiology

- Multiple mutations identified, though common feature to all subtypes involves abnormal collagen in connective tissues
  - Mutations in type V collagen (40–50 %)
  - Mutations in type III collagen
  - Mutation in collagen cross-linking enzyme, lysyl hydroxylase

Pathophysiology Laxity in multiple joints – shoulders, patellae, and ankles

- Kyphoscoliosis
- Loose, fragile skin with poor wound healing capability

Radiography

- Joint specific x-rays to rule out subluxations/dislocations
- PA/lateral spine radiographs to follow kyphoscoliosis

Classification
Villefranche (1998)

- Type I – Classic. Autosomal dominant. Mutations in type V collagen but no known universal cause. Major features: skin elasticity, wide scars, and joint hypermobility. Minor features: smooth skin, velvety skin, molluscoid pseudotumors, subcutaneous spheroids, muscle hypotonia, easy bruising, and positive family history
- Type II – Hypermobility. Autosomal dominant. Major features: skin involvement and joint hypermobility. Minor features: joint dislocations, chronic joint/limb pain, and positive family history
- Type III – Vascular. Autosomal dominant. Major features: thin, translucent skin and arterial/intestinal or uterine rupture, extensive bruising, and characteristic facial features (pinched nose, thin lips, tight skin, hollow cheeks). Minor features: small joint hypermobility, muscle/tendon rupture, clubfoot, varicose veins, pneumothorax, AV or carotid-cavernous sinus fistula, gingival recession, and positive family history
  - Col3A1 mutation results in abnormal procollagen III synthesis
- Type IV – Kyphoscoliosis. Autosomal recessive. Defect in lysyl hydroxylase, involved in collagen cross-linking. Major features: joint laxity, hypotonia at birth, progressive scoliosis, and globe ruptures. Minor features: tissue fragility, easy bruising, arterial rupture, microcornea, osteopenia, and positive family history
- Type V – Arthrochalasis. Autosomal dominant. Major features: extreme hyperlaxity, recurrent subluxations, and congenital hip dislocations. Minor features: hyperextensible skin, fragile tissues, atrophic scars, easy bruising, hypotonia, kyphoscoliosis, and osteopenia. Col1A1 or Col1A2
- Type VI – Dermatosparaxis. Autosomal recessive. Major features: skin fragility, sagging, or redundant skin. Minor features: soft skin, easy bruising, premature rupture of fetal membranes, and hernias

Treatment
No cure for underlying metabolic abnormalities of collagen production

- Nonoperative – mainstay of management
  - Reduce and immobilize joint dislocations
  - Physical therapy and orthotics
- Operative
  - Joint fusions for recalcitrant dislocations; soft tissue procedures alone have low success rate.
  - Posterior spinal fusion for kyphoscoliosis with long constructs.

Complications

- Joint dislocations
- Kyphoscoliosis
- Aortic dilatation
  - Cardiology consult
  - Echocardiogram
- Easy bruising and scarring
- Chronic pain

6.2 Marfan's Syndrome

Definition Connective tissue disorder with multiple manifestations: joint laxity, long limbs, scoliosis, cardiac valve abnormalities, aortic dilatation, etc.

Etiology Autonomic dominant mutation in fibrillin-1 gene and chromosome 15q21

Pathophysiology
Abnormal fibrillin-1 may also indirectly lead to increases in TGF-β which is implicated in the deleterious effects seen on heart valves and the aorta.

- Musculoskeletal findings – scoliosis, protrusio acetabula, pes planovalgus, tall, thin stature with long limbs (dolichostenomelia), and long fingers (arachnodactyly)
  - Steinberg sign – with the fingers clenched in a fist over an adducted thumb, the thumb tip protrudes out the ulnar aspect of the hand.
  - Walker sign – overlap of the thumb and little finger when attempting to encircle the contralateral wrist.
- Non-musculoskeletal findings
  - Cardiac abnormalities
    - Aortic root dilatation
    - Aortic dissection
    - Mitral valve prolapse

- Pectus excavatum
- Spontaneous pneumothoraces
- Ectopia lentis – superior lens dislocation

Radiography Scoliosis (PA and lateral spine films)

Classification

Revised Ghent system 2010

- Emphasizes presence of cardinal features of aortic root dilatation/dissection and ectopia lentis

Treatment

Diagnostic criteria for Marfan's syndrome
In the absence of family history:
1. Aortic dilatation/dissection AND ectopia lentis
2. Aortic dilatation/dissection AND FBN1 mutation
3. Aortic dilatation/dissection AND systemic score >7
4. Ectopia lentis AND FBN1 AND aortic dilatation/dissection
In the presence of family history:
5. Ectopia lentis AND positive family history
6. Systemic score ≥7 AND positive family history
7. Aortic dilatation/dissection AND positive family history
Systemic features
Assigned various points from 1 to 3, maximum score of 20, score greater than or equal to 7 indicates systemic involvement
Wrist AND thumb sign, pectus carinatum, pes planovalgus, pneumothorax, dural ectasia, protrusio acetabuli, scoliosis or thoracolumbar kyphosis, reduced elbow extension, facial features, skin striae, myopia, mitral valve prolapse

Adapted from revised Ghent nosology (2010)

- Nonoperative
  - Scoliosis – early bracing
  - Cardiac issues – beta-blockers for cardiac involvement
- Operative – scoliosis
  - Long posterior spinal fusion
  - Mandatory preoperative MRI
  - Cardiac consultation and echocardiogram
    - Pes planovalgus – flatfoot reconstruction
    - Protrusio acetabula – epiphysiodesis of triradiate cartilage (pediatric population); total hip arthroplasty for advanced joint degeneration

Complications

Scoliosis

- Higher complication rate than in adolescent idiopathic scoliosis
- 10–20 %, including pseudarthrosis, hardware failure, loss of correction, and infection

6.3 *Neurofibromatosis-1*

Definition Autosomal dominant disorder leading to hamartomatous proliferations

Etiology

- Mutation on chromosome 17 affecting the NF-1 gene.
- NF-1 is a tumor suppressor gene whose coded protein is implicated in cell growth and differentiation.

Pathophysiology

- Skeletal findings
  - Scoliosis
    - Thoracic spine involvement – short, sharply angled curves
    - Dystrophic subtype – likely to progress, risk of neurologic deficit
    - Non-dystrophic subtype – resembles AIS
  - Congenital pseudarthrosis of the tibia – anterolateral bowing of tibia often is present at birth
  - Hemihypertrophy – uncommon, unilateral, may involve bone and soft tissue
- Nonskeletal findings
  - Café au lait spots – hyperpigmented lesions with rounded borders
  - Axillary and inguinal freckling
  - Cutaneous neurofibromas – composed of axons and Schwann cells
  - Lisch nodules – pathognomonic dome-shaped elevations of the surface of the iris
  - Plexiform neurofibromas – subcutaneous lesions with "bag of worms" feel
    - 25% of patients with NF-1
    - 1–4 % risk of malignant degeneration – remove if lesions enlarge or become painful
    - Can lead to overgrowth of an extremity
  - Verrucous hyperplasia – thick overgrowth of skin with a soft, velvety feel that can form crevices predisposing to infections
  - Optic glioma – low-grade CNS tumor, present in 15–20 %

Diagnosis

Two of seven criteria as delineated by the NIH

Diagnostic criteria for neurofibromatosis
6 or more café au lait spots (>0.5 cm in children, >1.5 cm in adults)
2 or more cutaneous/subcutaneous neurofibromas or 1 plexiform neurofibroma
Optic glioma
Axillary/groin freckling
2 or more Lisch nodules
Bony dysplasia
First-degree relative with NF1
Clinical assessment and the presence of two of any of the above findings are diagnostic for NF-1

Radiography

- Tibia/fibula x-rays to monitor anterolateral bowing
- PA/Lateral spine radiographs to evaluate scoliosis
  - Sharp vertebral end plates
  - Rib penciling – central narrowing of rib shafts
- Preoperative spine MRI to rule out dural ectasia or intraspinal anomaly

Classification

- Neurofibromatosis-1
  - Autosomal dominant mutation of chromosome 17
  - Incidence 1/2,500–4,000
- Neurofibromatosis-2
  - Autosomal dominant mutation of chromosome 22
  - Incidence 1/25,000–40,000

Treatment

- Scoliosis
  - Attempt trial of bracing for non-dystrophic form
  - Posterior spinal fusion for management of dystrophic form and non-dystrophic form that has failed bracing
- Anterolateral bowing of tibia/Congenital pseudarthrosis
  - Brace with total contact orthosis prior to fracture
  - Surgical fixation once fracture or pseudarthrosis is present
  - Amputation for persistent pseudarthroses

Complications

- Scoliosis
  - Pseudarthrosis
- Anterolateral bowing of tibia/Congenital pseudarthrosis
  - Recurrent fracture in up to 50 % of individuals

6.4 Homocystinuria

Definition Inborn error of methionine metabolism resulting in mental retardation, thromboembolic events, inferior lens dislocation and skeletal manifestations similar to Marfan's syndrome

Etiology
Autosomal recessive mutation causing a deficiency in cystathionine synthetase

- Lack of cystathionine synthetase prevents conversion of homocysteine to cystathionine leading to homocystine accumulation.
- Homocystine is converted to homocystine.
- Homocystine accumulates in tissues and is excreted in the urine.
- Plasma methionine also becomes elevated.

Pathophysiology

- Skeletal manifestations
  - Tall, thin stature with long limbs (dolichostenomelia) and moderate arachnodactyly
  - Severe pes planovalgus
  - Thoracolumbar scoliosis
  - Osteoporosis
  - Pectus carinatum
- Nonskeletal manifestations
  - Venous/arterial thrombotic events
  - Inferior lens dislocations (ectopia lentis) from defective suspensory ligament

Radiography

- PA/lateral spine radiographs for thoracolumbar scoliosis with biconcave endplates and flattening (platyspondyly)
- Knee films – wide metaphyses and enlarged epiphyses

Diagnosis Screen for sulfur amino acid concentrations in urine (homocysteine)

Treatment Oral pyridoxine – 50 % of patients may respond.
Operative, scoliosis – posterior spinal fusion.

Complications

- Scoliosis
- Osteoporosis
- Pes planovalgus
- Blood clots
- Inferior lens dislocation

Bibliography

1. Bravo JF, Wolff C. Clinical study of hereditary disorders of connective tissues in a Chilean population: joint hypermobility syndrome and vascular Ehlers-Danlos syndrome. Arthritis Rheum. 2006;54(2):515–23.
2. Herring JA. Orthopaedic-related syndromes. In: Herring JA, editor. Tachdjian's pediatric orthopaedics. Dallas: Saunders Elsevier; 2008. p. 1795–913.
3. Kobayasi T. Dermal elastic fibres in the inherited hypermobile disorders. J Dermatol Sci. 2006;41(3):175–85.
4. Loeys BL, Dietz HC, Braverman AC, Callewaert BL, De Backer J, Devereux RB, et al. The revised Ghent nosology for the Marfan syndrome. J Med Genet. 2010;47(7):476–85.

Materials and Biomechanics

Brett D. Crist, Ajay Aggarwal, Charles Lewis, Ferris M. Pfeiffer, and Trent M. Guess

1 Biomaterials

Brett D. Crist and Ajay Aggarwal

1.1 Fracture Implants

Take-Home Message

- Modulus of elasticity for cortical bone is ~20 GPa, stainless steel ≈ 200 GPa, and titanium ≈ 100 GPa
- Bending stiffness of plates ≈ thickness of the plate^3
- Bending stiffness of intramedullary nails ≈ radius^4

Modulus of Elasticity

- Stress = force/area
- Strain = change in length/original length
- Modulus of elasticity (Young's modulus) = stress/strain. Most solid material has a linear portion of its stress-strain curve (Fig. 1). This portion is the slope of the

B.D. Crist, MD (✉) • A. Aggarwal, MD
F.M. Pfeiffer, PhD (✉) • T.M. Guess, PhD
Department of Orthopaedic Surgery, University of Missouri, Columbia, Missouri, USA
e-mail: cristb@health.missouri.edu; aggarwala@health.missouri.edu; pfeifferf@health.missouri.edu; guesstr@health.missouri.edu

C. Lewis, BSc, MSc, FRCS (✉)
Taranaki District Health Board, New Plymouth, New Zealand
e-mail: charliealewis7@gmail.com

C. Mauffrey, D.J. Hak (eds.), *Passport for the Orthopedic Boards and FRCS Examination*, DOI 10.1007/978-2-8178-0475-0_6

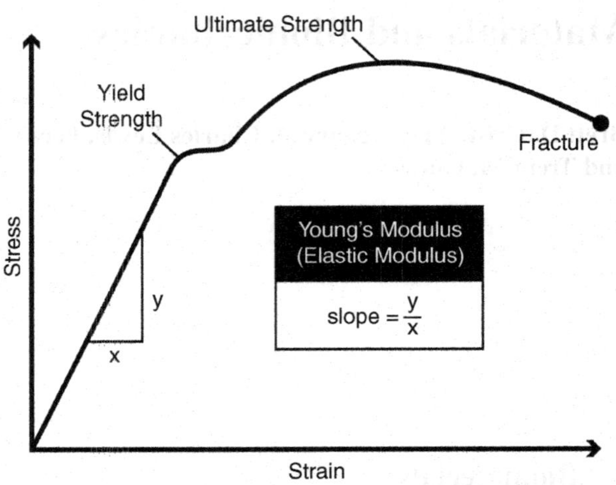

Fig. 1 Stress–strain curve (© Copyright 2014 by The Curators of the University of Missouri, a public corporation, with permission)

curve and the elastic modulus (*E*). Hooke's law of elasticity indicates that no permanent deformation/damage occurs within the linear area of the curve.

Yield and Ultimate Strength

- Once a material is loaded past the elastic portion of the stress-strain curve and there is permanent damage to the material (plastic deformation), it reaches its yield point.
- If loading continues past the yield point, the material will eventually catastrophically fail and that is the ultimate strength.
- Ductility: amount of plastic deformation tolerated before ultimate failure.
- Brittle materials: high elastic modulus, low ductility = stiff but fail at yield point
- Ductile materials: lower elastic modulus, larger area of plastic deformation before ultimate failure = flexible and deform prior to ultimate failure.

Fatigue Strength or Endurance Limit

- Materials can withstand cyclic loading until microdamage accumulates causing rapid failure. The fatigue strength/endurance limit is the maximum stress the material can withstand without failure after 10–100 million cycles.

Plates

- Extramedullary, usually load-bearing devices
- Bending stiffness ≈ to plate thickness^3
  - Ex: Increasing the thickness of a plate by 2 mm increases the bending stiffness eight times the original.

Intramedullary Nails

- Intramedullary, usually load-sharing devices
- Bending stiffness = $\pi \times$ radius^4
  - Ex: Increasing the radius of an IM nail by 2 mm increases the bending stiffness by 16 times.

Common Fracture Implant Materials

- Stainless steel: elastic modulus ~200 GPa, plates, and screws
  - Stiff and more brittle
  - Risk of rejection if patient has a nickel allergy
- Titanium: elastic modulus ~100 GPa, intramedullary nails, and plates and screws
  - Flexible and more ductile.
  - Titanium resists corrosion.
  - Titanium forms passivation layer to inhibit bacterial colonization.
  - Used in nickel-allergic patients.
  - Risk of cold welding that makes implant removal difficult.

1.2 *Arthroplasty*

Take-Home Message

- *Highly cross-linked polyethylene* liners have performed well in vivo. Wear is significantly lower compared to conventional polyethylene. Fracture of highly cross-linked polyethylene occurs and is multifactorial.
- *Metal-on-metal (MOM)*: Worldwide reduction in utilization of MOM is due to concerns about adverse local tissue reactions (ALTR) secondary to wear and/or corrosion of cobalt-chromium-based components. Elevated metal ions can cause pseudotumors and aseptic lymphocytic vasculitis-associated lesion (ALVAL).
- *Ceramic-on-ceramic*: Is an attractive option for young and active patients. The most significant disadvantage is the potential for fracture and squeaking.

Polyethylene Processing

Polyethylene is a long-chain hydrocarbon. When exposed to radiation, carbon–carbon and carbon–hydrogen bonds can be broken. As a result, chain scission or free radical formation can occur. Oxygen can bind at a free radical site, leading to oxidation. Both chain scission and oxidation have negative consequence for wear and mechanical properties.

Cross-linking involves formation of carbon–carbon bonds between two adjacent polyethylene polymers. Irradiation is the first step and produces free radicals. Free radicals then react and cross-link the polymer chains. The amount of cross-linking is proportional to the radiation dose. Doses of 50–100 kGy (5–10 mrads) are typically used. Heating is the second step, and it reduces the free radicals and thus decreases the risk of oxidation.

Conventional Polyethylene

- Radiation dose between 2.5 and 4.0 mrads.
  - Disadvantage: Higher linear and volumetric wear leading to increased incidence of osteolysis and loosening.

Highly Cross-Linked Polyethylene

- Radiation dose between 5.0 and 10.0 mrads.
  - Advantage: Markedly decreased linear (<0.004–0.25 mm/year) and volumetric wear. Smaller wear particles decrease the risk of osteolysis and loosening.
  - Disadvantage: Decreased mechanical properties leading to reduced strength, fatigue resistance, and fracture toughness. Fracture of polyethylene has been associated with suboptimal positioning of components, implant design with sharp corners at the locking mechanism, and thin polyethylene.

Vitamin E Polyethylene
Vitamin E helps in stabilizing the free radicals without postradiation melting and maintains the mechanical properties of polyethylene. Vitamin E highly cross-linked polyethylene demonstrates oxidative resistance, good strength, and low wear.

Metal-on-Metal (MOM)
MOM is characterized by higher wear during the run-in period (1–2 years) followed by substantially lower steady-state wear. Smaller <50 nm wear particles.

- Advantages: Low wear secondary to lower surface roughness and higher sphericity. Positioning of the acetabular component can influence wear and ion production. Wear decreases with increased head size and clearance decreases.
- Disadvantages: Local and systemic accumulation of metallic debris and ions. Elevated ions can cause ALVAL and pseudotumors.

  Factors associated with increased metal ions

- Small-diameter components implanted at higher abduction (>50–55°) and higher combined version are at increased risk of edge wear, elevated ions, and ALTR.
- Large diameter >36 mm MOM heads are at increased risk of head and neck taper and fretting corrosion.
- Serum ion levels (CO, Cr):
  - Low risk <3 ppb
  - Moderate risk 3–10 ppb
  - Higher risk >10 ppb.
  - Cross-sectional imaging with MARS MRI is indicated for symptomatic patients with elevated ions. CRP can be elevated.

Ceramic-on-Ceramic
Ceramics are stable, dense, and hard surfaces. They are scratch resistant and hydrophilic, have a low coefficient of friction, and create less reactive debris, making them an attractive option for young and active patients.

- Advantages: Low wear, hard, and scratch resistant.
- Disadvantages:
  - Brittle
  - Stripe wear due to localized edge loading in deep flexion.
  - Fracture in ceramics can be due to poor material, large grain size, small head size, incorrect component positioning, residual internal stress, and poor taper design.
  - Squeaking (incidence = 0.45–10.7 %)
  - Factors associated with squeaking include implant (stem) design, component malposition, edge loading, wear debris, disruption of lubrication film increasing the coefficient of friction, micro-separation, and stripe wear.

Bibliography

1. O'Keefe RJ, Jacobs JJ, Chu CR, Einhorn TA editors. Orthopaedic basic science. 4th ed. Rosemont: American Academy of Orthopaedic Surgeons; 2013.

2 Biomechanics: Free Body Analysis

Charles Lewis

Take-Home Message
- Force – is a load that acts on a body.
- JRF = force generated within a joint as a response to all forces acting on a joint.
- Moment – the effect of a force at a perpendicular distance from an axis.

2.1 Basic Definitions

Newton's Laws *First Law (Inertia)*

If there is no net force on an object, its velocity will remain constant.

Second Law (Action)

Force = mass × acceleration

Third Law (Reaction)

For every action, there is an equal and opposite reaction.

(This is important for the understanding of free body analysis.)

Force A push or pull on an object.

1 Newton = force required to give 1 kg mass an acceleration of 1 m/s^2.

Moment The tendency of a force to rotate a body around an axis
Moment = force × distance (perpendicular)

Torque Is the magnitude of a moment

Work When force acts upon an object to create displacement
Work = force × distance

Energy Ability of an object to perform work.
Kinetic energy = ½ mv^2
Potential energy = mass × gravity × height

Vector A quantity having direction as well as magnitude, especially as determining the position of one point in space relative to another.

2.2 *Hip Biomechanics and Free Body Analysis*

Static Analysis A method of determining forces and moments that act on a body by isolating that body part and ensuring it is in static equilibrium.

Forces and moments are vectors; they must = zero in all three perpendicular directions.

Free body analysis makes certain assumptions:

- Weight of the leg is 1/6 of total body weight

See Fig. 2 below:

W = gravitational force
M = abductor muscle force
R = joint reaction force

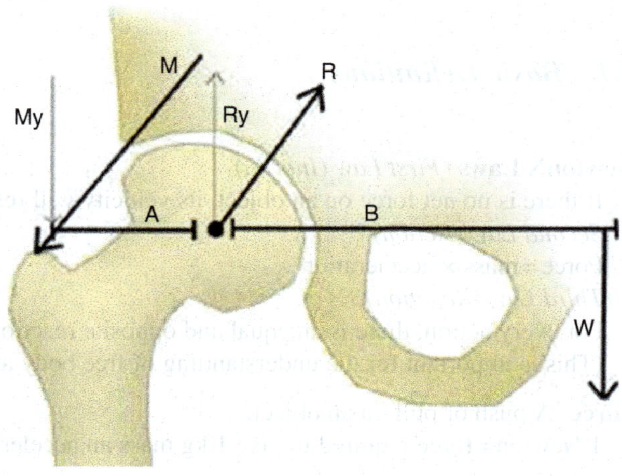

Fig. 2 Free body diagram for the human hip

To calculate JRF (R)
Sum of all moments = 0

$$(A \times \mathrm{My}) + (B \times W) = 0$$

Assume $A = 5$ cm and $B = 12.5$ cm
My = $2.5W$
Calculating Ry

$$\mathrm{Ry} = \mathrm{My} + W$$

$$\mathrm{Ry} = 2.5W + W$$

$$\mathrm{Ry} + 3.5W$$

Calculate R

$$R = \mathrm{Ry}(\text{cosine } 30°)$$

$$R = -4W$$

2.3 Strategies to Reduce JRF

Reduce Body weight

- Decrease lever arm
- Medialize axis or rotation
- Trendelenburg gait

Help Abductors

- Provide cane in opposite hand (reduces abductor muscle pull and decreases moment arm)
- Carrying load in ipsilateral hand
- Increase abductor lever arm by increasing offset/osteotomy/varus angulation of stem.

Bibliography

1. Nordin M, Frankel VH, editors. Basic biomechanics of the musculoskeletal system. 2nd ed. Philadelphia: Lea and Febriger; 1989.
2. Ramachandran M. Basic orthopaedic sciences – the Stanmore guide. 1st ed. London, UK: Edward Arnold Publishers Ltd; 2007.

3 Gait Cycle

Ferris M. Pfeiffer and Trent M. Guess

Take-Home Message

- Gait cycle – activity that occurs from heel strike to heel strike of one limb
- One complete gait cycle includes:
  - Stance phase – 60 % of walking cycle – foot of interest is in contact with the ground
  - Swing phase – 40 % of walking cycle – foot of interest is not in contact with the ground
- Pathologies induce alterations to "normal" gait through the nervous system and musculoskeletal system.
- Pathologies induce alterations to "normal" gait in an effort to translate the center of mass through space along a path of least energy [2].

Definitions

Stance phase: period of gait when the foot is on the ground, 60 % of gait cycle

Heel strike: start of the gait cycle, body's center of mass at lowest position
Foot flat: plantar foot surfaces touch the ground, body weight shifted from contralateral leg
Midstance: swinging contralateral foot passes the stance foot, body's center of mass at highest position
Heel-off: heel loses contact with ground, toes begin pushing off
Toe-off: toe loses contact with ground, ends the stance phase

Swing phase: period of gait when foot is not in contact with the ground, 40 % of gait cycle

Acceleration: leg is accelerating forward
Midswing: swing foot passes directly below the body
Deceleration: muscles slow limb in preparation for heel strike

Stride length: distance travelled in one gait cycle (heel strike to heel strike)
Double support: period when both feet are in contact with the ground
Single limb stance: period when only one foot is in contact with the ground

Etiology

Abnormal gait

Insufficiencies in nervous system – motor control, proprioception
Insufficiencies in musculoskeletal system – muscle, tendon, ligament, bone

Pathophysiology

Neuromuscular diseases affecting gait can arise from pathologies which affect the nerves, nervous junctions, and/or muscles. The effect of such pathologies on gait is often defined by the location of the pathology. Disorders such as cerebral palsy, traumatic brain injury, stroke, Parkinson's disease, and multiple sclerosis primarily affect upper motor neuron function Injuries/insufficiencies in the spinal nerves more often affect lower motor neuron function.

Musculoskeletal diseases such as muscular dystrophy, rheumatoid and osteoarthritis, tendon/ligament insufficiencies, and degenerative disc disease affect the ability of muscles and joints to stabilize and move the body in a controlled normal gait. This can be due to biomechanical limitations such as insufficient muscle force development (as is seen in muscular dystrophy) and excessive joint laxity (as is seen in ACL rupture).

Gait analysis: often performed with motion capture, force plates, and electromyography (EMG) sensors

Kinematic measures (motion) – joint rotations during movement (e.g., knee flexion/extension angle)
Kinetic measures (forces) – joint moments (e.g., hip adduction moment)
EMG – measures timing and magnitude of muscle activations

Classification

Phenomenologically classified as [1]:

Hemiparetic: extension and circumduction of unilateral leg
Paraparetic: extension, stiffness, adduction, scissoring of bilateral legs
Sensory: unsteady gait with lack of visual input
Steppage: foot drop, excessive hip and/or knee flexion to clear ground
Cautious: careful, wide based, and slow
Freezing: difficulty initiating steps, feet "stuck to floor"
Propulsive or retropulsive: center of gravity in front of (pro) or behind (retro) feet
Ataxic: wide based, uncoordinated
Waddling: wide based with swaying, symmetric bilaterally
Dystonic: hyperflexed hips
Choreic: irregular, spontaneous flexion of knees with raising of legs
Antalgic: limp

Vertiginous: unsteady with tendency to fall to one side
Hysteric: nonphysiologic

Anatomically classified as [1]:

Frontal gait disorders, corticobasal gait disorders, pyramidal gait disorders, cerebellar gait disorders, and cortical-subcortical gait disorders

Treatment
Surgical or medical intervention to remove pathology when possible. Physical therapy to improve balance, muscle function, and joint range of motion.

Bibliography

1. Jankovic J, Nutt JG, Sudarsky L. Classification, diagnosis, and etiology of gait disorders. Adv Neurol. 2001;87:119–33.
2. Saunders JB, Inman VT, Eberhardt HD. The major determinants in normal and pathological gait. J Bone Joint Surg Am. 1953;35-A(3):543–58.
3. Whittle M. Gait analysis: an introduction. 2nd ed. Oxford: Butterworth-Heinemann; 1996.

Statistics and Research & Diagnostic Imaging

David A. Volgas and Julia R. Crim

1 Statistics and Research

David A. Volgas

1.1 Definitions

Confounding Variable
a factor (such as educational level) not specifically assessed by a study, but which may influence outcome.

Bias
intentional or unintentional errors in assigning patients to treatment groups (selection bias) or in evaluating exposures or outcomes. These errors make the likelihood of making a type I or type II error more likely and thus diminish the value of a study.

Sensitivity
the probability that a test is positive when there is disease present (true positive/(true positive + false negative)).

Specificity
the probability that if a test is negative, then the disease will not be present (true negative/(true negative + false positive)).

D.A. Volgas, MD (✉)
Department of Orthopaedic Surgery, University of Missouri, Missour, Columbia, USA
e-mail: volgasd@health.missouri.edu

J.R. Crim, MD
Department of Radiology, University of Missouri, Missour, Columbi, USA

C. Mauffrey, D.J. Hak (eds.), *Passport for the Orthopedic Boards and FRCS Examination*, DOI 10.1007/978-2-8178-0475-0_7

Relative Risk
the probability that a patient who has a risk factor also has a disease or condition, compared to the probability that a patient who has the disease does not have the risk factor.

Given the following:

Risk factor	Disease present	Disease not present
Yes	*a*	*b*
No	*x*	*y*

$$\mathrm{RR} = \left(a/(a+b)\right)/\left(x/(x+y)\right)$$

Odds Ratio
if a patient has a disease or condition, what is the probability of having a given risk factor? (more commonly used in orthopedic literature than relative risk)

$$\mathrm{OR} = (a/x)/(b/y) \text{ or } ay/bx$$

Type I Error
an error in which the null hypothesis is true, but the statistics rejects this. Also known as "α" or false-positive rate. For example, a spam filter flags an email as spam, but in fact it is not.

Not to be confused with the significance level of a test, which is set by the researcher at a predetermined level (.05) and reflects the threshold at which he/she is willing to accept the likelihood of a type I error.

Type II Error
conversely, an error in which the null hypothesis is false, but the test statistics accepts it as true. Also known as "β" or false negative. For example, when a spam filter fails to catch a spam email.

***P*-Value**
the probability of the difference between two means is due to chance assuming that the null hypothesis is true.

Power
the ability of a study to correctly identify that the null hypothesis is false. Expressed as 1-β.

Effect Size
magnitude of the difference between the experimental group and the control group. Related to the concept of clinical significance in contrast to the statistical significance of a test.

Confidence Interval
a range which is likely to include the mean of a population for which the mean is unknown.

Incidence
the rate of having a given condition during a given time, e.g., the incidence of having a revision arthroplasty within 10 years from the index operation is 5 %.

Prevalence
a "snapshot" at a given point in time of how many subjects have a given condition, e.g., the prevalence of people of Asian ethnicity in San Francisco in the 1990 census was 29.1 %.

1.2 Statistical Inference

Statistical inference is the use of statistical tests to estimate the characteristics of the entire population based on the known characteristics of a limited sample.

Parametric tests are those which assume a normal population distribution. *Nonparametric tests* do not assume a normal population distribution.

Continuous data is numerical data which includes non-integer values. This data may be analyzed using a Student's *t*-test (parametric) or Mann–Whitney test (nonparametric).

Categorical data is data which has a limited set of values, e.g., male or female. This data may be analyzed using a chi-square test or, when there are less than five observations in a category, a Fisher's exact test. Proportions may also be analyzed with these methods.

Multiple regression analysis is a generic term encompassing several statistical methods which attempt to quantify the contribution of each of several variables to the observed outcome.

1.3 Study Design

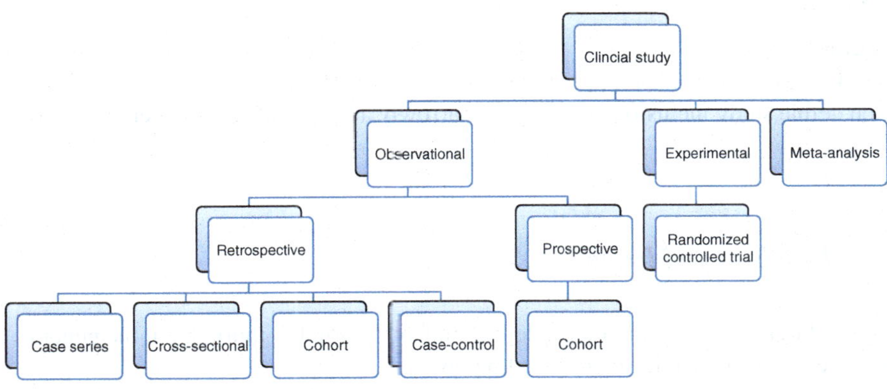

Experimental studies are those in which two (or more) treatment or exposure groups are selected by the investigator, usually assigned in a random fashion. These studies are potentially the most powerful studies since they may eliminate selection bias.

However, many clinical studies are not amenable to randomization because of ethical considerations (amputation vs. limb salvage) or group size considerations (rare diseases).

Observational studies are those in which the treatment or exposure is not selected by the researcher. This type of study may be very powerful if the researcher is careful to eliminate as many confounding variables and biases as possible prior to beginning the study.

Prospective Study
the outcome cannot occur until after the patient is enrolled.

Retrospective Study
the outcome has already occurred before the study begins. Generally is considered more prone to bias than prospective studies.

Cohort Study
a given outcome is correlated with a given treatment or exposure. A cohort study can be prospective or retrospective.

Case–Control Study
a retrospective study which has two groups, cases (subjects which received a given treatment) and controls (subjects which did not). These groups are compared for the presence or absence of risk factors.

Cross-sectional
a retrospective study which reports the prevalence of a condition. May be useful to determine if a condition warrants further study.

Case Series
a retrospective report of a group of patients who had the same treatment or exposure.

Meta-analysis
a study which combines similar outcomes from multiple studies. Meta-analyses often define study inclusion criteria very narrowly and exclude a large percentage of studies.

1.4 Levels of Evidence

Levels of evidence vary in precise definition from journal to journal, but the general characteristics of each level are listed below:

- High-quality randomized, prospective studies or high-quality meta-analyses with consistent results
- Lesser-quality randomized studies, high-quality prospective observational study, meta-analyses based on primarily level II studies
- Case–control study, retrospective cohort study

- Case series
- Expert opinion

Readers should be aware that levels of evidence do not necessarily take into consideration effect size, generalizability, assessment of bias, or handling of missing data.

1.5 Outcome Measures

Test Validity
the degree to which a test measures what it purports to measure.

Construct Validity
the degree to which test questions measure the outcome of interest completely but exclusively, a test which is designed to measure reading comprehension but is written in a foreign language would have poor construct validity.

Content Validity
the degree to which all aspects of the quality being measured are included, e.g., a scale measuring foot and ankle function should account for all aspects of function of the foot or ankle such as range of motion, pain, stability, etc.

Criterion-Based Validity
measures the degree to which a test agrees with other external measures of the same outcome.

2 Diagnostic Imaging

Julia R. Crim

Take-Home Message

- CT scan has advantages over MRI in rapidity of exam and visualization of fractures and their complications.
- Triple-phase technetium MDP bone scan is often viewed as a test specific for osteomyelitis, but yields positive results in cases of trauma, inflammatory, or crystal arthritis.
- MRI offers the most complete evaluation of soft-tissue and bony abnormalities.
- Ultrasound is increasingly used for targeted evaluation of the musculoskeletal system.

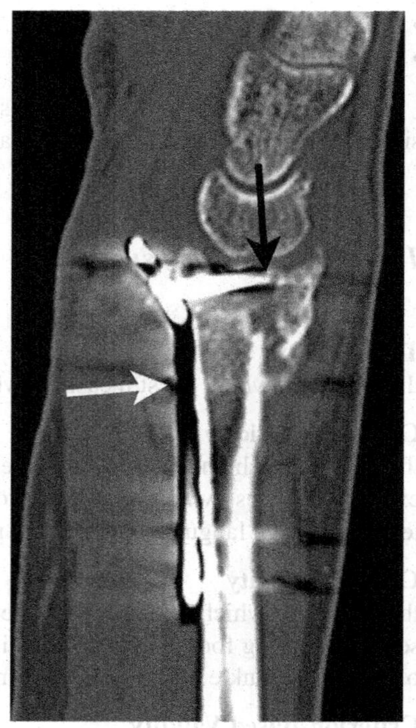

Fig. 1 Sagittal reformatted CT of distal radius hardware malposition. Hardware obscured the fracture line on routine radiographs (not shown). Sagittal reformatted CT scan shows the volar fixation plate and screws. One fixation screw (*black arrow*) is intra-articular, and there is separation of the fracture fragments. Three months after fixation, there is no central callus, although a small amount of peripheral callus is visible. Hardware was subsequently revised. *White arrow* shows artifact adjacent to the fixation plate. In most cases, artifact does not compromise CT diagnosis of fracture evaluation

CT (Computed Tomography) Scan

Current CT scanners obtain high-resolution images at submillimeter slices which can be reformatted in any plane. CT scan offers rapid evaluation of the trauma patient and has largely replaced trauma radiography of the cervical spine. CT scan can be performed with metallic hardware in place, although there is some degradation of image quality. CT scan is the modality of choice for evaluation of potential nonunion when radiographs and symptoms are inconclusive (Fig. 1). It is also useful to evaluate tumor matrix. It can be used to evaluate bone and soft-tissue infection, but is less sensitive than MRI. CT is used for guidance of biopsies and aspirations when fluoroscopy and ultrasound are not sufficient.

Coronal and sagittal reformatted images are standard in orthopedic imaging. Trauma imaging should never be considered complete unless reformatted images are obtained, since malalignment and fractures in the axial plane may be missed on axial images. 3D reformatted images are a useful adjunct in explicated complex fractures, especially in the pelvis.

Iodinated contrast agents are used with CT scan to assess vascularity of abnormalities. The contrast agent collects in areas of increased vascularity, a process known as tissue enhancement. Enhancement is seen in all vascularized tissues and is a very nonspecific process. Absence of enhancement can be used as a sign of necrosis. Contrast agents are not used in the setting of renal failure unless hemodialysis is planned.

The lifetime increased risk of cancer due to diagnostic imaging is widely debated. If there is a slight risk associated with low-dose radiation, it is a long-term increased risk of sarcoma, with a prolonged latency. Therefore, it is recommended that CT scans be limited in children and young adults when other imaging methods (primarily MRI and ultrasound) can be used instead.

Nuclear Medicine Scans

A variety of radionuclides are used to evaluate abnormalities of the musculoskeletal system. The most common is technetium 99 m-MDP, an agent which is injected intravenously and deposited in the soft tissues based on blood flow and osteoblastic activity. The triple-phase bone scan consists of an arterial phase obtained with multiple short images over the area of concern, a blood-pool phase several minutes after injection, and a delayed phase 4–6 h when the concentration of radionuclide is dependent primarily on osteoblastic activity. Although the triple-phase bone scan is often considered to be specific for osteomyelitis, it is also positive in inflammatory arthritis, gout and pseudogout, trauma, and neuropathic arthropathy. In the past, bone scans have been used to diagnose radiographically occult fractures in osteopenic patients. However, they have about a 10 % false-negative rate in the first 24 h after a fracture occurs and have been superseded by MRI for occult fracture. The primary use of bone scans currently is in the evaluation of metastatic disease (Fig. 2). Ninety percent of metastases and 50 % of myeloma lesions are positive on bone scans.

Gallium-67 scans and indium-111 scans are both performed for infection. Gallium scans can be false positive in noninfected nonunions. Indium scans may be false negative in chronic infections. Both are still used when MRI is not feasible because of metallic implants (Fig. 3).

Positron emission tomography (PET) scan is currently used primarily for tumor evaluation. Positron-labeled fluorodeoxyglucose (FDG) is injected intravenously and distributes in the body according to metabolic activity. Due to poor spatial resolution, PET scanning is almost always performed in conjunction with CT or MRI scan. It is important to know that not all sarcomas are FDG-avid. Inflammatory and infectious processes may also be PET-avid.

Magnetic Resonance Imaging (MRI)

MRI is the modality of choice for evaluation of internal derangements of joints, infection, and bone marrow abnormalities. It is more sensitive and specific than radionuclide scanning for diagnosis of stress fracture or occult fracture. Although metal causes MRI artifacts due to distortion of the magnetic field, diagnostic imaging quality can often be obtained adjacent to prostheses (Fig. 4).

MRI exploits the polarity of the hydrogen ion. In the normal resting state, hydrogen ions are randomly oriented. When the patient is placed in a strong magnetic field (0.3–3.0 tesla (T)), the hydrogen ions (protons) tend to align with the field. In MRI, various magnetic pulses are applied after the patient is placed in the static magnetic field. The magnetic signals emitted by protons are measured as the protons return to their resting state. The magnetic signal depends on the type of pulse applied, the number of free protons, and the characteristics of different tissue types. The pulses are described in terms of echo time (TE), repetition time (TR), inversion time (TI), and flip angle (FA). Many different types of MRI sequences are used. The most common sequences are fast spin echo (FSE). A T1-weighted FSE image (at 1.5 T,

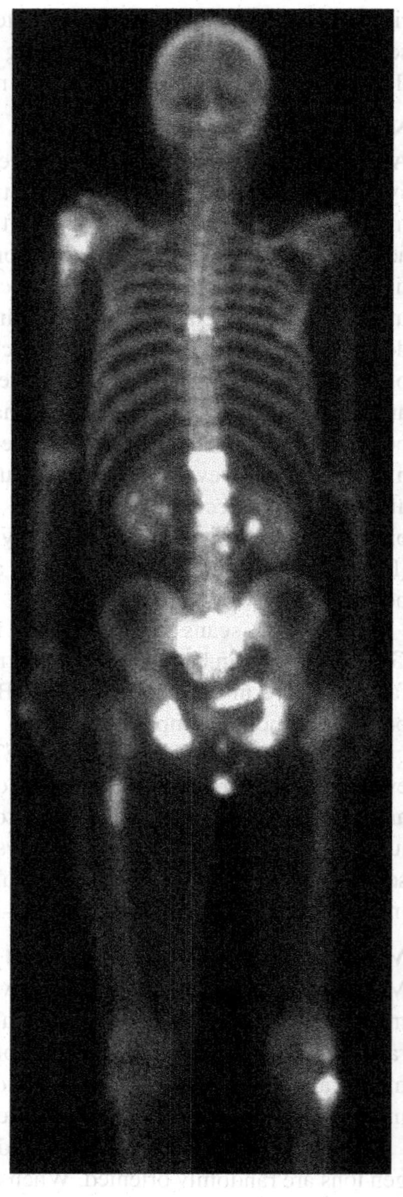

Fig. 2 Technetium bone scan in patient with metastatic prostate carcinoma. Multiple areas of increased radionuclide uptake are seen and are characteristic of metastases. The radionuclide is excreted by the kidneys, and activity in the kidneys and bladder is normal

TE<20, TR<600) shows fat and blood as white (high signal intensity). Cortical bone, tendons, calcifications, fluid, and fibrous tissue are black (low signal intensity). Muscle and many internal organs are gray (intermediate signal intensity.) Fluid-sensitive sequences show fluid as high signal intensity. They include T2-weighted (TE>60, TR>2,500), proton density (TE 20–60, TR>1,500), STIR (TE 30–45, TE 3,000–4,000, TI 110–150), and T2*gradient echo (variable parameters). Fat will also be

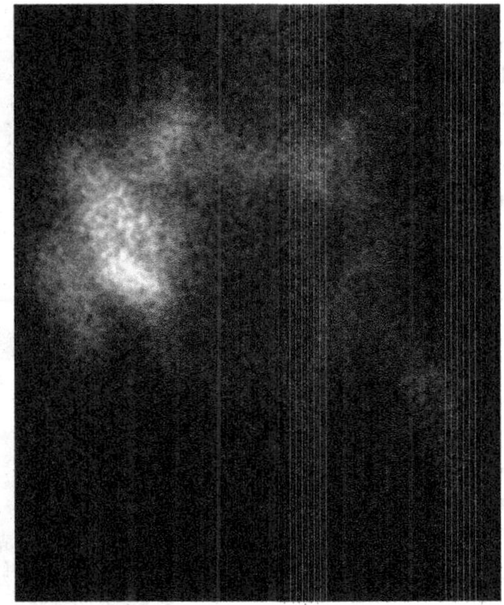

Fig. 3 Indium scan in patient with several years' history of aching hip pain after fracture. Extensive hardware precluded MRI. CT scan showed healed fracture and bone sclerosis. Indium scan showed increased radionuclide activity centered on the ischium. Surgery confirmed osteomyelitis

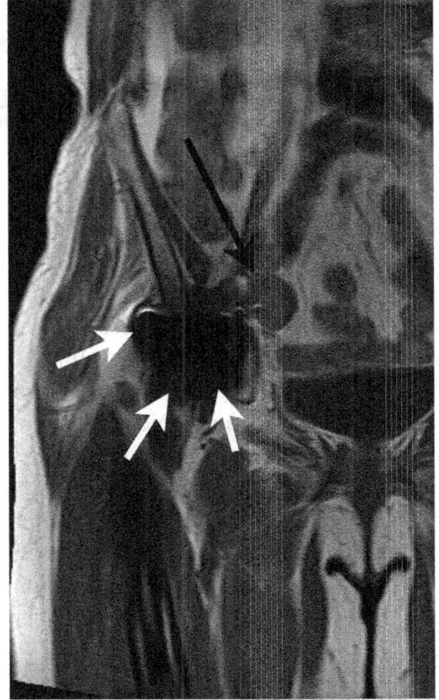

Fig. 4 T1-weighted coronal image shows metal artifact (*white arrows*) and focus of metallosis (*black arrow*). Metal artifact on MRI is larger than the metallic implant

high signal intensity, unless a fat suppression (also known as fat saturation or FS) technique is used. Fat suppression is important in musculoskeletal MRI because most abnormal fluid occurs in areas where fat is present. If fat suppression is not

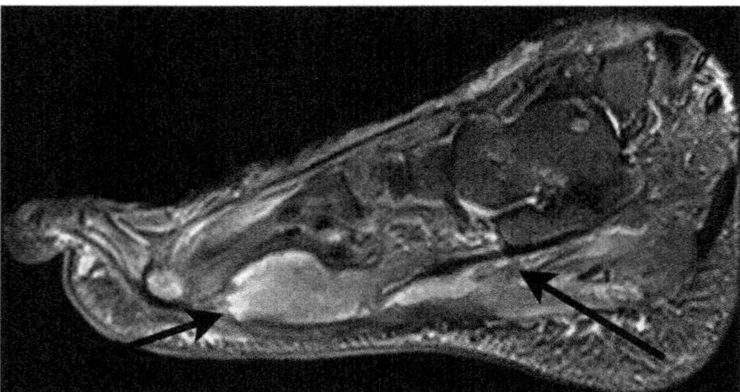

Fig. 5 Sagittal STIR image through the foot shows an elongated, nonanatomic region of high signal intensity (*arrows*). Gadolinium contrast (Fig. 6) is useful to distinguish phlegmon from abscess

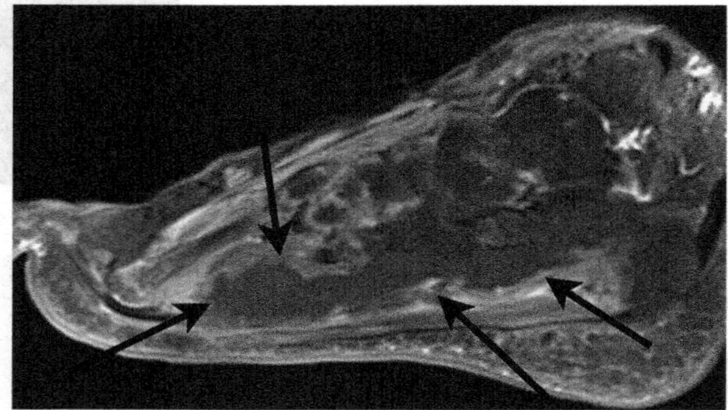

Fig. 6 Sagittal Gd-enhanced image through the foot in the same patient as Fig. 5 shows large deep abscess (*arrows*)

used, abnormalities are often masked by adjacent fat. Proton density sequences are intermediate between T1 and T2. STIR sequences use an inversion recovery (IR) pulse to suppress signal intensity from fat; fluid is high signal intensity on these sequences, and fat signal is more uniformly suppressed than on T2-weighted images with fat suppression (Fig. 5). Almost every disease process is characterized by increased tissue fluid. On MRI, the morphology and distribution of the fluid are analyzed together with anatomic features in order to reach a diagnosis.

Gadolinium is a rare earth which in chelated compounds is used to assess vascularity of tissues. Any process with increased vascularity will show increased signal intensity on T1-weighted images ("enhancement") following gadolinium administration. Abscesses and necrotic tumors show an enhancing rim around a central, nonenhancing rim (Fig. 6). Gadolinium is contraindicated in patients with poor renal function, as it can cause nephrogenic systemic fibrosis (NSF).

Ultrasound

Ultrasound is increasingly used in orthopedic imaging for evaluation of tendon and ligament injuries, as well as the initial evaluation of soft-tissue masses, and to guide aspiration and biopsy. It has considerable advantages over MRI in terms of cost and is accurate in experienced hands. Tissues are characterized on ultrasound based on their echogenicity. Simple fluid contains no echoes (anechoic, Fig. 7), while complex fluid contains low-level echoes. Tendons have a uniform, fine echotexture, while muscle has a looser architecture. A tendon tear on ultrasound shows both altered echogenicity and altered anatomy.

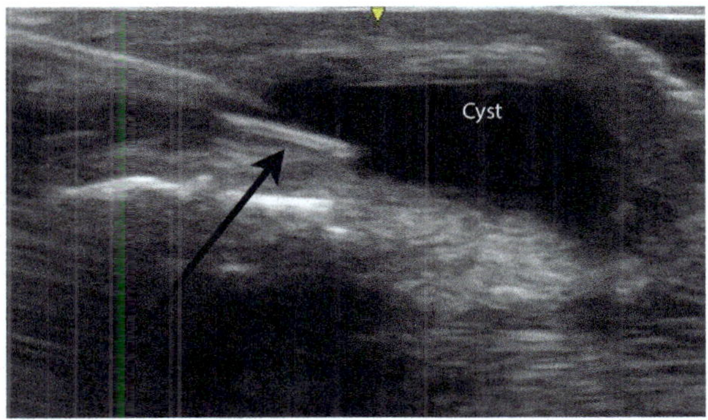

Fig. 7 Ultrasound can be used for both diagnosis and treatment. Image shows a painful cyst which has been punctured by a needle (*arrow*) for aspiration and steroid injection

Bone Densitometry

There are 2 methods of bone density measurement in common use today. Dual energy X-ray absorptiometry (DEXA) is more popular because of significantly lower cost. However, bone density as measured by DEXA can be artificially elevated in the presence of degenerative disc disease or chronic fractures.

Electrodiagnostic Studies

Nerve conduction studies are useful to assess the level and severity of nerve impingement. They are widely used to evaluate radiculopathies and nerve compression syndromes such as carpal tunnel syndrome. A transcutaneous electrode creates an action potential in the nerve, and velocity and signal amplitude is measured and compared to other nerves in the same region. Nerve velocity is measured as distance traveled/latency of pulse. Decreased nerve velocity and signal amplitude are a sign of nerve dysfunction, and the level of nerve injury can be fairly accurately determined. However, the sensitivity and specificity of nerve conduction studies for nerve compression compared to clinical exam is debated.

Electromyography utilizes an intramuscular electrode to evaluate electrical impulses at rest and during muscle contraction. It can determine acuity of neurogenic dysfunction and also distinguish between neurogenic and myopathic disease.

Bibliography

1. Bitar R, Leung G, Perng R, Tadros S, Moody AR, Sarrazin J, McGregor C, Christakis M, Symons S, Nelson A, Roberts TP. MR pulse sequences: what every radiologist wants to know but is afraid to ask. Radiographics. 2006;26(2):513–37.
2. Boland R, Kiernan M. Assessing the accuracy of a combination of clinical tests for identifying carpal tunnel syndrome. J Clin Neurosci. 2009;16(929):933.
3. Crim JR, Seeger LL. Imaging evaluation of osteomyelitis. Crit Rev Diagn Imaging. 1994;35(3):201–56.
4. Miller TT. Imaging of hip arthroplasty. Eur J Radiol. 2012;81(12):3802–12.
5. Palestro CJ, Love C. Radionuclide imaging of musculoskeletal infection: conventional agents. Semin Musculoskelet Radiol. 2007;11(4):335–52.
6. Roth TD, Buckwalter KA, Choplin RH. Musculoskeletal computed tomography: current technology and clinical applications. Semin Roentgenol. 2013;48(2):126–39.

Part III
Orthopaedic Trauma

Natalie Casemyr, Cyril Mauffrey, and David Hak

General Principles

Natalie Casemyr, Cyril Mauffrey, and David Hak

Take-Home Message

- ATLS protocol provides a systematic approach for assessing trauma patients to identify life-threatening injuries with simultaneous initiation of resuscitation
- Hemorrhagic shock: increased heart rate and increased systemic vascular resistance
- Neurogenic shock: decreased heart rate and decreased blood pressure
- Place pregnant women in the left lateral decubitus position to prevent vena cava compression

1 Epidemiology

- Traumatic injuries are the fifth most common cause of death
- The highest incidence in patients 12–24 years old
- Bimodal distribution of death by age:
  - 20s: motor vehicle accidents, firearms
  - 80s: falls, motor vehicle accidents

N. Casemyr, MD • C. Mauffrey, MD, FACS, FRCS (✉) • D. Hak, MD, FACS, MBA
Department of Orthopaedic Surgery, Denver Health Medical Center, 777 Bannock Street, Denver 80204, CO, USA
e-mail: cyril.mauffrey@dhha.org; cmauffrey@yahoo.com

C. Mauffrey, D.J. Hak (eds.), *Passport for the Orthopedic Boards and FRCS Examination*, DOI 10.1007/978-2-8178-0475-0_8

2 Trimodal Distribution of Mortality

- Immediate (50 %): massive hemorrhage, massive devastating neurologic injury
  - Prevention
- Early (30 %): often sequelae of neurologic injury
  - 62 % of in-hospital deaths occur in the first 4 h of admission
- Late (20 %): days to weeks, 80 % related to head injuries, 20 % related to multisystem organ failure and sepsis

3 Golden Hour

- Window to treat potentially survivable life-threatening injuries
- Approximately 60 % of preventable deaths occur in this time range

4 Advanced Trauma Life Support (ATLS)

- Primary Survey
  - Airway
    - Establish a secure airway for GCS < 8 and hemodynamic instability, consider in significant head and neck injuries
    - Always maintain c-spine precautions
  - Breathing
    - Identify and treat life-threatening injuries
    - Tension pneumothorax: urgent needle decompression at second intercostal space in midclavicular line followed by definitive chest tube placement
    - Open pneumothorax: "sucking chest wound," three-sided dressing
    - Positive pressure ventilation will worse a pneumothorax and possibly create a tension pneumothorax until a chest tube is placed
    - Flail chest: paradoxical chest wall motion creates a VQ mismatch with hypoxia
    - Massive hemothorax: >1,500 cc of blood or >200 cc/h for 4 h
  - Circulation
    - Average adult has 4.5–5 L circulating blood volume
    - Shock: compromise of circulation resulting in inadequate oxygen delivery to tissues

- Hypovolemic shock
  - Increased heart rate and increased systemic vascular resistance
  - Most commonly secondary to acute blood loss
  - Obvious external bleeding
  - Internal bleeding: chest, abdomen, retroperitoneum, pelvis, long bone
  - Classes of hemorrhagic shock
    - Class I: < 15 % blood loss, normal HR, normal BP, UOP >30 mL/h, pH normal, anxious, treat with fluid
    - Class II: 15–30 % blood loss, HR>100 bpm, normal BP, UOP 20–30 mL/h, pH normal, confused/irritable/combative, treat with fluid
    - Class III: 30–40 % blood loss, HR >120 bpm, decreased BP, UOP 5–15 mL/h, pH decreased, lethargic/irritable, treat with fluid and blood
    - Class IV: >40 % blood loss, HR >140 bpm, decreased BP, UOP minimal, pH decreased, lethargic/coma, treat with fluid and blood
- Neurogenic shock
  - Due to loss of sympathetic tone in spine cord injury
  - Decreased heart rate, decreased blood pressure, warm skin, failure to respond to crystalloids
  - Treat with dobutamine and dopamine
- Septic shock
  - Hyperdynamic state
  - Increased heart rate, massively decreased systemic vascular resistance, increased cardiac index
  - Treat with antibiotics and norepinephrine
- Cardiac tamponade more common with penetrating injuries
- Pregnant patients
  - Trauma is the most common cause of death in pregnant women
  - Place in the left lateral decubitus position to prevent vena cava compression by the uterus and reduces cardiac output
  - Radiation exposure from most x-ray studies does not pose a risk to the fetus

- Disability
- Exposure, environmental control, evaluation (neurologic status)

- Secondary Survey
  - Evaluation of injuries, interventions
- Tertiary Survey
  - Serial reevaluation

Bibliography

1. Browner BD, Jupiter JB, Levine AM, Trafton PG, Krettek C. Skeletal trauma. 4th ed. Philadelphia: Saunders; 2009. p. 177–92, 199–214.
2. Miller MD, Thompson SR, Hart JA. Review of orthopaedics. 6th ed. Philadelphia: Elsevier; 2012. p. 697–703.

Assessment and Principles of Treatment

Natalie Casemyr, Cyril Mauffrey, and David Hak

Take-Home Message

- Initiate blood product transfusion in patients who fail to respond to 2 l crystalloid bolus
- Massive transfusion protocol: 1:1:1 of pRBC:FFP:platelets
- Employ damage control orthopedics in severely injured patients with decreased base deficits and increased serum lactate levels
- Hemodynamic parameters are not sufficient end points to measure adequacy of resuscitation
- Base deficit and serum lactate levels are proxies for anaerobic metabolism and more accurately indicate adequacy of resuscitation
- Glasgow Coma Scale is predictive of injury severity and mortality

1 Radiologic Workup

- Trauma X-ray series
  - AP chest
    - Mediastinal widening, pneumothorax

N. Casemyr, MD • C. Mauffrey, MD, FACS, FRCS (✉) • D. Hak, MD, FACS, MBA
Department of Orthopaedic Surgery, Denver Health Medical Center, 777 Bannock Street, Denver 80204, CO, USA
e-mail: cyril.mauffrey@dhha.org; cmauffrey@yahoo.com

C. Mauffrey, D.J. Hak (eds.), *Passport for the Orthopedic Boards and FRCS Examination*, DOI 10.1007/978-2-8178-0475-0_9

- AP pelvis
  - Pelvic ring injury, acetabulum, proximal femur
- Lateral c-spine
  - Must visualize C7–T1 junction
  - Often replaced by CT c-spine
  - Valuable in patients going emergently to OR prior to CT scan

- CT scan
  - C-spine, chest, abdomen, pelvis
  - Increasingly used in the initial evaluation of the trauma patient
- Additional X-rays
  - Investigate potential injuries identified in secondary and tertiary surveys
  - Failure to image an extremity is the most common cause of delayed fracture diagnosis

2 Damage Control Orthopedics (DCO)

- Recognition of the impact of early definitive surgical care on resuscitation and brain injury lead to the concept of damage control orthopedics
- Subset of critically injured patients who may benefit from initial provisional stabilization to improve immediate survival with the least stress to the patient's physiologic condition
  - Minimize the second hit
  - Indicated for patients whose inflammatory response will be overwhelmed by further stimuli
- Stabilization of major fractures still imperative to decrease inflammatory mediators and catecholamine release, decrease analgesic requirements, and facilitate ICU care
  - Acute stabilization primarily achieved with external fixation, pelvic sheets/binders, and skeletal traction
  - Convert to definitive management of pelvic fractures within 7–10 days
  - Convert femur fractures to intramedullary nail fixation within 3 weeks
  - Convert tibia fractures to intramedullary nail fixation within 7–10 days

3 Systemic Effects of Trauma

- Systemic inflammatory response (SIR)
- Counter-regulatory anti-inflammatory response (CAR)

- Balance between SIR and CAR needed for homeostasis
- Parameters for DCO
  - ISS >40 (without thoracic trauma)
  - ISS >20 (with thoracic trauma)
  - Base deficit >5–6 (normal −2 to 2)
    - Best measure of resuscitation in the first 6 h after injury
    - Direct measure of metabolic acidosis, indirect measure of lactate levels
    - Correlates with organ dysfunction and mortality
  - Serum lactate >2–2.5 mmol/L
  - pH < 7.24
  - Hypothermia with temperature <35 °C
  - Coagulopathy, platelets <90,000
  - IL-6 >800 pg/mL
  - Bilateral femur fractures
  - Pulmonary contusion on chest X-ray
  - Multiple injuries with pelvic/abdominal trauma and hemorrhagic shock
- Acute inflammatory window from 2 to 5 days post-injury during which there is increased risk for ARDS and MSOF
  - Only potentially life-threatening injuries should be treated during this time

4 Resuscitation

- Immediate aggressive fluid resuscitation with placement of 2 large-bore IVs
- Crystalloid isotonic solutions to correct most extracellular volume deficits
  - 1–2 l
- Transfuse blood to patients who fail initial fluid boluses
  - Failure to respond to 2 l crystalloid bolus should be equated to estimated blood loss of >30 % of blood volume, or Class III–IV hemorrhagic shock, and blood product transfusion should be initiated
  - O-negative blood, type-specific blood, cross-matched blood
  - Massive transfusion protocol: 1:1:1 ratio of pRBC:FFP:platelets
  - Coagulopathy often develops after transfusion secondary to depletion of host clotting factors, platelets, and hypothermia and portends a worse prognosis
- Adequate resuscitation
  - Heart rate <100 bpm
  - Mean arterial pressure >60 mmHg
  - Urine output >0.5–1.0 mg/kg/h
  - Normalization of base deficit and lactate levels

5 Trauma Scoring Systems

- There are many trauma scoring systems which may be useful in triage and many of which have prognostic value
- Glasgow Coma Scale (GCS)
  - Quantifies severity of head injury with gross assessment of CNS function
  - Eye opening (4 pts), best verbal response (5 pts), best motor response (6 pts)
    - 3–9: severe head injury
    - 9–12: moderate head injury
    - 13–15: minor head injury
  - Predictive of injury severity and mortality
  - Patients with femur fracture, head injury, and hypotension have lower GCS on discharge
- Injury Severity Score (ISS)
  - Scoring system based on injury in nine anatomic regions
  - Calculate via sum of the squares for the highest-grade injury in three different anatomic regions
  - ISS > 15 associated with 10 % mortality rate
  - New Injury Severity Score (NISS) calculation uses the three highest-grade injuries regardless of anatomic region
    - More accurate scoring for patients with multiple injuries within a single anatomic region
    - NISS is a better predictor of complications and mortality than ISS
- Mangled Extremity Severity Score (MESS)
  - Predicts the need for amputation of a severely injured lower extremity
  - Points assigned for skeletal/soft tissue injury (1–4), ischemia time (1–3), patient age (1–3), and shock as defined by hypotension (0–2)
  - MESS > 7 predicts need for amputation

6 Open Fractures

- Require urgent and aggressive debridement and irrigation
  - Low-pressure lavage more effective at reducing bacterial counts than high-pressure lavage and does not impart additional trauma to compromised soft tissues
  - Saline is the irrigation fluid of choice
- Update tetanus prophylaxis as indicated

- Appropriate antibiotics based on grade and stabilization
  - Continue antibiotics until 24 h after the last surgical debridement
- Gustillo Anderson Open Fracture Classification
  - Type I: wound <1 cm, no periosteal stripping, first-generation cephalosporin
  - Type II: wound 1–10 cm, no or minimal periosteal stripping or soft tissue wound, first-generation cephalosporin
  - Type III: wound >10 cm or high-energy injury, periosteal stripping, possible segmental injury, first-generation cephalosporin, aminoglycoside, +/– penicillin for gross contamination (farm, bowel)
    - Type IIIA: adequate soft tissue for primary closure
    - Type IIIB: insufficient soft tissue for primary closure, flap required
    - Type IIIC: associated vascular injury requiring repair
- Antibiotics
  - First-generation cephalosporin: gram-positive coverage
  - Aminoglycosides: gram-negative coverage
  - Penicillin: anaerobic coverage (*Clostridium*)
  - Freshwater wounds: fluoroquinolones or ceftazidime
  - Saltwater wounds: doxycycline and ceftazidime or a fluoroquinolone

7 Compartment Syndrome

- Elevated fascial compartment pressures lead to decreased tissue perfusion
  - Local trauma and bleeding → increased interstitial pressure exceeds capillary pressure → vascular occlusion → myoneural ischemia
- Most commonly occurs in the leg, forearm, hand, foot, thigh, buttock, shoulder, and paraspinous muscles
- Etiology
  - Trauma: fractures, crush injury, contusion, gunshot injury
  - External compression: tight casts, dressings, or other wrappings
  - Vascular: arterial injury, reperfusion/post-ischemic injury
  - Burns
  - Bleeding disorders
  - Fluid extravasation
- Clinical assessment
  - 5 Ps
    - Pain out of proportion the most critical clinical sign
    - Pain with passive stretch the most critical clinical test
    - Paresthesias, pallor, and pulselessness are late findings

- Compartment pressure measurement
    - ΔP = diastolic pressure – compartment pressure
    - ΔP < 30 mmHg or absolute compartment pressure >30 mmHg indicate compartment syndrome
    - Intraoperative diastolic pressure decreased from baseline
        - Compare intraoperative compartment pressure measurements to preoperative diastolic pressure
- Maintain a high index of suspicion
    - Difficult to assess polytrauma patients and sedated patients
        - May need to rely on compartment pressure measurements with low threshold to proceed with fasciotomies

- Treatment
    - Emergent decompression with fasciotomy
        - Clinical presentation consistent with compartment syndrome
        - ΔP < 30 mmHg or absolute compartment pressure >30 mmHg
    - 4 Cs of viability: color, contractility, capacity to bleed, consistency
    - Serial exam of patients at risk for compartment syndrome
    - Foot compartment syndrome: nonoperative management vs. surgical fasciotomies debated
    - Nonoperative sequelae of claw toes is more easily treated; possible chronic nerve pain and hypersensitivity are especially difficult to treat
- Complications
    - Missed compartment syndrome results in permanent nerve and muscle injury with contractures and possible loss of the limb
        - Fasciotomies are generally contraindicated in missed compartment syndrome due to significantly increased risk of infection
        - May consider debridement in patients with organ failure secondary to metabolic waste from necrosed tissue

Bibliography

1. Browner BD, Jupiter JB, Levine AM, Trafton PG, Krettek C. Skeletal trauma. 4th ed. Philadelphia: Saunders; 2009. p. 177–92, 199–214, 367–396.
2. Hassinger SM, Harding G, Wongworawat MD. High-pressure pulsatile lavage propagates bacteria into soft tissue. Clin Orthop Relat Res. 2005;439:27–31.
3. Pape HC, et al. Epoff Study group. Systemic inflammatory response after extremity or truncal fracture operations. J Trauma. 2008;65(6):1379–84.
4. Sears BW, Stover MD, Callaci J. Pathoanatomy and clinical correlates of the immunoinflammatory response following orthopaedic trauma. J Am Acad Orthop Surg. 2009;17(4):255–65. Review.

Upper Extremity Trauma

Natalie Casemyr, Cyril Mauffrey, and David Hak

1 Sternoclavicular Dislocations

Take-Home Message

- Joint stability depends on the integrity of ligamentous structures.
- Anterior dislocation most common; majority remain unstable but asymptomatic.
- Posterior dislocation may present with dyspnea, dysphagia, tachypnea, or stridor.
- Assess for associated pneumothorax and injury to the trachea, esophagus, or major vascular structures.
- Imaging studies: serendipity view and CT scan.
- Thoracic surgery should be available prior to undertaking any closed or open reduction procedures.

- General
  - High-energy chest wall injury (MVA, contact sports).
  - Associated injuries: pneumothorax, nerve injury, injury to the trachea, esophagus, or major vascular structures.
  - Joint stability depends on the integrity of ligamentous structures.

N. Casemyr, MD • C. Mauffrey, MD, FACS, FRCS (✉) • D. Hak, MD, FACS, MBA
Department of Orthopaedic Surgery, Denver Health Medical Center, 777 Bannock Street, Denver 80204, CO, USA
e-mail: cyril.mauffrey@dhha.org; cmauffrey@yahoo.com

C. Mauffrey, D.J. Hak (eds.), *Passport for the Orthopedic Boards and FRCS Examination*, DOI 10.1007/978-2-8178-0475-0_10

- Posterior capsular ligament: anterior/posterior stability
- Anterior sternoclavicular ligament: primary restraint to superior displacement of the medial clavicle
- Costoclavicular ligaments: resist superior/inferior rotation and medial-lateral displacement
- Intra-articular disk ligament: prevents medial clavicle displacement, secondary restraint to superior clavicle displacement

- Imaging Studies
  - Serendipity view x-ray (40° cephalic tilt)
    - Anterior dislocation: affected clavicle above contralateral clavicle
    - Posterior dislocation: affected clavicle below contralateral clavicle
  - CT scan
    - Study of choice
    - Allows assessment of mediastinal structures
- Classification
  - Anterior dislocation
    - Deformity with palpable bump, prominence increases with abduction and elevation
  - Posterior dislocation
    - May compress mediastinal structures and present with dyspnea, tachypnea, dysphagia, stridor, or venous congestion or diminished pulse of the affected upper extremity
  - Chronic dislocation
    - Anterior or posterior sternoclavicular joint dislocations >3 weeks old
- Treatment
  - Nonoperative
    - Consider in atraumatic and chronic dislocations.
    - Accept deformity, local symptomatic treatment, sling for comfort, and return to unrestricted activity in 3 months.
  - Closed reduction under general anesthesia
    - Thoracic surgery should be available prior to any manipulation.
    - Acute anterior dislocations
      - Reduction maneuver: abduction, extension, and direct pressure over the medial clavicle.
      - Stable reduction: sling and swath for 6 weeks; return to activities at 3 months.
      - Unstable reduction: accept deformity (preferable) vs resect medial clavicle.

- Acute posterior dislocations
  - Reduction maneuver: abduction, extension, and anterior traction on the medial clavicle with towel clip.
  - Stable reduction: sling and swath for 6 weeks, consider figure of eight brace, and return to activities in 3 months.
  - Unstable reduction: resect medial clavicle (preferable) vs surgical stabilization.
- Operative
  - Thoracic surgery should be available prior to any open procedure.
  - Open reduction with soft tissue reconstruction vs surgical fixation
    - Consider in unstable posterior dislocations with compromise of mediastinal structures.
    - Smooth wires should not be used to stabilize the joint because of the risk of migration into the thorax.

- Complications
  - Recurrent instability of the SC joint: consider tendon graft reconstruction.
  - SC joint arthrosis: treat with medial clavicle excision.

Bibliography

1. Bicos J, Nicholson GP. Treatment and results of sternoclavicular joint injuries. Clin Sports Med. 2003;22(2):359–70. Review.
2. Browner BD, Jupiter JB, Levine AM, Trafton PG, Krettek C. Skeletal trauma. 4th ed. Philadelphia: Saunders; 2009. p. 1757–8.
3. Miller MD, Thompson SR, Hart JA. Review of orthopaedics. 6th ed. Philadelphia: Elsevier; 2012. p. 705.
4. Wirth MA, Rockwood Jr CA. Acute and chronic traumatic injuries of the sternoclavicular joint. J Am Acad Orthop Surg. 1996;4(5):268–78.

2 Clavicle Fractures

Take-Home Message

- Clavicle fractures are common injuries that most often occur in the middle third.
- Open clavicle fractures have high rates of associated pulmonary and closed head injuries.
- Treatment is controversial. The majority of clavicle fractures can be managed nonoperatively.
- Increased risk of nonunion in females, elderly, and fractures >100 % displacement or >2 cm shortening.
- Improved shoulder function and union rates for significantly displaced and shortened clavicle fractures.

- General
  - Clavicle fractures are common injuries, comprising 5–10 % of all fractures.
  - High-energy mechanisms may have associated ipsilateral scapula fractures, scapulothoracic dissociation, rib fracture, and pneumothorax and neurovascular injury.
    - Open clavicle fractures associated with high rates of pulmonary injury and closed head injuries
- Imaging
  - Clavicle fractures are often first identified on trauma series CXR.
  - AP view and 15° cephalad-oblique views: assess fracture location, configuration, and displacement.
  - CT scan: consider in medial third fractures; additionally may help evaluate displacement, comminution, and nonunion.
- Classification
  - Medial third (5 %)
    - Majority can be managed nonoperatively and are rarely symptomatic.
    - Assess for posterior displacement, and treat according to the principles for posterior sternoclavicular joint dislocation if present.
  - Middle third (80 %)
    - Majority can be managed nonoperatively.
    - Deforming forces in displaced fractures.
      - Medial fragment: the sternocleidomastoid and trapezius pull the medial fragment posterosuperiorly.
      - Lateral fragment: pectoralis major and weight of the arm pull the lateral fragment inferomedially.
    - Improved outcomes with ORIF for middle third clavicle fractures with 100 % displacement and >2 cm shortening.
      - Improved function with less pain and improved shoulder strength and endurance, increased union rates with faster time to union
      - Nonoperative management of fractures with 100 % displacement: 5–10 % nonunion
  - Lateral third (15 %)
    - Coracoclavicular ligaments provide superior/inferior stability.
      - Trapezoid ligament: 3 cm from the end of the clavicle
      - Conoid ligament: 4.5 cm from the end of the clavicle
    - Higher rates of nonunion compared to middle third clavicle fractures.

- Treatment
  - Treatment is controversial.
  - Nonoperative
    - Most clavicle fractures can be successfully treated nonoperatively.
    - Sling immobilization and figure-of-eight bandage have no difference in outcomes.
    - Begin range of motion exercises at 2–4 weeks.
  - Operative
    - Indications for surgical treatment continue to evolve.
    - Absolute indications: open fractures, associated vascular injury, skin tenting, floating shoulder, symptomatic nonunion, some significantly displaced fractures.
    - Relative indications: polytrauma patient, closed head injury, seizure disorder, brachial plexus injury.
    - Plate fixation
      - Superior plating: improved biomechanical strength, more symptomatic hardware, increased risk of neurovascular injury with drilling
      - Anterior plating: less symptomatic hardware
      - Hook plate: AC joint spanning fixation, indicated in lateral third clavicle fractures, requires plate removal
    - Intramedullary rod and screw
      - Percutaneous insertion possible, symptomatic hardware still possible
      - Increased complication rate, including migration
        - Avoid Steinmann pins for risk of migration into the thorax.
    - Coracoclavicular ligament repair/reconstruction
      - Consider in lateral third clavicle fractures.
      - Primary repair, suture supplementation.
    - Rehabilitation
      - Early active motion, strengthening at 6 weeks, return to activities at 3 months
        - Hook plate range of motion restriction: no forward flexion >90° or abduction >90° until plate is removed
- Complications
  - Hardware complications
    - Symptomatic hardware
      - 30 % of patients request hardware removal.
      - Superior plates associated with increased irritation.

    - Failure of fixation: 1.5 %

- Nonunion

    - Nonoperative management: 1–5 % overall

        - Asymptomatic: no treatment indicated
        - Symptomatic: consider nonunion take down and ORIF +/– bone graft (atrophic nonunions)

    - Risk factors: female, elderly, smoking, ≥100 % displacement, or ≥2 cm shortening

- Adhesive capsulitis

    - 4 % of patients who undergo surgical fixation

- Neurovascular injury

    - 3 %, increased risk with superior plating.
    - Acute neurovascular complications are rare, typically associated with scapulothoracic dissociation.

- Pneumothorax

    - A concern with operative fixation but actual case reports are rare

Bibliography

1. Browner BD, Jupiter JB, Levine AM, Trafton PG, Krettek C. Skeletal trauma. 4th ed. Philadelphia: Saunders; 2009. p. 1765–77.
2. Canadian Orthopaedic Trauma Society. Nonoperative treatment compared with plate fixation of displaced midshaft clavicular fractures. A multicenter, randomized clinical trial. J Bone Joint Surg Am. 2007;89(1):1–10.
3. Khan LA, Bradnock TJ, Scott C, Robinson CM. Fractures of the clavicle. J Bone Joint Surg Am. 2009;91(2):447–60.
4. Kim W, McKee MD. Management of acute clavicle fractures. Orthop Clin North Am. 2008;39(4):491–505.
5. McKee MD, et al. Deficits following nonoperative treatment of displaced midshaftclavicular fractures. J Bone Joint Surg Am. 2006;88(1):35–40.
6. Miller MD, Thompson SR, Hart JA. Review of orthopaedics. 6th ed. Philadelphia: Elsevier; 2012. p. 705–7.
7. Oh JH, et al. Treatment of distal clavicle fracture: a systematic review of treatment modalities in 425 fractures. Arch Orthop Trauma Surg. 2011;131(4): 525–33.
8. Robinson CM, Goudie EB, Murray IR, Jenkins PJ, Ahktar MA, Read EO, Foster CJ, Clark K, Brooksbank AJ, Arthur A, Crowther MA, Packham I, Chesser TJ. Open reduction and plate fixation versus nonoperative treatment for displaced midshaft clavicle fractures: a multicenter, randomized, controlled trial. J Bone Joint Surg Am. 2013;95:1576–84.

3 Acromioclavicular Injuries

Take-Home Message

- Acromioclavicular ligaments provide anterior/posterior stability.
- Coracoclavicular ligaments provide superior/inferior stability.
- Bilateral AP radiographs for comparison to contralateral side and zanca view.
- Nonoperative management: type I, II +/– III.
- Operative management: type IV, V, VI.
- AC joint arthrosis best treated with distal clavicle excision.

- General
  - Common injuries, comprise 9 % of shoulder girdle injuries
  - More common in males
  - Acromioclavicular ligament: provides anterior/posterior stability
  - Coracoclavicular ligaments: provide superior/inferior stability
- Imaging
  - Bilateral AP radiograph: compare distance from the top of the coracoid to the bottom of the clavicle to the contralateral side
  - Zanca view: 10° cephalic tilt and 50 % penetration, improved visualization of AC joint by eliminating overlying structures
  - Axillary view: assess for posterior clavicle displacement (type IV)
- Classification
  - Type I: AC ligament sprain, no displacement
  - Type II: AC ligament rupture, CC ligament sprain, vertical displacement with <25 % increase of CC interspace
  - Type III: AC and CC ligament ruptures, vertical displacement with 25–100 % increase of CC interspace
  - Type IV: AC and CC ligament ruptures, lateral clavicle buttonholed through trapezius posteriorly
  - Type V: AC and CC ligament ruptures, vertical displacement with >100 % increase of CC interspace and rupture of deltotrapezial fascia
  - Type VI: AC and CC ligament ruptures, distal clavicle translocated inferior to the coracoid
- Treatment
  - Nonoperative
    - Indicated in type I, II, and most type III injuries
    - Sling for 3 weeks, early range of motion, return to activities at 12 weeks

- Operative
  - Indicated in type IV, V, and VI injuries
  - Consider in type III injuries in laborers and elite athletes
  - ORIF or ligament reconstruction
    - ORIF with CC screw or suture fixation: beware of proximity of neurovascular structures inferior to the coracoid.
    - ORIF with hook plate: requires second surgery for plate removal.
    - CC ligament reconstruction: transfer of coracoacromial ligament to distal clavicle (modified Weaver-Dunn), free tendon graft.
    - Primary AC joint fixation: rarely performed.
  - Rehabilitation: sling without abduction, shoulder range of motion beginning at 6 weeks, return to activities at 4–6 months

- Complications
  - AC joint arthrosis: treat with open or arthroscopic distal clavicle excision.
  - Chronic instability: distal clavicle excision with stabilization of the stump.

Bibliography

1. Browner BD, Jupiter JB, Levine AM, Trafton PG, Krettek C. Skeletal trauma. 4th ed. Philadelphia: Saunders; 2009. p. 1759–60.
2. Clarke HD, McCann PD. Acromioclavicular joint injuries. Orthop Clin North Am. 2000;31(2):177–87.
3. Mazzocca AD, Arciero RA, Bicos J. Evaluation and treatment of acromioclavicular join injuries. Am J Sports Med. 2007;35:316–29.
4. Miller MD, Thompson SR, Hart JA. Review of orthopaedics. 6th ed. Philadelphia: Elsevier; 2012. p. 707.

4 Scapula Fractures

Take-Home Message

- High-energy injuries with high rates of associated injuries and 2–5 % mortality rate.
- Nonoperative management indicated for the majority of scapula fractures.
- Operative treatment indicated for glenoid fractures with significant articular involvement and displacement or humeral head instability and glenoid neck fracture with significant displacement and/or angulation.
- Consider fixation of floating shoulder injuries.

- General
  - Uncommon injuries associated with high-energy mechanisms
  - 80–90 % associated injuries: rib fractures, pulmonary injury, pneumothorax closed head injury, vascular injury, ipsilateral clavicle fracture, spine fracture, pelvis/acetabulum fracture, brachial plexus injury
  - 2–5 % associated mortality rate
- Imaging
  - True AP, scapular Y, and axillary lateral.
  - CT scan: assess for intra-articular involvement and displacement.
- Classification
  - Coracoid fractures
    - Type I: proximal to CC ligament
    - Type II: distal to CC ligament
  - Acromial fractures
    - Type I: nondisplaced or minimally displaced
    - Type II: displaced without compromise of subacromial space
    - Type III: displaced with compromise of subacromial space
  - Glenoid fractures
    - Type Ia/Ib: anterior/posterior rim fracture, respectively
    - Type II/III/IV: glenoid fossa fracture exiting scapula laterally/superiorly/medially, respectively
    - Type Va/Vb/Vc: combinations of types II, III, and IV
    - Type VI: severe comminution
  - Glenoid neck fractures
    - Assess for floating shoulder: associated AC joint separation or clavicle fracture.
    - Superior shoulder suspensory complex (SSSC): 2 struts comprised of the clavicle and lateral scapular body linked by a bony and soft tissue ring made up of the coracoid, acromion, AC and CC ligaments, distal clavicle, and glenoid process.
      - Disruption of the complex at two sites is more problematic than disruption at one site.
    - Many floating shoulder injuries are stable and can be managed nonoperatively with good outcomes.
    - Unstable injuries with disruption of the SSSC or >1 cm displacement may benefit from ORIF.

    - Fixation of clavicle alone is typically sufficient and may restore adequate alignment of the scapula fracture.

  - Scapular body fractures

- Treatment
  - Nonoperative
    - Indicated for the majority of scapula fractures.
    - Sling for 2 weeks, early range of motion; expect union at 6 weeks and not functional deficits.
  - Operative
    - Indications for surgical fixation
      - Glenoid fractures: involvement of >25 % glenoid with humeral head subluxation/instability, >5 mm glenoid articular step-off or major gap
      - Glenoid neck fractures: >40° of angulation, >1 cm translation, translation of the glenoid and humeral head anterior to the proximal fragment or excessive glenoid medialization
      - Coracoid fractures: >1 cm displacement in high-demand patients
      - Open fractures
    - Open reduction internal fixation may be combined with shoulder arthroscopy depending on the fracture pattern.
- Complications
  - Scapulothoracic crepitation: may develop as sequelae of scapular body fracture and cause pain.
  - Open treatment typically utilizes the posterior Judet approach, with risk of injury to the suprascapular nerve and artery and circumflex scapular artery.

Bibliography

1. Browner BD, Jupiter JB, Levine AM, Trafton PG, Krettek C. Skeletal trauma. 4th ed. Philadelphia: Saunders; 2009. p. 1760–5.
2. Miller MD, Thompson SR, Hart JA. Review of orthopaedics. 6th ed. Philadelphia: Elsevier; 2012. p. 707–9.
3. Van Noort A, van Kampen A. Fractures of the scapula surgical neck: outcome after conservative treatment in 13 cases. Arch Orthop Trauma Surg. 2005;123:696–700.
4. Veysi VT, Mittal R, Agarwal S, Dosani A, Giannoudis PV. Multiple trauma and scapula fractures: so what? J Trauma. 2003;55(6):1145–7.
5. Zlowodzki M, Bhandari M, Zelle BA, Kregor PJ, Cole PA. Treatment of scapula fractures: systematic review of 520 fractures in 22 case series. J Orthop Trauma. 2006;20(3):230–3.

5 Scapulothoracic Dissociation

Take-Home Message

- Maintain high index of suspicion for scapulothoracic dissociation with neurovascular injury and >1 cm lateral displacement of the scapula on AP CXR
- High incidence of associated trauma to the heart, chest wall, lungs, and ipsilateral shoulder girdle
- Functional outcome determined by the severity of the associated neurologic injury
- Mortality rate: 10 %

- General
  - High-energy injury with traumatic disruption of the scapulothoracic articulation
    - Typically caused by a lateral traction injury
  - High incidence of associated injuries
    - Trauma to the heart, chest wall, lungs
    - Neurologic injury (90 %): brachial plexus most common, poor outcomes, neurologic injury more common than vascular injury
    - Vascular injury: subclavian artery most common, axillary artery
  - Careful neurovascular exam is critical in patient assessment.
  - Mortality rate: 10 %.
- Imaging
  - AP CXR: >1 cm lateral displacement of the scapula from the spinous process compared to the contralateral side
    - Possible additional findings widely displaced clavicle fracture, AC separation, sternoclavicular dislocation
  - Angiogram: evaluate for injury to the subclavian and axillary artery.
  - EMG: consider 3 weeks after injury to further evaluate neurologic injury.
- Treatment
  - Nonoperative
    - Immobilization and supportive care
    - Indicated in hemodynamically stable patients without significant vascular injury

- Operative
    - Vascular repair indicated in hemodynamically unstable patients with significant vascular injury.
    - Consider ORIF of associated clavicle and AC joint injuries.
    - Forequarter amputation indicated for complete brachial plexus injury.
- Complications
  - Poor outcomes overall
    - Functional outcome largely determined by severity of neurologic injury
    - ~50 % of patients will have a flail extremity

Bibliography

1. Althausen PL, Lee MA, Finkemeier CG. Scapulothoracic dissociation: diagnosis and treatment. Clin Orthop Relat Res. 2003;416:237–44.
2. Clements RH, Reisser JR. Scapulothoracic dissociation: a devastating injury. J Trauma. 1996;40(1):146–9.
3. Miller MD, Thompson SR, Hart JA. Review of orthopaedics. 6th ed. Philadelphia: Elsevier; 2012. p. 709.
4. Zelle BA, Pape HC, Gerich TG, Garapati R, Ceylan B, Krettek C. Functional outcome following scapulothoracic dissociation. J Bone Joint Surg Am. 2004;86-A(1):2–8.

6 Glenohumeral Dislocations

Take-Home Message

- Shoulder dislocation must be evaluated with an axillary radiograph.
- Anterior glenohumeral dislocations are most common.
- Age at time of first dislocation is an important risk factor for recurrent instability and informs risk of associated injuries.
- Posterior shoulder dislocation is the commonly missed injury.
- Luxatio erecta has the highest risk of associated neurovascular injury.
- Assess for concurrent labral, cartilage, bony, and rotator cuff injuries which inform treatment options.
- Treatment of first time dislocators is controversial.

- General
  - The shoulder's extensive range of motion presents risk for instability, making it the most commonly dislocated joint in the body.
  - Direction of dislocation and age of onset key in determining risk of associated injuries and recurrent instability and in guiding treatment.

- Imaging
  - Standard x-ray series
    - True AP: unreliable, may see "lightbulb" sign with posterior dislocation.
    - Scapular Y.
    - Axillary: best view to demonstrate dislocation; consider Velpeau view if patient is unable to abduct.
  - Westpoint view: assess for glenoid fracture or bone loss (bony Bankart lesion).
  - Stryker notch view: assess posterior humeral head (Hill-Sachs lesion).
  - CT scan: may help assess location and extent of bony injuries/defects.
  - MRI: assess labral tears and rotator cuff tears.
- Anterior Dislocations
  - Typically traumatic and unilateral
  - Determinants of anterior static shoulder stability
    - SGHL: arm at side
    - MGHL: 45° abduction and external rotation
    - Anterior band of IGHL: 90° abduction and external rotation
  - Examination: apprehension sign, relocation sign, sulcus sign
  - Associated injuries
    - Labral and cartilage injuries
      - Bankart lesion: avulsion of the anterior inferior capsulolabral complex.
      - Humeral avulsion of the glenohumeral ligament (HAGL): increased risk of recurrent dislocation.
      - Glenoid labral articular defect (GLAD): sheared of articular cartilage with labrum.
      - Anterior labral periosteal sleeve avulsion (ALPSA): torn labrum may heal medially along the glenoid neck.
    - Bone injuries
      - Hill-Sachs lesion: anterior dislocations, clinically significant if it engages the glenoid
      - Bony Bankart lesion: fracture of the anterior inferior glenoid, present in 50 % of patients with recurrent anterior dislocations
      - Greater tuberosity fracture: anterior dislocations in patients >50
    - Nerve injuries
      - Axillary nerve injury: most common (5 %), transient neurapraxia
      - Musculocutaneous nerve injury second most common
    - Rotator cuff tears
      - Increasing incidence with increasing age
  - Bimodal distribution for risk of recurrent dislocation and associated injury

  - If <20 years old at time of first dislocation
    - High rate of recurrent dislocations
    - High rate of associated labral tears
  - If >40 years old at time of first dislocation
    - Lower rate of recurrent dislocations
    - High rate of associated rotator cuff tears

- Posterior Dislocations
  - Comprise 2–5 % of shoulder dislocations
  - Missed diagnosis in up to 50 % upon presentation to ED
  - May result from acute traumatic insult or microtrauma with labral injury and posterior capsule stretching (lineman, weight lifters, overhead athletes)
  - Associated with high-energy trauma, seizure and electrocution (internal rotators overpower external rotators), ligamentous laxity, glenoid retroversion, or hypoplasia
  - Examination: inability to externally rotate
  - Posterior shoulder stabilizers
    - Posterior band of IGHL: primary static restraint in internal rotation
    - Subscapularis: primary dynamic restraint in external rotation
    - Coracohumeral ligament: primary restraint to interior translation in adduction and external rotation, primary restraint to posterior translation in flexion, abduction, and internal rotation
  - Associated injuries
    - Labral and cartilage injuries
      - Reverse Bankart lesion: avulsion of posterior inferior capsulolabral complex
      - Posterior labral cyst
    - Bone injuries
      - Reverse Hill-Sachs lesion: present in 50 % of posterior dislocations
      - Reverse bony Bankart lesion: fracture of the posterior glenoid rim
      - Lesser tuberosity fracture: posterior dislocations

- Inferior Dislocations: Luxatio Erecta
  - Rare injuries, 0.5 % of all shoulder dislocations
  - Associated with MVAs and sports injuries
  - Examination: arm overhead in 100–160° abduction
  - Associated injuries
    - Highest incidence of neurovascular injury of all types of shoulder dislocation

  - Axillary nerve and artery most common
    - Axillary nerve palsy typically resolves with reduction.
    - May have diminished or absent pulses on presentation with return after reduction.
    - Axillary artery thrombosis may develop late.
- Glenohumeral ligament tears
- Capsulolabral tears possible
- Rotator cuff tears common

- Treatment
  - Nonoperative
    - Closed reduction, sling for 2–4 weeks and physical therapy with rotator cuff and periscapular muscle strengthening, activity modification
      - Immobilize posterior shoulder dislocation in neutral to external rotation.
    - Reduction maneuvers: many described, simple traction-countertraction most commonly used
  - Operative
    - Anterior dislocations
      - TUBS (traumatic unilateral Bankart surgery)
      - Open/arthroscopic Bankart repair +/– capsular shift: high success rate
      - Latarjet procedure: transfer of coracoid to address >20 % glenoid deficiency
      - Remplissage: posterior capsule and infraspinatus tendon advancement into >25 % Hill-Sachs lesion
      - Hill-Sachs bony reconstruction: allograft reconstruction, arthroplasty, or rotational osteotomy to address large engaging Hill-Sachs lesion
    - Posterior dislocations
      - Open/arthroscopic reverse Bankart repair +/– capsular shift: high success rate
      - McLaughlin: lesser tuberosity and subscapularis transfer to reverse Hill-Sachs defect <50 %
      - Hemiarthroplasty: reverse Hill-Sachs defect >50 %, chronic dislocations, severe humeral head arthrosis or collapse
      - Total shoulder arthroplasty: hemiarthroplasty indication with glenoid arthrosis
    - Inferior dislocations
      - Open/arthroscopic repair: indicated in young, active patients to address specific capsulolabral and rotator cuff pathology

- Complications
  - Recurrent instability: <10 % after operative treatment
  - Adhesive capsulitis
  - Capsular overtightening: may lead to subluxation or impingement
  - Posttraumatic arthrosis

Bibliography

1. Browner BD, Jupiter JB, Levine AM, Trafton PG, Krettek C. Skeletal trauma. Philadelphia: Saunders; 2009. p. 1717–35.
2. Lynch JR, Clinton JM, Dewing CB, Warme WJ, Matsen FA. Treatment of osseous defects associated with anterior shoulder instability. J Shoulder Elbow Surg. 2009;18(2):317–28.
3. Miller MD, Thompson SR, Hart JA. Review of orthopaedics. 6th ed. Philadelphia: Elsevier; 2012. p. 324–6, 711.
4. Millett PJ, Clavert P, Hatch 3rd GF, Warner JJ. Recurrent posterior shoulder instability. J Am Acad Orthop Surg. 2006;14:464–7.
5. Sewecke JJ, Varitimidis SE. Bilateral luxatio erecta: a case report and review of the literature. Am J Orthop. 2006;35(12):578–80.

7 Proximal Humerus Fractures

Take-Home Message

- Most proximal humerus fractures result from low-energy trauma in elderly patients.
- 85 % of proximal humerus fractures are minimally displaced and can be treated nonoperatively.
- Many patients will have significant residual functional deficits, irrespective of treatment.

- General
  - Comprise 5 % of all fractures
  - More common in women
  - Low-energy falls: osteoporosis, third most common fracture in elderly
  - High-energy trauma: young patients, increased incidence of neurovascular injures
  - Blood supply to the humeral head
    - Ascending branch of the anterior humeral circumflex artery, which runs in the lateral aspect of the bicipital groove, is classically described at the primary blood supply to the humeral head.

    - Posterior humeral circumflex artery shown to be the main supply to the humeral head in more recent studies.
    - Vascularity of the articular segment more likely to be preserved if >8 mm of calcar remains attached.
  - 45 % associated nerve injury
    - Axillary nerve injury most common
      - Distinguish from deltoid atony with pseudosubluxation of the humeral head.
    - Increased risk with fracture-dislocations
- Imaging
  - Trauma series x-rays: true AP, scapular Y, axillary.
  - CT scan: further assess fracture displacement, intra-articular involvement, and preoperative planning.
- Classification
  - Neer classification: part = displacement >1 cm or angulation >45° of the articular surface, greater tuberosity, lesser tuberosity, and shaft
  - One part
    - Nondisplaced or minimally displaced fracture, most commonly involving the surgical neck
  - Two part
    - Surgical neck: anteromedial displacement of the shaft from pull of pectoralis major
    - Greater tuberosity: posterosuperior displacement from pull of supraspinatus, infraspinatus, and teres minor
      - Displacement >5 mm may impinge and block external rotation and abduction.
    - Lesser tuberosity: posteromedial displacement from pull of subscapularis, associated with posterior shoulder dislocations
    - Anatomic neck: rare injury pattern
  - Three part
    - Displacement of greater or lesser tuberosity and articular surface
  - Four part
    - Displacement of shaft, articular surface, and both tuberosities
    - Head-splitting variant: split through articular surface
  - Valgus impaction
    - Posteromedial calcar typically intact: preserved blood supply to the articular segment, decreased risk of AVN

- Treatment
  - Nonoperative
    - Sling immobilization, early shoulder range of motion, and rehabilitation
    - Indicated for minimally displaced fractures, grater tuberosity fracture with <5 mm displacement and poor surgical candidates
      - Consider age, fracture characteristics, bone quality, medical comorbidities, and concurrent injuries.
  - Operative
    - Closed reduction percutaneous pinning
      - Two-part surgical neck fractures, some three-part and valgus impacted fractures
      - Consider bone quality, metaphyseal comminution, and involvement of medial calcar
    - Open reduction internal fixation
      - Greater tuberosity fracture with >5 mm displacement.
        - Techniques include screw fixation, nonabsorbable suture, and tension band wiring
      - Consider in two-, three-, and four-part fractures and head-splitting fractures in younger patients.
        - Lesser tuberosity component: large fragment amenable to ORIF; small fragments may be excised with cuff repair.
    - Intramedullary nailing
      - Consider in surgical neck fractures, some three-part fractures, and combined humeral shaft fractures.
      - Improved outcomes in younger patients.
    - Hemiarthroplasty
      - Anatomic neck fractures in the elderly or with significant comminution in younger patients, three- and four-part fractures not amenable to ORIF, fracture-dislocations, head-splitting fracture fractures, humeral head defect >40 %, loss of humeral head blood supply.
      - Consider in nonunions and malunions.
      - Requires an intact glenoid.
      - Humeral height, humeral version, and tuberosity reconstruction are important contributors to outcome.
        - Superior border of the pectoralis major insertion is a reliable landmark to determine height of the prosthesis.
      - In elderly patients, hemiarthroplasty may improve pain long term even if there is little functional benefit compared to nonoperative management.

- Total shoulder arthroplasty
  - Indications for hemiarthroplasty *plus* intact rotator cuff and glenoid compromise
- Reverse shoulder arthroplasty
  - Consider in elderly patients with nonreconstructable tuberosities
  - May result in improved outcomes when compared to hemiarthroplasty in elderly patients

- Complications
  - Avascular necrosis
    - 20–75 % in four-part fractures.
    - Risk of AVN increased with disruption of the medial periosteal hinge, medial metaphyseal extension less than 8 mm, increasing fracture complexity, displacement greater than 10 mm, angulation greater than 45°.
    - Incidence does not correlate with method of surgical fixation.
    - If symptomatic, treat with arthroplasty.
  - Nerve injury
    - Axillary nerve most commonly injured.
    - Suprascapular nerve and musculocutaneous nerve are also commonly injured.
    - Some specific risks for nerve injury pending type of surgical intervention and approach.
  - Hardware failure
    - Screw cutout, the most common complication following ORIF of the proximal humerus fractures with locking plates.
    - Inferomedial calcar screw in plate and screw constructs can help prevent varus collapse.
    - Intramedullary rods may migrate in the osteoporotic bone.
  - Nonunion
    - Most common after two-part fractures of the surgical neck.
    - If symptomatic, consider treatment with arthroplasty.
  - Malunion
    - Surgical neck fractures with varus and apex anterior deformity are poorly tolerated.
    - May consider osteotomy in symptomatic, young active patients.
  - Rotator cuff deficiencies
  - Adhesive capsulitis
  - Infection

Bibliography

1. Browner BD, Jupiter JB, Levine AM, Trafton PG, Krettek C. Skeletal trauma. Philadelphia: Saunders; 2009. p. 1643–712.
2. Cuff D, Pupello D. Comparison of hemiarthroplasty and reverse shoulder arthroplasty for the treatment of proximal humeral fractures in elderly patients. J Bone Joint Surg Am. 2013;95:2050–5.
3. Hettrich CM, Boraiah S, Dyke JP, Neviaser A, Helfet DL, Lorich DG. Quantitative assessment of the vascularity of the proximal part of the humerus. J Bone Joint Surg Am. 2010;92(4):943–8.
4. Jaberg H, Warner JJ, Jakob RP. Percutaneous stabilization of unstable fractures of the humerus. J Bone Joint Surg Am. 1992;74:508–15.
5. Konrad G, Bayer J, Hepp P, Voigt C, Oestern H, Kääb M, Luo C, Plecko M, Wendt K, Köstler W, Südkamp N. Open reduction and internal fixation of proximal humeral fractures with use of the locking proximal humerus plate. Surgical technique. J Bone Joint Surg Am. 2010;92(Suppl 1 Pt 1):85–95.
6. Miller MD, Thompson SR, Hart JA. Review of orthopaedics. 6th ed. Philadelphia: Elsevier; 2012. p. 709–11.
7. Olerud P, Ahrengart L, Ponzer S, Saving J, Tidermark J. Hemiarthroplasty versus nonoperative treatment of displaced 4-part proximal humerus fractures in elderly patients: a randomized controlled trial. J Shoulder Elbow Surg. 2011;20:1025–33.
8. Wijgman AJ, Roolker W, Patt TW, Raaymakers EL, Marti RK. Open reduction and internal fixation of three and four-part fractures of the proximal part of the humerus. J Bone Joint Surg Am. 2002;84-A(11):1919–25.

8 Humeral Shaft Fractures

Take-Home Message

- Nonoperative management with coaptation splint converted to functional bracing is indicated for the majority of humeral shaft fractures.
- Acceptable alignment: <30° varus/valgus angulation, <20° flexion/extension, <3 cm shortening.
- Absolute indications for surgical treatment: open fractures, associated vascular injury requiring repair, brachial plexus injury.
- Relative indications for surgical treatment: polytrauma, pathologic fractures, soft tissue injury that precludes bracing, some fracture patterns.
- Holstein-Lewis fracture: spiral distal 1/3 diaphyseal humerus fracture associated with increased risk of radial nerve injury.
- Intramedullary nail fixation has higher complication rates compared to plate osteosynthesis.
- The vast majority of radial nerve palsies resolve over time; observation is typically indicated as the initial treatment course.

- General
  - Comprise 3–5 % of all fractures
  - Associated radial nerve injury most common
    - Radial nerve courses through the spiral groove.
    - 20 cm proximal to the medial epicondyle.
    - 14 cm proximal to the lateral epicondyle.
    - Increased risk of radial nerve injury with Holstein-Lewis fracture patterns.
  - Careful neurovascular exam prereduction/splinting and preoperatively is critical
- Imaging
  - AP and lateral x-rays of the humerus, must include good visualization of the shoulder and elbow joints.
  - Traction views may be considered in some fracture patterns but are not required routinely.
- Classification
  - Descriptive
    - Fracture location: proximal, middle, distal 1/3
    - Fracture pattern: transverse, spiral, comminuted
  - Holstein-Lewis fracture
    - Spiral distal 1/3 diaphyseal humerus fracture
    - 22 % radial nerve injury
- Treatment
  - Nonoperative
    - Nonoperative management is the treatment of choice when possible.
    - Acceptable alignment: less than 30° of varus/valgus angulation, less than 20° flexion/extension, less than 3 cm of shortening.
    - Coaptation splint for 7–10 days followed by conversion to functional bracing.
    - Low nonunion rate
      - Proximal 1/3 diaphyseal humerus fracture have an increased risk of nonunion.
  - Operative
    - Absolute indications: open fracture, vascular injury requiring repair, brachial plexus injury
    - Relative indications: floating elbow, polytrauma (allow early weight bearing through humerus), pathologic fractures, soft tissues that preclude functional bracing, segmental fractures, neuromuscular conditions, some fracture patterns

- Plate fixation
  - Considered the gold standard for most humeral shaft fractures indicated for surgical fixation
  - High union rates
  - Decreased secondary operations
  - Safe to allow weight bearing to tolerance
- Intramedullary nailing
  - May be advantageous with pathologic fractures, segmental fractures, humeral shaft fractures combined with proximal humerus fractures, and poor soft tissues.
  - Antegrade or retrograde technique may be employed.
  - Higher total complication rates including nonunion, shoulder pain, and nerve injury
    - Early weight bearing does not affect union rate.
    - Radial nerve at risk with lateral to medial distal locking screw.
    - Musculocutaneous nerve at risk with anterior to posterior distal locking screw.

- Complications
  - Radial nerve palsy
    - Occurs in 5–10 % of humeral shaft fractures.
    - Increased incidence with distal 1/3 fractures and transverse fractures.
    - 85–90 % resolve over 3–4 months with observation
      - Wrist extension and radial deviation are expected to be regained first.
    - If not improving by 6–12 weeks, obtain EMG.
    - Radial nerve palsy in closed fracture after reduction: typically observe, and consider exploration for new pain.
    - Consider surgical exploration for open fractures with radial nerve palsy, closed fractures that fail to improve at 3–4 months, and fibrillations on EMG.
  - Nonunion
    - 2–10 % overall
      - Slightly higher rates of nonunion with surgical treatment
    - Risk factors: fracture distraction, open fractures, segmental fractures, infection, shoulder/elbow stiffness, patient factors (smoking, obesity, malnutrition, etc.).
    - Treat with compression plating with autogenous bone grafting.
  - Malunion
    - Varus angulation most common but typically asymptomatic

- Increased risk of malunion in proximal 1/3 diaphyseal fractures and transverse fractures.
- Pull of the deltoid on the proximal fragment contributes to varus malalignment.

Bibliography

1. Chapman JR, Henley MB, Agel J, Benca PJ. Randomized prospective study of humeral shaft fracture fixation: intramedullary nails versus plates. J Orthop Trauma. 2000;14(3):162–6.
2. DeFranco MJ, Lawton JN. Radial nerve injuries associated with humeral fractures. J Hand Surg Am. 2006;31(4):655–63. Review.
3. Heineman DJ, Poolman RW, Nork SE, Ponsen KJ, Bhandari M. Plate fixation or intramedullary fixation of humeral shaft fractures. Acta Orthop. 2010;81(2):216–23. Review.
4. McCormack RG, Brien D, Buckley RE, McKee MD, Powell J, Schemitsch EH. Fixation of fractures of the shaft of the humerus by dynamic compression plate or intramedullary nail. A prospective, randomised trial. J Bone Joint Surg Br. 2000;82(3):336–9.
5. Miller MD, Thompson SR, Hart JA. Review of orthopaedics. 6th ed. Philadelphia: Elsevier; 2012. p. 711–3.
6. Sarmiento A, Zagorski JB, Zych GA, Latta LL, Capps CA. Functional bracing for the treatment of fractures of the humeral diaphysis. J Bone Joint Surg Am. 2000;82(4):478–86.

9 Distal Humerus Fractures

Take-Home Message

- The majority of distal humerus fractures are indicated for surgical fixation.
- Distal intercondylar fractures are the most common variant.
- Maintain a high index of suspicion for nerve injury, brachial artery injury, and forearm compartment syndrome.
- Goal to restore functional elbow range of motion: 30–130°.
- For ORIF, both parallel plating and 90–90 plating configurations are supported.
- Triceps splitting, triceps sparring/paratricipital, and transolecranon osteotomies may be employed with different potential advantages and disadvantages pending fracture configuration.
- Ulnar nerve transposition not shown to decrease the incidence of ulnar nerve symptoms.
- Surgical fixation of comminuted, osteoporotic fractures is very challenging – consider total elbow arthroplasty.

- General
  - Most common in young males (high-energy falls) and elderly females (low-energy falls).
  - Distal intercondylar fractures are the most common variant.
  - Elbow position at injury impacts fracture pattern
    - Axial load with elbow flexed <90°: transcolumnar fracture
    - Axial load with elbow flexed >90°: intercondylar fracture more likely
  - Associated injuries include elbow dislocations, terrible triad injury, floating elbow, and forearm compartment syndrome.
  - Careful neurovascular exam to assess radial, ulnar, and median nerve as well as distal pulses
    - Maintain high index of suspicion for brachial artery injury and pursue further vascular work-up if there is any abnormality.
  - Injuries often complicated by low fracture lines, metaphyseal and articular comminution, and poor bone quality.
  - Goal to restore functional elbow range of motion: 30–130°
    - Poor outcomes in up to 25 % of patients
- Imaging
  - AP and lateral x-rays of the elbow, humerus, and forearm.
  - Obtain dedicated wrist views if additional elbow injury is identified or if there is wrist tenderness.
  - Consider oblique views and traction films for surgical planning.
  - CT scan often obtained for surgical planning, particularly helpful with coronal shear fractures of the capitellum and trochlea.
- Classification
  - Extra-articular supracondylar humerus fractures
    - Many variants: high extension, high flexion, low extension, low flexion, abduction, adduction.
    - 80 % are extension-type fractures.
  - Partial articular “single-column” fractures
    - Milch classification
      - May involve lateral or medial condyle but lateral is more commonly involved
      - Type I: lateral trochlear ridge intact
      - Type II: lateral trochlear ridge is violated
  - Complete articular “double-column” fractures

- Five major articular fragments: capitellum/lateral trochlea, lateral epicondyle, posterolateral epicondyle, posterior trochlea, and medial epicondyle/trochlea
- Jupiter classification
  - High T: transverse fracture proximal to or at the upper olecranon fossa with intercondylar split.
  - Low T: transverse fracture just proximal to the trochlea with intercondylar split.
  - Y: oblique fracture line through both columns with intercondylar split.
  - H: bicolumnar fracture with more than one fracture line extending to the articular surface where the trochlea is a free fragment; *increased risk of trochlear AVN.*
  - Medial lambda: proximal fracture line exits medially.
  - Lateral lambda: proximal fracture line exits laterally.
  - Multiplane T: T type with an additional fracture in the coronal plane.

- Treatment
  - Nonoperative
    - Nondisplaced single-column fractures with intact lateral trochlear ridge (Milch type I) may be considered for nonoperative management.
      - Lateral condyle fracture: immobilize in supination
      - Medial condyle fracture: immobilize in pronation
    - "Bag-of-bones" technique: consider in demented patients and patients with severe medical comorbidities.
  - Operative
    - The majority of distal humerus fractures are indicated for surgical fixation.
    - Surgical fixation in older patients with comminuted, osteoporotic bone is very challenging.
    - Closed reduction percutaneous pinning
      - Consider in some partial articular single-column fractures.
    - Open reduction internal fixation
      - Indicated in extra-articular, partial articular, and complete articular fractures.
      - For fractures involving both columns, ORIF with dual plating is typically performed.
      - Biomechanical studies support both parallel plating and 90–90 plating
        - Parallel plating: one plate medial, one plate lateral
        - 90–90 plating: one plate medially, one plate posterolaterally, interdigitating screws increases strength of construct

    - Triceps split and triceps sparring/paratricipital approaches best for extra-articular fracture and fractures with simple articular splits.
        - Triceps sparring/paratricipital approach may be converted into olecranon osteotomy if needed.
    - Transolecranon osteotomies provide the best exposure of the articular surface to facilitate joint reconstruction for complex intra-articular fractures and fractures with coronal shear components.
        - Avoid transolecranon osteotomy if total elbow arthroplasty is being considered.
    - Initiate early elbow range of motion.
    - Consider ulnar nerve transposition if in direct contact with implants.
        - Ulnar nerve transposition not shown to decrease the incidence of ulnar nerve symptoms
  - Total elbow arthroplasty
    - Consider in low bicolumnar fractures in elderly patients, particularly those with osteoporosis or rheumatoid arthritis
- Complications
  - Elbow stiffness is the most common complication
    - Contracture, fibrosis, and bone block may contribute to loss of motion.
    - Treat with static progressive splinting.
  - Ulnar nerve injury
    - Ulnar nerve a risk both from injury and surgical intervention
      - Critical to identify and protect the ulnar nerve throughout surgery.
      - Maintain blood supply to ulnar nerve when mobilizing.
  - Heterotopic ossification
    - Occurs in 4–8 % of patients, routine prophylaxis not recommended
  - Nonunion
    - Low incidence overall
  - Malunion
    - Lateral column fractures at risk for cubitus valgus
    - Medial column fractures at risk for cubitus varus
  - Avascular necrosis
    - Uncommon overall
    - Bicolumnar H-type fracture with free trochlear fragment at increased risk
  - Posttraumatic arthrosis

Bibliography

1. Frankle MA, Herscovici Jr D, DiPasquale TG, Vasey MB, Sanders RW. A comparison of open reduction and internal fixation and primary total elbow arthroplasty in the treatment of intraarticular distal humerus fractures in women older than age 65. J Orthop Trauma. 2003;17(7):473–80.
2. Galano GJ, Ahmad CS, Levine WN. Current treatment strategies for bicolumnar distal humerus fractures. J Am Acad Orthop Surg. 2010;18(1):20–30.
3. McKee MD, Jupiter JB, Bamberger HB. Coronal shear fractures of the distal end of the humerus. J Bone Joint Surg Am. 1996;78(1):49–54.
4. McKee MD, Veillette CJ, Hall JA, Schemitsch EH, Wild LM, McCormack R, Perey B, Goetz T, Zomar M, Moon K, Mandel S, Petit S, Guy P, Leung I. A multicenter, prospective, randomized, controlled trial of open reduction–internal fixation versus total elbow arthroplasty for displaced intra-articular distal humeral fractures in elderly patients. J Shoulder Elbow Surg. 2009;18(1):3–12.
5. Miller MD, Thompson SR, Hart JA. Review of orthopaedics. 6th ed. Philadelphia: Elsevier; 2012. p. 713–6.

10 Capitellum Fractures

Take-Home Message

- Simple coronal shear fractures of the capitellum are rare – these injuries are often more complex.
- High rates of elbow stiffness, but most patients are able to regain functional elbow range of motion.
- Nondisplaced and minimally displaced fracture amenable to nonoperative management with initial splint immobilization and early range of motion.
- Consider ORIF if fracture fragments are sufficiently large versus fragment excision if fracture fragments are too small or too comminuted to support fixation.
- Consider total elbow arthroplasty for unreconstructable capitellum fractures in elderly patients.

- General
  - Simple coronal shear fractures of the capitellum are rare – these injuries are often more complex.
  - Typically result from a fall on an outstretched hand.
  - More common in females, possibly related to greater carrying angle of the elbow in females.
  - May present with mechanical block to elbow flexion/extension.
  - ~20 % of capitellum fractures have an associated radial head fracture.

  - High rates of elbow stiffness but most patients are able to regain functional elbow range of motion.
  - High reoperation rates, up to 48 %.

- Imaging
  - AP and lateral x-rays of the elbow: double arc sign on lateral radiograph represents the overlap of the subchondral bone of the displaced capitellum and the lateral trochlea ridge; isolated effusion may represent a nondisplaced capitellum fracture.
  - Consider oblique view to better characterize the main fracture line and radiocapitellar view.
  - Maintain high index of suspicion for involvement of the trochlea, lateral condyle, and comminution.
  - CT scan: helpful to further characterize the injury and for surgical planning.
- Bryan-Morrey Classification
  - Type I (Hahn-Steinthal): complete fracture of the capitellum
  - Type II (Kocher-Lorenz): superficial shear fracture of the articular cartilage with little subchondral bone attached
  - Type III (Grantham): comminuted fracture
  - Type IV (McKee modification): coronal shear fracture involving the capitellum and portion of the trochlea
- Treatment
  - Nonoperative
    - Nondisplaced and minimally displaced (<2 mm) type I and type II fractures
      - Splint immobilization for 2–3 weeks and then early elbow range of motion
  - Operative
    - Open reduction internal fixation
      - Displaced (>2 mm) fractures with sufficient bone to allow fixation
        - Headless screw fixation.
        - Screw placement from posterior to anterior if capitellar fragment is sufficiently large.
        - Lateral approach often used; consider posterior approach to address concurrent elbow pathology.
    - Fragment excision
      - Fracture fragments that are too small or too comminuted to support fixation should be excised.

    - Total elbow arthroplasty
        - Consider in unreconstructable capitellar fractures in elderly patients with medial column instability.
- Complications
    - Nonunion
        - 1–11 % with ORIF
    - Heterotopic ossification
        - 4 % with ORIF
    - Avascular necrosis
        - Blood supply to the capitellum comes from the posterolateral aspect of the elbow.

Bibliography

1. Dushuttle RP, Coyle MP, Zawadsky JP, Bloom H. Fractures of the capitellum. J Trauma. 1985;25(4):317–21.
2. Frankle MA, Herscovici Jr D, DiPasquale TG, Vasey MB, Sanders RW. A comparison of open reduction and internal fixation and primary total elbow arthroplasty in the treatment of intraarticular distal humerus fractures in women older than age 65. J Orthop Trauma. 2003;17(7):473–80.
3. McKee MD, Jupiter JB, Bamberger HB. Coronal shear fractures of the distal end of the humerus. J Bone Joint Surg Am. 1996;78(1):49–54.
4. Miller MD, Thompson SR, Hart JA. Review of orthopaedics. 6th ed. Philadelphia: Elsevier; 2012. p. 715–6.

11 Radial Head Fractures

Take-Home Message

- Maintain high index of suspicion for Essex-Lopresti lesion: radial head fracture with concurrent DRUJ injury and interosseous membrane disruption, indicating length instability of the forearm ring.
- ORIF of displaced fractures when fixation is feasible.
- Keep forearm in pronation with ORIF to decrease risk of injury to posterior interosseous nerve.
- Safe zone for plates: 90–110° lateral arc from the radial styloid to Lister's tubercle with the forearm in neutral position.
- May consider partial excision of small fragments, but risk subsequent instability.
- Metallic radial head replacement recommended for fractures with three or more fragments and concurrent elbow pathology.
- Radial head resection alone may be considered in elderly, low-demand patients.

- General
  - One of the most common types of elbow fractures.
  - Associated injuries in 30 % of radial head fractures
    - DRUJ injuries, interosseous membrane disruption, coronoid fractures, MCL/LCL injury, elbow dislocation, terrible triad, carpal fractures
  - Mechanism of injury: axially load on an outstretched hand with pronated forearm.
  - Radial head is the secondary restraint to valgus force at the elbow.
  - Critical points of examination
    - Evaluate for mechanical block to motion with forearm pronation/supination and elbow flexion/extension.
      - Consider hematoma aspiration and injection of local anesthetic to facilitate examination.
    - Assess wrist for pain and DRUJ instability; compare to contralateral side.
- Imaging
  - AP and lateral elbow x-rays: isolated effusion may represent a nondisplaced radial head fracture.
  - Consider radiocapitellar view (oblique lateral) to further characterize fractures.
  - CT scan may be useful in comminuted fractures.
- Classification
  - Mason classification
    - Type I: nondisplaced or minimally displaced (<2 mm) partial articular or extra-articular radial head fracture with no mechanical block to forearm rotation
    - Type II: displaced (>2 mm) partial articular or extra-articular radial head fracture with possible mechanical block to forearm rotation
    - Type III: displaced complete articular radial head fracture or significantly displaced extra-articular radial head fracture with possible comminution and likely mechanical block to forearm rotation
    - Type IV (Hotchkiss modification): radial head fracture with elbow dislocation
  - Essex-Lopresti lesion: radial head fracture with DRUJ injury and interosseus membrane disruption
    - Indicates length instability of the forearm ring
    - Treatment with radial head resection alone contraindicated due to exacerbation of DRUJ instability and risk of proximal radial migration with resulting ulnocarpal impaction

- Treatment
  - Nonoperative
    - Short period of immobilization followed by early range of motion
      - Isolated minimally displaced fractures with no block to motion.
      - Elbow stiffness will result from prolonged immobilization.
  - Operative
    - Open reduction internal fixation
      - Displaced fractures where fixation is feasible, mechanical block to motion, concurrent elbow injuries.
      - Safe zone for plates: 90–110° lateral arc from the radial styloid to Lister's tubercle with the forearm in neutral position.
      - Countersink screws on articular surface or use headless compression screws.
      - With lateral and posterolateral approaches, keep forearm in pronation to decrease risk of injury to posterior interosseous nerve.
      - If three or more fragments, excision +/– radial head replacement is preferred.
    - Partial radial head excision
      - Consider in fragments <25 % of the radial head or <25–33 % of capitellar surface area.
      - May result in instability.
    - Radial head replacement
      - Displaced, comminuted fractures where ORIF is not feasible, Essex-Lopresti lesions with nonreconstructable radial head, elbow fracture-dislocations.
      - Good outcomes with metallic implants
        - Loose stemmed prostheses: act as spacers
        - Bipolar prostheses: cemented into the radial neck
      - Beware of "overstuffing the joint" which can lead to capitellar wear, malalignment, and instability.
      - Silastic radial head implants not recommended due to development of synovitis.
    - Radial head resection
      - Consider radial head resection alone in nonreconstructable radial head fractures in elderly, low-demand patients
        - Young active patients without an Essex-Lopresti lesion may still develop proximal radial migration (to a lesser degree) with symptomatic ulnocarpal impaction overtime.

    - Contraindicated with concurrent elbow instability with coronoid fracture, MCL deficiency, or interosseous membrane disruption
    - May be performed in a delayed fashion for pain control following radial head fracture
    - Risk of subsequent elbow instability, proximal radial migration, cubitus valgus, decreased strength and pain

- Complications
  - Elbow stiffness
  - Decreased forearm rotation
  - Posterior interosseous nerve injury with operative management
    - Pronate the forearm to increase the distance between the operative site and PIN to help prevent injury.
  - Proximal radial migration with ulnocarpal impaction in unrecognized Essex-Lopresti lesions with radial head excision
  - Radiocapitellar joint arthritis

Bibliography

1. Herbertsson P, Josefsson PO, Hasserius R, Besjakov J, Nyqvist F, Karlsson MK. Fractures of the radial head and neck treated with radial head excision. J Bone Joint Surg Am. 2004;86-A(9):1925–30.
2. Herbertsson P, Josefsson PO, Hasserius R, Karlsson C, Besjakov J, Karlsson M. Uncomplicated Mason type-II and III fractures of the radial head and neck in adults. A long-term follow-up study. J Bone Joint Surg Am. 2004;86-A(3): 569–74.
3. Miller MD, Thompson SR, Hart JA. Review of orthopaedics. 6th ed. Philadelphia: Elsevier; 2012. p. 719.
4. Paschos NK, Mitsionis GI, Vasiliadis HS, Georgoulis AD. Comparison of early mobilization protocols in radial head fractures. A prospective randomized controlled study. The effect of fracture characteristics on outcome. J Orthop Trauma. 2013;27(3):134–9.
5. Ring D, Quintero J, Jupiter JB. Open reduction and internal fixation of fractures of the radial head. J Bone Joint Surg Am. 2002;84-A(10):1811–5.
6. Tejwani NC, Mehta H. Fractures of the radial head and neck: current concepts in management. J Am Acad Orthop Surg. 2007;15(7):380–7.

12 Coronoid Fractures

Take-Home Message

- Rarely occur as isolated injuries, typically associated with elbow dislocations with risk for recurrent elbow instability.
- Coronoid is the primary restraint to elbow subluxation/dislocation.
- Anteromedial coronoid facet fractures may result in posteromedial rotatory instability.
- Coronoid fractures with a stable elbow are amenable to nonoperative management with a short period of immobilization and early elbow range of motion.
- Coronoid fractures with elbow instability or current elbow pathology should undergo ORIF with a variety of techniques described pending the specific fracture pattern and associated pathology.

- General
  - Rare as isolated injuries, typically associated with elbow dislocations with increased risk of recurrent instability.
  - Coronoid acts as an anterior buttress and is the primary restraint to elbow subluxation/dislocation.
  - Mechanism of injury: traumatic shear injury as the distal humerus is driven against the coronoid.
  - Assess elbow flexion/extension and pronation/supination, and perform varus/valgus stress testing.
  - Fractures at the base of the coronoid are particularly prone to elbow instability as the anterior capsule inserts 6 mm distal to the tip of the coronoid and the anterior bundle of the MCL inserts on the sublime tubercle 18 mm distal to the tip.
  - Associated injuries/conditions
    - Terrible triad of the elbow: transverse coronoid fracture, radial head fracture, and elbow dislocation
    - Olecranon fracture-dislocation: often with a large coronoid fragment
    - Posteromedial rotatory instability: varus force with fracture of the anteromedial facet of the coronoid and LCL disruption
    - Posterolateral rotatory instability: coronoid tip fracture, radial head fracture, LCL injury

- Imaging
  - AP and lateral elbow x-rays.
  - CT scan may be helpful.
- Regan and Morrey Classification
  - Type I: fracture of the tip of the coronoid process
  - Type II: fracture ≤50 % of the coronoid height
  - Type III: fracture >50 % of the coronoid height
  - Anteromedial facet coronoid fractures: caused by varus posteromedial rotatory force
- Treatment
  - Nonoperative
    - Brief immobilization with early range of motion
      - Minimally displaced coronoid fractures with stable elbow
  - Operative
    - Open reduction internal fixation
      - Coronoid fractures with elbow instability, anteromedial facet fractures with posteromedial rotatory instability, olecranon fracture-dislocations, and terrible triad of the elbow
      - May secure coronoid with cerclage wire or suture fixation through drill holes, retrograde screws, or plate fixation
      - Ligament repair as indicated
      - Early active motion in the postoperative period; consider restricting shoulder abduction to prevent varus moment on the elbow
    - Hinged elbow external fixation
      - Consider for coronoid fractures with elbow instability in patients with compromised soft tissues, poor bone quality, and complex revision cases.
- Complications
  - Recurrent elbow instability
  - Elbow stiffness
  - Heterotopic ossification
  - Posttraumatic arthrosis

Bibliography

1. McKee MD, Pugh DM, Wild LM, Schemitsch EH, King GJ. Standard surgical protocol to treat elbow dislocations with radial head and coronoid fractures. Surgical technique. J Bone Joint Surg Am. 2005;87(Suppl 1(Pt 1)):22–32.
2. Miller MD, Thompson SR, Hart JA. Review of orthopaedics. 6th ed. Philadelphia: Elsevier; 2012. p. 718–9.

3. Ring D. Fractures of the coronoid process of the ulna. J Hand Surg Am. 2006;31:1679–89.
4. Ring D, Doornberg JN. Fracture of the anteromedial facet of the coronoid process. J Bone Joint Surg Am. 2006;88(10):2216–24.
5. Steinmann SP. Coronoid process fracture. J Am Acad Orthop Surg. 2008;16:519–29.
6. Tashjian RZ, Katarincic JA. Complex elbow instability. J Am Acad Orthop Surg. 2006;14(5):278–86.

13 Olecranon Fractures

Take-Home Message

- Consider nonoperative management for fractures with no articular incongruity and intact elbow extensor mechanism.
- Recommend surgical fixation for all displaced fractures and all patients without active extension.
- Tension band wiring converts dorsal distractive forces into compressive forces at the articular surface and fracture site; best for transverse noncomminuted fractures proximal to the coronoid.
- Tension band constructs: wire loops should be dorsal to the mid-axis of the ulna, and K-wires should engage but not protrude beyond the anterior cortex to prevent loss of forearm rotation and injury to the AIN.
- Plate fixation indicated in comminuted fractures and fractures that extend distal to the coronoid process.
- Consider excision and triceps advancement of up to 50 % of the proximal ulna in elderly, low-demand patients with nonreconstructable comminuted proximal ulna fractures.

- General
  - Result from high-energy injuries in the young and low-energy falls in the elderly.
  - Assess ulnar nerve function and integrity of the elbow extensor mechanism (palpable gap may be present).
- Imaging
  - AP and lateral elbow x-rays: true lateral needed to best delineate the fracture.
  - CT scan may be useful for very comminuted fractures and aid preoperative planning.

- Colton Classification
  - Type I: avulsion fracture
  - Type IIA-D: oblique and transverse fractures, +/– comminution
  - Type III: fracture-dislocations
  - Type IV: high-energy comminuted, multisegmented fractures
- Treatment
  - Nonoperative
    - Immobilization at 60–90° for 2–3 weeks and then gentle early elbow range of motion
      - Consider in fractures with no articular incongruity (<1–2 mm displacement)
  - Operative
    - Tension band fixation
      - Best employed in transverse displaced fractures proximal to the coronoid without articular surface comminution or dorsal cortex comminution
      - Converts distractive forces at the dorsal cortex into compression forces at the articular surface and fracture
        - Wire loops should be dorsal to the mid-axis of the ulna to facilitate transformation of tensile forces into compressive forces.
        - K-wires should be anchored in the anterior cortex to prevent migration; however, proud K-wires may injure the anterior interosseous nerve or block forearm rotation.
      - May combine with lag screw fixation for noncomminuted oblique fractures proximal to the coronoid
    - Plate and screw fixation
      - Comminuted fractures, fractures extending distal to the coronoid process, oblique fracture lines.
      - Plate is placed on the dorsal (tension) side of the ulna.
      - May combine with lag screw fixation for oblique fractures.
    - Intramedullary fixation
      - Best employed in noncomminuted and oblique fractures.
      - Partially threaded intramedullary screw must engage the distal intramedullary canal to provide sufficient fixation but may generate more torque than compression.
      - Higher rate of fixation failure compared to tension banding
        - Considered insufficient fixation when used in isolation by many
        - May be combined with tension banding

- Excision and triceps advancement
  - Consider in elderly, low-demand patients with poor bone quality and comminuted, nonreconstructable proximal olecranon fractures.
  - Excise portion of the olecranon fracture, repair triceps tendon with non-absorbable sutures passed through drill holes in the proximal ulna so insertion point is close to the articular surface.
  - Do not excise >50 % of the olecranon and this may cause subsequent elbow instability.

- Complications
  - Painful hardware the most common complication
    - Hardware removal undertaken in 40–80 % of cases
  - Elbow stiffness
    - Occurs in 50 % of patients.
    - Majority of patients are able to regain functional elbow range of motion even if they develop some residual stiffness.
  - Nonunion
  - Nerve injury
    - Ulnar nerve
    - Anterior interosseous nerve
  - Posttraumatic arthrosis

Bibliography

1. Bailey CS, MacDermid J, Patterson SD, King GJ. Outcome of plate fixation ofolecranon fractures. J Orthop Trauma. 2001;15(8):542–8.
2. Candal-Couto JJ, Williams JR, Sanderson PL. Impaired forearm rotation after tension-band-wiring fixation of olecranon fractures: evaluation of the transcortical K-wire technique. J Orthop Trauma. 2005;19(7):480–2.
3. Duckworth AD, Bugler KE, Clement ND, Court-Brown CM, McQueen MM. Nonoperative management of displaced olecranon fractures in low-demand elderly patients. J Bone Joint Surg Am. 2014;96(1):67–72.
4. Hak DJ, Golladay Jr G. Olecranon fractures: treatment options. J Am Acad Orthop Surg. 2000;8:266–75.
5. Miller MD, Thompson SR, Hart JA. Review of orthopaedics. 6th ed. Philadelphia: Elsevier; 2012. p. 716–8.
6. Parker JR, Conroy J, Campbell DA. Anterior interosseus nerve injury following tension band wiring of the olecranon. Injury. 2005;36(10):1252–3.
7. van der Linden SC, van Kampen A, Jaarsma RL. J Shoulder Elbow Surg. K-wire position in tension-band wiring technique affects stability of wires and long-term outcome in surgical treatment of olecranon fractures 2012;21(3):405–11.

14 Elbow Dislocations

Take-Home Message

- Elbow dislocations are the second most common joint dislocation.
- 80 % are posterolateral dislocations.
- Simple elbow dislocations have no associated fractures and are typically stable and amenable to nonoperative management.
- Complex elbow dislocations have associated fractures and often represent unstable injuries for which surgical intervention is warranted.
- Anterior and divergent elbow dislocations represent high-energy injuries with increased risk of open wounds, neurovascular injury, associated fractures, recurrent instability, and compartment syndrome.
- Elbow stiffness with loss of terminal extension is the most common complication of simple elbow fractures.

- General
  - Elbow dislocations are the second most common major joint dislocation, following shoulder dislocation.
  - Posterolateral dislocations most common: 80 % of elbow dislocations.
  - Typically occur in young patients 10–20 years old.
  - Elbow functional range of motion: 30–130° flexion/extension, 50–50° pronation/supination (100° arc).
  - Elbow stabilizers
    - Primary stabilizers: ulnar lateral collateral ligament (varus stress), anterior band of the medial collateral ligament (valgus stress), coronoid/ulnohumeral joint
    - Secondary elbow stabilizer: radiocapitellar joint (valgus stress), capsule, flexor and extensor tendon origins
  - Mechanism of injury: commonly axial loading with supination of the forearm and a posterolaterally based valgus force
    - Progression of injury from lateral to medial: LCL failure (avulsion at lateral epicondylar origin > midsubstance ruptures, possible MCL failure depending on energy of injury
  - Associated injuries: medial and lateral epicondyle avulsion fractures, radial head fractures, coronoid fractures, osteochondral injuries.
  - Careful neurovascular examination.
  - Maintain a high index of suspicion for compartment syndrome.
  - Assess elbow stability following reduction to help guide treatment.

- Imaging
  - AP and lateral elbow x-rays: best to assess joint congruency.
  - Consider oblique views to assess for periarticular and avulsion fractures.
  - CT scan may be useful when complex injury pattern is suspected.
- Classification
  - Simple vs complex
    - Simple: no associated fractures, 50–60 % of elbow dislocations
    - Complex: associated fracture(s) present, may represent terrible triad of the elbow or varus posteromedial rotatory instability, increased risk of recurrent elbow instability
  - Anatomic
    - Posterolateral dislocation: 80 %
    - Other variants: direct posterior, anterior, medial, lateral, divergent
      - Anterior and divergent dislocations typically result from high-energy mechanisms and have a higher incidence of open wound, neurovascular injury, associated fractures, recurrent instability, and compartment syndrome.
- Treatment
  - Nonoperative
    - Brief splint immobilization in 90° elbow flexion with forearm rotation guided by assessment of postreduction stability, followed by early active motion.
    - Reduce with inline traction and supination followed by elbow flexion with pressure on the olecranon
      - Elbow may be unstable in extension postreduction.
      - LCL disruption: splint in pronation.
      - MCL disruption: splint in supination.
    - Indicated for acute stable simple elbow dislocations.
    - If simple elbow fracture is unstable in extension following reduction, consider treatment in a hinged elbow brace.
  - Operative
    - Open reduction internal fixation
      - Fixation of associated coronoid, radial and olecranon fractures, LCL and MCL repair as indicated
      - Indicated for acute complex elbow dislocations with instability following reduction, dislocations not amenable to closed reduction, and incarcerated osteochondral fragments

- Open reduction, capsular release, and hinged external fixator
  - Hinged external fixator protects repair while allowing early motion.
  - Indicated for chronic elbow dislocations.

- Complications
  - Elbow stiffness with flexion contracture/loss of terminal extension is the most common complication of simple elbow dislocations
    - Severity of contracture correlates with length of immobilization.
  - Chronic instability
  - Varus posteromedial instability: associated with anteromedial facet coronoid fracture and LCL injury
  - Neurovascular injury
    - Ulnar and median nerve injuries
    - Brachial artery injury
    - Anterior and divergent elbow dislocations: increased risk of associated neurovascular injury
  - Compartment syndrome
  - Heterotopic ossification: often involves the collateral ligaments

Bibliography

1. Cohen MS, Hastings 2nd H. Acute elbow dislocation: evaluation and management. J Am Acad Orthop Surg. 1998;6(1):15–23. Review.
2. Josefsson PO, Gentz CF, Johnell O, Wendeberg B. Surgical versus nonsurgical treatment of ligamentous injuries following dislocation of the elbow joint. A prospective randomized study. J Bone Joint Surg Am. 1987;69(4):605–8.
3. McKee MD, Schemitsch EH, Sala MJ, O'driscoll SW. Pathoanatomy of lateral ligamentous disruption in elbow instability. J Shoulder Elbow Surg. 2003;12:391–6.
4. Miller MD, Thompson SR, Hart JA. Review of orthopaedics. 6th ed. Philadelphia: Elsevier; 2012. p. 719.
5. Ring D, Doornberg JN. Fracture of the anteromedial facet of the coronoid process. J Bone Joint Surg Am. 2006;88(10):2216–24.
6. Ross G, McDevitt ER, Chronister R, Ove PN. Treatment of simple elbow dislocation using immediate motion protocol. Am J Sports Med. 1999;27:308–11.

15 Terrible Triad of the Elbow

Take-Home Message

- Terrible triad of the elbow: posterolateral elbow dislocation with associated coronoid fracture and radial head fracture with high coincidence of LCL disruption.
- Nearly all terrible triad injuries are unstable and warrant surgical intervention with radial head ORIF/replacement, coronoid ORIF, LCL repair, and +/– MCL repair.
- Fracture-dislocations of the elbow are difficult to manage with high rate of both persistent instability and elbow stiffness.

- General
  - Posterolateral elbow dislocation with associated coronoid fracture, radial head fracture
  - High coincidence of LCL disruption, typically avulsion from the lateral epicondylar origin
  - Mechanism of injury: axial loading with supination of the forearm and a valgus force
    - Structures fail from lateral to medial: LCL typically disrupted, anterior bundle of MCL the last to fail
  - Inherently unstable injuries that require surgical treatment
    - Varus instability common, may have valgus instability with MCL disruption
- Imaging
  - AP and lateral elbow x-rays best to assess joint congruency.
  - CT scan may be helpful to further evaluate coronoid and radial head fractures.
- Classification
  - Terrible triad
    - Historically, elbow dislocations with combined radial head and coronoid fractures had consistently poor outcomes, leading to the name “terrible triad.”

- Treatment
  - Nonoperative
    - Brief immobilization in 90° of elbow flexion followed by early active motion with terminal extension restrictions.
    - Rarely indicated: nearly all terrible triad injuries are unstable and warrant surgical intervention.
    - May consider nonoperative management for elbows that are concentrically reduced, remain stable up to 30° of extension, and have minor radial head fractures with no block to motion and coronoid fractures involving only the tip.
  - Operative
    - Radial head fixation/replacement, coronoid ORIF, LCL repair, +/– MCL repair.
    - Indicated for all unstable terrible triad injuries.
    - The primary goal of surgical fixation is to stabilize the elbow to permit early motion.
    - *See sections on radial head fractures and coronoid fractures for further details.*
- Complications
  - Persistent instability: more common following type I and type II coronoid fractures.
  - Elbow stiffness: very common; early range of motion and rehabilitation are crucial.
  - Heterotopic ossification.
  - Failure of fixation.
  - Posttraumatic arthrosis.

Bibliography

1. Forthman C, Henket M, Ring DC. Elbow dislocation with intra-articular fracture: the results of operative treatment without repair of the medial collateral ligament. J Hand Surg Am. 2007;32(8):1200–9.
2. Mathew PK, Athwal GS, King GJ. Terrible triad injury of the elbow: current concepts. J Am Acad Orthop Surg. 2009;17(3):137–51.
3. Miller MD, Thompson SR, Hart JA. Review of orthopaedics. 6th ed. Philadelphia: Elsevier; 2012. p. 719.
4. Pugh DM, Wild LM, Schemitsch EH, King GJ, McKee MD. Standard surgical protocol to treat elbow dislocations with radial head and coronoid fractures. J Bone Joint Surg Am. 2004;86-A(6):1122–30.
5. Ring D, Jupiter JB, Zilberfarb J. Posterior dislocation of the elbow with fractures of the radial head and coronoid. J Bone Joint Surg Am. 2002;84:547–51.

16 Monteggia Fractures

Take-Home Message

- Proximal 1/3 ulna fractures with radial head dislocation in the direction of the apex of the ulna fracture.
- 10–20 % associated PIN injury, usually resolve with observation for 3 months.
- Monteggia fractures are inherently unstable injuries that warrant surgical fixation in all adults.
- Radial head will typically reduce and be stable with ORIF of the ulna.
- Radial head may remain unreduced or be irreducible with malreduction of the ulna or soft tissue interposition (annular ligament most common).
- Posterior radial head dislocations (type II) and injuries with associated radial head fractures have higher complication rates.

- General
  - Proximal 1/3 ulna fracture with associated radial head dislocation.
  - Radial head dislocates in the direction of the apex of the ulna fracture.
  - Rare in adults, most common in children.
  - Posterior interosseous nerve injury: 20 %.
  - Associated injuries: radial head fracture, coronoid fracture, olecranon fracture-dislocation, LCL injury, terrible triad of the elbow, interosseous membrane disruption, TFCC injury.
  - Most Monteggia fractures are unstable injuries that warrant surgical fixation.
- Imaging
  - AP and lateral x-rays of the elbow, forearm, and wrist.
  - CT scan may be helpful to further assess associated coronoid, olecranon, and radial head fractures when present.
- Bado Classification
  - Type I (60 %): apex anterior proximal 1/3 ulna fracture with anterior radial head dislocation
  - Type II (15 %): apex posterior proximal 1/3 ulna fracture with posterior radial head dislocation
  - Type III: proximal 1/3 ulna fracture with lateral radial head dislocation
  - Type IV: proximal ulna *and* radius fractures with radial head dislocation in any direction
  - "Monteggia equivalent/variant": proximal 1/3 ulnar fracture with radial head fracture

- Treatment
  - Nonoperative
    - Closed reduction and supination splint/cast mobilization
      - May consider in children where closed reduction can be obtained and ulnar length maintained.
      - Malreduction leads to poor outcomes.
  - Operative
    - Open reduction internal fixation
      - Open reduction with plate fixation of the ulna fracture.
      - Radial head will typically reduce indirectly with reduction and stabilization of the ulna fracture.
      - If radial head fails to reduce, reassess ulna reduction
        - Malreduction of the ulna is the most common cause for failure of radial head reduction.
      - If radial head fails to reduce and ulna fracture is confirmed to be anatomic, open reduction of the radial head may be required to address an interposed annular ligament, capsule, biceps tendon, or brachial fascia.
      - If there is an associated radial head fracture, repair is preferred over replacement when feasible.
- Complications
  - Higher complication rates described for Bado type II injuries and Monteggia equivalent injuries
  - PIN injury
    - 10–20 % of Monteggia fractures.
    - Usually resolves with observation over 3–4 months.
    - If no improvement, obtain EMG.
  - Malunion with radial head dislocation/subluxation
    - Perform corrective ulna osteotomy +/– open radial head reduction.
  - Elbow stiffness
  - Synostosis

Bibliography

1. Bado JL. The Monteggia lesion. Clin Orthop Relat Res. 1967;50:71–86.
2. Eglseder WA, Zadnik M. Monteggia fractures and variants: review of distribution and nine irreducible radial head dislocations. South Med J. 2006;99(7):723–7.
3. Konrad GG, Kundel K, Kreuz PC, Oberst M, Sudkamp NP. Monteggia fractures in adults: long-term results and prognostic factors. J Bone Joint Surg Br. 2007; 89(3):354–60.

4. Miller MD, Thompson SR, Hart JA. Review of orthopaedics. 6th ed. Philadelphia: Elsevier; 2012. p. 720.
5. Ring D, Jupiter JB, Waters PM. Monteggia fractures in children and adults. J Am Acad Orthop Surg. 1998;6(4):215–24. Review.

17 Radius and Ulna Shaft Fractures

Take-Home Message

- Both-bone forearm fractures typically result from high-energy mechanisms, are often open, and are at risk for compartment syndrome.
- All both-bone forearm fractures should undergo ORIF; utilize two-incision approach to decrease the risk of synostosis.
- Isolated nondisplaced or distal 2/3 ulna fractures with <50 % translation and <10° angulation are amenable to trial of nonoperative management.
- Isolated proximal 1/3 and distal 2/3 ulna fractures with greater displacement should undergo ORIF.

- General
  - "Both-bone forearm fractures": diaphyseal fractures of the radius and ulna.
  - More common in men.
  - High incidence of open fractures.
  - The ulna acts as an axis around which the radius rotates.
  - Interosseous membrane is comprised of five ligaments: central band, accessory band, distal oblique bundle, proximal oblique cord, and dorsal oblique accessory cord.
  - Typically result from direct trauma high-energy mechanisms: motor vehicle accidents, falls from height, athletics.
  - Maintain a high index of suspicion for compartment syndrome.
  - Careful neurovascular exam critical in patient evaluation.
- Imaging
  - AP and lateral x-rays of the forearm.
  - Consider ipsilateral dedicated wrist and elbow x-rays if not well visualized on forearm films or suspected associated injury.
- Classification
  - Both-bone forearm fractures
    - Descriptive: closed vs open, location, comminuted/segmental/bone loss, displacement, angulation, rotation

- Isolated ulna fractures
  - "Nightstick fractures"
  - Stable: <25–50 % translation and <10–15° angulation
  - Unstable: >50 % translation or >10–15° angulation

- Treatment
  - Nonoperative
    - Short arm cast to functional fracture brace with interosseous mold
      - Isolated nondisplaced or distal 2/3 ulna fractures with <50 % translation and <10° angulation
      - Union rates >96 %
  - Operative
    - Open reduction internal fixation of the radius and ulna +/− bone grafting
      - Plate fixation of the radius and ulna via dual-incision approach to decrease the risk of synostosis.
      - Indicated in all both-bone forearm fractures, displaced distal 2/3 ulna fractures, proximal 1/3 isolated ulna fractures, radial shaft fractures.
      - Restoration of the lateral radial bow is important for pronation/supination and directly relates to functional outcome
        - Radial styloid should be 180° from the bicipital tuberosity.
      - Acute bone grafting indicated for segmental bone loss >2 cm and bone loss with associated open
        - Routine bone grafting for closed, comminuted fracture no longer indicated
      - Initiate immediate range of motion postoperatively.
    - External fixation
      - May consider with temporizing or definitive treatment in Gustilo IIIb and IIIc open fractures and injuries with severely compromised soft tissue envelope
    - Intramedullary nailing
      - May consider with severely compromised soft tissue envelope
      - Difficult to maintain axial and rotational stability
        - Increased risk of malunion and nonunion

- Complications
  - Synostosis
    - Occur in 3–9 % of both-bone forearm fractures

    - Increased risk with ORIF >2 weeks after injury, single-incision approach, fractures at the same level, closed head injury, high-energy mechanisms, infection, long screws, screws or bone graft on the interosseous membrane
    - Treat with early excision and irradiation and/or indomethacin

  - Refracture

    - Increased risk if hardware is removed <12–18 months postoperatively.
    - After hardware removal, recommend functional forearm brace for 6 weeks and restricted activity for 3 months.

  - Nonunion

    - Increased risk with intramedullary fixation.
    - Treat with revision ORIF and autogenous cancellous bone grafting.
    - Vascularized fibula grafts may be used for large defects.

  - Malunion

    - Increased risk with definitive external fixation, intramedullary fixation, segmental bone loss, and extensively comminuted fractures
    - Restoration of lateral radial bow most important for functional outcome

  - Compartment syndrome

    - Increased risk with high-energy mechanisms, crush injuries, open fractures, low-velocity gunshot wounds, associated vascular injuries, and coagulopathy

Bibliography

1. Bauer G, Arand M, Mutschler W. Post-traumatic radioulnar synostosis after forearm fracture osteosynthesis. Arch Orthop Trauma Surg. 1991;110(3):142–5.
2. Beingessner DM, Patterson SD, King GJ. Early excision of heterotopic bone in the forearm. J Hand Surg Am. 2000;25(3):483–8.
3. Miller MD, Thompson SR, Hart JA. Review of orthopaedics. 6th ed. Philadelphia: Elsevier; 2012. p. 720–2.
4. Ring D, Allende C, Jafarnia K, Allende BT, Jupiter JB. Ununited diaphyseal forearm fractures with segmental defects: plate fixation and autogenous cancellous bone-grafting. J Bone Joint Surg Am. 2004;86-A(11):2440–5.
5. Rumball K, Finnegan M. Refractures after forearm plate removal. J Orthop Trauma. 1990;4(2):124–9.
6. Schemitsch EH, Richards RR. The effect of malunion on functional outcome after plate fixation of fractures of both bones of the forearm in adults. J Bone Joint Surg Am. 1992;74(7):1068–78.
7. Wright RR, Schmeling GJ, Schwab JP. The necessity of acute bone grafting in diaphyseal forearm fractures: a retrospective review. J Orthop Trauma. 1997;11(4):288–94.

18 Galeazzi Fractures

Take-Home Message

- Distal 1/3 radial shaft fracture with associated DRUJ injury.
- Incidence of DRUJ instability correlates with proximity of the radius fracture to the wrist.
- DRUJ is most stable in supination.
- Galeazzi fractures are unstable injuries that should undergo surgical fixation of the radius with subsequent assessment and treatment of the DRUJ as indicated.

- General
  - Distal 1/3 radial shaft fracture with associated DRUJ injury.
  - Incidence of DRUJ instability correlates with proximity of radius fracture to the wrist
    - Radius fracture <7.5 cm from articular surface: 55 % unstable
    - Radius fracture >7.5 cm from articular surface: 6 % unstable
  - Mechanism of injury: fall onto outstretched hand with forearm pronation, direct wrist trauma.
  - Primary stabilizers of the DRUJ: volar and dorsal radioulnar ligaments.
  - DRUJ is most stable in supination.
  - DRUJ dislocation is almost always dorsal but may be palmar.
- Imaging
  - AP and lateral forearm, wrist, and elbow x-rays
    - Signs of DRUJ instability: associated ulnar styloid fracture, DRUJ widening on AP view, DRUJ dislocation on lateral view, ≥5 mm of radial shortening
- Classification
  - Rettig and Raskin classification
    - Type I: radius fracture ≤7.5 cm from the midarticular surface of the distal radius, significantly increased risk of DRUJ instability after fixation of the radius
    - Type II: radius fracture >7.5 cm from the midarticular surface of the distal radius, decreased risk of DRUJ instability after fixation of the radius
  - Bruckner classification
    - Simple: DRUJ easily reduced after fixation of the radius
    - Complex: DRUJ unstable or irreducible after fixation of the radius

– Galeazzi equivalent: distal 1/3 radius fracture with associated distal ulna fracture

- Treatment
  - Nonoperative
    - Not indicated
  - Operative
    - Open reduction internal fixation of the radius followed by DRUJ assessment
      - Anatomic reduction and plate fixation of the radius with care to restore/maintain the radial bow.
      - If DRUJ remains reduced and stable following fixation of the radius, splint in supination and initiate early range of motion.
      - If DRUJ is reduced but unstable following radius fixation, closed reduction and percutaneous cross-pinning of the ulna to the radius is indicated.
      - If DRUJ is irreducible following radius fixation, suspect interposed ECU tendon
        - Proceed with dorsal approach to DRUJ to remove interposed soft tissue precluding reduction.
        - Subsequent DRUJ stabilization as indicated.
      - Large associated ulnar styloid fractures benefit from fixation with pinning or supination immobilization of the DRUJ as indicated.
- Complications
  - Compartment syndrome: may occur with high-energy injuries
  - Malunion
  - Nonunion
  - DRUJ subluxation
    - Consider bracing versus further surgical intervention with pinning/repinning +/– radioulnar ligament repair or dorsal capsulodesis
  - DRUJ arthrosis
    - Consider resection arthroplasty/Darrach procedure (elderly, low demand), hemiresection or interposition arthroplasty, Sauve-Kapandji procedure, ulnar head prosthetic replacement

Bibliography

1. Budgen A, Lim P, Templeton P, Irwin LR. Irreducible Galeazzi injury. Arch Orthop Trauma Surg. 1998;118(3):176–8.
2. Giannoulis FS, Sotereanos DG. Galeazzi fractures and dislocations. Hand Clin. 2007;23(2):153–63. Review.

3. Korompilias AV, Lykissas MG, Kostas-Agnantis IP, Beris AE, Soucacos PN. Distal radioulnar joint instability (Galeazzi type injury) after internal fixation in relation to the radius fracture pattern. J Hand Surg Am. 2011;36(5):847–52.
4. Miller MD, Thompson SR, Hart JA. Review of orthopaedics. 6th ed. Philadelphia: Elsevier; 2012. p. 720.
5. Paley D, McMurtry RY, Murray JF. Dorsal dislocation of the ulnar styloid and extensor carpi ulnaris tendon into the distal radioulnar joint: the empty sulcus sign. J Hand Surg Am. 1987;12:1029–32.
6. Rettig ME, Raskin KB. Galeazzi fracture-dislocation: a new treatment-oriented classification. J Hand Surg Am. 2001;26(2):228–35.

19 Distal Radius Fractures

Take-Home Message

- Most common upper extremity fracture, high-energy trauma in young patients, low-energy fall in elderly/osteoporotic patients.
- Maintain a high index of suspicion for acute carpal tunnel syndrome and treat with emergent carpal tunnel release.
- Treatment guided by radiographic parameters, fracture pattern stability, and patient age and functional demands.
- Increased risk of attritional EPL rupture with nondisplaced distal radius fractures.
- Many methods of surgical fixation may be successfully employed pending specific fracture characteristics.
- High coincidence of ulnar-sided wrist pathology.
- Malunions are common; revision is recommended for young patients and symptomatic patients as indicated by the nature of the malunion.

- General
  - Most common fracture of the upper extremity
    - Greatest incidence in Caucasian women >50 years old
    - DEXA scan for all women who sustain distal radius fractures
  - High-energy trauma in young, open fractures more common.
  - Low-energy trauma in elderly/osteoporotic.
  - 50 % intra-articular.
  - Always assess for anatomic snuffbox tenderness, ulnar-sided wrist pain, median and ulnar nerve function, DRUJ injury, and TFCC injury.
  - Associated ulnar styloid fracture indicative of higher-energy injury with greater initial displacement.

    - Ulnar styloid base fracture associated with TFCC injury
  - Distal radius fractures are a predictor for sustaining subsequent fractures.
- Imaging
  - AP x-ray: 12 mm radial height, 23° radial inclination.
  - Lateral x-ray: 11° volar tilt.
  - Acceptable parameters: <5 mm radial shortening, <5° loss of radial inclination, volar tilt within 10–20° of contralateral side or <5° dorsal angulation, <1–2 mm articular step-off.
  - CT scan may be useful to assess intra-articular involvement and preoperative planning.
  - MRI may be warranted in some cases to assess TFCC and intercarpal ligaments.
- Classification
  - Frykman classification
    - Joint involvement +/– radial styloid fracture.
    - Type I/II*: extra-articular fracture.
    - Type III/IV*: radiocarpal extension.
    - Type V/VI*: radioulnar extension.
    - Type VII/VIII*: radiocarpal and radioulnar extension.
    - ** Types II, IV, VI, and VIII have concurrent ulnar styloid fractures.*
  - Melone classification
    - Describes four fragments of the radiocarpal joint: radial styloid, radial shaft, volar medial, volar dorsal
    - Types I–IV: increasingly comminuted and displaced fractures of the four fragments
    - Type V: severe comminution without identifiable fragments
  - Fernandez classification
    - Based on mechanism of injury, designed to guide treatment decision making
    - Type I: bending fractures
    - Type II: articular shear fractures, associated with perilunate injuries
    - Type III: compression fractures
    - Type IV: fracture-dislocations with associated ligamentous injury
    - Type V: combined mechanism
  - Eponyms
    - Colles' fracture: apex anterior, dorsally angulated fracture
    - Smith's fracture: apex dorsal, volarly angulated fracture
    - Barton's fracture: volar or dorsal lip fractures
    - Chauffer's fracture: radial styloid fracture
    - Die-punch fracture: depressed fracture of the lunate facet

- Treatment
  - Outcomes correlate with restoration of anatomic alignment with radial height and volar tilt of greater importance than radial inclination, good articular congruency, and early wrist and digit motion.
  - Radiographic parameters shown to have less importance in management of distal radius fractures in the elderly.
  - Prereduction radiographs are the best predictor of instability
  - Nonoperative
    - Closed reduction and cast immobilization
      - Indicated for distal radius fractures with acceptable parameters (detailed above).
      - Monitor closely for loss of reduction.
      - Nondisplaced distal radius fractures have increased risk of attritional EPL rupture.
  - Operative
    - Indicated for fractures that fail to meet acceptable parameters, unstable fracture patterns (articular shear, volar/dorsal lip fractures, metadiaphyseal extension, associated distal ulnar shaft fracture, etc.), and loss of reduction following closed reduction and casting
    - Percutaneous pinning
      - Most effective in maintaining sagittal alignment in extra-articular fractures with stable volar cortex
      - Unable to maintain sagittal alignment with volar or bicortical comminution
      - 80–90 % good outcomes with appropriate indications
    - External fixation
      - Relies on ligamentotaxis to maintain reduction
        - Difficult to restore volar tilt with external fixation alone, may combine with percutaneous pinning or plate fixation
      - Radial shaft pins should be placed under direct visualization to protect the superficial radial nerve.
      - Associated increased risk of malunion/nonunion, stiffness, pin-site complications, injury to superficial radial nerve, median neuropathy, RSD/CRPS.
    - ORIF
      - Volar plating most commonly performed
        - Increased risk of FPL rupture
        - Flexor and extensor tendon irritation possible

   - Dorsal plating
     - May be beneficial in fractures with dorsal comminution, dorsal lip fractures, and dorsal shear patterns
     - Historically associated with increased risk of extensor tendon irritation and rupture, less common today with low-profile plates
   - Radial column plating
     - Consider with unstable radial column injuries and radial styloid fractures.
   - Complex intra-articular fractures may benefit from arthroscopically assisted reduction and fragment specific fixation.
   - May be combined with other fixation techniques.
   - ORIF of ulnar styloid fracture may be indicated in cases with associated instability.
- Complications
  - Median nerve neuropathy
    - Occurs 1–12 % of distal radius fractures, up to 30 % in high-energy injuries
    - Carpal tunnel pressure lowest with neutral wrist position
    - Treat acute carpal tunnel syndrome with emergent carpal tunnel release
    - Carpal tunnel release recommended for progressive paresthesias and persistent paresthesias that fail to improve with fracture reduction
  - Ulnar nerve neuropathy
    - Associated with DRUJ injuries
  - Reflex sympathetic dystrophy/chronic regional pain syndrome
    - Postoperative vitamin C supplementation may help prevent RSD/CRPS.
  - Attritional EPL rupture
    - Increased risk in nondisplaced distal radius fractures treated with cast immobilization.
    - Treat with EIP to EPL transfer.
  - DRUJ injuries, TFCC injuries, late ulnar-sided wrist pain, tenosynovitis
    - Poor fracture reduction is the primary contributor to DRUJ pathology in distal radius fractures.
      - Incongruity of the DRUJ with >20° of dorsal tilt
    - ECU or EDM may be entrapped in the DRUJ.
  - Malunion and nonunion

- Intra-articular malunion: malunion takedown and ORIF.
- Extra-articular malunion: opening wedge osteotomy with ORIF and bone grafting.
- Significant radial shortening may lead to ulnar impaction syndrome.
  - 2 mm of shortening increases ulnar force transmission by 42 %.
  - If unable to restore radial height, consider ulnar shortening osteotomy.

- Weakness
- Radiocarpal posttraumatic arthrosis
  - Develops in 2–30 % of patients, increased risk in young patients with >1–2 mm of articular incongruency
  - May be asymptomatic

Bibliography

1. Dyer G, Lozano-Calderon S, Gannon C, Baratz M, Ring D. Predictors of acute carpal tunnel syndrome associated with fracture of the distal radius. J Hand Surg Am. 2008;33(8):1309–13.
2. Fernandez DL. Correction of post-traumatic wrist deformity in adults by osteotomy, bone-grafting, and internal fixation. J Bone Joint Surg Am. 1982;64(8):1164–78.
3. Harness NG, Jupiter JB, Orbay JL, Raskin KB, Fernandez DL. Loss of fixation of the volar lunate facet fragment in fractures of the distal part of the radius. J Bone Joint Surg Am. 2004;86-A(9):1900–8.
4. Ilyas AM, Jupiter JB. Distal radius fractures–classification of treatment and indications for surgery. Orthop Clin North Am. 2007;38(2):167–73, v. Review.
5. Kim JK, Koh YD, Do NH. Should an ulnar styloid fracture be fixed following volar plate fixation of a distal radial fracture? J Bone Joint Surg Am. 2010;92(1):1–6.
6. Lafontaine M, Hardy D, Delince P. Stability assessment of distal radius fractures. Injury. 1989;20(4):208–10.
7. Lichtman DM, Bindra RR, Boyer MI, Putnam MD, Ring D, Slutsky DJ, Taras JS, Watters III WC, Goldberg MJ, Keith M, Turkelson CM, Wies JL, Haralson III RH, Boyer KM, Hitchcock K, Raymond L. Treatment of distal radius fractures. J Am Acad Orthop Surg. 2010;18(3):180–9.
8. Miller MD, Thompson SR, Hart JA. Review of orthopaedics. 6th ed. Philadelphia: Elsevier; 2012. p. 722–5.
9. Roth KM, Blazar PE, Earp BE, Han R, Leung A. Incidence of extensor pollicis longus tendon rupture after nondisplaced distal radius fractures. J Hand Surg Am. 2012;37(5):942–7.
10. Yu YR, Makhni MC, Tabrizi S, Rozental TD, Mundanthanam G, Day CS. Complications of low-profile dorsal versus volar locking plates in the distal radius: a comparative study. J Hand Surg Am. 2011;36(7):1135–41.
11. Zollinger PE, Tuinebreijer WE, Breederveld RS, Kreis RW. Can vitamin C prevent complex regional pain syndrome in patients with wrist fractures? A randomized, controlled, multicenter dose–response study. J Bone Joint Surg Am. 2007;89(7):1424–31.

20 Carpal Fractures

Take-Home Message

- Primary scaphoid blood supply has retrograde flow (distal to proximal) with significantly increased risk of AVN in proximal pole fractures.
- Nondisplaced, stable scaphoid fractures are treated with thumb spica cast immobilization, the duration of which depends of fracture location.
- Displaced, unstable, and proximal pole scaphoid fractures as well as fractures with delayed diagnosis should undergo operative fixation.
- Scaphoid nonunion can lead to advanced collapse with progressive arthritis (SNAC wrist) with treatment options guided by the severity of involvement.
- Lunate fractures of the volar pole are most common and may involve the blood supply.
- Lunate fractures may progress to osteonecrosis with collapse and ultimate radiocarpal arthrosis.
- Dorsal shear triquetral fractures should undergo a trial of nonoperative management with fragment excision for persistent symptoms.
- Pisiform fractures are uncommon injuries that should almost universally undergo nonoperative management with excision for persistent symptoms.
- Trapezium fractures must be assessed for associated Bennett fracture and first carpometacarpal dislocation.
- Capitate fracture rarely occurs in isolation, and surgical fixation is recommended to address displaced fractures and associated injuries.
- Hook of hamate fractures are best visualized on the carpal tunnel view and are treated acutely with cast immobilization with excision for persistently symptomatic chronic fractures.
- Hamate fractures may be associated with ulnar nerve paresthesias and intrinsic motor weakness due to compression at Guyon's canal and occasionally result in flexor tendon synovitis with attritional rupture.

- Scaphoid Fractures
  - General
    - Common fracture with acute wrist injuries.
    - >75 % of the scaphoid is covered by cartilage.
    - Blood supply
      - Major blood supply: a dorsal carpal branch of the radial artery enters at the dorsal ridge and perfuses 80 % of the scaphoid from distal to proximal (retrograde flow).

    - Minor blood supply: a branch of superficial palmar arch enters the distal tubercle.
    - Watershed at the scaphoid waist.

  - Mechanism of injury: fall onto a hyperextended and radially deviated wrist.
  - Assess for anatomic snuffbox tenderness, scaphoid tubercle tenderness, and pain with resisted pronation.
  - Time to union correlates with fracture location with longer healing times for more proximal fractures.
  - Increased risk of AVN in proximal pole fractures.

- Imaging

  - AP and lateral wrist x-rays.
  - Scaphoid view: 30° wrist extension, 20° ulnar deviation.
  - Clenched fist view.
  - If initial films are negative and clinical suspicion remains high, repeat imaging in 2–3 weeks.
  - MRI: most sensitive to diagnose occult fractures within 24 h; assess ligamentous injury and vascularity of the proximal pole.
  - Bone scan: highly sensitive and specific in identifying occult fractures at 72 h.
  - Fine cut CT scan: further characterize fracture, collapse, and progression to union.

- Anatomic Classification

  - Waist: 65 %
  - Proximal pole: 25 %, increased risk of AVN

    - Proximal 1/5: 100 % AVN
    - Proximal 1/3: 30 % AVN

  - Distal pole: 10 %, most common in children

- Treatment

  - Nonoperative

    - Thumb spica cast immobilization.
    - Indicated for stable nondisplaced scaphoid fractures.
    - If high index of suspicion for occult fracture with negative initial imaging, immobilize in short arm thumb spica cast until definitive diagnosis is made.
    - Short arm vs long arm thumb spica casting is debated

      - No consensus.
      - Long arm casting may have shorter time to union, and decreased nonunion rate, however, risks elbow stiffness.

- Fracture location guides recommendations for duration of casting
  - Distal fractures: 8–12 weeks
  - Waist fractures: 12–16 weeks
  - Proximal fractures: 16+ weeks, consider casting until union, may opt for surgical fixation to facilitate earlier motion
- 90 % union rate for fractures with appropriate indications for treatment with cast immobilization.

- Operative
  - Open reduction internal fixation vs percutaneous fixation
    - Indicated in displaced fractures, unstable fractures, proximal fractures, and delayed diagnosis.
    - Dorsal approach: proximal pole fracture; limit exposure of the proximal scaphoid to protect the blood supply entering at the dorsal ridge.
    - Volar approach: waist and distal pole fractures, humpback flexion deformity.
    - Screw should be placed through the central axis of the scaphoid to optimize construct rigidity.
    - Increased risk of screw penetration with percutaneous technique.
    - Surgical fixation facilitates earlier range of motion.
    - 90–95 % union rates.

- Complications
  - Scaphoid nonunion
    - CT scan is the best imaging modality to assess progression to union.
    - Vascularized bone graft: 1,2 intercompartmental supraretinacular artery, good option for proximal pole fracture with osteonecrosis.
    - Inlay (Russe) bone graft: minimal deformity and no associated carpal collapse.
    - Intercalary bone graft with internal fixation: humpback scaphoid deformity, may combine with radial styloidectomy for isolated radioscaphoid arthrosis.
    - If left untreated, scaphoid nonunion can progress to carpal collapse and degenerative arthritis.
  - Scaphoid nonunion advanced collapse (SNAC wrist)
    - Progressive degenerative changes: (1) radial styloid, (2) capitate, (3) capitolunate articulation, spares the lunate fossa
    - Treatment options guided by severity of degenerative changes
      - Proximal row carpectomy: preserved capitolunate articulation
      - Scaphoid excision and four-corner fusion: preserved or arthrosed capitolunate articulation

        - Wrist arthrodesis: arthrosed capitolunate articulation and pancarpal arthritis, provides good pain relief and grip strength with sacrifice of wrist motion

- Lunate Fractures
  - General
    - Lunate considered the "carpal keystone."
    - Mechanism of injury: direct trauma, axial load on a hyperextended wrist.
    - Typically present with volar wrist pain.
    - Lunate fractures must be distinguished from Kienböck disease.
  - Imaging
    - AP and lateral wrist x-rays.
    - Oblique views may help to further delineate fracture.
    - CT scan, MRI, and bone scan may be needed to confirm diagnosis and/or further characterize injury.
  - Anatomic classification
    - Volar pole coronal fracture (most common, may involve nutrient arteries)
    - Dorsal pole coronal fracture
    - Transarticular coronal fracture of the body
    - Transverse body fractures
    - Osteochondral fractures of the proximal articular surface
  - Treatment
    - Nonoperative
      - Cast immobilization
        - Nondisplaced fractures, requires close follow up to monitor healing
    - Operative
      - Open reduction internal fixation
        - Displaced fractures, may be advantageous for maintaining vascularity to the lunate
  - Complications
    - Lunate osteonecrosis and collapse
      - May progress to radiocarpal arthrosis
- Triquetral Fractures
  - General
    - Third most common carpal fracture, following scaphoid and lunate fractures

    - Multiple mechanisms of injury described: fall onto an extended and ulnarly deviated wrist, fall onto a flexed wrist, direct trauma

  - Imaging

    - AP and lateral wrist radiographs: dorsal aspect of the triquetrum is best seen on the lateral view.
    - Oblique views may help to further characterize body fractures.

  - Anatomic classification

    - Dorsal shear/avulsion fractures: most common
    - Body fractures: rare

  - Treatment

    - Nonoperative

      - Splint/cast immobilization for 4–6 weeks followed by range of motion

        - Dorsal shear injuries, nondisplaced body fractures

    - Operative

      - Fragment excision

        - Dorsal shear injuries with persistent symptoms following trial of nonoperative management

      - Open reduction internal fixation

        - Displaced body fractures

  - Complications

    - Rare

- Pisiform Fractures

  - General

    - Uncommon injuries, comprise 1–3 % of all carpal fractures.
    - Pisiform is a sesamoid bone located within the FCU tendon and is the origin of abductor digiti minimi.
    - The pisiform contributes to stability of the ulnar column but resisting triquetral subluxation and fulcrum for force transmission from the forearm to the hand.
    - Associated injuries in 50 %: distal radius fracture, hamate fracture, triquetrum fracture.

  - Imaging

    - AP, lateral, and oblique wrist x-rays.
    - Lateral view with 30° wrist supination: best visualization of the pisotriquetral joint.

        - Consider carpal tunnel view.
    - Classification
        - Avulsion fractures
        - Transverse body fractures
        - Comminuted fractures
    - Treatment
        - Nonoperative
            - Short arm cast immobilization with 30° wrist flexion and ulnar deviation for 6 weeks
                - Nearly all pisiform fractures are recommended to undergo conservative treatment with cast immobilization.
    - Complications
        - Symptomatic nonunion
            - Pisiform excision provides reliable pain relief without impacting wrist function.
- Trapezium Fractures
    - General
        - Uncommon injuries
        - May occur in isolation or in combination with other carpal bone injuries
            - Assess for concurrent fracture of the base of the first metacarpal and/or subluxation or dislocation of the first carpometacarpal joint.
            - Trapezial ridge fractures have an increased coincidence of distal radius fractures.
    - Imaging
        - AP and lateral wrist x-rays
            - Robert's AP view: hand in full pronation
        - Consider carpal tunnel view
    - Classification
        - Body fracture: vertically oriented, comminuted
        - Trapezial ridge fracture
            - Type I: base of ridge
            - Type II: tip of ridge
    - Treatment
        - Nonoperative

    - Thumb spica cast immobilization for 6 weeks
      - Trapezial ridge fractures and nondisplaced body fractures.
      - Type II trapezial ridge fractures should have molded abduction of the first ray.
  - Operative
    - Open reduction internal fixation
      - Displaced body fractures
      - Volar approach, K-wire fixation often used
- Complications
  - Symptomatic nonunion of trapezial ridge fractures
    - Treat with excision.

- Capitate Fractures
  - General
    - Rarely occur in isolation
    - Associated injuries: perilunate dislocations, scaphoid fracture, carpometacarpal fracture-dislocation
  - Imaging
    - AP, lateral, and oblique wrist radiographs
    - CT scan often helpful
  - Classification
    - Isolated capitate fracture
    - Scaphocapitate syndrome: scaphoid fracture with proximal capitate fracture
  - Treatment
    - Nonoperative
      - Cast immobilization
        - Nondisplaced, isolated capitate fractures
    - Operative
      - Open reduction internal fixation
        - Displaced capitate fractures, fractures with associated scaphoid fractures, perilunate dislocation, and carpometacarpal fracture-dislocations
        - Typically approached dorsally with screw and/or K-wire fixation

- Complications
    - Osteonecrosis
    - Nonunion
        - May be treated with fusion of the capitate, scaphoid, and lunate
- Hamate Fractures
    - General
        - Hook of hamate fractures are common in golf, baseball, hockey, and racquet sports.
        - Body fractures are associated with fourth and fifth carpometacarpal fracture-dislocation.
        - Must distinguish from bipartite hamate.
        - Present with hypothenar pain, decreased grip strength, possible ulnar nerve paresthesias and intrinsic motor weakness (compression at Guyon's canal), and possible median nerve paresthesias (compression at the carpal tunnel).
    - Imaging
        - AP and lateral wrist x-rays: difficult to visualize on AP
        - Carpal tunnel view: best visualization of the hamate
    - Classification
        - Hook of hamate fractures: most common
        - Body fractures: uncommon
    - Treatment
        - Nonoperative
            - Cast immobilization for 6 weeks
                - Acute hook of hamate fractures, nondisplaced body fractures
        - Operative
            - Open reduction internal fixation
                - Displaced and unstable body fractures
                - Rarely performed in hook of hamate fractures
            - Excision
                - Persistently symptomatic, chronic hook of hamate fractures
    - Complications
        - Ulnar nerve symptoms
            - May have ulnar nerve paresthesias and/or intrinsic motor weakness secondary to compression at Guyon's canal
        - Flexor tendon synovitis and attritional rupture
            - Described following hook of hamate fractures

Bibliography

1. Bishop AT, Beckenbaugh RD. Fracture of the hamate hook. J Hand Surg Am. 1988;13(1):135–9.
2. Bond CD, Shin AY, McBride MT, Dao KD. Percutaneous screw fixation or cast immobilization for nondisplaced scaphoid fractures. J Bone Joint Surg Am. 2001;83-A(4):483–8.
3. Kawamura K, Chung KC. Treatment of scaphoid fractures and nonunions. J Hand Surg Am. 2008;33(6):988–97.
4. Lam KS, Woodbridge S, Burke FD. Wrist function after excision of the pisiform. J Hand Surg Br. 2003;28(1):69–72.
5. Miller MD, Thompson SR, Hart JA. Review of orthopaedics. 6th ed. Philadelphia: Elsevier; 2012. p. 725–7.
6. O'Shea K, Weiland AJ. Fractures of the hamate and pisiform bones. Hand Clin. 2012;28(3):287–300. Review.
7. Trumble TE, Salas P, Barthel T, Robert 3rd KQ. Management of scaphoid nonunions. J Am Acad Orthop Surg. 2003;11(6):380–91.

21 Lunate and Perilunate Dislocations

Take-Home Message

- High-energy injuries with high incidence of associated median nerve injury and acute carpal tunnel syndrome.
- Imaging may show "spilled teacup sign," loss of greater and lesser carpal arcs (disruption of Gilula's lines), overlapping carpal bones, and loss of sagittal colinearity between the radius, lunate, and capitate.
- Treat with emergent closed reduction followed by ORIF with ligament repair +/– carpal tunnel release.
- Chronic injuries (>8 weeks) may be treated with proximal row corpectomy, triscaphe fusion, or wrist arthrodesis.
- Poor functional outcomes are common with decreased wrist motion, decreased grip strength, possible persistent carpal instability, chondrolysis, and ultimate posttraumatic arthrosis.

- General
  - High-energy injuries with poor functional outcomes
  - ~25 % missed on presentation
  - Mechanism of injury: wrist hyperextension and ulnar deviation leading to intercarpal supination and dislocation
  - Associated median nerve injury

  - 25 % of patients have median nerve symptoms on presentation.
  - Increased risk of median nerve injury and acute carpal tunnel syndrome with volar lunate dislocation.

- Imaging
  - AP and lateral wrist x-rays
    - AP view: "spilled teacup sign" (rotation of lunate so concavity tipped proximally), loss of greater and lesser carpal arcs (disruption of Gilula's lines), overlapping carpal bones
      - Great arc disruption: ligamentous disruption with associated fractures of the radius, ulna, and carpal bones
      - Lesser arc disruption: purely ligamentous
    - Lateral view: loss of colinearity between radius, lunate, and capitate, scapholunate angle >70°.
    - Assess for associated fractures.
- Classification
  - Lunate dislocation
    - Lunate dislocates volar (via space of Poirier, most common) or dorsal to the intact carpus.
  - Perilunate dislocation
    - Carpus dislocates around the intact lunate.
    - Types: transscaphoid-perilunate, perilunate, transradial-perilunate, transscaphoid-trans-capitate-perilunar.
  - Mayfield classification
    - Stage I: scapholunate dissociation
    - Stage II: plus lunocapitate disruption (via space of Poirier)
    - Stage III: plus lunotriquetral disruption
    - Stage IV: lunate dislocation
- Treatment
  - Nonoperative
    - Emergent closed reduction and splinting
      - Decreases risk of permanent median nerve injury and subsequent chondrolysis
      - Follow with early surgical fixation

  - No role for definitive nonoperative management with universally poor outcomes and high risk of recurrent dislocation
- Operative
  - Open reduction internal fixation and ligament repair +/– carpal tunnel release
    - Indicated for all acute injuries (<8 weeks)
    - Volar and dorsal approaches described and may be combined
    - Follow with thumb spica splinting/casting for 6 weeks postoperatively
  - Salvage procedures
    - Indicated for chronic injuries (>8 weeks)
    - Proximal row carpectomy
    - Triscaphe fusion
    - Wrist arthrodesis: for chronic injury with associated degenerative changes

- Complications
  - Median nerve injury
  - Acute carpal tunnel syndrome
    - Emergent carpal tunnel release for symptoms that persist following emergent closed reduction
  - Poor functional outcomes
    - 50 % loss of wrist motion, 60 % loss of grip strength
  - Chondrolysis
  - Persistent carpal instability
  - Posttraumatic arthrosis
  - Nonunion/malunion

Bibliography

1. Kozin SH. Perilunate injuries: diagnosis and treatment. J Am Acad Orthop Surg. 1998;6:114–20.
2. Miller MD, Thompson SR, Hart JA. Review of orthopaedics. 6th ed. Philadelphia: Elsevier; 2012. p. 727.
3. Sawardeker PJ, Kindt KE, Baratz ME. Fracture-dislocations of the carpus: perilunate injury. Orthop Clin North Am. 2013;44(1):93–106.
4. Stanbury SJ, Elfar JC. Perilunate dislocation and perilunate fracture-dislocation. J Am Acad Orthop Surg. 2011;19(9):554–62. Review.

22 Metacarpal Fractures

Take-Home Message

- Treatment of metacarpal fractures depends on which metacarpal is involved and location of fracture with acceptable angulation and shortening varying by location.
- Malrotation is never acceptable.
- 7° degree extensor lag for every 2 mm of shortening.
- Maintain a high index of suspicion for compartment syndrome with multiple metacarpal fractures and crush injuries.
- Open wounds overlying the metacarpal head should be considered to be "fight bites" until proven otherwise.
- Bennett fracture deforming forces: volar oblique ligament hold volar lip fragment in place, metacarpal shaft pulled proximally, dorsally and radially by APL and adductor pollicis.
- Fractures with deformity greater than acceptable parameters allowed should undergo reduction and surgical fixation.
- Stiffness is the most common complication and is best prevented with early motion with both nonoperative and operative management.

- General
  - Metacarpal fractures comprise 40 % of hand injuries and are most common in men 10–29 years old
    - Most common fracture site: metacarpal neck
    - Most common metacarpal injured: fifth metacarpal
    - Most common thumb base fracture: Bennett fracture
  - First, fourth, and fifth metacarpals for the mobile borders while second and third metacarpals form the stiffer central pillar.
  - Acceptable alignment parameters depend on fracture location and the metacarpal involved.
  - Malrotation is never acceptable
    - Assess malrotation with finger cascade (fingertips should point to scaphoid, no scissoring), parallel nail plates
  - 7° extensor lag for every 2 mm of shortening
    - "Shortening" may be secondary to flexion/extension deformity.
  - Associated injuries: dorsal wounds common and almost always represent open fractures, tendon laceration, and neurovascular injury.
  - Maintain high index of suspicion for compartment syndrome with multiple metacarpal fractures and crush injuries.

- Imaging
  - AP, lateral and oblique hand x-rays.
  - 30° pronated lateral: assess fourth and fifth CMC joints.
  - 30° supinated view: assess second and third CMC joints.
  - Brewerton view: metacarpal head fractures.
  - Robert's view (AP hand in full pronation): thumb CMC joint.
  - Hyperpronated thumb view: thumb base fractures.
  - Semi-pronated, semi-supinated, traction films: small metacarpal base fractures.
  - CT scan: further evaluation of CMC fracture-dislocations and complex metacarpal head fractures.
- Classification
  - Metacarpal head fractures
    - Vertical, horizontal, oblique, comminuted.
    - Any associated wound should be considered an open fracture ("fight bite") until proven otherwise.
  - Metacarpal neck fractures
    - "Boxer's fracture": fifth metacarpal neck fracture.
    - Assessment of rotational deformity is critical.
  - Metacarpal shaft fractures
    - Transverse, oblique, spiral, comminuted
  - Acceptable alignment
    - Index and long finger: 10–20° shaft angulation, 2–5 mm shortening, 10–15° neck angulation
    - Ring finger: 30° shaft angulation, 2–5 mm shortening, 30–40° neck angulation
    - Small finger: 40° shaft angulation, 2–5 mm shortening, 50–60° neck angulation
  - Thumb base fractures
    - Bennett fracture: intra-articular volar ulnar lip fracture of the thumb metacarpal base, most common thumb base fracture
      - Volar ulnar lip fragment held in place by volar oblique ligament (volar beak ligament).
      - Metacarpal shaft is pulled proximally, dorsally, and radially from deforming forces of APL and adductor pollicis.
    - Rolando fracture: complete articular thumb metacarpal base fracture
      - "Y" fracture, "T" fracture, comminuted fracture

        - Extra-articular fracture: transverse, oblique
            - Acceptable alignment: < 30°angulation
    - Small metacarpal base fractures
        - Reverse Bennett (baby Bennett) fractures: epibasal, two-part, three-part, comminuted
            - Nonoperative vs CRPP/ORIF controversial.
            - Fracture fragment may be displaced by ECU.
            - Assess for possible associated carpometacarpal fracture-dislocation.
    - Nonoperative
        - Immobilization with 70–90° MCP flexion and PIP extension for 4 weeks
            - Stable injury pattern with acceptable angulation and shortening, no rotational deformity, may consider in severely comminuted thumb base fractures
            - Angulated metacarpal neck fractures may be amenable to closed reduction and casting
                - Jahss technique: 90° MCP flexion, dorsal pressure through proximal phalanx while stabilizing the metacarpal shaft
    - Operative
        - General indications: intra-articular fractures, angulation and/or shortening outside acceptable parameters, malrotation, multiple metacarpal shaft fractures, loss of inherent stability from border digit, open fractures
        - Initiate early motion in the postoperative period
        - Open reduction internal fixation vs closed reduction percutaneous fixation
            - Techniques include antegrade and retrograde pinning, pinning to adjacent metacarpal (comminuted metacarpal shaft fractures), lag screw fixation (ideal for long spiral fractures), and plating (ideal for transverse fracture and bridging of comminuted fractures).
                - Ideal fixation allows for early motion.
            - Dorsal approach with central extensor mechanism split or sagittal band takedown and repair.

  - External fixation
    - Consider in severely comminuted metacarpal head fractures and severely comminuted thumb base fractures.
  - MCP arthroplasty
    - Consider in severely comminuted metacarpal head fractures.
- Complications
  - Stiffness
    - The most common complication
    - Prevent with early motion
  - Tendon hardware irritation
    - Cover plates with periosteum when possible; initiate early motion.
  - Malunion
    - Malrotation poorly tolerated; treat with osteotomy and ORIF.
  - Posttraumatic arthrosis
    - Metacarpal head fractures: MCP arthroplasty, MCP arthrodesis.
    - Thumb base metacarpal fractures: relationship of postoperative joint congruency to posttraumatic arthrosis is controversial.
    - Small metacarpal base fractures.

Bibliography

1. Henry MH. Fractures of the proximal phalanx and metacarpals in the hand: preferred methods of stabilization. J Am Acad Orthop Surg. 2008;16(10):586–95.
2. Kawamura K, Chung KC. Fixation choices for closed simple unstable oblique phalangeal and metacarpal fractures. Hand Clin. 2006;22(3):287–95.
3. Miller MD, Thompson SR, Hart JA. Review of orthopaedics. 6th ed. Philadelphia: Elsevier; 2012. p. 729–34.
4. Souer JS, Mudgal CS. Plate fixation in closed ipsilateral multiple metacarpal fractures. J Hand Surg Eur Vol. 2008;33(6):740–4.
5. Soyer AD. Fractures of the base of the first metacarpal: current treatment options. J Am Acad Orthop Surg. 1999;7(6):403–12.

23 Phalanx Fractures

Take-Home Message

- Diaphyseal proximal phalanx fractures often present with apex volar angulation due to proximal fragment flexion from pull of interossei and distal fragment extension from pull of central slip.
- Diaphyseal middle phalanx fractures may present with volar angulation, dorsal angulation, or no angulation pending fracture location with respect to FDS insertion.
- Compression (pilon) fractures of the base of the middle phalanx are unstable with greater than 42 % joint involvement and may subluxate with as little as 10–15 % joint involvement.
- Distal phalanx fracture often has associated nail bed injuries.
- Regardless of treatment modality, initiate motion within 3–4 weeks to prevent stiffness.
- Fractures with deformity greater than acceptable parameters allowed should undergo reduction and surgical fixation.
- Malunions with functional impairment should undergo corrective osteotomy.
- Symptomatic posttraumatic DIP and PIP arthrosis should undergo arthrodesis with position determined by digit and joint involvement; silicone arthroplasty may be used for PIP arthrosis with good bone stock and no deformity.

- General
  - Phalanx fractures are common injuries that account for 10 % of all fractures.
    - Distal phalanx is the most commonly fractured bone in the hand.
  - Mechanism of injury: sports (young patients), machinery (middle-aged patients), falls (elderly patients).
  - Distal phalanx fracture frequently has associated nail bed injuries and often results from crush injuries.
- Imaging
  - Dedicated finger AP and lateral x-rays: must get true lateral of any involved joint
  - AP and lateral hand x-rays to assess for associated fractures
- Classification
  - Proximal and middle phalanx fractures

- Diaphyseal fractures: transverse, oblique, spiral, comminuted
  - Proximal phalanx fractures deformity
    - Apex volar angulation: proximal fragment flexion (interossei) and distal fragment extension (central slip)
  - Middle phalanx fracture deformity
    - Apex volar *or* dorsal deformity.
    - Apex dorsal angulation: fracture proximal to FDS insertion with proximal fragment extension (central slip).
    - Apex volar angulation: fracture distal to FDS insertion.
    - Fractures through the middle third may exhibit volar angulation, dorsal angulation, or no angulation.
- Intra-articular base fractures
  - Collateral ligament avulsion.
  - Vertical shear: typically involve volar shear fracture of the middle phalanx with dorsal subluxation/dislocation, dorsal shear with volar subluxation/dislocation, and lateral shear with lateral subluxation/dislocation also possible.
  - Compression (pilon): typically involve the base of the middle phalanx; joint will be stable with involvement of up to 42 % of the volar half of base of the middle phalanx; however subluxation can occur with only 10–15 % joint surface involvement.
- Other variants: neck, condylar, and extra-articular base fractures
- Acceptable alignment parameters for extra-articular proximal and middle phalanx fractures: <10° angulation, <2 mm shortening, and no rotational deformity

– Distal phalanx fractures
  - Transverse, longitudinal, comminuted
  - High coincidence of nail bed injuries

- Treatment
  - Regardless of treatment modality, initiate motion within 3–4 weeks to prevent stiffness
  - Nonoperative
    - Buddy taping for 3–4 weeks followed by aggressive motion
      - Stable diaphyseal phalanx fractures, nondisplaced collateral ligament avulsions, nondisplaced neck, condylar and extra-articular base
    - Digital splint +/– nail bed repair
      - Nondisplaced condylar fractures, distal phalanx fractures.

    - Treat nail bed injuries as open fractures with appropriate irrigation and debridement.
    - Nail matrix may be incarcerated within the distal phalanx fracture.

  - Operative

    - Open reduction internal fixation vs closed reduction percutaneous pinning

      - Unstable or malrotated diaphyseal phalanx fractures, displaced collateral ligament fractures (may also tension band), intra-articular compression fractures (+/– bone grafting), intra-articular shear fractures, displaced neck, condylar and extra-articular base.
      - Techniques include minifragment lag screw fixation (may be used alone in long oblique fractures), plate fixation, crossed K-wires, and Eaton-Belsky pinning (transarticular pinning through metacarpal head for extra-articular proximal phalanx base fractures).
      - Minimize extent of surgical dissection to decrease risk of stiffness.

    - Dynamic external fixation

      - May be utilized in some PIP joint fracture-dislocations

    - Hemi-hamate arthroplasty

      - May be utilized in unstable middle phalanx pilon fractures or as a salvage option following failed external fixation or ORIF of PIP joint fracture-dislocations

- Complications

  - Stiffness

    - Most common complication
    - Flexor tendon adhesions, flexion contractures
    - Increased risk with prolonged immobilization, associated joint injury and extensive surgical dissection

  - Malunion

    - Malrotation, volar/dorsal angulation, lateral translation, shortening
    - Corrective surgery indicated for functional impairment

      - Osteotomy at malunion site preferred over metacarpal osteotomy

  - Nonunion

    - Uncommon overall
    - Treat symptomatic nonunions with nonunion takedown and ORIF +/– bone grafting or ray amputation or arthrodesis in salvage situations.
    - Treatment of symptomatic distal phalanx fractures with percutaneous compression screw is described.

- Posttraumatic arthrosis
  - Observation and NSAIDS for mild symptoms
  - Symptomatic DIP arthrosis: arthrodesis
    - Index and long finger: extension
    - Ring and small finger: 10–20° flexion
  - Symptomatic PIP arthrosis
    - Arthrodesis
      - Index finger: 30° flexion
      - Long finger: 35° flexion
      - Ring finger: 40° flexion
      - Small finger: 45° flexion
    - Silicone arthroplasty
      - Indicated for long and ring finger PIP arthrosis with good bone stock and no significant deformity

Bibliography

1. Calfee RP, Kiefhaber TR, Sommerkamp TG, Stern PJ. Hemi-hamate arthroplasty provides functional reconstruction of acute and chronic proximal interphalangeal fracture-dislocations. J Hand Surg Am. 2009;34(7):1232–41.
2. Freeland AE, Orbay JL. Extraarticular hand fractures in adults: a review of new developments. Clin Orthop Relat Res. 2006;445:133–45.
3. Henry MH. Fractures of the proximal phalanx and metacarpals in the hand: preferred methods of stabilization. J Am Acad Orthop Surg. 2008;16(10):586–95.
4. Kawamura K, Chung KC. Fixation choices for closed simple unstable oblique phalangeal and metacarpal fractures. Hand Clin. 2006;22(3):287–95. Review.
5. Meijs CM, Verhofstad MH. Symptomatic nonunion of a distal phalanx fracture: treatment with a percutaneous compression screw. J Hand Surg Am. 2009;34(6):1127–9.
6. Miller MD, Thompson SR, Hart JA. Review of orthopaedics. 6th ed. Philadelphia: Elsevier; 2012. p. 734.

Pelvis and Lower Extremity Trauma

Natalie Casemyr, Cyril Mauffrey, and David Hak

1 Pelvic Ring Injuries

Take-Home Message

- Pelvic ring injuries are most commonly described using the Young-Burgess classification.
- Hemodynamically unstable patients require emergent intervention with pelvic binder/sheet, volume resuscitation, possible external fixation and pelvic packing, possible angiographic embolization, skeletal traction in vertically unstable patterns, and possible C clamp.
- Anterior pelvic ring injuries commonly treated with plate fixation. External fixation may be favorable in some patients, and injury patterns place the lateral femoral cutaneous nerve at risk.
- Posterior pelvic ring injuries require anatomic reduction and stabilization with anterior plating, SI screws, or posterior tension band plating.
- Placement of percutaneous sacroiliac screws requires meticulous fluoroscopic visualization with appropriate inlet, outlet, and lateral sacral views.
- Vertical sacral fractures are at increased risk for loss of fixation/reduction.
- Vertically unstable pelvic ring injuries should be treated with stabilization of the anterior and posterior pelvic ring; consider lumbopelvic fixation.

N. Casemyr, MD • C. Mauffrey, MD, FACS, FRCS (✉) • D. Hak, MD, FACS, MBA
Department of Orthopaedic Surgery, Denver Health Medical Center,
777 Bannock Street, Denver 80204, CO, USA
e-mail: cyril.mauffrey@dhha.org; cmauffrey@yahoo.com

C. Mauffrey, D.J. Hak (eds.), *Passport for the Orthopedic Boards and FRCS Examination*, DOI 10.1007/978-2-8178-0475-0_11

- High incidence of thromboembolic disease and urogenital injuries.
- Increased risk of mortality with blood transfusion requirement in the first 24 h, open fractures, associated bladder ruptures, and more severe/unstable fracture patterns.

General

- Mechanism of injury: typically high-energy blunt trauma
- High mortality rates
  - Closed fracture: 15–25 % mortality
  - Open fractures: up to 50 % mortality
    - Complete examination of the perineum, vagina, and rectum to rule out occult open injuries.
    - Open pelvis fractures may require a diverting colostomy.
- High incidence of associated injuries
  - Chest, head, abdominal, long bone fractures, spine fractures, internal iliac vessels and branches, lumbosacral plexus (L5 and S1 most common), urogenital injuries.
  - Urogenital injuries: blood at the urethral meatus, high-riding prostate, significant displacement of the anterior pelvic ring.
    - Males (21 %) > females (8 %).
    - If retrograde urethrogram is negative and there is persistent hematuria, obtain a cystogram.
  - Fracture patterns with significant ilium/crescent components have increased risk of soft tissue degloving and bowel injury or entrapment.
  - Mortality usually results from sequelae of nonpelvic-associated injuries.
- Hemorrhage is the leading cause of death
  - Internal pudendal artery injuries associated with the most significant intrapelvic hemorrhage
  - Must evaluate for nonpelvic sources of bleeding
    - Binders, sheeting, external fixation, pelvic clamp, and pelvic packing: decrease the volume of the pelvis and tamponade bleeding
  - Good for venous hemorrhage
  - Less effective for arterial hemorrhage
    - Angiography with embolization for ongoing arterial hemorrhage

Imaging

- AP pelvis: assess each hemipelvis for asymmetry, rotation, and displacement and for possible associated fracture of the L5 transverse process, ischial spine, and ischial tuberosity.

- Inlet view: 25–45° caudad angulation; S1 should overlie S2; assess anteroposterior displacement of the sacroiliac joint, sacroiliac joint widening, rotational deformity, and sacral ala impaction fracture.
- Outlet view: 45–60° cephalad angulation; pubic symphysis shoulder overlies S2; assess vertical displacement of the sacroiliac joint and flexion/extension of the hemipelvis and disruption of sacral foramina.
- CT scan: should be obtained routinely to further evaluate pelvic ring injuries
  - Better characterization of posterior ring injuries, involvement of sacral foramina, comminution, and rotation

Young and Burgess Classification

- Anteroposterior compression injuries
  - High incidence of associated visceral injuries and retroperitoneal injuries
  - APC I: symphyseal diastasis <2.5 cm, posterior pelvic ring intact
  - APC II: symphyseal diastasis >2.5 cm, disruption of the sacrotuberous, sacrospinous, and anterior sacroiliac ligaments; posterior sacroiliac ligaments intact
  - APC III: symphyseal diastasis >2.5 cm, complete separation of the hemipelvis from the pelvic ring with disruption of the sacrotuberous, sacrospinous, and anterior and posterior sacroiliac ligaments
- Lateral compression injuries
  - High incidence of closed head injury and intra-abdominal injury.
  - LC I: pubic ramus fracture with sacral compression fracture.
  - LC II: pubic ramus fracture with posterior iliac wing fracture-dislocation (crescent fracture).
  - LC III: pubic ramus fracture with ipsilateral lateral compression injury and contralateral APC injury (windswept pelvis); common mechanisms include rollover MVC and auto vs pedestrian.
- Vertical shear injuries
  - Highest incidence of intrapelvic hemorrhage with resulting hemorrhagic shock (~65 %)
  - Posterior and superior directed force, common mechanism with fall from height
- Combined mechanism injuries

Tile Classification

- Stable (posterior arch intact)
  - A1: fracture not involving the pelvic ring (avulsion, iliac wing)
  - A2: minimally displaced, stable ring fracture
  - A3: transverse sacral fracture
- Rotationally unstable, vertically stable
  - B1: anteroposterior compression injury (external rotation)
  - B2: lateral compression injury (internal rotation)

- B2-1: anterior ring rotation with displacement through the ipsilateral rami
- B2-2: anterior ring rotation with displacement through the contralateral rami

– B3: bilateral

- Rotationally and vertically unstable (complete disruption of the posterior arch)
  - C1: unilateral
    - C1-1: iliac fracture
    - C1-2: sacroiliac fracture-dislocation
    - C1-3: sacral fracture
  - C2: bilateral with one side B type and one side C type
  - C3: bilateral C type

Treatment

- Emergent volume resuscitation and hemorrhage control
  - Massive transfusion protocol: PRBC-FFP-platelets in 1:1:1 ratio improves mortality.
  - Bleeding sources: intra-abdominal, intrathoracic, retroperitoneal, extremity, pelvic
    - Pelvic sources of hemorrhage
      - Venous plexus hemorrhage: 80–85 %
      - Bleeding cancellous bone
      - Arterial injury 15–20 %
        - Superior gluteal > internal pudendal > obturator > lateral sacral
  - Reduce pelvic volume and stabilize fracture.
    - Pelvic binder/sheet centered over greater trochanters, may internal rotate lower extremities and bind ankles together; prolonged pressure from binder or sheet can cause skin necrosis.
    - External fixation, skeletal traction (vertically unstable injuries), pelvic C clamp (rarely used) to decrease pelvic volume and tamponade bleeding and to stabilize fracture allowing clot to form over bleeding bone and venous plexus.
      - External fixator should be placed before pelvic packing (if performed) or laparotomy.
    - Angiographic embolization may be considered if there is ongoing arterial hemorrhage with the goal to selectively embolize bleeding sources, risk of gluteal necrosis, and impotence.
  - Nonoperative
    - Mobilization with weight bearing as tolerated indicated for mechanically stable pelvic ring injuries

  - LC I and APC I pelvis fractures, isolated pubic ramus fractures
- May consider protected weight bearing for some anterior injuries with ipsilateral partial posterior ring injuries

- Operative
  - Open reduction internal fixation
    - Indicated for symphyseal diastasis >2.5 cm, complete sacroiliac joint disruption, displaced sacral fractures, vertically unstable fractures, displacement or rotation of hemipelvis.
    - Anterior injuries: anterior plate fixation most common, external fixation with supra-acetabular pins or iliac wing pins (lateral femoral cutaneous nerve at risk, indicated with suprapubic catheter placement).
    - Posterior injuries: sacroiliac joint dislocations and fracture-dislocations require anatomic reduction.
      - Open reduction and anterior plating of the sacroiliac joint via lateral window, L4 and L5 nerve roots at greatest risk with retractor placement.
      - Sacroiliac screws: L5 nerve root at greatest risk; ensure screws are posterior to the iliac cortical density on the lateral sacral view and appropriately positioned on inlet and outlet pelvis views.
      - Posterior tension band plating: risk of prominent hardware and wound healing problems.
    - Vertically unstable injury patterns should be treated with anterior and posterior ring stabilization to decrease risk of loss of reduction; consider lumbopelvic fixation.

Complications

- Poor outcomes associated with SI joint incongruity, increased injury severity and initial displacement, malunion with residual displacement >1 cm, nonunion, leg length discrepancy >2 cm.
  - Vertical sacral fractures have the highest risk of loss of fixation/reduction.
- Neurologic injury
  - L5 nerve root at greatest risk as it courses over the sacral ala.
  - L4 and S1 nerve roots at lesser risk.
  - Additional sacral nerve root may be compromised at the time of injury, reduction of sacral fracture, or overcompression of transforaminal sacral fractures.
- High risk of thromboembolic disease
  - Pharmacologic prophylaxis, mechanical prophylaxis, IVC filters in patients otherwise contraindicated for chemical anticoagulation

- Urogenital injuries
  - Present in 10–20 % of pelvic ring injuries, more common in males.
  - Urethral tear, bladder rupture (increased risk of mortality).
    - May result in urethral stricture, impotence, incontinence, and increased risk of anterior pelvic ring infection.
  - Dyspareunia, possible need for cesarean section.
- Chronic instability is a rare complication.
  - Assess with single-leg stance pelvis x-rays.
- Increased risk of mortality associated with blood transfusion requirement in the first 24 h, open fractures, associated bladder ruptures, and more severe/unstable fracture patterns.

Bibliography

1. Barei DP, Bellabarba C, Mills WJ, Routt ML Jr. Percutaneous management of unstable pelvic ring disruptions. Injury. 2001;32(Suppl 1):SA33–44.
2. Burgess AR, Eastridge BJ, Young JW, Ellison TS, Ellison PS Jr, Poka A, Bathon GH, Brumback RJ. Pelvic ring disruptions: effective classification system and treatment protocols. J Trauma. 1990;30(7):848–56.
3. Croce MA, Magnotti LJ, Savage SA, Wood GW 2nd, Fabian TC. Emergent pelvic fixation in patients with exsanguinating pelvic fractures. J Am Coll Surg. 2007;204(5):935–9.
4. Griffin DR, Starr AJ, Reinert CM. Vertically unstable pelvic fractures fixed with percutaneous iliosacral screws: does posterior injury pattern predict fixation failure? J Orthop Trauma. 2006;20:S30–6.
5. Hak DJ, Smith WR, Suzuki T. Management of hemorrhage in life-threatening pelvic fracture. J Am Acad Orthop Surg. 2009;17(7):447–57.
6. Karadimas EJ, Nicolson T, Kakagia DD, Matthews SJ, Richards PJ, Giannoudis PV. Angiographic embolisation of pelvic ring injuries. Treatment algorithm and review of the literature. Int Orthop. 2011;35(9):1381–90.
7. Krieg JC, Mohr M, Ellis TJ, Simpson TS, Madey SM, Bottlang M. Emergent stabilization of pelvic ring injuries by controlled circumferential compression: a clinical trial. J Trauma. 2005;59(3):659–64.
8. Miller MD, Thompson SR, Hart JA. Review of orthopaedics. 6th ed. Philadelphia: Elsevier; 2012. p. 735–8.
9. Routt ML Jr, Simonian PT, Agnew SG, Mann FA. Radiographic recognition of the sacral alar slope for optimal placement of iliosacral screws: a cadaveric and clinical study. J Orthop Trauma. 1996;10(3):171–7.
10. Siegel J, Templeman DC, Tornetta P III. Single-leg-stance radiographs in the diagnosis of pelvic instability. J Bone Joint Surg Am. 2008;90(10):2119–25.
11. Smith W, Williams A, Agudelo J, Shannon M, Morgan S, Stahel P, Moore E. Early predictors of mortality in hemodynamically unstable pelvis fractures. J Orthop Trauma. 2007;21(1):31–7.
12. Starr AJ, Walter JC, Harris RW, Reinert CM, Jones AL. Percutaneous screw fixation of fractures of the iliac wing and fracture-dislocations of the sacro-iliac joint (OTA Types 61-B2.2

and 61-B3.3, or Young-Burgess "lateral compression type II" pelvic fractures). J Orthop Trauma. 2002;16(2):116–23.
13. Tile M. Acute pelvic fractures: I. Causation and classification. J Am Acad Orthop Surg. 1996;4(3):143–51.
14. Tile M. Acute pelvic fractures: II. Principles of management. J Am Acad Orthop Surg. 1996;4(3):152–61.

2 Acetabular Fractures

Take-Home Message

- Bimodal distribution with high-energy blunt trauma in the young and low-energy fall in the elderly.
- Corona mortis is an anastomosis between the external iliac (or deep epigastric) vessels and the obturator vessels.
- Corona mortis present in ~30 % of patients, risk life-threatening hemorrhage if injured.
- Six cardinal lines on the AP pelvis: iliopectineal line, ilioischial line, anterior wall, posterior wall, sourcil, teardrop.
- Iliac oblique profiles the anterior column and posterior wall.
- Obturator oblique profiles the posterior column and anterior wall.
- Fractures with roof arc angle >45° on AP; obturator and iliac oblique views do not involve the weight-bearing dome.
- On axial CT scan, vertical fracture lines represent transverse or T-type fractures, while horizontal line represents column fractures.
- Letournel classification divides acetabular fractures into five elementary and five associated types.
- Associated both-column fractures: complete dissociation of the articular surface of the acetabulum from the axial skeleton; the spur sign on obturator oblique represents the undisplaced intact posterior ilium.
- Nonoperative management of minimally displaced fractures, fractures outside the weight-bearing dome, and fractures with secondary congruence.
- Surgical fixation indicated for displaced fractures, fractures with roof arc angle <45° on any view, incarcerated intra-articular fragments, irreducible fracture-dislocations, and unstable hips with associated wall fractures.
- Posterior wall fractures: <20 % presumed to be stable, 20–40 % perform dynamic fluoroscopic EUA to determine stability, >40 % presumed to be unstable.
- ORIF and acute total hip arthroplasty for patients >60 years with superomedial dome impact (gull sign), significant osteopenia and/or comminution, and associated femoral neck fractures

- Posttraumatic arthrosis is the most common complication.
- Heterotopic ossification is common; increased risk with extensile and posterior approaches.
- High risk of thromboembolic disease; all patients should receive DVT prophylaxis and/or IVC filter.
- Risk of iatrogenic sciatic nerve injury can be decreased by maintaining hip extension and knee flexion to reduce tension on the nerve.
- Quality of reduction is the most important determinant of outcome; increased risk of malreduction with delay to surgery.

General

- Bimodal distribution
  - High-energy blunt trauma in young patients
  - Low-energy falls in elderly patients
- Fracture pattern determined by position of the hip and force vector
  - Flexed hip with axial load most common (dashboard injury)
- Associated injuries: hip dislocation, sciatic nerve injury, other lower extremity injuries (35 %), additional organ system injury (50 %)
- Acetabulum supported by two columns of bone in an "inverted Y" and connected to the sacrum through the sciatic buttress
  - Posterior column: ischial tuberosity, greater and lesser sciatic notches, posterior wall and dome, and quadrilateral surface
  - Anterior column: lateral superior pubic ramus, iliopectineal eminence, anterior wall and dome, anterior ilium
- Corona mortise: anastomosis of external iliac (or deep epigastric) vessels and the obturator vessels (arising from the internal iliac vessels)
  - Present in 30 % of patients
  - At risk with lateral dissection along the superior pubic ramus
    - Typically located ~3 cm from the symphysis pubis.
    - Variable anomalous branches may be present.
  - Risk of life-threatening hemorrhage if injured

Imaging Studies

- AP pelvis: six cardinal lines
  - Iliopectineal line: radiographic representation of the anterior column
  - Ilioischial line: radiographic representation of the posterior column
  - Teardrop: radiographic representation of the medial acetabular wall

- Sourcil
- Anterior wall
- Posterior wall
- Shenton's line: not a cardinal line, helps detect occult hip dislocation

- Judet views (45° oblique views)
  - Obturator oblique: involved obturator foramen en face, anterior column, posterior wall
  - Iliac oblique: involved iliac wing en face, posterior column, anterior wall

- Roof arc angles: angle from a vertical line to the geometric center of the acetabulum to the point where the fracture line intersects the acetabulum on AP, obturator and iliac oblique views
  - If roof arc angle is >45°, fracture does not involve the weight-bearing dome.
  - CT correlate: fracture line >10 mm from the apex of the dome does not involve the weight-bearing surface
  - Cannot be applied to associated both-column fractures or posterior wall fractures (no intact portion of the acetabulum on which to base measurements).

- CT scan: assess articular surface involvement, marginal impaction, posterior wall size, incarcerated intra-articular fragments, preoperative planning
  - Vertical fracture line on axial CT: transverse or T-type fracture.
  - Horizontal fracture line on axial CT: column fracture.
  - 3D reconstruction with femoral head subtraction is a useful adjunct for some.

Letournel Classification

- Elementary
  - Posterior wall: most common acetabular fracture, gull sign on obturator oblique
  - Posterior column: increased risk of injury to superior gluteal neurovascular bundle
  - Anterior wall: rare
  - Anterior column: more common with low-energy fractures in the elderly
  - Transverse: only elementary fracture pattern that involves both columns, anterior to posterior directed fracture line on axial CT

- Associated
  - Posterior column posterior wall: only associated fracture pattern that does not involve both columns.
  - Anterior column posterior hemi-transverse: common in elderly patients.
  - Transverse posterior wall: most common associated fracture pattern.
  - T type: anterior to posterior fracture line on proximal axial CT scan with medial extension through the quadrilateral surface and the ischium distally.

- Associated both columns: most commonly associated acetabular fracture pattern; no part of the articular surface of the acetabulum remains in contact with the axial skeleton (via the sacroiliac joint), spur sign on obturator oblique represents the undisplaced intact posterior ilium.

Treatment

- Nonoperative management
  - Touchdown versus protected weight bearing for 8 weeks
    - Indications: nondisplaced and minimally displaced fracture (<1 mm step, <2 mm gap), roof arc angle >45°, posterior wall fragment <20 %, associated both columns with secondary congruence, severe comminution in the elderly with plan for total hip arthroplasty following fracture consolidation
  - Skeletal traction rarely indicated as definitive management
- Operative
  - Open reduction internal fixation
    - Indications: displacement with >1 mm step or 2 mm gap with roof arc angle <45° on any view, instability on stress exam of the hip, marginal impaction, incarcerated intra-articular fragments, irreducible fracture-dislocations
      - Posterior wall fracture 20–40 %: dynamic fluoroscopic examination under anesthesia to assess hip stability
      - Posterior wall fracture >40 %: presumed to be unstable
    - Relative contraindications: morbid obesity, low-demand elderly and nonambulatory patients, known DVT with contraindication to IVC filter, delay to surgery >3 weeks.
    - Approach determined by fracture pattern, may be combined.
    - Risks specific to surgical approach for ORIF
      - Kocher-Langenbeck: sciatic nerve injury, avascular necrosis of the femoral head
      - Ilioinguinal: femoral nerve injury, LFCN injury, femoral vessel thrombosis, corona mortis laceration
      - Extensile (extended iliofemoral, triradiate): heterotopic ossification, gluteal necrosis
    - Outcomes correlate with quality of articular reduction, hip muscle strength, and restoration of gait.
  - ORIF and acute total hip arthroplasty
    - Relative indications: age >60 years with superomedial dome impaction (gull sign), significant osteopenia and/or comminution, associated displaced femoral neck fracture, significant preexisting hip arthrosis

    - Up to 80 % construct survival at 10 years
    - Worse outcomes in males, patients <50 or >80 years of age, and significant acetabular defects
  - Percutaneous fixation with column screws
    - Indications: minimally displaced column fractures, column fractures in elderly and low-demand patients to facilitate early mobilization and weight bearing
    - Imaging
      - Obturator oblique: best to assess joint penetration.
      - Iliac oblique: assess clearance of the sciatic notch and start point for supra-acetabular screws on the apex of the posterior inferior iliac spine (PIIS).
      - Inlet iliac oblique: assess position of screw in the pubic ramus.
      - Inlet obturator oblique: assess position of screw within tables of the ilium.
      - Obturator outlet: assess start point for supra-acetabular screws.

Complications

- Posttraumatic arthrosis is the most common complication
  - Total hip arthroplasty, hip arthrodesis
    - Worse outcomes for total hip arthroplasty following acetabular fracture as compared to osteoarthritis
- Heterotopic ossification
  - Greatest risk with extensile surgical approaches, lowest risk with ilioinguinal approach.
    - Extended approaches: 20–50 %
    - Kocher-Langenbeck: 8–25 %
    - Anterior approach: 2–10 %
  - Prophylaxis: indomethacin ×5 weeks post-op, low-dose external-beam radiation of 600 cGy within 48 h of surgery.
  - Excision of the devitalized gluteal muscle at time of surgery may help decrease incidence and severity.
  - In severe cases where heterotopic ossification interferes with hip function, may consider excision once mature.
- Avascular necrosis
  - Increased risk with posterior fractures and approaches, fracture-dislocations, and iatrogenic injury to the medial femoral circumflex artery
- Thromboembolic disease
- High risk of DVT and PE

  - Chemical prophylaxis recommended for all patients unless specific contraindications exist
    - Place IVC filter if not contraindicated.
- Infection
  - Increased risk with associated Morel-Lavellée lesions (internal degloving)
- Bleeding
  - Early surgery may have greater blood loss; however increased delay to surgery results in longer operative times (reduction more difficult to obtain) with resulting increased blood loss.
  - Significant, potentially life-threatening, bleeding possible with injury to corona mortis vessels.
- Neurologic injury
  - Sciatic nerve injury
    - Increased risk of sciatic nerve injury (especially peroneal division) with associated posterior hip dislocation.
    - Maintain hip extension and knee flexion intraoperatively to reduce tension on the sciatic nerve.
  - Lateral femoral cutaneous nerve injury
    - Anterior approaches
- Hardware malposition
  - Intra-articular hardware, violation of sciatic notch
- Abductor muscle weakness
  - Posterior approach > anterior approach
- Chondrolysis
- Malreduction
  - Associated with increased delay to surgery
- Nonunion
  - Very rare

Bibliography

1. Engsberg JR, Steger-May K, Anglen JO, Borrelli J Jr. An analysis of gait changes and functional outcome in patients surgically treated for displaced acetabular fractures. J Orthop Trauma. 2009;23(5):346–53.
2. Gardner MJ, Nork SE. Stabilization of unstable pelvic fractures with supraacetabular compression external fixation. J Orthop Trauma. 2007;21(4):269–73.

3. Grimshaw CS, Moed BR. Outcomes of posterior wall fractures of the acetabulum treated nonoperatively after diagnostic screening with dynamic stress examination under anesthesia. J Bone Joint Surg Am. 2010;92(17):2792–800.
4. Jimenez ML, Tile M, Schenk RS. Total hip replacement after acetabular fracture. Orthop Clin North Am. 1997;28:435–46.
5. Kazemi N, Archdeacon MT. Immediate full weightbearing after percutaneous fixation of anterior column acetabular fractures. J Ortho Trauma. 2012;26(2):73–9.
6. Letournel E. Acetabulum fractures: classification and management. Clin Orthop Relat Res. 1980;151:81–106.
7. Miller MD, Thompson SR, Hart JA. Review of orthopaedics. 6th ed. Philadelphia: Elsevier; 2012. p. 738–43.
8. Starr AJ, Reinert CM, Jones AL. Percutaneous fixation of the columns of the acetabulum: a new technique. J Ortho Trauma. 1998;12(1):51–8.
9. Tornetta P 3rd. Displaced acetabular fractures: indications for operative and nonoperative management. J Am Acad Orthop Surg. 2001;9(1):18–28.
10. Tornetta P 3rd. Non-operative management of acetabular fractures. The use of dynamic stress views. J Bone Joint Surg Br. 1999;81(1):67–70.

3 Sacral Fractures

Take-Home Message

- Sacral fractures commonly comprise part of a pelvic ring injury.
- ~25 % associated neurologic injury with increased risk in transforaminal, medial/spinal canal, transverse, and U-type sacral fractures.
- Lower sacral nerve roots control the anal sphincter, bulbocavernosus reflex, and perianal sensation.
- Unilateral sacral nerve root function sufficient for bowel and bladder control.
- Vertical sacral fractures at increased risk for loss of reduction/fixation with resulting nonunion, malunion, and poor functional outcomes
- Sacral U fractures are unstable injuries that represent spinopelvic dissociation and require stabilization.
- Stable injuries with incomplete sacral fractures can mobilize as tolerated.
- Minimally displaced complete sacral fractures may be treated with protected weight bearing or surgical stabilization.
- Unstable, displaced sacral fractures should undergo reduction and stabilization ± decompression with careful technique to avoid iatrogenic nerve injury.

General

- Bimodal distribution, common in pelvic ring injuries
  - Young adults: high-energy trauma with MVC and fall from height most common
  - Elderly: low-energy falls, insufficiency fractures
- Neurologic injury in 25 %
  - Lower sacral root function: anal sphincter, bulbocavernosus reflex, perianal sensation.
  - Neurologic deficit is the most important predictor of outcome.
    - Unilateral sacral nerve root function sufficient for bowel and bladder control.

Imaging

- Radiographs demonstrate 30 % of sacral fractures.
  - AP pelvis: symmetry of foramina, associated L4 and L5 transverse process fractures.
  - Inlet view: sacral spinal canal, S1 body.
  - Outlet view: true AP of the sacrum; assess symmetry of the foramina.
  - Lateral view: kyphosis.
- CT scan study of choice to further delineate fracture pattern and help guide treatment.
- MRI is for cases with concern for neural compromise.

Denis Classification

- Zone I: alar fracture (lateral to the foramina)
  - 5 % neurologic injury, most commonly L5
- Zone II: transforaminal
  - 30 % neurologic injury, most commonly L5, S1, S2.
  - Vertical and shear-type fractures are highly unstable with increased risk of poor functional outcome.
- Zone III: medial to the foramina into the spinal canal
  - 60 % neurologic injury, most commonly the caudal nerve roots with bowel, bladder, and sexual dysfunction.
  - Unilateral sacral root preservation is sufficient for bowel/bladder control.

Transverse Fractures

- High incidence of neurologic injury

Sacral U Fracture

- High incidence of neurologic injury
- Typically results from axial loading
- Unstable injuries, often with kyphosis through the fracture, that represent spino-pelvic dissociation and require surgical stabilization

Treatment Principles

- Nonoperative: stable and minimally displaced fractures
  - Weight bearing as tolerated: incomplete sacral fractures where the intact sacrum remains in continuity with the ilium, neurologically intact
    - Anterior impaction sacral fractures with LC mechanism, isolated sacral ala fractures
  - Toe-touch weight bearing: consider in complete sacral fractures with minimal displacement.
  - Post-mobilization x-rays to assess for subsequent displacement.
- Operative
  - Open reduction internal fixation ± decompression
    - Displaced fractures (>1 cm), displacement of fracture with trial of non-operative management, foraminal compromise, unstable fracture patterns
    - Percutaneous sacroiliac screws, posterior tension band plating, transiliac sacral bars, lumbopelvic fixation
    - Open decompression considered for transforaminal fractures with neurologic injury and sacral U fractures with kyphosis and compromise of the spinal canal

Complications

- Neurologic deficit is the most important predictor of outcome
  - Lower extremity deficits, bowel/bladder dysfunction, sexual dysfunction
  - Nerve compromise at the time of injury
  - Risk of iatrogenic nerve injury with implant malposition and overcompression of fractures involving the sacral foramina
- Malunion/nonunion
  - Vertical sacral fractures at increased risk for loss of fixation/reduction with resulting malunion, nonunion, and poor functional outcomes
- Thromboembolic disease
- Chronic low back pain

Bibliography

1. Denis F, Davis S, Comfort T. Sacral fractures: an important problem. Retrospective analysis of 236 cases. Clin Orthop Relat Res. 1988;227:67–81.
2. Mehta S, Auerbach JD, Born CT, Chin KR. Sacral fractures. J Am Acad Orthop Surg. 2006;14(12):656–65 (Review).
3. Miller MD, Thompson SR, Hart JA. Review of orthopaedics. 6th ed. Philadelphia: Elsevier; 2012. p. 738.
4. Robles LA. Transverse sacral fractures. Spine J. 2009;9(1):60–9. Epub 2007 Nov 5. Review.

4 Hip Dislocations

Take-Home Message

- High-energy trauma; position of the hip at the time of injury determines the direction of the dislocation and risk of associated injuries.
- Hip dislocations require emergent closed reduction within 6 h to decrease the risk of avascular necrosis.
- If closed reduction is not possible, proceed to the operating room in urgent fashion for open reduction.
- Obtain a postreduction CT scan to assess for associated fracture and incarcerated fragments.
- Commonly associated injuries include acetabular fractures, femoral head fractures, labral tears, sciatic nerve injury, and ipsilateral knee injuries.

General

- Typically occur in young adults following high-energy trauma.
  - Axial loading; position of the hip determines the direction of the dislocation.
  - 90 % of hip dislocations are posterior.
- High incidence of associated injuries
  - Acetabular fractures (posterior wall fracture, marginal impaction), femoral head fractures, chondral injury, labral tears (30 %), sciatic nerve injury, ipsilateral knee injuries (25 %)

Imaging

- AP pelvis: dislocated femoral head appears smaller than the contralateral side (posterior dislocation); discontinuity of Shenton's line; carefully assess femoral neck for possible fracture.
- Lateral hip: confirm direction of dislocation.

- Postreduction AP pelvis and lateral hip to confirm reduction; consider Judet views to further evaluate for possible associated acetabular fracture.
- Postreduction CT scan mandatory: assess for loose bodies, incarcerated fragments, femoral head fracture, and acetabular fracture.
- MRI may be useful in follow-up to further evaluate concern for subsequent avascular necrosis or labral injury.

Classification

- Simple: hip dislocation with no associated fracture
- Complex: hip dislocation with associated acetabular or proximal femur fracture
- Anatomic classification
  - Posterior dislocation (90 %)
    - Hip flexed, adducted, and internally rotated
    - "Dashboard injury"
    - Associated injuries: posterior wall fracture, anterior femoral head fracture, ipsilateral knee injury
      - Increased hip flexion and internal rotation at the time of injury decreases the risk of associated fracture.
  - Anterior dislocation
    - Hip extended, abducted, and externally rotated
    - Associated injuries: impaction fracture, chondral injury
  - Obturator dislocation

Treatment

- Nonoperative
  - Emergent closed reduction within 6 h; evaluate hip stability postreduction
    - Closed reduction contraindicated with ipsilateral femoral neck fractures
  - Weight bearing as tolerated vs protected weight bearing for 4–6 weeks: stable hip without associated injuries.
  - Consider traction and/or abduction pillow for unstable hips or associated injuries requiring further intervention.
- Operative
  - Open reduction ± removal of incarcerated fragments
    - Irreducible hip dislocation, incarcerated fragments, incongruent reduction
  - Open reduction internal fixation
    - Associated acetabular, femoral head, and femoral neck fractures.
      - Femoral neck fracture should be stabilized prior to reduction.

  - Hip arthroscopy
    - May be used to remove incarcerated fragments

Complications

- Avascular necrosis: 10–20 %
  - Increased risk with delay to reduction
- Posttraumatic arthritis
- Sciatic nerve injury: 10–20 %
  - Peroneal division most common
  - Increased risk with delay to reduction
- Rare recurrent dislocation

Bibliography

1. Miller MD, Thompson SR, Hart JA. Review of orthopaedics. 6th ed. Philadelphia: Elsevier; 2012. p. 743–4.
2. Schmidt GL, Sciulli R, Altman GT. Knee injury in patients experiencing a high-energy traumatic ipsilateral hip dislocation. J Bone Joint Surg Am. 2005; 87:1200–4.
3. Tornetta P 3rd, Mostafavi HR. Hip dislocation: current treatment regimens. J Am Acad Orthop Surg. 1997;5(1):27–36.

5 Femoral Head Fractures

Take-Home Message

- Typically associated with hip dislocations with position of the hip at the time of dislocation, determining the location and size of the femoral head fracture.
- Treatment goals are to restore congruity of the weight-bearing portion of the femoral head, restore hip stability, remove incarcerated fragments, and address associated femoral head and acetabular fractures appropriately.
- Smith-Peterson approach favored when possible for not increasing the risk of AVN and providing good access to most femoral head fractures.
- Risk of AVN greatest in Pipkin III fractures as related to the degree of displacement of the associated femoral neck fracture.
- Increased risk of AVN with delay to reduction of associated hip dislocation.
- May consider arthroplasty in older patients and significantly comminuted fractures not amenable to primary reconstruction.

General

- Femoral head fractures are rare injuries that typically occur in combination with hip dislocations,
  - High-energy mechanism: MVC, fall from height.
  - The position of the hip at the time of dislocation determines the location and size of the femoral head fracture.
- Posterior hip dislocations: 5–15 % associated femoral head fracture
- Anterior hip dislocations: associated with impaction fractures of the femoral head
- Associated injuries: femoral neck fracture, acetabular fracture, sciatic nerve injury, femoral head avascular necrosis, ipsilateral knee injury (dashboard)
- Primary blood supply to the femoral head in adults: medial femoral circumflex artery

Imaging

- AP pelvis and lateral hip: assess for symmetry, femoral head fracture, and hip dislocation; obtain pre- and postreduction.
- Judet views: assess for associated acetabular fracture.
- Postreduction CT scan: assess for concentric reduction, incarcerated fragments, associated femoral neck, and acetabular fractures.

Pipkin Classification

- Type I: infrafoveal fracture, below the weight-bearing surface of the femoral head
- Type II: suprafoveal fracture, involves the weight-bearing surface of the femoral head
- Type III: type I or II plus femoral neck fracture
- Type IV: type I, II, or III plus acetabular fracture

Treatment

- Nonoperative
  - Emergent closed reduction of hip fractures within 6 h (see Sect. 4 above)
  - Touchdown weight bearing for 4–6 weeks, hip dislocation precautions
    - Pipkin I fractures, nondisplaced Pipkin II fractures
      - Follow closely with serial radiographs to assess for subsequent displacement of initially nondisplaced Pipkin II fractures.
- Operative
  - Open reduction internal fixation
    - Displaced Pipkin II fractures ± associated acetabular or femoral neck fractures (Pipkin III, Pipkin IV), irreducible fracture-dislocation, incarcerated fragments.

    - Smith-Peterson approach preferred, no associated increased risk of AVN, facilitates reduction and fixation as femoral head fractures are often anteromedial.
        - Worse outcomes for fractures addressed via a Kocher-Langenbeck approach.
    - Treat associated acetabular fractures according to the type of acetabular fracture.
  - Arthroplasty
    - Consider in femoral head fractures in older patients, particularly with significant displacement, comminution, and osteoporosis.

Complications

- Avascular necrosis in up to 25 %
  - Highest incidence of AVN in Pipkin III injuries
    - Rate of AVN increases with increasing displacement of the femoral neck fracture.
  - Increased risk with delay to reduction of dislocated hip
- Sciatic nerve injury in 10–25 %
  - Related to associated hip dislocation
  - Involvement of peroneal division most common
- Posttraumatic arthritis in 10–75 %
  - Cartilage damage at the time of injury
  - Joint incongruity/imperfect reduction
- Heterotopic ossification in 5–65 %
  - May consider adjunctive therapy (radiation, indomethacin) at time of surgery in patients at increased risk (head injury)

Bibliography

1. Droll KP, Broekhuyse H, O'Brien P. Fracture of the femoral head. J Am Acad Orthop Surg. 2007;15(12):716–27 (Review).
2. Miller MD, Thompson SR, Hart JA. Review of orthopaedics. 6th ed. Philadelphia: Elsevier; 2012. p. 744–6.

6 Femoral Neck Fractures

Take-Home Message

- High-energy femoral neck fractures are more likely to be vertical and associated with femoral shaft fractures.
- Depending on fracture characteristics, patient age, functional status, and comorbidities, femoral neck fractures may be treated with cannulated screws, sliding hip screw, hip hemiarthroplasty, and total hip arthroplasty.
- Increased risk of avascular necrosis with increased initial displacement, nonanatomic reduction, and increasing patient age.
- Increased risk of nonunion with displaced fractures, vertically oriented fractures, varus malreduction, and cannulated screw fixation.
- Quality of reduction is more important than time to reduction.
- Cannulated screws should begin above the lesser trochanter to decrease the risk of peri-implant subtrochanteric fracture.
- Hemiarthroplasty has a lower risk of dislocation compared to total hip arthroplasty.
- Active elderly patients have improved functional outcomes with total hip arthroplasty.
- Mortality at 1 year in elderly patients is 15–35 %.
- Pre-injury cognitive function and mobility are the more important determinants of postoperative functional outcome.

General

- Bimodal distribution
  - Young: high-energy injuries
    - More likely to have a vertically oriented fracture and associated femoral shaft fracture
  - Elderly: low-energy injuries
    - Increasing incidence with the aging population.
    - More common in women and Caucasians.
    - Elderly patients should proceed to the OR as soon as medically ready to allow early mobilization.
- Associated injuries
  - 5–10 % of femoral shaft fractures have an associated femoral neck fracture.
  - ~30 % of femoral neck fractures associated with femoral shaft fractures are missed upon initial presentation.

- Healing potential
  - Intracapsular fractures bathed in synovial fluid with no periosteum.
  - Displaced femoral neck fractures will disrupt the blood supply.
    - Primary blood supply: lateral epiphyseal artery arising from the medial femoral circumflex artery.
  - Impact of intracapsular hematoma is debated.

Imaging

- AP pelvis, AP and cross-table lateral of the hip, full-length femur films
  - Obtain AP films with the legs in internal rotation to adjust for femoral neck anteversion.
  - Assess orientation of trabecular lines and displacement.
- Consider contralateral hip films for arthroplasty templating.
- Traction views may be helpful in some cases.
- CT scan is helpful to further assess displacement and comminution in some cases.
- MRI is the study of choice to evaluate for occult fracture.

Classification

- Garden classification
  - Type I: incomplete, valgus impacted
  - Type II: complete, nondisplaced
  - Type III: complete, 50 % displaced
  - Type IV: complete, >50 % displaced
- Pauwels classification
  - Increasing vertical orientation increases shear forces across the fracture, which increases the risk of nonunion and fixation failure.
  - Type I: <30° verticality
  - Type II: 30–50° verticality
  - Type III: >50° verticality
- Stress fractures
  - Tension side (superior neck): high risk for fracture completion; treat with surgical stabilization.
  - Compression side (inferior neck): lower risk for fracture completion, may treat with protected weight bearing.

Treatment

- Nonoperative
  - Observation
    - May consider in valgus impacted fractures in older patients, nonambulators, and patients at excessively high surgical risk

- Leadbetter maneuver for closed reduction of femoral neck fractures
  - Hip flexion to 90°, adduction, traction.
  - Then internally rotate to 45° while maintaining traction.
  - Then bring the leg into slight abduction and full extension while maintaining traction and internal rotation.
  - Typically proceed with surgical fixation and formal open reduction if fracture is not adequately reduced.

- Operative
  - Open reduction internal fixation
    - Indications: young (<50) and physiologically young patients with nondisplaced and displaced fractures, older patients with nondisplaced fractures
      - Considered a surgical emergency in young patients.
      - Quality of reduction is the most important factor impacting outcome.
        - Posterior translation or angulation of the femoral head leads to increased reoperation rates.
    - Cannulated screws
      - Start point at or above the level of the lesser trochanter to avoid generating a stress riser that propagates into a subtrochanteric femur fracture.
      - Minimize cortical passes when placing guide wires to minimize additional lateral stress risers.
      - 3-screw inverted triangle along calcar; consider 4 screws for posterior comminution.
    - Sliding hip screw ± derotational screw
      - Sliding permits dynamic compression of the fracture with axial loading and can facilitate fracture healing.
      - Sliding/compression may result in shortening of the femoral neck and may make implants prominent and/or affect joint biomechanics.
  - Hip hemiarthroplasty
    - Advocated for displaced fractures in older debilitated patients, demented patients (unable to comply with hip precautions), patients with neuromuscular disorders.
    - Outcomes for cemented technique superior to uncemented.
    - Posterior approach has increased risk of dislocation, while approach has increased risk of abductor weakness.
  - Total hip arthroplasty
    - Advocated for displaced fractures in older active patients, patients with preexisting hip arthropathy
    - Higher risk of dislocation

Complications

- Avascular necrosis in 10–40 %
  - Increased risk with increased initial displacement, nonanatomic reduction, and increasing patient age.
  - Quality of reduction is more important than time to reduction.
  - Importance of decompressing intracapsular hematoma is controversial.
  - Treatment
    - Young symptomatic patients: core decompression (controversial), free vascularized fibula graft, total hip arthroplasty, hip arthrodesis
    - Elderly symptomatic patients: prosthetic replacement
- Nonunion in 10–30 %
  - Increased risk with displaced fractures, varus malreduction, and cannulated screw fixation.
  - Tend to be more symptomatic than AVN and will require intervention.
  - Consider MRI to evaluate for concurrent AVN.
  - Treatment
    - Young patients: valgus intertrochanteric osteotomy (converts shear forces into compression forces across the fracture), free vascularized fibula graft, total hip arthroplasty, hip arthrodesis
    - Elderly patients: prosthetic replacement
- Dislocation
  - Higher risk of dislocation for THA vs hemiarthroplasty
  - ~10 % incidence for THA performed for femoral neck fracture
- Mortality
  - 1-year mortality 15–35 %.
  - Pre-injury cognitive function and mobility are the most important determinants of postoperative functional outcome and survival.
  - Increased mortality in patients to undergo surgical fixation/replacement >48 h after injury.

Bibliography

1. Dedrick DK, Mackenzie JR, Burney RE. Complications of femoral neck fracture in young adults. J Trauma. 1986;26(10):932–7.
2. Gurusamy K, Parker MJ, Rowlands TK. The complications of displaced intracapsular fractures of the hip: the effect of screw positioning and angulation on fracture healing. J Bone Joint Surg Br. 2005;87(5):632–4.
3. Haidukewych GJ, Rothwell WS, Jacofsky DJ, Torchia ME, Berry DJ. Operative treatment of femoral neck fractures in patients between the ages of fifteen and fifty years. J Bone Joint Surg Am. 2004;86:1711–6.

4. Holt EM, Evans RA, Hindley CJ, Metcalfe JW. 1000 femoral neck fractures: the effect of pre-injury mobility and surgical experience on outcome. Injury. 1994; 25(2):91–5.
5. Keating JF, Grant A, Masson M, Scott NW, Forbes JF. Randomized comparison of reduction and fixation, bipolar hemiarthroplasty, and total hip arthroplasty. Treatment of displaced intracapsular hip fractures in healthy older patients. J Bone Joint Surg Am. 2006;88(2):249–60.
6. Miller MD, Thompson SR, Hart JA. Review of orthopaedics. 6th ed. Philadelphia: Elsevier; 2012. p. 746–7.
7. Peljovich AE, Patterson BM. Ipsilateral femoral neck and shaft fractures. J Am Acad Orthop Surg. 1998;6:106–13.

7 Intertrochanteric Hip Fractures

Take-Home Message

- Fragility fractures in the elderly typically resulting from low-energy falls, sequelae of high-energy trauma in the young.
- MRI is the study of choice to evaluate for occult fracture.
- Stability related to size and location of lesser trochanteric fragment and integrity of the lateral femoral cortex.
- Sliding hip screw indicated for fixation of most intertrochanteric fractures; expectations include reverse obliquity fracture, subtrochanteric fractures, and fractures with disruption of the lateral femoral cortex.
- Cephalomedullary nails indicated for fixation of most intertrochanteric fractures; long nails should be used for reverse obliquity and subtrochanteric fractures.
- Lowest risk of implant failure/cutout with tip-apex distance <25 mm.
- Sliding hip screws more likely to have excessive collapse and medialization which can alter hip mechanics.
- Cephalomedullary nails associated with increased risk of peri-implant fracture, although less common with modern designs.
- Mortality rates of 15–35 % at 1 year.
- Delay to surgery >48 h associated with increased risk of mortality at 1 year.
- ASA classification predicts mortality.

General

- Extracapsular hip fractures between the greater and lesser trochanters
- Bimodal distribution
  - Elderly: low-energy falls, osteoporosis
    - More common in women
    - Increased risk with osteoporosis, history of prior hip fracture, and history of falls
    - Patients typically older than those sustaining femoral neck fractures
  - Young: high-energy trauma

Imaging

- AP pelvis, AP hip, cross-table lateral of the hip, full-length femur films.
- Traction views may be helpful to further delineate fracture pattern in some cases.
- Isolated fracture of the lesser trochanter should be considered pathologic until proven otherwise.
- MRI is the study of choice to evaluate for occult fracture.

Classification

- Stability (once reduced)
  - Stable: resist medial compressive loads
  - Unstable: risk of varus collapse, medial shaft translation
- Number of parts
  - Two-part fracture: typically stable, low risk of collapse.
  - Three-part fracture: intermediate stability determined by size and location of lesser trochanter fragment; large posteromedial fragments are less stable.
  - Four-part fracture: comminuted, unstable fractures at increased risk for shortening, varus collapse, and nonunion.

Treatment

- Nonoperative
  - Touchdown weight bearing for 6–8 weeks, early mobilization
    - Nonambulatory patients, excessively high perioperative mortality risk, patients who desire comfort measures only.
    - High rates of pneumonia, thromboembolic disease, urinary tract infections, and decubitus ulcers.
    - Surgical fixation may be considered in nonambulatory patients for pain control and/or palliation.
- Operative
  - Internal fixation is indicated for nearly all intertrochanteric fractures.
  - Goal of operative management is to restore neck-shaft alignment and translation.

- Medial displacement osteotomy has no proven benefit.
- Sliding hip screw
  - Dynamic interfragmentary compression with axial loading
  - Goal for center-center screw position, tip-apex distance <25 mm associated with lowest screw failure rate
    - Consider mild valgus overreduction for unstable fracture patterns.
    - Risk of extension deformity when fixing left hip fractures from torque forces on screw insertion.
  - Contraindicated in reverse obliquity fractures, subtrochanteric fractures, and fractures without an intact lateral femoral cortex.
- Cephalomedullary nail
  - Resists excessive fracture collapse and medicalization as the IM nail reconstitutes the lateral buttress
  - Short nails indicated for standard obliquity fractures
  - Long nails indicated for standard obliquity fractures, reverse obliquity fractures, and subtrochanteric fractures
  - Goal for center-center position with tip-apex distance <25 mm for single lag screw or helical blade
  - Increased risk of peri-implant fracture and screw cutout compared to sliding hip screws
- 95 blade plate/proximal femoral locking plate
  - Indicated for reverse obliquity fractures, severely comminuted fractures, and nonunion repair.
    - Proximal femoral locking plates have an increased risk of nonunion when used for primary fracture repair.
- Arthroplasty
  - May consider in severely comminuted fractures, preexisting hip arthropathy, salvage of failed surgical fixation
  - Typically requires a calcar replacing prosthesis
  - Attempt fixation of the greater trochanter to the shaft

Complications

- Excessive collapse with limb shortening and medicalization
  - Reduces abductor moment arm, alters hip mechanics, and may result in functional deficits
  - More collapse with sliding hip screws compared to cephalomedullary nails and with greater displacement of the lesser trochanter
- Implant failure and cutout
  - Most common complication, typically within 3 months of surgical fixation

  - Young: revision ORIF, corrective osteotomy
  - Elderly: arthroplasty

- Peri-implant fracture
  - More common with cephalomedullary nail fixation compared to sliding hip screws.
  - Implant design changes have decreased the risk of peri-implant fractures
    - Tapered end of the nail, smaller distal interlock screws, reduced trochanteric bend
  - Anterior perforation of the distal femoral cortex with cephalomedullary nail
    - Radius of curvature mismatch between the femur and the implant
- Nonunion in <2 %
  - Treat with revision ORIF ± bone grafting, arthroplasty ±.
  - Calcar replacing prosthesis or proximal femoral replacement
- Malunion
  - Varus and rotational deformity
  - May consider corrective osteotomy if very symptomatic
- Mortality
  - 1-year mortality rate 20–30 %.
  - Surgery within 48 h provided medically ready improves 1-year mortality outcomes.
  - ASA classification predicts mortality.

Bibliography

1. Barton TM, Gleeson R, Topliss C, Greenwood R, Harries WJ, Chesser TJ. A comparison of the long gamma nail with the sliding hip screw for the treatment of AO/OTA 31-A2 fractures of the proximal part of the femur: a prospective randomized trial. J Bone Joint Surg Am. 2010;92(4):792–8.
2. Baumgaertner MR, Curtin SL, Lindskog DM, Keggi JM. The value of the tip-apex distance in predicting failure of fixation of peritrochanteric fractures of the hip. J Bone Joint Surg Am. 1995;77(7):1058–64.
3. Bolhofner BR, Russo PR, Carmen B. Results of intertrochanteric femur fractures treated with a 135-degree sliding screw with a two-hole side plate. J Orthop Trauma. 1999;13:5–8.
4. Gotfried Y. The lateral trochanteric wall: a key element in the reconstruction of unstable peritrochanteric hip fractures. Clin Orthop Relat Res. 2004;425:82–6.
5. Miller MD, Thompson SR, Hart JA. Review of orthopaedics. 6th ed. Philadelphia: Elsevier; 2012. p. 747–8.
6. Mohan R, Karthikeyan R, Sonanis SV. Dynamic hip screw: does side make a difference? Effects of clockwise torque on right and left DHS. Injury. 2000;31(9):697–9.

7. Sadowski C, Lübbeke A, Saudan M, Riand N, Stern R, Hoffmeyer P. Treatment of reverse oblique and transverse intertrochanteric fractures with use of an intramedullary nail or a 95 degrees screw-plate: a prospective, randomized study. J Bone Joint Surg Am. 2002;84-A(3):372–81.
8. Zuckerman JD, Skovron ML, Koval KJ, Aharonoff G, Frankel VH. Postoperative complications and mortality associated with operative delay in older patients who have a fracture of the hip. J Bone Joint Surg Am. 1995;77(10):1551–6.

8 Subtrochanteric Femur Fractures

Take-Home Message

- Proximal fragment pulled into abduction, flexion, and external rotation by the gluteus medius and minimus, iliopsoas, and short external rotators, respectively.
- Bisphosphonate-associated fractures may have preceding thigh pain and are characterized by beaking of the lateral femoral cortex, transverse fracture patterns, and a medial spike. Consider screening and even prophylactic fixation of the contralateral side in bisphosphonate-associated fractures.
- Varus and procurvatum (flexion) is the most pattern of malreduction.
- Piriformis entry nails better resist varus deformity compared to lateral entry nails.
- Increased risk of nonunion in bisphosphonate-associated fractures and varus malreduction.
- Nonunions often treated with conversion to fixed-angle plate with compression.

General

- Proximal femur fractures from the lesser trochanter to 5 cm distally
  - Proximal fragment deforming forces: gluteus medius and minimus → abduction, iliopsoas → flexion, short external rotators → external rotation
  - Distal fragment deforming forces: adductors → adduction and shortening
- Bimodal distribution
  - Young: high-energy trauma
  - Elderly: low-energy falls

- May be associated with prolonged bisphosphonate use
  - "Fosamax fractures," beaking of lateral femoral cortex, transverse fracture pattern, medial spike, history of preceding thigh pain
  - Screen for involvement of the contralateral side and consider prophylactic fixation if there is concern for bisphosphonate-associated fractures

Imaging

- AP pelvis, AP/lateral hip, AP/lateral femur films
- Dedicated films of the contralateral side warranted if bisphosphonate-associated fracture is suspected

Russell-Taylor Classification

- Type IA: fracture below the lesser trochanter
- Type IB: fracture involves the lesser trochanter, greater trochanter intact
- Type IIA: greater trochanter involved, lesser trochanter intact
- Type IIB: greater and lesser trochanters involved

Treatment

- Nonoperative
  - Observation, comfort care
    - Nonambulatory patients who have exceedingly high risk of perioperative mortality
- Operative
  - Surgical fixation indicated in nearly all patients
  - Intramedullary nail
    - Load-sharing implant, stronger construct for unstable fractures.
    - Intramedullary fixation has a lower reoperation rate at 1 year than fixed-angle plate fixation.
    - Stand proximal locking for fractures with intact lesser trochanter.
    - Reconstruction interlocking for fracture with involvement of the lesser trochanter.
    - Piriformis entry nails better resist varus malreduction; contraindicated in fractures involving the piriformis fossa.
    - Lateral nailing: easier reduction of flexion deformity, facilitates obtaining start point – particularly for piriformis entry nails.
    - Supine nailing: may be indicated in spine-injured and polytrauma patients, easier to assess correction of external rotation deformity.

  Fixed-angle device with side plate

    - Weaker construct, increased risk of varus collapse.
    - Blade plate may function as a tension band construct, converting tensile forces on the lateral cortex to compressive forces on the medial cortex.
    - May consider in fractures with significant proximal comminution, preexisting femoral shaft deformity, or nonunion.

Complications

- High rates of implant failure
- Nonunion
  - Increased risk in bisphosphonate-associated fractures and varus malreduction
  - Often treated with conversion to fixed-angle plate with compression
- Malunion: varus and procurvatum (flexion)

Bibliography

1. Bellabarba C, Ricci WM, Bolhofner BR. Results of indirect reduction and plating of femoral shaft nonunions after intramedullary nailing. J Orthop Trauma. 2001;15(4):254–63.
2. Kinast C, Bolhofner BR, Mast JW, Ganz R. Subtrochanteric fractures of the femur. Results of treatment with the 95 degrees condylar blade-plate. Clin Orthop Relat Res. 1989;238:122–30.
3. Lundy DW. Subtrochanteric femoral fractures. J Am Acad Orthop Surg. 2007;15(11):663–71 (Review).
4. Miller MD, Thompson SR, Hart JA. Review of orthopaedics. 6th ed. Philadelphia: Elsevier; 2012. p. 748–9.
5. Ricci WM, Bellabarba C, Lewis R. Angular malalignment after intramedullary nailing of femoral shaft fractures. J Orthop Trauma. 2001;15(2):90–5.
6. Weil YA, Rivkin G, Safran O, Liebergall M, Foldes AJ. The outcome of surgically treated femur fractures associated with long-term bisphosphonate use. J Trauma. 2011;71(1):186–90.

9 Femoral Shaft Fractures

Take-Home Message

- Reamed intramedullary nails are the treatment of choice for nearly all femoral shaft fractures.
- Anterior start point in piriformis entry nails increases hoop stresses and risk of iatrogenic fracture. Piriformis entry nail contraindicated in skeletally immature patients (increased risk of osteonecrosis) and in fractures that involves the piriformis fossa.
- Maintain a high index of suspicion for associated femoral neck fracture – present in up to 10 % of femoral shaft fractures, often nondisplaced, vertical, and basicervical.
- Prioritize fixation of associated femoral neck fractures, when present. Fixation of combined femoral neck and shaft fractures with separate

devices recommended as fixation with a single device increases the risk of malreduction of at least one of the fractures.
- Polytrauma patients, particular those with significant head and chest injuries, may benefit from damage control strategies with initial external fixation and safe conversion to intramedullary nail up to 3 weeks later.
- Comminuted femur fractures are at increased risk for malrotation and leg length discrepancy – compare to the contralateral limb.
- Nonunions may be treated with exchange reamed nailing or conversion to plate fixation ± bone grafting.

General

- Mechanism
  - High-energy injuries in young patients are most common.
    - High incidence of associated injuries.
    - Ipsilateral femoral neck fracture in 5–10 % of femoral shaft fractures, increased incidence in comminuted midshaft fractures; up to 30 % of these are missed on presentation.
      - Prioritize treatment of neck fractures.
        - Often nondisplaced, vertical, and basicervical.
        - Decreased risk of malunion of concurrent ipsilateral femoral neck and shaft fractures when separate devices are used for fixation.
        - Favored constructs include cannulated screw or sliding hip screw fixation of the femoral neck fracture with retrograde nail of plate fixation of the femoral shaft fracture.
    - Bilateral femur fractures have increased risk of complications.
    - Critical to avoid hypotension in patients with closed head injuries to prevent second hit. May benefit from delay to definitive fixation.
  - Low-energy injuries in the elderly
    - Fall from standing
- Early stabilization associated with: decreased pulmonary and thromboembolic complications, improved rehabilitation, decreased hospital costs

Imaging

- AP and lateral femur
- AP and lateral hip: assess for associated femoral neck fractures AP and lateral knee.
- CT scan: frequently obtained in the work-up of polytrauma patients; assess carefully for occult femoral neck fracture.

Winquist-Hansen Classification

- Based on degree of comminution and cortical continuity
- Type 0: no comminution
- Type I: comminution <25 %
- Type II: comminution 25–50 %, >50 % cortical contact
- Type III: comminution >50 %, <50 % cortical contact
- Type IV: segmental fracture with no contact between proximal and distal fragments

Treatment

- Nonoperative
  - Splint or cast immobilization
    - Rarely indicated; consider in nonambulatory patients and patients with excessively high risk of perioperative mortality
- Operative
  - External fixation
    - Indicated as a damage control measure in polytrauma patients (particularly with head and/or pulmonary injuries), open fractures with severe soft tissue injury, fractures with associated vascular injury
    - May be safely converted to intramedullary fixation without increased risk of infection or nonunion up to 3 weeks from the time of external fixation
  - Plate fixation
    - May elect to employ in specific circumstances (neck-shaft fractures, periprosthetic fractures)
    - Increased risk of infection, nonunion, and implant failure, delay to weight bearing
  - Intramedullary nailing
    - Treatment of choice for nearly all femoral shaft fractures is a reamed intramedullary nail.
    - Unreamed nails associated with increased time to union and increased risk of nonunion.
    - Piriformis entry nails contraindicated when fracture extends into the piriformis fossa and in skeletally immature patients (increased risk of osteonecrosis).
      - Anterior start point increases hoop stresses and risks iatrogenic comminution.
    - In polytrauma patients, there is no specific relationship between pulmonary complications and timing of femur fracture fixation.

    - The severity of injury, not the time of femur fracture fixation, determines pulmonary outcome.

  - Retrograde nailing

    - Indications: obesity, ipsilateral femoral neck fracture/knee arthrotomy/tibial shaft fracture, bilateral femur fractures

Complications

- Infection

  - Rare, <1 % of closed fractures
  - Intramedullary reaming with exchange nail or removal of implants pending status of fracture healing
  - No increased risk of infection with immediate nailing of open fractures following debridement

- Nonunion

  - Rare, <2 % of closed fractures
  - Increased risk in smokers and heavy postoperative use of NSAIDS
  - Exchange reamed nailing, conversion to plate fixation ± bone grafting

- Malunion

  - Nailing technique associated with specific malunion risk

    - Supine: increased risk of internal rotation
    - Lateral: increased risk of external rotation
    - Traction/fracture table: increased risk of lengthening and internal rotation
    - No traction: increased risk of shortening in comminuted fractures

  - Increased risk of malreduction with

    - Retrograde nailing of proximal fractures
    - Antegrade nailing of distal fractures

  - Malrotation difficult to assess, particularly with comminuted fractures

    - Compare to contralateral side (when intact).

  - Leg length discrepancy more likely in comminuted fractures

    - Compare to contralateral side (when intact).
    - Lengthening or shortening along the anatomical axis leads to mechanical axis deviation.

- Delayed union

  - Exchange reamed nailing has higher success rate than dynamization.

- Heterotopic ossification
  - ~25 %, rarely of clinical significance
  - Typically involves the abductors with reaming for antegrade nail insertion
- Pudendal nerve palsy
  - Perineal post pressure
  - Prolonged traction

Bibliography

1. Bedi A, Karunakar MA, Caron T, Sanders RW, Haidukewych GJ. Accuracy of reduction of ipsilateral femoral neck and shaft fractures – an analysis of various internal fixation strategies. J Orthop Trauma. 2009;23(4):249–53.
2. Canadian Orthopaedic Trauma Society. Nonunion following intramedullary nailing of the femur with and without reaming. Results of a multicenter randomized clinical trial. J Bone Joint Surg Am. 2003;85-A(11): 2093–6.
3. Hak DJ, Lee SS, Goulet JA. Success of exchange reamed intramedullary nailing for femoral shaft nonunion or delayed union. J Orthop Trauma. 2000;14(3): 178–82.
4. Jaarsma RL, van Kampen A. Rotational malalignment after fractures of the femur. J Bone Joint Surg Br. 2004;86(8):1100–4.
5. Kobbe P, Micansky F, Lichte P, Sellei RM, Pfeifer R, Dombroski D, Lefering R, Pape HC, TraumaRegister DGU. Increased morbidity and mortality after bilateral femoral shaft fractures: myth or reality in the era of damage control? Injury. 2013;44(2):221–5.
6. McKee MD, Schemitsch EH, Vincent LO, Sullivan I, Yoo D. The effect of a femoral fracture on concomitant closed head injury in patients with multiple injuries. J Trauma. 1997;42(6):1041–5.
7. Miller MD, Thompson SR, Hart JA. Review of orthopaedics. 6th ed. Philadelphia: Elsevier; 2012. p. 749–51.
8. Ostrum RF, Agarwal A, Lakatos R, Poka A. Prospective comparison of retrograde and antegrade femoral intramedullary nailing. J Orthop Trauma. 2000; 14(7):496–501.
9. Peljovich AE, Patterson BM. Ipsilateral femoral neck and shaft fractures. J Am Acad Orthop Surg. 1998;6(2):106–13.
10. Stephen DJ, Kreder HJ, Schemitsch EH, Conlan LB, Wild L, McKee MD. Femoral intramedullary nailing: comparison of fracture-table and manual traction. a prospective, randomized study. J Bone Joint Surg Am. 2002; 84-A(9):1514–21.

10 Distal Femur Fractures

Take-Home Message

- Obtain CT scan if concerned for intercondylar extension or to further characterize fracture with obvious intercondylar extension.
- Coronal plane fractures (Hoffa fractures) present in 40–30 % of intercondylar fractures; 80 % of these involved the lateral condyle.
- Most distal femur fractures are stabilized with fixed-angle plates. Retrograde intramedullary nails may be used for extra-articular fractures and simple intra-articular fractures.
- Slight compression and shortening through the metaphysis and/or metadiaphysis may help decrease the risk of nonunion in osteoporotic bone.
- Prominent medial screws are poorly tolerated. As the distal femur narrows posteriorly, obtain a 30° internal rotation view to ensure proper screw length.

General

- Femur fracture from 5 cm above the distal metaphyseal flare to the distal articular surface
- Bimodal distribution
  - Young: high-energy injury, typically more displaced
  - Elderly: low-energy injury, typically less displaced
- Increased risk for vascular injury with increased fracture displacement
  - Low threshold to initiate further vascular work-up with asymmetric pulses, abnormal ABIs, or other findings concerning for vascular injury

Imaging

- AP and lateral femur x-rays.
- AP and lateral knee x-rays.
- Traction views may be helpful to further delineate fracture pattern in some cases.
- CT scan: concern for intra-articular extension, further characterize fractures with obvious intra-articular extension for operative planning.
  - Hoffa fragment: coronal plane fracture present in 30–40 % of distal femur fractures with an intercondylar split.
    - 80 % of these involve the lateral condyle.
  - Important to recognize Hoffa fragments for effective preoperative planning – will not be effectively captured by commonly used lateral to medial directed screws.

Classification

- Supracondylar: no intercondylar extension
- Intercondylar: associated intercondylar split, possible associated coronal plane fracture (Hoffa fragment)

Treatment

- Nonoperative
  - Non-weight bearing, early knee range of motion with hinged knee brace.
  - Consider in nondisplaced fractures, nonambulatory patients, and patients with excessively high perioperative mortality risk.
- Operative
  - Principles of surgical fixation
    - Indicated in displaced fractures
    - Anatomic reduction of articular surface (when involved), restoration of length, alignment, and rotation
      - Varus malalignment poorly tolerated
    - Initiate early knee range of motion
  - Non-fixed-angle plates
    - Historically considered in severely comminuted fractures
    - Increased risk of varus malalignment
    - Largely replaced by fixed-angle constructs
  - Fixed-angle plates
    - Options include blade plates, dynamic condylar screw plates, and a multitude of locked plates.
    - Options for direct open reduction and indirect reduction with MIPO technique
      - Indirect reduction: high union rate >80 %
      - Increased risk of nonunion with locking condylar plates compared to blade plates
    - Frequently combined with lag screws and positional screws for intercondylar fractures and coronal plane fractures.
  - Retrograde intramedullary nail
    - Consider in supracondylar fractures without significant comminution, fractures without intra-articular involvement, or fractures with a simple articular split and in obese patients.
    - Good option for osteoporotic bone and many periprosthetic fractures (provided sufficiently large intercondylar box).

    - Blocking screws may help facilitate reduction and improve stability.
    - May allow for early weight bearing.
  - Arthroplasty
    - Typically requires distal femoral replacement.
    - May consider if reconstruction and stable fixation is not possible.
    - In setting of preexisting knee arthropathy, typically proceed with ORIF to constitute bone stock and consider arthroplasty at a later date.

Complications

- Nonunion
  - Treat with revision ORIF ± bone grafting.
  - Slight shortening/compression through the metaphysis and metadiaphysis may be desired at the time of initial fixation in osteoporotic bone to help decrease the risk of nonunion.
- Malunion
  - May be symptomatic with >5° of malalignment in any plane.
  - Plate fixation prone to valgus malalignment.
  - Increased overall risk of malalignment with intramedullary nails.
  - Effects of malunion may be particularly deleterious in patients with periprosthetic fractures.
- Failure of fixation
  - Varus collapse most common, increased risk with non-fixed-angle plates
- Symptomatic hardware
  - Lateral plate
    - Irritation from motion of the IT band over the plate with knee range of motion
  - Medial screw prominence
    - Long screws that protrude through the medial cortex are poorly tolerated.
    - As the distal femur narrows posteriorly, screw length should be assessed on a 30° internal rotation view intraoperatively.
- Arthrofibrosis
- Knee pain

Bibliography

1. Gwathmey FW Jr, Jones-Quaidoo SM, Kahler D, Hurwitz S, Cui Q. Distal femoral fractures: current concepts. J Am Acad Orthop Surg. 2010;18(10):597–607 (Review).
2. Miller MD, Thompson SR, Hart JA. Review of orthopaedics. 6th ed. Philadelphia: Elsevier; 2012. p. 751–3.

3. Nork SE, Segina DN, Aflatoon K, Barei DP, Henley MB, Holt S, Benirschke SK. The association between supracondylar-intercondylar distal femoral fractures and coronal plane fractures. J Bone Joint Surg Am. 2005;87:564–9.
4. Vallier HA, Immler W. Comparison of the 95-degree angled blade plate and the locking condylar plate for the treatment of distal femoral fractures. J Orthop Trauma. 2012;26(6):327–32.

11 Knee Dislocations

Take-Home Message

- Orthopedic emergency that requires urgent reduction.
- Importance of exam to identify occult injury.
- High rates of associated neurovascular injury.
- Physical exam with ABIs and selective arteriography is the standard of care.
- If ABI is <0.9 or exam is abnormal but limb is perfused, initiate further vascular injury work-up with arterial duplex ultrasound or CT angiography.
- Serial exam critical to assess for changes in the neurovascular status of the limb and compartment syndrome.
- Early reconstruction/repair when possible.

General

- Rare, potentially limb-threatening injuries.
- Estimated 20–50 % of knee dislocations spontaneously reduce in the field.
  - True incidence is likely underreported.
- Injury to 3 or more ligaments should be considered a knee dislocation equivalent.
- High overall incidence of associated injury.
- Low energy: fall, sports injuries, obesity
  - Lower incidence of associated soft tissue, cartilage, and neurovascular injury
- High energy: vehicular trauma, fall from height
  - More severe soft tissue injury, increased incidence of neurovascular injury.
  - ~25 % will have associated severe head, chest, and abdominal trauma
    - Increased risk of delayed diagnosis and management in the polytrauma patients.

Vascular Injury

- ~20 % risk of vascular injury across all knee dislocations.
- 40–50 % risk of vascular injury in anterior/posterior dislocations.
  - Anterior dislocation: traction/bowstringing of the popliteal artery, more likely to result in an intimal tear
  - Posterior dislocation: more likely to result in complete arterial tears/disruptions
- Assess distal pulses, capillary refill, popliteal fossa, and ankle-brachial index
  - Collateral circulation may maintain distal pulses and capillary refill initially but cannot sustain limb viability.
- Hard signs of vascular injury: absent pulses, bleeding, expanding hematoma, bruit, thrill.
- Soft signs of vascular injury: diminished pulses, delayed capillary refill.
- Physical exam with ABI and selective arteriography is the standard of care.
  - If ABI >0.9 and exam is normal, monitor with serial exam.
    - Arteriogram does not have an advantage over serial exam in patients with normal exam and ABIs upon presentation.
    - If the vascular status of the limb changes on serial exam, then pursue further work-up.
  - If ABI is <0.9 or exam is abnormal but the limb is perfused, pursue further work-up with arterial duplex ultrasound or CT angiography with vascular surgery consultation if vascular injury is confirmed.
    - When hard signs of vascular injury are present, the patient should proceed directly to the OR.
    - Revascularize within 6–8 h to minimize the risk of amputation.
    - Ischemia time of >3 h increased the risk of reperfusion injury.
      - Perform prophylactic fasciotomies after vascular repair.
- Late presentation of vascular injury is possible.
  - Intimal tears and partial arterial injuries may develop late thrombosis with complete arterial occlusion and limb ischemia hours or even days after injury.
  - Popliteal artery aneurysm may also develop in a delayed fashion.
  - Highlights the importance of serial exam.

Nerve Injury

- 10–40 % peroneal nerve injury
  - Increased risk with lateral and posterolateral dislocations
  - Neuropraxia common, transection rare
  - Tibial nerve injured less frequently

Serial Exam

- Critical for assess changes in vascular and neurologic status of the limb.
- Serial compartment checks are warranted.
  - Compartment syndrome may occur in the absence of vascular injury.

Imaging

- AP and lateral knee x-rays: assess for asymmetric or irregular joint space, avulsion fractures, and osteochondral defects.
  - X-rays may be normal in multiligamentous injury.
  - Physical exam is paramount.
- MRI obtained after acute treatment to assess soft tissue injury and for surgical planning.

Classification

- Directional classification (Kennedy)
  - Describes the position of the tibia relative to the femur, suggestive of ligament involvement
  - Anterior (30–50 %): knee hyperextension >30°, associated PCL and possible ACL tear, increasing incidence of popliteal artery injury with increased hyperextension
  - Posterior (25 %): posterior force against the proximal tibia of a flexed knee, "dashboard injury," associated with ACL and PCL disruption, increased risk of popliteal artery injury with increased tibial displacement
  - Lateral (13 %): vagus force, medial supporting structures disrupted, both the cruciate ligaments often involved
  - Medial (3 %): varus force, lateral and posterolateral structures disrupted
  - Rotational (4 %): varus/valgus force with rotatory component, may see buttonholing of the femoral condyle through the articular capsule
- Anatomic knee dislocation classification (Schenck)
  - KDI: one cruciate plus one or both collaterals
  - KDII: ACL and PCL, collaterals intact (rare)
  - KDIIIM: ACL, PCL, and MCL (most common)
  - KDIIIL: ACL, PCL, and LCL, often PLC (higher incidence of peroneal nerve injury)
  - KDIV: ACL, PCL, MCL, and LCL, often PLC (less common, high-energy mechanism, higher incidence of vascular injury)
  - KDV: fracture-dislocation
  - C (added to above): associated arterial injury
  - N (added to above): associated nerve injury

Treatment

- Initial treatment
  - Considered an orthopedic emergency.
  - Treat with emergent reduction and neurovascular examination.
    - If the limb is grossly deformed upon presentation, do not delay reduction to obtain radiographs.
    - "Dimple sign" – buttonholing of medial femoral condyle through the medial capsule
      - May represent an irreducible posterolateral dislocation
- Nonoperative
  - Historically treatment with closed reduction and immobilization which frequently resulted in late instability.
  - With advanced instrumentation and techniques, these injuries are now typically managed surgically.
- Operative
  - Emergent surgical intervention
    - Vascular injury repair
    - Open fracture and dislocations
    - Irreducible dislocations
    - Compartment syndrome
  - Delayed reconstruction
    - Paucity of high-level evidence on which to base treatment decisions
    - Controversies regarding early versus delayed surgical treatment, use of joint spanning external fixation, and simultaneous versus staged reconstruction of cruciates and/or PLC and PMC
      - Outcomes may be improved with early treatment (within 3–4 weeks), provided the condition of the patient and the limb allows.
    - Improved outcomes in patients <40 years old, low-energy mechanism of injury, and functional rehabilitation (vs immobilization)
      - Surgical repair/reconstruction of the cruciate ligaments needed to achieve sufficient stability for functional rehabilitation

Complications

- Vascular injury
  - Claudication, skin changes, and muscle atrophy may develop as sequelae of vascular injury.

  - Popliteal artery aneurysm may develop as a late sequelae of popliteal vessel injury
    - May present with swelling in the popliteal fossa and knee flexion deformity to accommodate the mass
- Nerve injury
  - The peroneal nerve is most commonly injured in knee dislocations.
    - Increased incidence with posterolateral dislocation.
    - Poor prognosis with ~50 % partial to full recovery.
    - Outcomes not improved with acute, subacute, or delayed nerve explorations.
    - Neurolysis, tendon transfers, and bracing comprise the primary treatment options.
- Arthrofibrosis
  - Stiffness is the most common complication (38 %).
  - Increased incidence with delayed mobilization.
- Instability and laxity
  - Occurs in 37 % of patients.
  - Redislocation is uncommon.

Bibliography

1. Harner CD, Waltrip RL, Bennett CH, Francis K, Cole B, Irrgang J. Surgical management of knee dislocations. JBJS. 2004;86-A(2):262–73.
2. Levy BA, Fanelli GC, Whelan DB, Stannard JP, MacDonald PA, Boyd JL, Marx RG, Stuart MJ. Knee Dislocation Study Group. Controversies in the treatment of knee dislocations and multiligament reconstruction. J Am Acad Orthop Surg. 2009;17(4):197–206 (Review).
3. Miller MD, Thompson SR, Hart JA. Review of orthopaedics. 6th ed. Philadelphia: Elsevier; 2012. p. 753.
4. Mills WJ, Barei DP, McNair P. The value of the ankle-brachial index for diagnosing arterial injury after knee dislocation: a prospective study. J Trauma. 2004;56:1261–65.
5. Stannard JP, Sheils TM, Lopez-Ben RR, McGwin G Jr, Robinson JT, Volgas DA. Vascular injuries in knee dislocations: the role of physical examination in determining the need for arteriography. J Bone Joint Surg Am. 2004;86-A(5): 910–5.
6. Wascher DC. High-velocity knee dislocation with vascular injury. Treatment principles. Clin Sports Med. 2000;19(3):457–77.

12 Patella Fractures

Take-Home Message
- Inability to actively extend the knee indicates a clinically significant extensor mechanism injury.
- Fracture displacement correlates with retinacular disruption.
- Nonoperative management of nondisplaced and minimally displaced fractures with intact extensor mechanism.
- Operative fixation of displaced fractures commonly performed with tension band fixation ± cerclage ± ORIF of comminuted segments.
- Partial patellectomy may be used when reconstructing distal pole fractures and severely comminuted fractures.
- Preserve the patella whenever possible – complete patellectomy is contraindicated.

General

- Common fractures most common in patients 20–50 years of age.
- Mechanism of injury
  - Direct blow
  - Eccentric contraction
- Inability to actively extend the knee indicates a clinically significant extensor mechanism injury.
- The patella has the thickest articular cartilage in the body.

Imaging

- AP and lateral knee x-rays: fracture displacement best evaluated on the lateral
  - Displacement correlates with retinacular disruption.

Descriptive Classification

- Transverse
- Vertical
- Comminuted (stellate)
- Proximal pole
- Distal pole
- Osteochondral

Treatment

- Nonoperative
  - Weight bearing as tolerated in a knee immobilizer or hinged knee brace locked in extension for 6 weeks
  - Indicated in nondisplaced and minimally displaced fractures with intact extensor mechanism

- Operative
  - Tension band fixation
    - Indicated with simple fracture patterns
    - Converts tensile forces into compressive forces
    - May use k-wires or cannulated screws, wire, or braided nonabsorbable suture
  - Open reduction internal fixation, cerclage, and tension band fixation
    - Comminuted stellate fractures with varying degrees of displacement
    - May use minifrag or fine k-wire fixation of independent fragments
  - Partial patellectomy
    - Preserve patella whenever possible.
    - Consider partial patellectomy in extra-articular distal pole fractures and several comminuted fractures.
    - Preserve the largest fragments for reconstruction of the extensor mechanism.
    - Complete patellectomy is contraindicated.
      - Reduces quadriceps torque by 50 %.

Complications

- Symptomatic hardware
- Failure of fixation (up to 20 %)
  - Technical error
  - Patient noncompliance
- Nonunion <5 %
- Arthrofibrosis
- Infection
- Osteonecrosis of the proximal fragment
  - Observe; most spontaneously revascularize.

Bibliography

1. Eggink KM, Jaarsma RL. Mid-term (2–8 years) follow-up of open reduction and internal fixation of patella fractures: does the surgical technique influence the outcome? Arch Orthop Trauma Surg. 2011;131(3):399–404. Epub 2010 Dec 15.
2. Kastelec M, Veselko M. Inferior patellar pole avulsion fractures: osteosynthesis compared with pole resection. J Bone Joint Surg Am. 2004;86-A(4): 696–701.
3. Melvin JS, Mehta S. Patellar fractures in adults. J Am Acad Orthop Surg. 2011;19(4):198–207 (Review).
4. Miller MD, Thompson SR, Hart JA. Review of orthopaedics. 6th ed. Philadelphia: Elsevier; 2012. p. 753–5.

13 Quadriceps Tendon Rupture

Take-Home Message

- Typically occurs in patients >40 years of age, more common in males, more common in the nondominant limb.
- Increased risk with chronic renal disease, diabetes, rheumatoid arthritis, gout, hyperparathyroidism, connective tissue disorders, steroid use, and fluoroquinolones.
- Patients with bilateral ruptures must be worked up for underlying medical disorder and should receive DVT prophylaxis.
- Assess for patella baja on lateral knee x-ray with 30° of flexion: Insall-Salvati ratio <0.8, inferior pole of patella below Blumensaat's line.
- Tendon rupture occurs most commonly ~2 cm proximal to the superior pole of the patella.
- Treat partial tears with intact extensor mechanism with immobilization and progressive weight bearing; counsel on increased future risk of complete rupture.
- Complete tears with disruption of the extensor mechanism should undergo early primary repair.
- Tendon reconstruction may be required for severely degenerated quadriceps tendon, failed prior repairs, and chronic injuries. Complicated by contracture of the quadriceps and may require tendon lengthening and/or allograft.
- Weakness and knee stiffness are common complications.

General

- Typically occur in adults >40 years old, often with medical comorbidities, males>>females, nondominant limb>dominant limb.
- Quadriceps tendon rupture is more common than patella tendon rupture.
- Increased risk with chronic renal disease, diabetes, rheumatoid arthritis, hyperparathyroidism, connective tissue disorders, steroid use – oral and corticosteroid injection – gout, and fluoroquinolones.
- Bilateral ruptures: assess for underlying medical problem, treatment follows guidelines for unilateral injuries but will require period of non-weight bearing and DVT prophylaxis.
- Mechanism: eccentric loading often with the foot planted and knee slightly bent, direct trauma.
- On exam, unable to perform straight leg raise or maintain knee extension, palpable gap at superior pole of the patella.

Imaging

- AP and lateral x-rays: patella baja (complete rupture), Insall-Salvati ratio <0.8, inferior pole of the patella below Blumensaat's line
  - Insall-Salvati ratio: ratio of patella tendon length over length of the patella (TL/PL)
    - Calculate from lateral knee x-ray with 30° of knee flexion
  - Blumensaat's line: corresponds to roof of the intercondylar notch of the distal femur on a lateral knee x-ray, should intersect the inferior pole of the patella
- Ultrasound: not reliable to establish diagnosis in equivocal cases, particular in obese and very muscular patients
- MRI: adjunct to delineate partial and complete injuries in equivocal cases

Classification

- Partial rupture.
- Complete rupture.
- Tendon rupture occurs most commonly ~2 cm proximal to the superior pole of the patella (relative watershed area).

Treatment

- Nonoperative
  - Immobilization with progressive weight bearing
    - Partial tear with intact knee extensor mechanism, risk of future complete rupture
- Operative
  - Primary repair
    - Complete quadriceps tendon ruptures that can be reapproximated.
    - Transosseous tendon repair: nonabsorbable suture through drill hole construct.
    - End-to-end repair.
    - Suture anchor tendon repair (advocated by some).
    - Repair retinaculum; knee should flex to 90° after repair.
    - Rehabilitation: promote motion while protecting repair
      - Prone knee flexion with passive extension
      - Heel slides with active flexion and passive extension
  - Tendon reconstruction
    - Severely degenerated quadriceps tendon, failure of prior repair, delayed presentation/chronic injuries

- V-Y lengthening (Codivilla procedure)
- Quadriceps tendon lengthening
- Quadriceps turndown
- Allograft reconstruction

Complications

- Weakness: 30–50 %
- Extensor lag
- Stiffness
- Inability to return to pre-injury level of activity: 50 % of patients
- Worse outcomes with delayed reconstruction
  - Quadriceps can retract 5 cm in as little as 2 weeks, requiring mobilization and/or quadriceps tendon lengthening to facilitate reconstruction.
  - Increased risk of failure of reconstruction.

Bibliography

1. Ciriello V, Gudipati S, Tosounidis T, Soucacos PN, Giannoudis PV. Clinical outcomes after repair of quadriceps tendon rupture: a systematic review. Injury. 2012;43(11):1931–8.
2. Hak DJ, Sanchez A, Trobisch P. Quadriceps tendon injuries. Orthopedics. 2010;33(1):40–6.
3. Miller MD, Thompson SR, Hart JA. Review of orthopaedics. 6th ed. Philadelphia: Elsevier; 2012. p. 755–6.
4. Pocock CA, Trikha SP, Bell JS. Delayed reconstruction of a quadriceps tendon. Clin Orthop Relat Res. 2008;446(1):221–4.

14 Patellar Tendon Rupture

Take-Home Message

- Injury typically occurs in the 3rd and 4th decade of life, more common in males.
- Risk factors include patellar tendinitis, diabetes, rheumatologic disease, renal disease, corticosteroid injections, and fluoroquinolones.
- May occur as an avulsion from the inferior pole of the patella (most common), midsubstance tear, or tibial tubercle avulsion (rare).
- Assess for patella alta on lateral knee x-ray with 30° of flexion: Insall-Salvati ratio >1.2, inferior pole of patella above Blumensaat's line.
- Treat partial tears with intact extensor mechanism with initial immobilization followed by progressive weight bearing and range of motion.

- Complete tears may undergo primary repair via transosseous tunnels, suture anchors, or end-to-end repair.
- Tendon reconstruction with autograft (local hamstring) or allograft if insufficient tendon for primary repair, failed prior repair, and delayed presentation.
- Rehabilitate with prone knee flexion and heel slides to promote knee range of motion while not stressing the repair.
- Knee stiffness and extensor lag are the most common complications.

General

- Typically occur in active adults <40 years old, male > female
- Increased risk with patellar tendinitis, diabetes, rheumatologic disease, chronic renal disease, corticosteroid injection, infection, and fluoroquinolones
- Mechanism: tensile overload of extensor mechanism, frequently with eccentric contraction, often the result of chronic tendon degeneration
- Avulsion from the distal pole of the patella more common than midsubstance tendon tears
- On exam, unable to perform straight leg raise or maintain knee extension, palpable gap at inferior pole of patella

Imaging

- AP and lateral knee x-rays: patella alta (complete rupture), Insall-Salvati ratio >1.2, inferior pole of patella above Blumensaat's line
  - Insall-Salvati ratio: ratio of patella tendon length over length of the patella (TL/PL)
    - Calculate from lateral knee x-ray with 30° of knee flexion.
  - Blumensaat's line: corresponds to roof of the intercondylar notch of the distal femur on a lateral knee x-ray, should intersect the inferior pole of the patella
- Ultrasound: may be useful to further evaluate equivocal presentations and chronic injuries
- MRI: adjunct to delineate partial and complete injuries in equivocal cases

Classification

- Inferior pole of patella avulsion (most common)
- Midsubstance tear
- Tibial tubercle avulsion (rare)

Treatment

- Nonoperative
  - Immobilization in extension with progressive weight bearing
    - Partial tears, intact extensor mechanism

- Operative
  - Primary repair
    - Complete patella tendon ruptures that can be reapproximated.
    - Transosseous tendon repair: nonabsorbable suture through drill hole construct.
    - End-to-end repair
    - Suture anchor tendon repair (advocated by some).
    - Consider supplementation with cerclage wire or tape.
    - Rehabilitation: promote motion while protecting repair
      - Prone knee flexion with passive extension
      - Heel slides with active flexion and passive extension
  - Tendon reconstruction
    - Severely degenerated patella tendon, failure of prior repair, delayed presentation
    - Semitendinosus or gracilis tendon harvested (leaving tendon insertion intact) and passed transosseously through patella and tibial tubercle
    - Allograft may be considered in salvage situation or absence of autograft options (prior hamstring ACL reconstruction, etc.)

Complications

- Extensor lag
- Stiffness
- Superior patella tilt
  - Reinsert the patellar tendon anteriorly to prevent superior tilt of the patella

Bibliography

1. Casey MT Jr, Tietjens BR. Neglected ruptures of the patellar tendon. A case series of four patients. Am J Sports Med. 2001;29(4):457–60.
2. Marder RA, et al. Effects of partial patellectomy and reattachment of the patella tendon on patellofemoral contact areas and pressures. J Bone Joint Surg Am. 1995;75:35–45.
3. Matava MJ. Patellar tendon ruptures. J Am Acad Orthop Surg. 1996;4(6): 287–96.
4. Miller MD, Thompson SR, Hart JA. Review of orthopaedics. 6th ed. Philadelphia: Elsevier; 2012. p. 775.

15 Tibial Plateau Fractures

Take-Home Message

- Usually occur with axial compression and varus/valgus loading.
- Associated soft tissue injuries in 50–90 % of cases, meniscal tears most common, typically in the periphery, lateral > medial.
- Medial tibial plateau fractures should be considered knee dislocation equivalents.
- Goal of treatment is to restore normal alignment and bicondylar width; restoration of the articular surface is of secondary importance.
- Knee spanning temporary external fixation with compromised soft tissue and polytrauma.
- Locked plate technology advantageous in condylar fractures and poor bone quality.
- Posteromedial fragments may not be captured by standard lateral plates; use a separate posteromedial plate when needed.
- Calcium phosphate bone void filler has superior compressive strength and resists subsidence better than autologous iliac crest bone grafting.
- Posttraumatic arthritis correlates with initial severity of injury, axial injury, and meniscal injury; quality of articular reduction does not directly correlate with development of posttraumatic arthritis.
- Maintain a high index of suspicion for compartment syndrome – most common in the anterior and lateral compartments in the setting of tibial plateau fracture.

General

- Typical mechanism of axial compression with varus/valgus loading
- Bimodal distribution
  - High-energy trauma: adult and middle-aged patients, more common in males
  - Low-energy falls: osteoporotic insufficiency fractures, more common in women
- Lateral plateau fractures most common, followed by bicondylar, followed by medial plateau fractures
  - Medial plateau fractures should be considered knee dislocation equivalents.

- Associated soft tissue injury in 50–90 % of cases
  - Meniscus tears most common, lateral meniscus injury > medial meniscus injury, peripheral tears most common
    - Lateral plateau fractures: lateral meniscal pathology
    - Medial plateau fractures: medial meniscal pathology
  - ACL injuries most common in bicondylar fractures
- Condition of soft tissue envelope critical in determining timing and type of definitive treatment

Imaging

- AP and lateral x-rays of the knee and tibia
  - Carefully assess for posteromedial fracture lines.
- Oblique knee x-rays may help assess joint depression.
- CT scan useful to characterize articular depressions, comminution, and involvement of the tibial tubercle and for preoperative planning.
- MRI best to evaluate associated soft tissue injury (meniscus, ligamentous).

Classification

- Schatzker classification
  - Type I: lateral split
  - Type II: lateral split depression
  - Type III: lateral depression
  - Type IV: medial plateau, possible knee dislocation equivalent
  - Type V: bicondylar
  - Type VI: metaphyseal-diaphyseal dissociation
- Moore classification: better characterizes proximal tibia fracture-dislocations
  - Type I: coronal split
  - Type II: entire condylar fractures
  - Type III: lateral plateau rim avulsion
  - Type IV: rim compression fracture
  - Type V: 4 part fractures

Treatment

- Nonoperative
  - Non-weight bearing in hinged knee brace with early range of motion and progressive weight bearing at 8–12 weeks.
    - Consider with <3 mm articular step-off, <10° varus/valgus with knee in extension and overall stable fracture pattern, and nonambulatory patients.

- Operative
  - Indications
    - Articular step-off >3 mm, condylar widening >5 mm, all medial plateau and bicondylar plateau fractures (inherently unstable fracture patterns).
    - Overall alignment is the most important determinant of outcome
      - Varus malalignment poorly tolerated
  - Bridging external fixation
    - Temporary stabilization to restore length, alignment, and rotation while allowing the soft tissue envelope to improve
    - Soft tissue injury, polytrauma
  - Fine wire frame ± percutaneous reduction techniques
    - Good option for patients with compromised soft tissue envelope.
    - Thin wires should be placed >14 mm from the joint to ensure extra-articular position and decrease the risk of septic arthritis.
  - Open reduction internal fixation
    - Typically performed with plate fixation with the goal to achieve direct anatomic reduction of the articular surface.
    - Critical to respect soft tissues, particularly with combined medial and lateral approaches.
    - Posteromedial fragment may not be captured by lateral plate; recommended to use posteromedial plate when needed.
    - Locked plate technology for poor quality bone.
    - Calcium phosphate cement to fill bone voids has the highest compressive strength and less subsidence than autogenous iliac crest bone graft.

Complications

- Posttraumatic arthritis
  - Increased risk with increased severity of initial injury, varus/valgus malalignment, failure to restore bicondylar width, significant meniscal injury and ligament instability
- Compartment syndrome
  - Maintain a high index of suspicion of compartment syndrome.
  - Most common in the anterior and lateral compartments.
  - Increased risk with higher-energy injuries and more proximal fractures.
  - Treat with emergent fasciotomies.
- Malunion
  - Increased risk of varus collapse with nonoperative management and severe bicondylar fractures treated with conventional plating

- Infection
  - Surgical approach is the most significant risk factor.
- Wound healing complications
  - Assess soft tissue envelope for timing of ORIF.
  - Carefully plan incisions and skin bridges when more than one incision is used; do not undermine skin; meticulous soft tissue handling.
- Peroneal nerve injury

Bibliography

1. Barei DP, Nork SE, Mills WJ, Coles CP, Henley MB, Benirschke SK. Functional outcomes of severe bicondylar tibial plateau fractures treated with dual incisions and medial and lateral plates. J Bone Joint Surg Am. 2006;88(8):1713–21.
2. Bhattacharyya T, McCarty LP III, Harris MB, Morrison SM, Wixted JJ, Vrahas MS, Smith RM. The posterior shearing tibial plateau fracture: treatment and results via a posterior approach. J Orthop Trauma. 2005;19(5):305–10.
3. Gardner MJ, Yacoubian S, Geller D, Suk M, Mintz D, Potter H, Helfet DL, Lorich DG. The incidence of soft tissue injury in operative tibial plateau fractures: a magnetic resonance imaging analysis of 103 patients. J Orthop Trauma. 2005;19(2):79–84.
4. Miller MD, Thompson SR, Hart JA. Review of orthopaedics. 6th ed. Philadelphia: Elsevier; 2012. p. 757–60.
5. Russell TA, Leighton RK, Alpha-BSM Tibial Plateau Fracture Study Group. Comparison of autogenous bone graft and endothermic calcium phosphate cement for defect augmentation in tibial plateau fractures. A multicenter, prospective, randomized study. J Bone Joint Surg Am. 2008;90(10):2057–61.
6. Trenholm A, Landry S, McLaughlin K, Deluzio KJ, Leighton J, Trask K, Leighton RK. Comparative fixation of tibial plateau fractures using alpha-BSM, a calcium phosphate cement versus cancellous bone graft. J Orthop Trauma. 2005;19:698–702.

16 Tibial Shaft Fractures

Take-Home Message

- Tibia shaft fractures are the most common long bone fracture.
- Associated soft tissue injury is critical to guiding treatment and risk of complications.
- Nonoperative management considered for low-energy, closed tibia fractures with varus/valgus angulation <5°, sagittal plane angulation <10°, cortical apposition >50 %, shortening <1–2 cm, rotational alignment within 10°. Shortening and translation on injury films is the expected position at union.

- Early antibiotic administration is the most important factor in decreasing the risk of infection in open tibia fractures.
- Reamed IM nailing of fractures is the gold standard for treating indicated tibia fractures.
- Proximal third tibia fractures at risk for valgus and apex anterior deformity, may utilize lateral start point, blocking screws in the concavity of the deformity, provisional unicortical plates, semiextended nailing and/or universal distractor/traveling traction.
- Distal third fractures are at increased risk for rotational malalignment.
- Anterior knee pain occurs in >30 % of patients who undergo IM nailing of tibia fractures; resolution of pain is unpredictable with hardware removal.
- Risk factors for reoperation within 1 year to achieve bony union include open fractures, transverse fracture patterns, and cortical contact <50 %.
- Maintain a high index of suspicion for compartment syndrome in all tibia fractures, including open fractures.

General

- Most common long bone fracture
- Mechanism correlates with fracture pattern
  - Low-energy fracture patterns
    - Spiral, tibia, and fibula fractures at different levels, minor soft tissue injury
  - High-energy fracture patterns
    - Comminuted, transverse, segmental, tibia and fibula fractures at same level, diastasis between tibia and fibula, significant soft tissue injury
- Associated soft tissue injury is critical in guiding treatment and risk of complications.
- Fractures of the posterior malleolus are commonly associated with distal third spiral tibia fractures.

Imaging

- AP and lateral x-rays of the tibia, knee, and ankle.
- CT scan: further evaluate intra-articular extension.

Classification

- Winquist-Hansen classification for femoral shaft fractures is sometimes applied to tibial shaft fractures.
- Rockwood classification based on fracture location, pattern, fibula fracture characteristics, position, and number of fragments and soft tissues.
- Gustillo classification of open tibia fractures
  - Initially described open fractures of the tibia, now commonly applied to most open fractures

Treatment

- Nonoperative
  - Initial long leg cast with non-weight bearing and conversion to patellar tendon-bearing cast or functional brace at 6 weeks
    - Long leg cast can control varus/valgus, flexion/extension, and rotation.
    - Shortening and translation on injury films is the expected position at union with nonoperative management.
    - Increased risk of shortening with oblique fracture patterns.
    - Increased risk of varus malunion with midshaft tibia fracture and intact fibula.
  - Indicated in low-energy fractures with acceptable alignment
    - Varus/valgus angulation <5°
    - Sagittal plane angulation <10°
    - Cortical apposition >50 %
    - Shortening <1–2 cm
    - Rotational alignment within 10°
- Operative
  - Open tibia fractures
    - Prompt administration of antibiotics and tetanus
      - Early antibiotic administration is the most important factor in decreasing the risk of infection.
    - Urgent and thorough surgical debridement within 6–8 h of injury
      - Excise all devitalized tissue, including the cortical bone.
    - BMP-2 may be used as an adjuvant in treating type III open tibia fractures to promote union.
  - Intramedullary nailing
    - Indications: acceptable parameters for nonoperative management, significant soft tissue injury, segmental fractures, ipsilateral limb injury, polytrauma, bilateral tibia fractures, morbid obesity.
    - Intramedullary nailing considered the treatment of choice for high-energy and unstable tibia fractures
      - Decreased risk of malalignment, decreased time to union, and decreased time to weight bearing
    - Reamed technique is considered the gold standard with increased union rate, decreased time to union, and lower rates of hardware failure
      - Union >80 % for closed injuries

- Proximal third tibia fractures: fractures proximal to the isthmus of the tibial shaft are at increased risk for valgus and apex anterior deformity with IM nail fixation
  - Avoid malreduction using
    - Laterally based start point and anterior insertion angle
    - Blocking screws placed posteriorly and laterally in the proximal segment (place in the concavity of the deformity)
    - Provisional unicortical plates
    - Semiextended position for nailing, suprapatellar nail insertion technique
    - Use of femoral distractor or traveling traction
- External fixation
  - Applications for temporary stabilization in polytrauma patients or in patients with proximal and distal metadiaphyseal fractures to allow improvement of the soft tissue envelope.
    - May consider definitive treatment in a circular frame for very proximal and distal tibia fractures with poor soft tissue envelope.
  - Pin tract infections are common.
  - Definitive treatment with external fixation associated with longer time to union, higher rates of malunion, and worse functional outcome compared to intramedullary nailing.
  - Safely convert to IM nail within 7–21 days.
- Plate fixation
  - Indications: extreme proximal and distal tibia shaft fractures with inadequate fixation available with IM nailing.
  - Higher risk of infection and wound healing problems in open fractures compared to IM nailing.
  - Use of a long percutaneous plates risk injury to the superficial peroneal nerve at holes 11, 12, and 13. Larger incision with screw placement under direct visualization recommended in this zone.

Complications

- Knee and ankle stiffness most common
- Anterior knee pain
  - >30 % of patients who undergo intramedullary nailing.
  - Ensure the nail is not proud on lateral view.
  - Resolution of knee pain unpredictable with nail removal.
  - No difference in incidence or duration of knee pain with transtendinous versus paratendinous nail insertion.

- Nonunion and delayed union
  - ~6–9 months.
  - Risk factors for reoperation within 1 year to achieve bony union include open fractures, transverse fracture patterns, and cortical contact <50 %.
  - Always assess for possible underlying infection.
  - May treat with nail dynamization (axially stable fractures), exchange nailing, bone grafting, BMP-7, or noninvasive approaches (electrostimution, ultrasound).
- Malunion
  - Proximal third tibia fractures: valgus and apex anterior deformity, most common malunion in tibia fractures.
  - Distal third tibia fractures: increased risk of rotational malalignment.
  - Malunion increases the risk of arthrosis, ankle > knee, especially with varus malunion.
- Infection
  - Increased risk with increasing severity of soft tissue injury and time to soft tissue coverage
- Compartment syndrome
  - Occurs in 1–9 % of tibia fractures
  - Maintain a high index of clinical suspicion for all tibia fractures, including open fractures
  - Treat with emergent fasciotomies
- Nerve injury
  - Superficial peroneal nerve at risk at holes 11–13 in long percutaneous plates
  - Transient peroneal nerve palsy described following closed IM nailing, conservative treatment recommended

Bibliography

1. Boraiah S, Gardner MJ, Helfet DL, Lorich DG. High association of posterior malleolus fractures with spiral distal tibial fractures. Clin Orthop Relat Res. 2008;466(7):1692–8.
2. Finkemeier CG, Schmidt AH, Kyle RF, Templeman DC, Varecka TF. A prospective, randomized study of intramedullary nails inserted with and without reaming for the treatment of open and closed fractures of the tibial shaft. J. Orthop Trauma. 2000;14:187–93.
3. Govender S, Csimma C, Genant HK, et al. Recombinant human bone morphogenetic protein-2 for treatment of open tibial fractures: a prospective, controlled, randomized study of four hundred and fifty patients. J Bone Joint Surg Am. 2002;84-A(12):2123–34.

4. Miller MD, Thompson SR, Hart JA. Review of orthopaedics. 6th ed. Philadelphia: Elsevier; 2012. p. 760–2.
5. Puloski S, Romano C, Buckley R, et al. Rotational malalignment of the tibia following reamed intramedullary nail fixation. J Orthop Trauma. 2004;18: 397–402.
6. Templeman D, Thomas M, Varecka T, Kyle R. Exchange reamed intramedullary nailing for delayed union and nonunion of the tibia. Clin Orthop Relat Res. 1995;315:169–75.
7. Toivanen JA, Väistö O, Kannus P, Latvala K, Honkonen SE, Järvinen MJ. Anterior knee pain after intramedullary nailing of fractures of the tibial shaft. A prospective, randomized study comparing two different nail-insertion techniques. J Bone Joint Surg Am. 2002;84-A(4):580–5.

17 Tibial Plafond Fractures

Take-Home Message

- Most commonly occur with high-energy axial loading.
- Increasing incidence with improved survival following MVC.
- Injury severity related to degree of articular impaction and comminution, metaphyseal comminution, and associated soft tissue injury.
- Three main fracture fragments with intact ankle ligaments: medial fragment (deltoid ligament), posterolateral/Volkmann fragment (posterior inferior tibiofibular ligament), anterolateral/Chaput fragment (anterior inferior tibiofibular ligament).
- Nonoperative management for nondisplaced fractures, patients with significant perioperative risk or increased risk of wound breakdown.
- Most commonly treated with temporizing external fixation with delayed open reduction internal fixation.
- Limited internal fixation combined with external fixation may decrease the risk of wound breakdown; however it may not be possible to anatomically reduce the joint surface.
- High rates of wound breakdown: delay ORIF until soft tissue envelope improves, meticulous soft tissue handling; free flap may be required.
- Nonunion most commonly involves the metaphyseal region and is more common following hybrid fixation.
- Worse outcomes associated with lower level of education, lower income, male sex, work-related injuries, medical comorbidities.
- Clinical improvement may continue for up to 2 years.
- Posttraumatic arthrosis is common.

General

- Account for 10 % of lower extremity trauma.
  - Increasing incidence attributed to improved vehicle safety and trauma systems resulting in increased survivorship of high-energy accidents.
- Male > female, patients 30–40 years of age.
  - High-energy trauma with axial loading: motor vehicle accident, fall from height.
    - May also result from high-energy sheer/torsion injuries.
- More severe injuries have a greater degree of articular impaction and comminution, metaphyseal comminution, and more severe associated soft tissue injury.
- Typical fracture pattern attributed to intact ankle ligaments.
  - Medial fragment: deltoid ligament.
  - Posterolateral/Volkmann fragment: posterior inferior tibiofibular ligament.
  - Anterolateral/Chaput fragment: anterior inferior tibiofibular ligament.
  - Die punch: central impaction.
- Associated injuries: 75 % ipsilateral fibula fracture, frequently have other ipsilateral and/or contralateral lower extremity injury and possible spine injury.
- Increased risk of poor outcome with lower level of education, medical comorbidities, male sex, work-related injuries, and lower-income levels.
- Tibial plafond fractures may show continued clinical improvement for up to 2 years.

Imaging

- AP, lateral, and mortise views of the ankle.
- Full-length tibia and foot x-rays.
- CT scan: assess fracture pattern and surgical planning; most useful after overall length and alignment restored with bridging external fixation (when indicated).

Ruëdi-Allgöwer Classification

- Type I: nondisplaced
- Type II: simple displacement of the articular surface
- Type III: comminution of the articular surface

Treatment

- Nonoperative
  - Long leg cast immobilization for 6 weeks followed by fracture brace and ROM
    - Stable fracture patterns with no displacement of the articular surface, excessively high perioperative risk, nonambulatory patients, high risk of wound healing problems (diabetes, peripheral vascular disease); consider in severe neuropathy.

- Operative
  - Surgery indicated for displaced fractures
  - Bridging external fixation
    - Restore length, alignment, and rotation to allow soft tissue envelope to improve
    - May consider ORIF of the fibula acutely
    - May consider for definitive treatment with critical soft tissues
      - Decreased incidence of wound complications and deep infection compared to ORIF
  - Temporizing external fixation with delayed ORIF
    - Goal is to achieve anatomic reduction of the articular surface.
    - Surgical approach depends on the specific fracture pattern.
    - High rate of soft tissue complications
      - Meticulous soft tissue handling and development of full-thickness flaps are critical.
      - Maintain skin bridges of at least 7 cm.
      - Wound breakdown may require free flap.
    - May combine limited internal fixation with external fixation, including hybrid fixators.
      - May decrease risk of wound breakdown and infection.
      - Anatomic reconstruction of the joint surface may not be possible.

Complications

- Wound breakdown in 10–30 %
  - Delay conversion to ORIF until soft tissue envelope is improved
  - May require free flap for soft tissue coverage
- Deep infection in 5–15 %
- Malunion
  - Varus malunion
- Nonunion
  - Most commonly involved the metaphyseal region
  - Increased risk with hybrid fixation
  - Treat with bone grafting and plate fixation
- Posttraumatic arthrosis
- Chondrolysis
- Stiffness

Bibliography

1. Bartlett CS, Winer LS. Fractures of tibial plafond. In: Browner BD, Jupiter JB, Levine AM, et al., editors. Skeletal trauma: basic science, management, and reconstruction. 2nd ed. Philadelphia: WB Saunders; 2003. p. 2257–306.
2. Miller MD, Thompson SR, Hart JA. Review of orthopaedics. 6th ed. Philadelphia: Elsevier; 2012. p. 262–4.
3. Pollak AN, McCarthy ML, Bess RS, Agel J, Swiontkowski MF. Outcomes after treatment of high-energy tibial plafond fractures. J Bone Joint Surg Am. 2003;85-A(10):1893–900.
4. Sirkin M, Sanders R, DiPasquale T, Herscovici D Jr. A staged protocol for soft tissue management in the treatment of complex pilon fractures. J Orthop Trauma. 2004;18(8 Suppl):S32–8.
5. Williams TM, Nepola JV, DeCoster TA, Hurwitz SR, Dirschl DR, Marsh JL. Factors affecting outcome in tibial plafond fractures. Clin Orthop Relat Res. 2004;423:93–8.

18 Ankle Fractures

Take-Home Message

- Often low-energy twisting injuries.
- Many types of fracture patterns and classifications; Lauge-Hansen classification is based on the foot's position and motion at injury.
- Assess for associated deltoid ligament and syndesmotic disruption with stress radiographs.
- Bosworth ankle fracture-dislocations are typically irreducible posterior ankle fracture-dislocations with incarceration of fibula on the posterolateral ridge of the distal tibia; associated compartment syndromes have been reported.
- Goal of treatment is anatomic reduction of the talus in the mortise: 1 mm lateral talar shift increases tibiotalar contact stress by 42 %.
- Surgical constructs depend on fracture pattern and location and may include lag screws ± neutralization plates, bridge plates, buttress plates, and tension band construction.
- Wound healing problems in 5 % and deep infection in ~2 %.
- Timing of surgery dictated by condition of the soft tissue envelope; meticulous soft tissue handling is critical.
- Diabetics are at increased risk for complications with both operative and nonoperative management of ankle fractures.

General

- Often lower-energy injuries with twisting or rotational mechanism.
- Always assess for associated syndesmotic injury and associated deltoid ligament incompetence.
- Deep portion of the deltoid ligament is the primary restraint to anterolateral translation of the talus.
- The fibula serves as a buttress to prevent lateral displacement of the talus.
- Clinical improvement may be continued up to 2 years following injury.
- Worse outcomes with lower level of education, smoking, alcohol abuse, and medial malleolus fracture.

Imaging

- AP, lateral, and mortise x-rays of the ankle: medial clear space <4 mm, talocrural angle $83 \pm 4°$, talar tilt <2 mm, syndesmotic tibial clear space <5 mm, tibiofibular overlap <10 mm.
- External rotation stress and gravity stress radiographs: assess competency of the deltoid ligament; medial clear space >5 mm predictive of deep deltoid disruption.

Classification

- Lauge-Hansen classification
  - Supination-adduction
    - Stage I: talofibular sprain or distal fibula avulsion fracture
    - Stage II: vertical medial malleolus with impaction of the anteromedial plafond in 50 %
  - Supination-external rotation
    - Stage I: anterior inferior tibiofibular ligament sprain.
    - Stage II: lateral short oblique fibula fracture (anteroinferior to posterosuperior).
    - Stage III: posterior inferior tibiofibular ligament rupture or fracture of the posterior malleolus.
    - Stage IV: transverse medial malleolus fracture or deltoid ligament disruption.
    - Perform stress test to differentiate SER-II from SER-IV.
  - Pronation-abduction
    - Stage I: transverse medial malleolus fracture or deltoid ligament disruption
    - Stage II: anterior and posterior inferior tibiofibular ligament disruption
    - Stage III: transverse comminuted fracture of the fibula above the level of the syndesmosis

- Pronation-external rotation
    - Stage I: transverse medial malleolus fracture or deltoid ligament disruption
    - Stage II: anterior and posterior inferior tibiofibular ligament disruption
    - Stage III: lateral short oblique or spiral fracture of the fibula above level of the joint
    - Stage IV: posterior inferior tibiofibular ligament rupture or posterior malleolus fracture

- Danis-Weber classification
  - A: infrasyndesmotic fibula fracture (stable)
  - B: transsyndesmotic fibular fracture
  - C: suprasyndesmotic fibula fracture
- Bosworth fracture-dislocation of the ankle
  - Posterior ankle fracture-dislocation with incarceration of the fibular shaft behind the posterolateral ridge of the distal tibia.
  - Typically irreducible by closed means due to intact interosseous membrane.
  - Associated compartment syndromes have been reported.
- Other fracture patterns
  - Isolated medial malleolus, lateral malleolus, or posterior malleolus
  - Bimalleolar, bimalleolar equivalent, trimalleolar fractures
  - Associated syndesmotic injuries

Treatment

- Goal of treatment is anatomic reduction of the talus in the mortise.
  - 1 mm lateral talar shift increases tibiotalar contact stress by 42 %.
- Nonoperative
  - Short leg walking cast or boot for 6 weeks
    - Indicated for isolated lateral malleolus fracture with intact deltoid ligament, isolated nondisplaced medial malleolus fracture and medial malleolus tip avulsion fractures, and some nondisplaced bimalleolar ankle fracture (require close follow-up)
- Operative
  - ORIF
    - Indicated for displaced bimalleolar, bimalleolar equivalent, and trimalleolar ankle fractures, displaced medial malleolus fractures, syndesmotic disruptions and some posterior malleolus fractures, Bosworth fracture-dislocations, open fractures
    - Timing of surgery determined by soft tissue envelope

- Unstable fracture-dislocations may require temporizing external fixation with delayed ORIF.

- Construct depends on the specific fracture pattern and location
  - Fibular fixation
    - Anteroposterior lag screw with lateral neutralization plate
    - Posterolateral plate: increased biomechanical stability but with a risk of peroneal tendon irritation
    - Intramedullary retrograde screw, pin, or nail
    - Assess fibular length: anatomic reduction of simple fibula fractures, talocrural angle, realignment of the medial fibular prominence with the tibiotalar joint, "dime sign"/Shenton's line
  - Medial malleolar fixation
    - Medial lag screws: transverse fractures
    - Tension band: transverse fracture (especially very distal), comminuted fractures, osteoporotic bone
    - Medial buttress plate: vertical fractures, must reduce any associated plafond impaction
  - Posterior malleolar fixation
    - Anteroposterior lag screws, posterior buttress plate.
    - Indications for surgical fixation of the posterior malleolus are debated. Widely accepted indications include involvement of >25 % of the articular surface and >2 mm step-off.
  - Assess syndesmotic stability after ORIF
    - External rotation stress fluoroscopy, dynamic fluoroscopy, cotton test
      - Compare to lateral view of the contralateral side as needed.
    - Common with fibular fractures ≥6 cm above the ankle joint.
    - Uncommon with low-fibula fractures.
    - Malreduction of the syndesmosis leads to poor functional outcomes.

Complications

- Wound healing problems in ~5 %.
  - Meticulous soft tissue handling is paramount.
- Deep infection in ~2 %.
- Posttraumatic arthritis.
  - May treat with injections, bracing, ankle arthrodesis.
  - Ankle arthrodesis often leads to ipsilateral hindfoot and midfoot arthrosis.

- Stiffness.
- Diabetics have higher rates of complication with both operative and nonoperative management of ankle fractures.
  - Recommend prolonged period of non-weight bearing for diabetics up to 3–6 months.
  - Consider augmenting fixation heavier plates, quadricortical screws and syndesmotic fixation, and/or transarticular screws or pins.
  - Concomitant peripheral neuropathy further increases risk of complications
    - Cast treatment: increased risk skin breakdown, loss of reduction, and nonunion
    - ORIF: increased risk of wound complications, deep infection (up to 20 %), failure of fixation, and loss of reduction
  - Up to 30 % amputation rate
- Compartment syndrome
  - Has been described in association with Bosworth ankle fracture-dislocations

Bibliography

1. Beekman R, Watson JT. Bosworth fracture-dislocation and resultant compartment syndrome. J Bone Joint Surg Am. 2003;85:2211–4.
2. Chaudhary SB, Liporace FA, Gandhi A, Donley BG, Pinzur MS, Lin SS. Complications of ankle fracture in patients with diabetes. J Am Acad Orthop Surg. 2008;16(3):159–70.
3. Egol KA, Amirtharajah M, Tejwani NC, Capla EL, Koval KJ. Ankle stress test for predicting the need for surgical fixation of isolated fibular fractures. J Bone Joint Surg Am. 2004;86-A(11):2393–8.
4. Gardner MJ, Demetrakopoulos D, Briggs SM, Helfet DL, Lorich DG. Malreduction of the tibiofibular syndesmosis in ankle fractures. Foot Ankle Int. 2006;27(10):788–92.
5. Hak DJ, Lee MA. Ankle fractures: open reduction internal fixation. In: Wiss DA, editor. Master techniques in orthopaedic surgery: fractures. 2nd ed. Philadelphia: Lippincott Williams & Wilkins; 2006. p. 551–67.
6. Herscovici D Jr, Anglen JO, Archdeacon M, et al. Avoiding complications in the treatment of pronation-external rotation ankle fractures, syndesmotic injuries, and talar neck fractures. J Bone Joint Surg Am. 2008;90:898–908.
7. Leeds HC, Ehrlich MG. Instability of the distal tibiofibular syndesmosis after bimalleolar and trimalleolar ankle fractures. J Bone Joint Surg Am. 1984; 66:490–503.
8. Miller MD, Thompson SR, Hart JA. Review of orthopaedics. 6th ed. Philadelphia: Elsevier; 2012. p. 764–9.

19 Syndesmotic Disruption

Take-Home Message

- Syndesmosis injuries may occur in isolation or as part of an ankle sprain or fracture injury pattern.
- Common associated injuries include osteochondral lesions, 5th metatarsal base fractures, talar process fractures, and deltoid ligament injury.
- The syndesmosis is comprised of the AITFL, PITFL, transverse tibiofibular ligament, and interosseous membrane.
- The syndesmosis maintains integrity between the tibia and fibula, resisting axial, rotational, and translational forces.
- Syndesmotic sprains with instability should undergo reduction and screw vs suture button fixation.
- Excellent outcomes with anatomic reduction of syndesmosis.
- Risk of posttraumatic ankle arthrosis increased in missed injuries; risk of posttraumatic tibiofibular synostosis.

General

- May occur in isolation, as a Maisonneuve fracture, or in association with an ankle fracture.
  - 0.5 % of ankle sprains without fracture.
  - 13 % of all ankle fractures, most common in Weber C-type fractures.
- Syndesmosis is comprised of the AITFL, PITFL, transverse tibiofibular ligament, and interosseous membrane.
- Syndesmosis maintains integrity between the tibia and fibula, resisting axial, rotational, and translational forces.
- Mechanism: external rotation forces the talus laterally against the fibula with resulting dissociation of the distal tibiofibular joint.
- Associated injuries: osteochondral lesions (20 %), peroneal tendon injuries (up to 25 %), ankle fracture, proximal fibula fracture (Maisonneuve type injury), 5th metatarsal base fracture, talar process fractures, deltoid ligament injury.
- Identification and treatment with anatomic reduction leads to excellent functional outcomes
  - Hopkin's squeeze test: compression of the tibia and fibula in the mid-calf elicits pain as the syndesmosis.
  - External rotation test: pain at syndesmosis with external rotation of the foot with hip and knee in 90° of flexion.
- Failure to treat may result in ankle arthrosis.

Imaging

- AP, lateral, and mortise ankle x-rays.
- AP and lateral tibia x-rays: assess for proximal fibula fracture.
- Stress views
  - External rotation stress AP view: decreased tibiofibular overlap (normal > 6 mm), increased tibiofibular clear space (normal < 6 mm).
  - External rotation stress mortise view: commonly obtained, decreased tibiofibular overlap (normal > 1 mm), increased tibiofibular clear space (normal < 6 mm).
  - External rotation stress lateral view is also described and has better interobserver reliability; instability of the syndesmosis greatest in the AP direction.
- CT scan: further assess suspected syndesmotic injury with normal radiographs, postoperatively to assess reduction of syndesmosis following fixation.
- MRI: suspected syndesmotic injury with normal radiographs, highly sensitive and specific.
- Intraoperative assessment: external rotation stress views, dynamic fluoroscopy, cotton test.

Classification

- Syndesmotic sprain without instability
- Syndesmotic sprain with instability

Treatment

- Nonoperative
  - Non-weight bearing in cast or boot for 2–3 weeks, or until pain-free
    - Syndesmotic sprains without instability
    - Anticipate prolonged and highly variable recovery period
- Operative
  - Indicated for syndesmotic sprains with instability, refractory syndesmotic sprains, syndesmotic injuries with associated fracture that remain unstable following fracture fixation
  - Syndesmotic screw fixation
    - Fixation with 1 vs 2 cortical position screws 2–4 cm above the joint, angled 20–30° posterior to anterior and traversing 3 vs 4 cortices
      - Restore length and rotation of the fibula
      - Low threshold to perform open reduction to confirm quality of reduction
      - Maximum ankle dorsiflexion during screw placement *not* required
  - Syndesmotic suture button fixation
    - Fiber wire suture through buttons tensioned over the syndesmosis

    - May help achieve more perfect reduction, possible earlier return to activity

  - Rehabilitation
    - Non-weight bearing for 8–12 weeks.
    - May consider screw removal at 3–6 months.
      - Equivalent outcomes with hardware retention and removal.
    - Suture button fixation does not require removal.

Complications

- Posttraumatic tibiofibular synostosis
  - Occurs in ~10 % of injuries with associated Weber C-type fractures
    - If symptomatic, consider surgical excision once ossification in mature.
- Posttraumatic ankle arthrosis
  - Significant risk with missed syndesmotic injuries

Bibliography

1. Egol KA, Amirtharajah M, Tejwani NC, Capla EL, Koval KJ. Ankle stress test for predicting the need for surgical fixation of isolated fibular fractures. J Bone Joint Surg Am. 2004;86-A(11):2393–8.
2. Herscovici D Jr, Anglen JO, Archdeacon M, et al. Avoiding complications in the treatment of pronation-external rotation ankle fractures, syndesmotic injuries, and talar neck fractures. J Bone Joint Surg Am. 2008;90:898–908.
3. Leeds HC, Ehrlich MG: Instability of the distal tibiofibular syndesmosis after bimalleolar and trimalleolar ankle fractures. J Bone Joint Surg Am. 1984; 66:490–503.
4. Miller MD, Thompson SR, Hart JA. Review of orthopaedics. 6th ed. Philadelphia: Elsevier; 2012.
5. Nielson JH, Sallis JG, Potter HG. Correlation of interosseous membrane tears to the level of the fibular fracture. J Orthop Trauma. 2004;18:68–74.
6. Summers HD, Sinclair HK, Stover MD. J Orthop Trauma. A reliable method for intraoperative evaluation of syndesmotic reduction. 2013;24(4):196–200.
7. Wikerøy AK, Høiness PR, Andreassen GS, Hellund JC, Madsen JE. No difference in functional and radiographic results 8.4 years after quadricortical compared with tricortical syndesmosis fixation in ankle fractures. J Orthop Trauma. 2010;24(1):17–23.
8. Xenos JS, Hopkinson WJ, Mulligan ME, Olson EJ, Popovic NA. The tibiofibular syndesmosis. Evaluation of the ligamentous structures, methods of fixation, and radiographic assessment. J Bone Joint Surg Am. 1995;77(6): 847–56.
9. Zalavras C, Thordarson D. Ankle syndesmotic injury. J Am Acad Orthop Surg. 2007;15(6):330–9.

20 Achilles Tendon Rupture

Take-Home Message

- Achilles tendon blood supply comes from the posterior tibial artery.
- Achilles tendon ruptures most commonly occur during a sport event in the non-insertional watershed region ~4 cm proximal to the calcaneal insertion.
- ~25 % of injuries are missed upon presentation.
- Consider ultrasound and MRI to further evaluate suspected Achilles tendon ruptures with equivocal exams.
- All acute Achilles tendon ruptures are amenable to nonoperative management with plantar flexion immobilization and rehabilitation protocol.
- Improved outcome with early weight bearing for Achilles tendon ruptures managed nonoperatively.
- Percutaneous Achilles tendon repair has decreased strength and increased risk of sural nerve injury compared to open repair, however with lower risk of wound healing complications.
- Consider V-Y advancement for chronic injuries with <4 cm defect.
- Consider FHL transfer ± V-Y advancement for chronic injuries with >4 cm defect.
- New evidence challenges prior assertion of increased risk of re-rupture and plantar flexion weakness with nonoperative management compared to operative management.

General

- Achilles tendon is the largest tendon in body, formed the confluence of the soleus and gastrocnemius tendon.
- Blood supply comes from the posterior tibial artery.
- More common in men and patients 30–40 years of age.
- Mechanism: traumatic injury during sport event with sudden forced plantar flexion or dorsiflexion of a plantar-flexed foot.
- Increased risk with episodic athletes, fluoroquinolones, and steroid injections.
- ~25 % missed diagnosis upon presentation.
  - Thompson test: lack of plantar flexion with calf squeeze.
  - Increased resting ankle dorsiflexion, palpable gap, weak ankle plantar flexion, inability to single-toe raise.

Imaging

- Ankle and/or foot radiographs.
- Consider ultrasound: further assess partial versus complete rupture.
- MRI: suspected rupture with equivocal exam, chronic presentation.

Classification

- Rupture severity
  - Partial rupture
  - Complete rupture
- Rupture location
  - Non-insertional: most common, disruption 2–4 cm above the calcaneal insertion, watershed region
  - Insertional: disruption at the calcaneal insertion

Treatment

- Nonoperative
  - Functional bracing/casting in resting equinus with rehabilitation protocol
    - Initiate plantar flexion immobilization within 48 h.
  - Acute injuries with decision for nonoperative management, non-athletes, sedentary patients, medical comorbidities
  - Higher risk of re-rupture and lower risk of skin complications compared to surgical repair
    - Decreased risk of re-rupture with early weight bearing compared to nonoperative management with prolonged non-weight bearing
  - Decreased plantar flexion strength compared to surgical repair challenged in newer studies
- Operative
  - High-demand patients, athletes, chronic injuries
  - Open end-to-end Achilles tendon repair
    - Acute ruptures, likely decreased risk of re-rupture and increased plantar flexion strength compared to nonoperative management
    - May reinforce with turndown
  - Percutaneous Achilles tendon repair
    - Weaker repair and increased risk of sural nerve injury compared to open repair
    - Lower risk of wound healing problems
  - V-Y advancement
    - Chronic ruptures with <4 cm defect
  - Flexor hallucis transfer ± V-Y advancement
    - Chronic ruptures with >4 cm defect

Complications

- Wound healing complications in 5–10 %
  - Increased risk with smoking, female sex, steroids, and diabetes
  - Increases risk of infection
- Sural nerve injury
  - Percutaneous repair > open repair
- Re-rupture and weakness
  - New evidence challenges prior assertion of increased risk of re-rupture and plantar flexion weakness with nonoperative management of Achilles tendon ruptures compared to operative management

Bibliography

1. Bruggeman NB, Turner NS, Dahm DL, Voll AE, Hoskin TL, Jacofsky DJ, Haidukewych GJ. Wound complications after open Achilles tendon repair: an analysis of risk factors. Clin Orthop Relat Res. 2004;427:63–6.
2. Chiodo CP, Glazebrook M, Bluman EM, Cohen BE, Femino JE, Giza E, Watters WC 3rd, Goldberg MJ, Keith M, Haralson RH 3rd, Turkelson CM, Wies JL, Raymond L, Anderson S, Boyer K, Sluka P, American Academy of Orthopaedic Surgeons. Diagnosis and treatment of acute Achilles tendon rupture. J Am Acad Orthop Surg. 2010;18(8):503–10.
3. Keating JF, Will EM. Operative versus non-operative treatment of acute rupture of tendon Achilles: a prospective randomised evaluation of functional outcome. J Bone Joint Surg Br. 2011;93(8):1071–8.
4. Khan RJ, Fick D, Keogh A, Crawford J, Brammar T, Parker M. Treatment of acute achilles tendon ruptures. A meta-analysis of randomized, controlled trials. J Bone Joint Surg Am. 2005;87(10):2202–10.
5. Weber M, Niemann M, Lanz R, Müller T. Nonoperative treatment of acute rupture of the achilles tendon: results of a new protocol and comparison with operative treatment. Am J Sports Med. 2003;31(5):685–91.
6. Willits K, Amendola A, Bryant D, Mohtadi NG, Giffin JR, Fowler P, Kean CO, Kirkley A. Operative versus nonoperative treatment of acute Achilles tendon ruptures: a multicenter randomized trial using accelerated functional rehabilitation. J Bone Joint Surg Am. 2010;92(17):2767–75.

21 Talus Fractures

Take-Home Message

- High-energy injuries, frequently open.
- Talar neck fractures most common.
- The talus has a tenuous blood supply; the primary blood supply to the talar body is from the artery of the tarsal canal; secondary blood supply is from the artery of the sinus tarsi.
- Increasing risk of AVN with increased initial fractures displacement and associated dislocation.
- Hawkins sign represents intact vascularity/revascularization of the talus after injury; however, absence of Hawkins sign does not predict AVN.
- Associated dislocation must undergo emergent closed vs open reduction to prevent skin necrosis and relieve neurovascular stretch injury.
- Most advocate reinsertion of an extruded talus.
- Nondisplaced talus fractures amenable to nonoperative management in short leg cast ± supplementation with percutaneous fixation for talar neck and body fractures.
- Displaced talus fractures should undergo operative fixation.
- Dual incisions decrease risk of varus malreduction in talar neck fractures with dorsomedial comminution.
- Posterolateral to anteromedial directed screws provide the strongest fixation in talar neck fractures.
- Outcomes vary widely and are most dependent on the region of the talus involved, initial displacement, presence of associated dislocation, and quality of reduction.
- Posttraumatic arthrosis is common, subtalar > tibiotalar.
- AVN of the talus is a devastating complication with poor outcomes.

General

- Talus fractures are uncommon injuries, comprising <1 % of all fractures.
- High-energy injuries with 16–44 % open fractures.
  - Primarily divided into talar neck fractures, talar body fractures, and talar process fractures.
- Tenuous blood supply to the talus.
  - No muscular attachments, 60 % covered with articular cartilage.
  - Blood supply enters via ligament and capsular attachments to the neck, medial body, and posterior process.
  - Primary blood supply: artery of the tarsal canal (branch of posterior tibial artery), main supply to talar body.

- Secondary blood supply: artery of the sinus tarsi (branch of peroneal artery).
- Deltoid branches from the posterior tibial artery.

- High rates of associated injuries: ipsilateral lower extremity fractures, spine injuries.
- Outcomes vary widely and depend most on the region of the talus involved, degree of initial displacement, presence of associated dislocation, and quality of reduction.

Imaging

- AP, lateral, and mortise ankle x-rays
- Canale view: visualizes talar neck; obtain with plantar flexion, 15° pronation, and 15° cephalic tilt.
- CT scan helpful to further characterize injuries; in cases of talar body dislocation, obtain CT scan after talar body is reduced.
  - X-rays often underestimate the extent of injury.

Classification

- Talar neck fractures: 50 % of talus fractures.
  - Mechanism of injury: forced dorsiflexion and axial load cause talar neck impingement on the anterior distal tibia; supination drives the neck into the medial malleolus, causing medial neck comminution and rotatory displacement of the head; continued force can lead to talar body dislocation.
    - Comminution is an important predictor of outcome with respect to both malunion and posttraumatic arthrosis.
  - Hawkins classification
    - Hawkins I: nondisplaced, 0–13 % AVN.
    - Hawkins II: displaced with subtalar dislocation, 20–50 % AVN.
    - Hawkins III: displaced with talar body dislocation, 20–100 % AVN,
    - Hawkins IV: displaced with talar body and head dislocation, 100 % AVN.
      - Hawkins types III and IV are devastating injuries that nearly always lead to long-term functional impairment.
  - Hawkins sign
    - Subchondral lucency of the talar dome appreciated 6–8 weeks after talus fracture.
    - Presence of Hawkins sign is indicative of intact vascularity/revascularization of the talus.
    - Absence of Hawkins sign does *not* predict AVN.
- Talar body fractures: 13–26 % of talus fractures
  - Typically involve the tibiotalar joint and posterior facet of subtalar joint

- Frequently have medial and dorsal comminution, disruption of talocalcaneal ligament, possible subluxation/dislocation of tibiotalar and subtalar joints
  - Typically posteromedial dislocation of the posterior talus
  - High rates of AVN with talar body dislocation
- Classification
  - Group I: talar body cleavage fractures (horizontal, sagittal, coronal, or shear)
  - Group II: talar process or tubercle fractures
  - Group III: compression/impaction fractures

- Talar process fractures: 10–24 % of talus fractures
  - Lateral process > posterior process > medial process fractures
  - Lateral process fractures
    - “Snowboarder’s fracture.”
    - Lateral process articulates with the fibula and subtalar joint.
    - Mechanism of injury: inversion (avulsion) or eversion and axial loading (impaction).
  - Posterior process fractures
    - Posterior process composed of lateral tubercle (Stieda process/os trigonum) and medial tubercle with FHL passing in groove between lateral and medial processes
    - Lateral tubercle fracture: avulsion of posterior talofibular ligament
    - Medial tubercle fracture: avulsion of posterior tibiotalar ligament or posterior deltoid ligament
    - Must differentiate posterior process fracture from os trigonum (present in up to 50 %)
- Talar head fractures
  - Least common talus fracture
- Talus osteochondral injuries
  - Frequently occur in combination with talar neck and body fractures
  - Berndt and Hardy classification
    - Type I: subchondral compression fracture
    - Type II: partially detached osteochondral fragment
    - Type III: completely detached osteochondral fragment without displacement
    - Type IV: detached and displaced osteochondral fragment
    - Type V (Loomer): associated subchondral cyst
- Extruded talus
  - May occur with partial or complete talus extrusion

- Wounds most commonly in the anterolateral region of the ankle
- Often have associated soft tissue injuries, tendon injuries, and lateral malleolus fractures
- Reinsert vs discard
  - Most advocate cleansing and reinserting the talus.
  - Preservation of the talus may help to facilitate later reconstruction and preserve limb length.
- High rates of infection: 25–50 %

Treatment

- Nonoperative
  - Immobilization in short leg cast for 6 weeks
    - Nondisplaced lateral talar process fractures, posterior process fractures, nondisplaced talar head fractures; consider in nondisplaced talar neck and body fractures.
  - Emergent closed reduction for all dislocated joints
    - Reduction maneuver for talar body dislocation: with flexed knee, apply longitudinal traction on plantar-flexed forefoot to realign head with body and correct varus/valgus.
    - If unable to obtain closed reduction, proceed to OR urgently to achieve reduction and prevent skin necrosis.
- Operative
  - Open reduction internal fixation
    - Displaced talar neck fractures (urgent fashion as soft tissues allow), displaced talar body fractures (>2 mm), subluxation of tibiotalar or subtalar joints, malalignment (varus), displaced lateral talar process fractures (>2 mm), unstable osteochondral fragments of sufficient size to support fixation.
    - Anatomic reduction maximizes potential for improved outcome.
    - Talar neck fractures
      - Dorsomedial comminution of the talus is common and predisposes to varus malreduction.
        - Combined medial and lateral approaches to the talar neck decreases risk of varus malreduction.
        - Medial plate prevents loss of medial length; lateral plate acts as a tension band to resist fracture gapping.
        - Avoid stripping dorsal neck vessels to decrease the risk of AVN.
        - Maintain sufficient skin bridge.

- Posterolateral to anteromedial directed screws provide the strongest fixation.
  - Withstand shear forces of active motion, screws perpendicular to fracture.
  - Screw heads may impinge in plantar flexion.
- Talar body fractures
  - Medial or lateral malleolar osteotomy may be necessary to access some talar body fractures.
  - Posterolateral or posteromedial approach can provide access to a large portion talar body with ankle dorsiflexion/plantar flexion.
- Talar process and osteochondral fractures
  - Small implants, headless screws
- Non-weight bearing for 12–16 weeks

- Closed reduction percutaneous fixation
  - Consider in nondisplaced talar neck and talar body fractures
- Fragment excision
  - Small (up to 1 cm) and heavily comminuted lateral process fractures, symptomatic posterior process fractures, small unstable osteochondral fragments not amenable to fixation
    - Excision of 1 cm of the lateral process leads to incompetence of the lateral talocalcaneal ligament without biomechanical sequelae.
- External fixation
  - Limited role, polytrauma
  - Temporizing measure to stabilize reduced joints

Complications

- Posttraumatic arthrosis
  - 30–90 % overall
    - Subtalar arthrosis, 50 %
      - 2 mm displacement alters subtalar contact pressures; greatest at the posterior facet.
      - Worse with dorsomedial and varus displacement and lateral process fractures.
    - Tibiotalar arthrosis: 33 %
    - Talonavicular arthrosis
  - Increased risk with increased severity of Hawkins type
  - Conservative management with bracing

- Surgical treatment with arthrodesis
  - Assess for concurrent AVN.
  - Subtalar arthrodesis, tibiotalar arthrodesis, talonavicular arthrodesis, triple arthrodesis, tibiotalocalcaneal fusion, or pan-talar fusion (avoid when possible)

- Malunion
  - Varus malunion of talar neck fractures
    - 30 % of talar neck fractures.
    - Shortening of the medial column limits hindfoot eversion, leading to symptomatic overloading of the lateral border of the foot.
    - Increased risk with medial neck comminution in talar neck fractures and with increased severity of Hawkins type.
    - Conservative treatment: footwear modification.
    - Surgical treatment: talar neck osteotomy, medial column lengthening, lateral column shortening, or triple arthrodesis.
  - Dorsal malunion
    - Talar head dorsal to talar neck leads to impingement of the distal tibia and restricted ankle dorsiflexion.
    - In the absence of arthrosis, resect dorsal prominence of the talar neck.
- Delayed union and nonunion
  - Nonunion uncommon, even with AVN: 2.5 %.
  - Delayed union very common: allow up to 8–9 months for healing; frequently results in late malalignment.
- Avascular necrosis of the talus
  - A devastating complication with poor outcome
  - Increased risk with increased initial displacement and associated dislocation
  - Precollapse treatment
    - Modified weight bearing, patellar tendon-bearing cast
  - Postcollapse treatment
    - Observation and bracing, Blair fusion, tibiotalocalcaneal fusion, talectomy ± fusion
- Skin necrosis
  - Increased risk with high-energy injuries, greater displacement of fragments, and frank talar body dislocation
- Arthrofibrosis
- Chondrolysis
- Infection

Bibliography

1. Canale ST, Kelly FB Jr. Fractures of the neck of the talus. Long-term evaluation of seventy-one cases. J Bone Joint Surg Am. 1978;60(2):143–56.
2. Fortin PT, Balazsy JE. Talus fractures: evaluation and treatment. J Am Acad Orthop Surg. 2001;9(2):114–27.
3. Halorson JJ, Winter SB, Teasdall RD, Scott AT. Talar neck fractures: a systematic review of the literature. J Foot Ankle Surg. 2013;52(1):56–61.
4. Hawkins LG. Fractures of the neck of the talus. J Bone Joint Surg Am. 1970;52(5):991–1002.
5. Langer P, Nickisch F, Spenciner D, Fleming B, DiGiovanni CW. In vitro evaluation of the effect lateral process talar excision on ankle and subtalar joint stability. Foot Ankle Int. 2007;28(1):78–83.
6. Lindvall E, Haidukewych G, DiPasquale T, Herscovici D Jr, Sanders R. Open reduction and stable fixation of isolated, displaced talar neck and body fractures. J Bone Joint Surg Am. 2004;86-A(10):2229–34.
7. Miller MD, Thompson SR, Hart JA. Review of orthopaedics. 6th ed. Philadelphia: Elsevier; 2012. p. 769–70.
8. Sanders DW, Busam M, Hattwick E, et al. Functional outcomes following displaced talar neck fractures. J Orthop Trauma. 2004;18:265–70.
9. Tezval M, Dumont C, Sturmer KM. Prognostic reliability of the Hawkins sign in fractures of the talus. J Orthop Trauma. 2007;21:538–43.
10. Vallier HA, Nork SE, Barei DP, Benirschke SK, Sangeorzan BJ. Talar neck fractures: results and outcomes. J Bone Joint Surg Am. 2004;86-A(8):1616–24.
11. Van Opstal N, Vandeputte G. Traumatic talus extrusion: case reports and literature review. Acta Orthop Belg. 2009;75(5):699–704.

22 Subtalar Dislocations

Take-Home Message

- High-energy injuries that are open in 25–40 % of cases.
- Medial subtalar dislocations exceedingly more common than lateral subtalar dislocations.
- High incidence of associated tarsal fractures.
- Medial subtalar dislocation block to reduction: extensor digitorum brevis, extensor retinaculum, capsule, osteochondral talar head fracture, navicular fracture.
- Lateral subtalar dislocation block to reduction: posterior tibial tendon, flexor hallucis longus, flexor digitorum longus.
- Perform urgent closed reduction; successful in 60–90 % of patients.

- Proceed to OR for open reduction (± debridement) for irreducible dislocations and open injuries.
- Worse outcomes with high-energy mechanisms, open injuries, and lateral subtalar dislocations *with* associated injuries.
- Posttraumatic subtalar arthrosis develops in up to 90 % of patients; treat symptomatic patients with subtalar arthrodesis.

General

- Typically high-energy injuries
  - 25–40 % open injuries.
  - Lateral dislocations are more likely to be open.
- Medial>>lateral
- Associated tarsal fractures in 45–90 %
  - Medial subtalar dislocations: dorsomedial talar head, posterior process of talus, lateral navicular
  - Lateral subtalar dislocations: cuboid, anterior process of calcaneus, lateral process of talus, lateral malleolus

Imaging

- AP, lateral, and mortise ankle x-rays
- AP, lateral, and oblique foot x-rays
- Consider postreduction CT scan to further assess for associated injuries or subtalar debris

Classification

- Medial subtalar dislocation: 65–85 %
  - Block to reduction: extensor digitorum brevis, capsule, extensor retinaculum, osteochondral talar head fracture, navicular fracture
- Lateral subtalar dislocation: 15–35 %
  - Higher-energy injury, increased rate of associated injuries
  - Block to reduction: posterior tibial tendon, flexor hallucis longus, flexor digitorum longus

Treatment

- Nonoperative treatment
  - Urgent closed reduction, non-weight bearing in short leg cast for 6 weeks

- Closed subtalar dislocations.
- Reduction maneuver: with knee flexed and longitudinal traction applied to the foot, first accentuate and then reverse the deformity
  - Successful in 60–90 % of patients

- Operative treatment
  - Open reduction (± debridement)
  - Irreducible dislocations, open injuries
  - Consider placing subtalar transarticular pins if the joint remains unstable after reduction

Complications

- Direction of dislocation does not impact outcome in isolated subtalar dislocations.
  - Worse outcomes with high-energy mechanisms, open injuries, and lateral subtalar dislocation *with* associated injuries.
  - Absence of associated bony injuries leads to best long-term outcomes.
- Hindfoot stiffness
  - Most common complication, usually asymptomatic
- Posttraumatic arthrosis
  - Develops in up to 90 % of patients, symptomatic in 63 % of patients
  - Subtalar fusion in symptomatic patients

Bibliography

1. Bibbo C, Anderson RB, Davis WH. Injury characteristics and the clinical outcomes of subtalar dislocations: a clinical and radiographic analysis of 25 cases. Foot Ankle Int. 2003;24:158–63.
2. Bohay DR, Manoli A 2nd. Subtalar joint dislocations. Foot Ankle Int. 1995; 16(12):803–8.
3. Heppenstall RB, Farahvar H, Balderston R, Lotke P. Evaluation and management of subtalar dislocations. J Trauma. 1980;20(6):494–7.
4. Miller MD, Thompson SR, Hart JA. Review of orthopaedics. 6th ed. Philadelphia: Elsevier; 2012. p. 270.
5. Saltzman C, Marsh JL. Hindfoot dislocations: when are they not benign? J Am Acad Orthop Surg. 1997;5:192–8.
6. Van Opstal N, Vandeputte G. Traumatic talus extrusion: case reports and literature review. Acta Orthop Belg. 2009;75(5):699–704.
7. Wagner R, Battert TR, Weckback A. Talar dislocations. Injury. 2004;35: SB36–45.

23 Calcaneus Fractures

Take-Home Message

- Commonly results from high-energy axial loading injuries.
- Low-energy injuries with gastrocnemius contraction and avulsion are common with osteoporosis and diabetes, challenging to fix and have high rates of wound complications.
- "Best" treatment controversial with consideration of many patient factors and fracture characteristics guiding decision-making.
- Primary fracture line in axial load injuries, a superolateral to inferomedial oblique shear fracture that creates the sustentacular constant fracture and tuberosity fragment.
- Typical deformity with heel shortening, widening, and varus.
- Special imaging considerations: assess Bohler angle, angle of Gissane, and lateral wall blowout and obtain Harris heel and Broden views.
- Nonoperative management with closed reduction cannot restore articular congruity but may help with heel position.
- Goals of surgery: restore height, restore width, correct varus, ± reconstruct joint.
- Poor prognosis with 40 % complication rate and substantial risk of long-term morbidity.
- Lateral extensile approach has high rates of wound complications and apical necrosis.
- Malunion often involves lateral exostosis, loss of height, and heel deformity.
- Subtalar arthrosis occurs in 25–50 % of patients.

General

- The calcaneus is the most frequently fractured tarsal bone.
- Mechanism of injury
  - High-energy axial loading: fall from height, MVC
    - 17 % open fractures, medial shear wound over sustentaculum most common
  - Low energy
    - Gastrocnemius contraction with avulsion
    - Osteopenic bone, diabetics
- Primary fracture line in axial load injuries represents an oblique shear fracture that runs from superolateral to inferomedial

- Creates the sustentacular constant fragment (remains in its anatomic position) and tuberosity fragments and frequently involves the articular surface of the posterior facet

- Typical deformity: heel shortening, widening, and varus
- Associated injuries with high-energy fractures: 10 % lumbar spine fractures, 10 % contralateral calcaneus fracture, extension to the calcaneocuboid joint in 60 %
- Poor prognosis with up to 40 % complication rate

Imaging

- AP, lateral, and oblique foot x-rays.
  - Bohler angle (20–40°)
    - Flattening (decreased angle) represents collapse of the posterior facet; double density indicates subtalar incongruity.
  - Angle of Gissane (130–145°)
    - Increased angle represents collapse of the posterior facet.
- AP ankle: may better demonstrate lateral wall blowout.
- Harris heel view: assess heel widening and varus/valgus alignment and shortening; obtain with foot in maximal dorsiflexion and beam angled 45°.
- Broden's view: assess posterior facet subtalar joint; useful intraoperatively; obtain with ankle in neutral dorsiflexion; and x-rays taken at 40°, 30°, 20°, and 10° of internal rotation.
- CT scan: assess articular involvement and displacement; facilitates operative planning.
- MRI: evaluate suspected calcaneal stress fracture.

Classification

- Sanders classification: based on degree of posterior facet involvement on CT scan
  - Type I: nondisplaced posterior facet
  - Type II: single fracture line through posterior facet with 2 posterior facet fragments
  - Type III: 2 fracture lines with 3 posterior facet fragments
  - Type IV: 3 fracture lines with 4+ posterior facet fragments
- Essex-Lopresti classification: based on location of the secondary fracture line
  - Tongue type
    - Secondary fracture line in the axial plane beneath the facet, exits posteriorly
    - 21 % posterior skin compromise

- Joint depression type
    - Secondary fracture line behind the posterior facet.
    - More likely to have varus deformity.
    - Anterior process is tethered to the bifurcate ligament.

- Beak fractures
  - Concern for skin necrosis
- Avulsion fractures
  - Increased risk in osteopenic and diabetic patients
- Sustentaculum tali fractures
  - Increased risk of FHL adhesions
- Anterior process fractures
  - Inversion and plantar flexion of the foot lead to avulsion of the bifurcate ligament

Treatment

- Treatment decisions informed by patient factors and fracture characteristics
  - Patient factors: age, sex, type of work, workers' compensation status, smoking, diabetes
  - Fracture patterns: degree of articular involvement and displacement, Bohler's angle, heel morphology
  - Factors associated with improved outcomes with operative treatment: female, age <29 years, nonworkers' compensation status, sedentary/light work load, Bohler's angle 0–14°, comminuted fractures
  - Factors associated with poor outcomes: male, >50 years, obesity, manual labor, workers' compensation, smoking, bilateral calcaneus fracture, polytrauma, vasculopathy
  - Relative contraindications to ORIF: peripheral vascular disease, poorly controlled diabetes, heavy smoking, neuropathy, noncompliance, psychiatric disorders, elderly sedentary patients
- Nonoperative
  - Cast immobilization (± closed reduction), non-weight bearing for 10–12 weeks, early range of motion exercises
    - Nondisplaced fractures, some extra-articular fractures.
    - Closed reduction cannot restore articular congruity but may help with heel position.
  - Short leg walking cast vs boot
    - Anterior process fractures with <25 % joint involvement and minimal displacement

- Operative
  - Goals of surgery: restore height, restore width, correct varus, ± reconstruct joint
    - Outcomes correlate with degree of articular involvement and quality of reduction.
  - Postoperatively: non-weight bearing for 10–12 weeks, early motion, may see clinical improvement for up to 2 years
  - Open reduction internal fixation
    - The goal is to achieve anatomic reduction.
    - Large extra-articular fractures, posterior facet displacement >2–3 mm, flattened Bohler's angle, varus malalignment, anterior process fracture with >25 % joint involvement, and incongruity.
    - Time of surgery: typically 1–3 weeks following injury once swelling subsides and + wrinkle sign.
    - Low-profile implants.
    - Extensile lateral approach with "no touch" technique or limited subtalar approach
      - Up to 20 % wound healing complications
    - Subchondral screws across the posterior facet may exit medially at the FHL groove and cause FHL triggering
      - Take care when drilling through the medial cortex to not injure the FHL tendon and medial neurovascular bundle.
    - No strong evidence to support use of bone graft/substitute
      - Advocates argue that use of calcium phosphate to fill voids will resist compression and loss of Bohler's angle and may allow for earlier weight bearing.
  - Closed reduction percutaneous fixation
    - Tongue-type fractures, beak fractures, large extra-articular fractures, or fractures with minimal joint involvement, soft tissue envelope that prohibits formal open approach.
    - Essex-Lopresti maneuver: manipulate to increase varus deformity, plantar flex forefoot, correct varus deformity with valgus reduction, and stabilize with k-wires (or open fixation).
    - Can restore hindfoot morphology and provide stability for early ROM.
    - Timing of surgery depends on fracture and soft tissues.
      - Urgent reduction and fixation in tongue-type and beak fractures to prevent posterior skin necrosis.
      - Earlier surgery facilitates reduction with percutaneous techniques.

- Primary subtalar arthrodesis
  - Consider in Sanders type IV calcaneus fractures and other severely comminuted fractures.
  - May combine with ORIF to restore height and heel morphology.

Complications

- Subtalar arthrosis
  - Occurs in 25–50 % of patients.
  - Treat symptomatic patients with subtalar arthrodesis (and associated procedures as indicated)
    - Increased risk of delayed subtalar fusion in males, workers' compensation patients, manual laborers, and patients with initial Bohler's angle <0°
  - Delayed subtalar fusion: patient with prior ORIF and subsequent subtalar fusion have improved outcome measures and fewer wound complications compared to patients with prior nonoperative management and subsequent subtalar fusion.
- Malunion
  - Lateral exostosis: causes lateral impingement.
  - Loss of height: decreased Bohler's angle decreases the talar declination angle and results in relative dorsiflexion of the talus with tibiotalar impingement.
  - Heel deformity: widening, shortening, and varus.
    - Shoe wear difficult.
  - Treatment options guided by nature of the malunion: subtalar arthrodesis versus subtalar distraction bone block arthrodesis ± lateral wall resection, ± valgus osteotomy.
- Tendon complications
  - Peroneal tendon dislocation and/or impingement
    - Nonoperative management with lateral wall blowout
  - FHL adhesions and hardware irritation
- Neurologic complications
  - Sural nerve pathology
    - Seen with both operative and nonoperative management
    - 10 % sural nerve complications with ORIF
  - Tibial nerve entrapment

- Wound healing complications
  - 10–20 % of patients who undergo operative fixation
  - Apical wound necrosis of lateral extensile approach most common
  - Increased risk in smokers and diabetics
- Infection
  - 1–2 % overall
  - Treat with debridement, antibiotics ± soft tissue coverage.
- Chondrolysis
- Gait problems
- Compartment syndrome 10 %

Bibliography

1. Bajammal S, Tornetta P 3rd, Sanders D, Bhandari M. Displaced intra-articular calcaneal fractures. J Orthop Trauma. 2005;19(5):360–4.
2. Buckley R, Tough S, McCormack R, Pate G, Leighton R, Petrie D, Galpin R. Operative compared with nonoperative treatment of displaced intra-articular calcaneal fractures: a prospective, randomized, controlled multicenter trial. J Bone Joint Surg Am. 2002;84-A(10):1733–44.
3. Csizy M, Buckley R, Tough S, Leighton R, Smith J, McCormack R, Pate G, Petrie D, Galpin R. Displaced intra-articular calcaneal fractures: variables predicting late subtalar fusion. J Orthop Trauma. 2003;17(2):106–12.
4. Folk JW, Starr AJ, Early JS. Early wound complications of operative treatment of calcaneus fractures: analysis of 190 fractures. J Orthop Trauma. 1999;13:369–72.
5. Gehrmann RM, Renard RL. Current concepts review: stress fractures of the foot. Foot Ankle Int. 2006;27(9):750–7 (Review).
6. Miller MD, Thompson SR, Hart JA. Review of orthopaedics. 6th ed. Philadelphia: Elsevier; 2012. p. 770–1.
7. Myerson M, Quill GE Jr. Late complications of fractures of the calcaneus. J Bone Joint Surg Am. 1993;75(3):331–41.
8. Radney CS, Clare MP, Sanders RW. Subtalar fusion after displaced intra-articular calcaneal fractures: does initial operative treatment matter? J Bone Joint Surg Am. 2009;91(3):541–6.
9. Rammelt S, Grass R, Zawadski T, Biewener A, Zwipp H. Foot function after subtalar distraction bone-block arthrodesis. A prospective study. J Bone Joint Surg Br. 2004;86(5):659–68.
10. Sanders R. Displaced intra-articular fractures of the calcaneus. JBJS Am. 2000;82:225–50.

24 Midfoot Tarsal Fractures (Navicular and Cuboid)

Take-Home Message

- The navicular and its articulations play an important role in hindfoot biomechanics.
- Navicular stress fractures should be treated with short leg cast immobilization and non-weight bearing ×6 weeks.
- Navicular stress fractures are at increased risk for AVN and nonunion.
- Navicular dorsal lip avulsion fractures result from plantar flexion; symptomatic treatment is recommended.
- Navicular tuberosity fractures occur at the site of the posterior tibial tendon insertion; fixation of fractures with >5 mm displacement and large intra-articular fragments.
- Navicular body fractures result from axial load with compression of the medial column; ORIF is recommended for fractures with articular incongruity.
- Type III navicular body fractures may require external fixation or primary fusion; goal is to maintain medial column length.
- The calcaneocuboid joint does not contribute significantly to hindfoot function; arthrodesis results in no loss of hindfoot motion. However, maintaining lateral column length is very important for foot shape and function.
- Cuboid stress fractures should be treated with immobilization, non-weight bearing, and gradual return to activities.
- Cuboid avulsion fractures should undergo symptomatic treatment with immediate weight bearing in a walking boot.
- Cuboid body fractures result from axial load with compression of the lateral column; goal is to maintain lateral column length with ORIF, external fixation, or arthrodesis ± bone grafting.

Navicular fractures

- The tarsal navicular and its articulations play an important role in complex hindfoot biomechanics.
- Navicular stress fracture
  - Mechanism: repetitive trauma and overuse, especially running, jumping, and baseball.
  - Typically occurs in the central third of the navicular, which has limited blood supply.
  - CT scan is the gold stand for diagnosis.
  - MRI and bone scan may also aid in establishing diagnosis.
  - Short leg cast immobilization and non-weight bearing ×6 weeks.

  - Risk of AVN.
  - Increased risk of nonunion without conservative period of restricted weight bearing
    - Delayed union and nonunion are the most common complications and may require ORIF.
- Navicular dorsal lip avulsion fracture
  - Mechanism: plantar flexion
  - Symptomatic treatment for most injuries
  - Weight bearing as tolerated in short leg cast or removable boot
  - Fragment excision for recalcitrant symptoms
- Navicular tuberosity fractures
  - Site of the posterior tibial tendon insertion.
  - Mechanism: eversion with simultaneous contraction of PTT.
  - May represent acute diastasis of an accessory navicular.
  - Oblique 45° radiograph best visualizes tuberosity fractures.
  - ORIF for fractures with >5 mm displacement or large intra-articular fragments.
- Navicular body fractures
  - Mechanism: axial loading with compression of the medial column, "nutcracker."
  - Sangeorzan classification of navicular body fractures
    - Type I: transverse dorsal fracture involving <50 % of the bone
    - Type II: oblique fracture usually from dorsolateral to plantar medial, may have forefoot adduction deformity
    - Type III: central or lateral comminution, abduction deformity
  - ORIF indicated for intra-articular fractures with incongruity.
  - Type III navicular body fractures may require external fixation versus primary arthrodesis
    - Goal is to maintain medial column length.

Cuboid Fractures

- The calcaneocuboid joint does not contribute significantly to normal hindfoot function
  - Arthrodesis results in no loss of hindfoot motion.
- Maintaining lateral column length is very important for foot shape and function.
- Cuboid stress fracture
  - Mechanism: repetitive trauma and overuse, especially running, jumping, and dancing.
  - CT scan, MRI, and bone scan may help confirm diagnosis.
  - Treat with immobilization, non-weight bearing, and gradual return to activities.

- Cuboid avulsion fractures
  - Symptomatic treatment
  - Weight bearing as tolerated with short leg cast or removable boot, if needed
- Cuboid body fractures
  - Mechanism: axial loading with compression of the lateral column with cuboid between the anterior process of the calcaneus and bases of the 4th and 5th metatarsals, "nutcracker"
    - Often associated with jumping sports, such as basketball
  - If there is significant shortening of the lateral column or articular incongruity >2 mm, treat with ORIF vs external fixation vs arthrodesis with the goal of reconstituting the lateral column; bone graft may be required.
  - Short leg cast, non-weight bearing for 6–8 weeks.

Bibliography

1. Lee S, Anderson RB. Stress fractures of the tarsal navicular. Foot Ankle Clin. 2004;9(1):85–104.
2. Miller MD, Thompson SR, Hart JA. Review of orthopaedics. 6th ed. Philadelphia: Elsevier; 2012. p. 771.
3. Torg JS, Moyer J, Gaughan JP, Boden BP. Management of tarsal navicular stress fractures: conservative versus surgical treatment: a meta-analysis. Am J Sports Med. 2010;38(5):1048–53.

25 Tarsometatarsal Fracture-Dislocations (Lisfranc Injury)

Take-Home Message

- Lisfranc ligament is a plantar structure that runs from the base of the second metatarsal to the medial cuneiform.
- AP radiographs: medial bases of first and second metatarsal should align with respective cuneiforms.
- Oblique radiographs: medial base of fourth metatarsal should align with medial edge of cuboid.
- Lateral: dorsal surfaces of tarsals and metatarsals should align.
- Fleck sign represents avulsion of the Lisfranc ligament from the base of the 2nd metatarsal and is diagnostic of Lisfranc injury.
- Obtain stress views, weight-bearing views, and/or comparison views of the contralateral side to further evaluate equivocal cases.
- Contiguous proximal metatarsal base or tarsal fractures may represent Lisfranc-equivalent injuries.

- Operative treatment is recommended for any displaced Lisfranc injury.
- ORIF is preferred for bony fracture-dislocations, while primary arthrodesis may be advantageous in pure ligamentous injuries.
- Posttraumatic midfoot arthrosis is the most common complication and may cause chronic pain, disability, and/or altered gait.

General

- High energy: axial load of a hyperplantar flexed forefoot.
- Low energy: dorsiflexion, twisting.
  - Subtle injuries may be misdiagnosed as a foot sprain.
  - Maintain high index of suspicion when assessing midfoot swelling and/or tenderness.
- Lisfranc joint is comprised of the tarsometatarsal articulations, intermetatarsal articulations, and intertarsal articulations
  - Bony stability, "keystone" configuration with second metatarsal sitting in mortise of the medial cuneiform and recessed middle cuneiform.
- Lisfranc ligament is a plantar structure running from the medial cuneiform, the base of the 2nd metatarsal.
  - Tightens with pronation and abduction of the foot.
  - This maneuver causes pain in acute injuries.
  - Critical for stabilizing the second metatarsal and maintain the arch of the foot.
- Dorsal tarsometatarsal ligaments are weaker than plantar tarsometatarsal ligaments.
- Intermetatarsal ligaments connect the 2nd through 5th metatarsal bases
  - No direct ligament between the 1st and 2nd metatarsal
- Associated proximal metatarsal tarsal fractures are common
  - Contiguous proximal metatarsal base or tarsal fractures may represent Lisfranc-equivalent injuries.
- Clinical improvement may continue for >1 year.

Imaging

- AP foot x-ray: assess alignment of the medial bases of the first and second metatarsals with respective cuneiforms; assess for widening of interval between 1st and 2nd rays and fleck sign (bony fragment in this region that represents avulsion of the Lisfranc ligament from the base of the 2nd metatarsal).
- Oblique foot x-ray: assess alignment medial border of the third metatarsal with medial border of the lateral cuneiform and medial base of the 4th metatarsal with medial border of cuboid.

- Lateral foot x-ray: asses for metatarsal base dorsal subluxation.
- In equivocal cases, consider stress views, weight-bearing views, and comparison views of the contralateral side.
- CT scan may help to further delineate the injury and facilitate operative planning.
- MRI may be helping in confirming diagnosis of pure ligamentous injury.

Classification

- Homolateral: all joints displaced in the same direction, medial or lateral
- Isolated (Partial): first tarsometatarsal joint or rays 2–5
- Divergent: first tarsometatarsal joint displaced medially and rays 2–5 displaced laterally

Treatment

- Goals of treatment: maintain anatomic reduction of all affected joints, avoid soft tissue complications
- Nonoperative
  - Cast immobilization and non-weight bearing ×8 weeks.
  - Isolated dorsal sprains, no subluxation on weight bearing and stress radiographs, no bony injury on CT scan.
  - Consider nonoperative management in nonambulatory patients, severe peripheral vascular disease, and peripheral neuropathy.
- Operative
  - Open reduction internal fixation
    - The goal is to achieve anatomic reduction and stable fixation.
    - Indicated for injuries with any evidence of instability.
    - Preferred in bony fracture-dislocations (as opposed to pure ligamentous injuries)
      - Screw fixation of medial joints
      - Temporary k-wire fixation of the lateral column with removal at 6–8 weeks to preserve motion
    - Delay operative treatment until soft tissue envelop improves (2–3 weeks)
      - Early external fixation or k-wire fixation may be required to temporize grossly unstable injuries.
  - Primary arthrodesis of the first, second, and third tarsometatarsal joints
    - Consider in purely ligamentous injuries and injuries with significant articular comminution.
    - Equivalent functional outcome compared to ORIF with decreased rates of hardware removal and revision surgery.

    - Maintain motion of lateral column.

  - Midfoot arthrodesis
    - Consider in chronic Lisfranc injuries with progressive arch collapse, forefoot abduction, and advanced midfoot arthrosis with failure of conservative management.

  - Rehabilitation
    - Non-weight bearing for 10–12 weeks, early midfoot range of motion.
    - Screws may be removed at 3–6 months.

Complications

- Posttraumatic midfoot arthrosis
  - Most common complication.
  - May cause altered gait, chronic pain, and/or disability.
  - Treat cases refractory to conservative management with midfoot arthrodesis.
- Traumatic planovalgus deformity
  - May develop with missed diagnosis or improper treatment
- Fractured implants
  - Remove only if symptomatic.
- Compartment syndrome
  - Maintain high index of suspicion for foot compartment syndrome.
- Nonunion
  - Uncommon; however revision surgery recommended unless patient is very low demand

Bibliography

1. Henning JA, Jones CB, Sietsema DL, Bohay DR, Anderson JG. Open reduction internal fixation versus primary arthrodesis for Lisfranc injuries: a prospective randomized study. Foot Ankle Int. 2009;30(10):913–22.
2. Ly TV, Coetzee JC. Treatment of primarily ligamentous Lisfranc joint injuries: primary arthrodesis compared with open reduction and internal fixation. A prospective, randomized study. J Bone Joint Surg Am. 2006;88(3):514–20.
3. Miller MD, Thompson SR, Hart JA. Review of orthopaedics. 6th ed. Philadelphia: Elsevier; 2012. p. 771–3.
4. Thompson MC, Mormino MA. Injury to the tarsometatarsal joint complex. J Am Acad Orthop Surg. 2003;11(4):260–7 (Review).
5. Watson TS, Shurnas PS, Denker J. Treatment of Lisfranc joint injury: current concepts. J Am Acad Orthop Surg. 2010;18(12):718–28.

26 Metatarsal Fractures

Take-Home Message

- Assess for Lisfranc-equivalent injury with contiguous metatarsal base fractures.
- The goal is to maintain the transverse and longitudinal arches of the forefoot and proper metatarsal declination angles.
- Most injuries are treated nonoperatively.
- Surgical treatment indicated for displaced first metatarsal fractures; contiguous 2nd, 3rd, and 4th metatarsal fractures; metatarsal fractures with >10° sagittal plane deformity or skin tenting; and some 5th metatarsal base fractures.
- Maintain high index of suspicion for underlying metabolic disorder or foot deformity in patients with metatarsal stress fractures in the absence of increased training or new activities.
- Malunion with prominence on the plantar or dorsal aspect of the foot can lead to pain, plantar callous, ulceration, transfer metatarsalgia, and difficulty with shoe wear.

General

- Common injuries
  - First and fifth metatarsals are more mobile and the most commonly injured.
- Common mechanisms include rotation of hindfoot or leg with fixed forefoot (most common) and crush injury (may have significant associated soft tissue injury).
- The goal is to maintain the transverse and longitudinal arches of the forefoot.
- Critical to assess for the presence of a Lisfranc-equivalent injury with contiguous metatarsal base fractures.

Imaging

- AP, lateral, and oblique views of the foot.
- Stress views, weight-bearing views, and comparison views of the contralateral foot may be helpful in select cases.
- CT scan: may be helpful to assess delayed healing or nonunion.
- MRI: may be helpful to confirm diagnosis of stress fractures and to assess delayed healing or nonunion.
- Bone scan: may be helpful to confirm diagnosis of stress fractures.

First Metatarsal Fractures

- First metatarsal bears 30–50 % of body weight during gait
  - Important to maintain normal declination angle of the first metatarsal for proper forefoot loading
- Nondisplaced fractures: weight bearing as tolerated in hard-soled shoe or low boot.
- Displaced fractures: ORIF with lag screws and/or plate fixation.

Second, Third, and Fourth Metatarsal Fractures

- Metatarsal shaft fractures
  - Majority of these fractures are nondisplaced due to bony architecture and ligamentous attachments in the midfoot
    - Isolated fractures are stable due to intermetatarsal ligaments at the metatarsal base and neck.
    - Isolated fractures of the 3rd metatarsal are rare
      - 70 % have associated 2nd or 4th metatarsal fracture.
  - Most fractures should be weight bearing as tolerated in a hard-soled shoe with arch support or low boot.
  - Surgical fixation recommended for fractures with >10° sagittal plane deformity and concurrent fractures of the 2nd, 3rd, and 4th metatarsals (intermetatarsal ligaments cannot provide inherent stability) and fractures with >4 mm translation
    - ORIF with antegrade-retrograde pinning, lag screws, and/or minifragment plates.
    - Maintain proper metatarsal length and declination angle to prevent transfer metatarsalgia and plantar callous.
- Metatarsal neck fractures
  - Most fractures weight bearing as tolerated in hard-soled shoe or low boot.
  - Consider reduction and pinning of multiple metatarsal neck fractures and fractures with complete displacement.
- Metatarsal shaft fractures
  - The majority of metatarsal shaft fractures are managed nonoperatively.
- Metatarsal base fractures
  - Occur in metaphyseal region, heal quickly.
  - Assess carefully for presence of Lisfranc injury.

- Metatarsal stress fractures
  - Common fractures that result from repetitive stress, overuse, and cavovarus foot
    - Second metatarsal stress fracture most common, seen in amenorrheal dancers
  - Diagnosis with periosteal reaction on x-ray, MRI, or bone scan.
  - Evaluate for metabolic bone disease, especially with insidious onset and absence of increased training or new activities.
  - Weight bearing as tolerated in hard-soled shoe, activity modification.
  - Recurrent stress fractures secondary to cavovarus foot may require alignment reconstruction.

Fifth Metatarsal Fractures

- Subset of metatarsal fractures with special consideration
- Anatomic classification
  - Zone I: pseudo-Jones fracture
    - Avulsion fracture of proximal 5th metatarsal tuberosity.
    - Mechanism: hindfoot inversion with pull on the lateral band of plantar fascia and/or peroneal brevis tendon
      - Avulsion of plantar ligaments more common than avulsion of peroneal brevis insertion
    - May extend into the cubometatarsal joint.
    - Assess lateral ankle ligamentous complex.
    - High rates of union.
    - Symptomatic treatment with weight bearing as tolerated vs initial protected weight bearing in hard-soled shoe or low boot
      - Symptoms may persist for up to 6 months.
    - Consider lag screw fixation for significant displacement of the metatarsocuboid joint, significant malrotation, or skin tenting.
  - Zone II: Jones fracture
    - 5th metatarsal base fracture at the metadiaphysis with extension into the fourth-fifth intermetatarsal joint.
    - Mechanism: forefoot adduction.
    - Vascular watershed area, higher incidence of nonunion.
    - Acute injuries: non-weight bearing in short leg cast for 6–8 weeks.
    - Consider surgical fixation with intramedullary screw for recurrent fracture following conservative treatment and treatment of elite athletes (faster healing and return to sport).

- Zone III: proximal diaphyseal fractures
  - Proximal 5th metatarsal diaphyseal fractures distal to the fourth-fifth inter-metatarsal joint
  - Commonly represent stress fractures
    - Slower healing time and risk of nonunion
  - Mechanism: repetitive microtrauma
  - High risk of refracture of stress fractures with nonoperative management
    - Surgical fixation with intramedullary screw ± bone grafting (may have significant resorption with nonunion).
    - If cavovarus foot position is a contributing factor, consider concurrent foot realignment procedure.

Complications

- Nonunion
  - Most common with Zone II and Zone III 5th metatarsal base fractures due to vascular watershed; treat with screw fixation ± bone grafting.
- Malunion
  - Prominence on the plantar or dorsal surface of the foot can lead to pain, ulceration, transfer metatarsalgia, and difficulty with shoe wear.
  - Failure of conservative treatment (modified shoe wear, etc.) may require osteotomy to correct deformity
- Failure of fixation
  - Increased risk in elite athletes, return to sport prior to radiographic union, and screws that perforate the metatarsal shaft due to radius of curvature mismatch.

Bibliography

1. Buddecke DE, Polk MA, Barp EA. Metatarsal fractures. Clin Podiatr Med Surg. 2010;27(4):601–24 (Review).
2. Miller MD, Thompson SR, Hart JA. Review of orthopaedics. 6th ed. Philadelphia: Elsevier; 2012. p. 490–1, 773.
3. Nunley JA. Fractures of the base of the fifth metatarsal: the jones fracture. Orthop Clin North Am. 2001;32(1):171–80 (Review).
4. O'Malley MJ, Hamilton WG, Munyak J, DeFranco MJ. Stress fractures at the base of the second metatarsal in ballet dancers. Foot Ankle Int. 1996;17(2): 89–94.
5. Roche AJ, Calder JD. Treatment and return to sport following a Jones fracture of the fifth metatarsal: a systematic review. Knee Surg Sports Traumatol Arthrosc. 2013;21(6):1307–15.

27 Phalangeal Fractures

Take-Home Message

- Phalangeal fractures commonly result from crush injuries (dropping heavy object) and axial load injuries (stubbing toe).
- Associated nail bed injury in distal phalanx fracture may represent open fracture.
- The vast majority of phalangeal fractures can be managed nonoperatively with buddy tapping, weight bearing as tolerated, and range of motion.
- Consider ORIF for displaced intra-articular hallux fractures involving >25 % of the joint or with associated instability.
- Phalangeal fractures with significant abduction/adduction deformity not amenable to conservative management may benefit from ORIF as malunion may cause difficulty with shoe wear.
- Stiffness is the most common complication.

General

- Common injuries: hallux > fifth toe > middle toes
- Mechanism
  - Crush: dropping heavy object, comminuted or transverse fracture patterns
  - Axial load: stubbing toes, oblique or spiral fracture
- Assess for nail bed injury and possible open fracture with distal phalanx fractures
  - Irrigate and treat with appropriate antibiotics and tetanus.

Imaging

- AP, oblique, and lateral foot x-rays.
- Dedicated foots of the forefoot may be helpful.

Treatment

- Nonoperative
  - Buddy tapping, weight bearing as tolerated in hard-soled shoe, range of motion
    - Indicated for the vast majority of phalangeal fractures, including intra-articular fractures of the lesser toes

- Operative
  - Reduction and internal fixation versus pinning
    - Consider for displaced intra-articular fractures of the hallux involving >25 % of the joint or with associated instability.
    - Grossly unstable fractures.
    - Phalangeal fractures with significant abduction/adduction deformity not amenable to closed reduction and buddy taping.
      - Significant malunion may cause difficulty with shoe wear.

Complications

- Stiffness is the most common complication.

Bibliography

1. Galant JM, Spinosa FA. Digital fractures. A comprehensive review. J Am Podiatr Med Assoc. 1991;81(11):593–600 (Review).
2. Miller MD, Thompson SR, Hart JA. Review of orthopaedics. 6th ed. Philadelphia: Elsevier; 2012. p. 490, 773.
3. Van Vliet-Koppert ST, Cakir H, Van Lieshout EM, De Vries MR, Van Der Elst M, Schepers T. Demographics and functional outcome of toe fractures. J Foot Ankle Surg. 2011;50(3):307–10.
4. Won SH, Lee S, Chung CY, Lee KM, Sung KH, Kim TG, Choi Y, Lee SH, Kwon DG, Ha JK, Lee SY, Park MS. Buddy tapping: is it a safe method for treatment of finger and toe injuries? Clin Orthop Surg. 2014;6(1): 26–31.

Complications of Trauma

Natalie Casemyr, Cyril Mauffrey, and David Hak

Take-Home Message

- Early stabilization of long bone fractures significantly decreases the risk of pulmonary complications, ARDS, fat embolism, and thromboembolic disease
- DVT prophylaxis must balance the risk of bleeding with the risk of thromboembolic disease
- No regimen of DVT prophylaxis has been shown to decrease the rate of fatal pulmonary embolism

1 Nonunions

- Arrest in the fracture healing process with no evidence of progression in bone healing over 4–6 months
- Risk factors: inadequate fracture stabilization, poor blood supply (scaphoid, distal tibia, fifth metatarsal, intercalary fragments in segmental fractures), infection, smoking, poor nutritional status, immunocompromise

N. Casemyr, MD • C. Mauffrey, MD, FACS, FRCS (✉) • D. Hak, MD, FACS, MBA
Department of Orthopaedic Surgery, Denver Health Medical Center,
777 Bannock Street, Denver 80204, CO, USA
e-mail: cyril.mauffrey@dhha.org; cmauffrey@yahoo.com

C. Mauffrey, D.J. Hak (eds.), *Passport for the Orthopedic Boards and FRCS Examination*, DOI 10.1007/978-2-8178-0475-0_12

- Classification
  - Hypertrophic nonunion: inadequate fracture stability with adequate blood supply, elevated type II collagen, typically heals with improved mechanical stability
  - Oligotrophic nonunion: poor reduction with fracture fragment displacement
  - Atrophic nonunion: inadequate immobilization and inadequate blood supply
  - Septic nonunion
  - Pseudarthrosis
- Presentation
  - Pain with mechanical loading
  - Failure of fracture fixation
  - Radiographs are the primary study to assess fracture healing
  - May consider CT scan if the presence of union is unclear
- Treatment
  - Identify and treat infection, if present
    - May require staged approach
  - Provide stability for hypertrophic nonunions
  - Provide biology for atrophic nonunions
    - Remove dysvascular bone
    - Autologous iliac crest bone graft (gold standard, osteogenic), BMPs (osteoinductive), osteoconductive agents
  - No strong evidence for the use of ultrasound or electromagnetic devices to stimulate bone healing

2 Heterotopic Ossification (HO)

- Ectopic bone that forms in soft tissues
  - Most commonly occurs as a sequelae of trauma or surgical dissection
  - Closed head injury significantly increases the risk of HO
- Risk factors: male, closed head injury, increased ISS, spinal cord injury, ankylosing spondylitis, DISH, Paget's disease
- Common in hip, elbow, and shoulder fractures and any fracture with extensive muscle injury
- Presentation
  - Loss of range of motion, ankylosis, contractures
  - Chronic regional pain syndrome symptoms
  - Inflammation with warm, swollen painful joint or fever
  - Labs: elevated serum alkaline phosphatase, CRP, and CK

- Prophylaxis
  - Radiation: 700 rad 4 h preoperatively or within 72 h postoperatively
    - Inhibits the differentiation and proliferation of osteoprogenitor cells
  - NSAIDS: Indomethacin 75 mg/day ×6 weeks
  - Bisphosphonates: inhibit mineralization but not osteoid matrix formation, HO may become evident with discontinuation of bisphosphonates
- Treatment
  - Sufficiently symptomatic HO may be excised once mature
    - Timing of resection is controversial
    - May consider bone scan or stable appearance of disease on serial radiographs to determine maturity of heterotopic bone
    - Risk of recurrent HO

3 Acute Respiratory Distress Syndrome (ARDS)

- Acute lung injury leads to non-cardiogenic pulmonary edema, respiratory distress, refractory hypoxemia with poor gas exchange, and decreased lung compliance
  - Ultimately results in acute respiratory failure
- Presents with tachypnea, dyspnea, and hypoxemia
- Diagnostic work-up: CXR with bilateral diffuse fluffy infiltrates, arterial blood gas measurements
- Supportive care with high PEEP ventilation and treatment of the underlying pathology
  - Risk of pneumothorax with high PEEP ventilation
  - Steroids not proven to be effective
- Associated with late sepsis and MSOF
- High mortality of 50 % despite critical care
- Early stabilization of long bone fractures significantly decreases the risk of pulmonary complications

4 Fat Embolism

- Inflammatory response to embolized fat and marrow elements
- Incidence: 1–4 % of isolated long bone fractures, 10–15 % of polytrauma patients

- Onset: 24–48 h post-injury
- Diagnostic criteria
  - Major: hypoxemia (PaO_2 <60), CNS confusion/depression, petechial rash, pulmonary edema
  - Minor: tachycardia, pyrexia, retinol emboli, fat in urine or sputum, thrombocytopenia, decreased hematocrit
- Supportive care with high PEEP ventilation
- 10–15 % mortality rate
- Early stabilization of long bone fractures is the most important factor in prevention

5 Systemic Inflammatory Response Syndrome (SIRS)

- Generalized response to trauma with increased cytokines, complement, and hormones
- SIRS criteria
  - Heart rate >90 bpm
  - WBC <4 or >10
  - Respirations <20 breaths per minute with $PaCO_2$ <32 mm
  - Temperature <36 °C or >38 °C
- Associated with disseminated intravascular coagulopathy (DIC), ARDS, renal failure, shock, and multisystem organ failure

6 Thromboembolic Disease

- Virchow's Triad: venous stasis, hypercoagulability, intimal injury
- Risk factors: history of thromboembolism, obesity, malignancy, oral contraceptives, smoking, blood disorders that create a hypercoaguable state, immobilization, paralysis, pregnancy
- Thromboplastin triggers the coagulation cascade and is released in large amounts during orthopedic procedures
- High incidence of DVT in trauma patients not receiving prophylaxis
  - Pelvis/acetabular fractures: 20 %
  - Polytrauma patients: 35 %
  - Hip fractures: 60 %
  - Spine fracture with paralysis: 100 %
- Early fracture stabilization lowers incidence

- Prophylaxis
  - Mechanical prophylaxis prevents venous stasis and increases fibrinolytic activity
  - Many options for chemical prophylaxis
  - Prophylactic treatment should be determined by balancing the risk of bleeding with risk of thromboembolic disease
  - Consider vena cava filter in high-risk patients (pelvic trauma, polytrauma, bleeding diathesis) with contraindication to chemical prophylaxis
- Diagnosis
  - Clinical suspicion: extremity pain, swelling, and Homan's sign
  - Assess with venography, duplex ultrasonography, CT scan
- Pulmonary embolus
  - Symptoms: tachypnea 90 %, tachycardia 60 %, EGC changes 25 %, pleuritic chest pain
  - Diagnostic studies: ECG, CXR, arterial blood gas, ventilation-perfusion scan, pulmonary angiography (gold standard)
  - Risk of upper extremity DVT embolization: ~5 %
  - Risk of lower extremity DVT embolization: ~20 %
  - No regimen of DVT prophylaxis has been shown to lower the incidence of *fatal* PE

Bibliography

1. Browner BD, Jupiter JB, Levine AM, Trafton PG, Krettek C. Skeletal trauma. 4th ed. Philadelphia: Saunders; 2009. p. 177–92, pp 199–214.
2. Falck-Ytter Y, Francis CW, Johanson NA, Curley C, Dahl OE, Schulman S, Ortel TL, Pauker SG, Colwell CW Jr, American College of Chest Physicians. Prevention of VTE in orthopedic surgery patients: Antithrombotic Therapy and Prevention of Thrombosis, 9th ed: American College of Chest Physicians Evidence-Based Clinical Practice Guidelines. Chest. 2012;141(2 Suppl):e278S–325.
3. Knudson MM, Collins JA, Goodman SB, McCrory DW. Thromboembolism following multiple trauma. J Trauma. 1992;32(1):2–11.
4. Miller MD, Thompson SR, Hart JA. Review of orthopaedics. Philadelphia: Elsevier; 2012. p. 20, 105–109, 698–703.
5. Pape HC, Lehmann U, van Griensven M, Gänsslen A, von Glinski S, Krettek C. Heterotopic ossifications in patients after severe blunt trauma with and without head trauma: incidence and patterns of distribution. J Orthop Trauma. 2001;15(4):229–37.

Part IV
Spine

Samuel E. Smith

General Topics

Samuel E. Smith

1 Spinal Biomechanics

Samuel E. Smith

Take-Home Message

- Motion segment – disc and paired facet joints
- Must have at least 50 % of the facet joints intact for stability:
- White and Panjabi criteria for stability

- Spinal stability: general definition is that motion segment provides mobility while at the same time protecting neurologic structures and function and implies non-painful movement.
- White and Panjabi.
- Cervical spine stability when less than 3.5 mm of translation at each segment and less than 11° of flexion relative to adjacent motion segments.
- Motion at each segment of the spine largely defined by facet joint orientation.
- Occiput-C1 provides for flexion/extension.
- C1/C2 provides for rotation due to unique anatomy.
- Subaxial cervical spine provides flexion/extension and lateral bending coupled with rotation.
- Thoracic motion is rotational.

S.E. Smith, MD
Department of Orthopaedics, Denver Health Medical Center,
777 Bannock Street, Denver 80204, CO, USA
e-mail: samuel.smith@dhha.org

C. Mauffrey, D.J. Hak (eds.), *Passport for the Orthopedic Boards and FRCS Examination*, DOI 10.1007/978-2-8178-0475-0_13

- Lumbar motion is combined. Flexion and extension with lateral bending and rotation which are limited by the unique orientation of the lumbar facet joints, lateral bending, and rotation are coupled.
- Instantaneous axis of rotation is the posterior half of the disc.
- In general, the anterior column experiences compression forces; cages and structural grafts best resist this compression; anterior plates confer some advantage but do not resist flexion well.
- Lateral plates are a little better.
- In general, the posterior column experiences tension forces, and a screw and rod construct resists this best and also resists shear forces.

Bibliography

1. White 3rd AA, Johnson RM, Panjabi MM, Southwick WO. Biomechanical analysis of clinical stability in the cervical spine. Clin Orthop Relat Res. 1975;109:85–96.

2 Degenerative Cascade

Samuel E. Smith

Take-Home Message
- Read Kirkaldy-Willis
- Represents the continuum of degenerative changes in the motion segment of the spine

Definition

- The degenerative changes over time which occur in the motion segment of each spinal level
- Involves both disc and facet joint degenerative changes

Etiology

- Chondrocyte degeneration
- Water loss and disc desiccation
- Instability
- Hypertrophic change

Pathophysiology

- A continuum of degenerative changes which start with chondrocyte degeneration of the surrounding cartilage matrix
- Leads to instability and the natural process of hypertrophic change – Mother Nature's attempt at stability

- Leads to stenosis, deformity, slip, etc.
- Inflammatory changes ensue

Radiographs

- Marginal osteophytes causing a change in the surface area of disc and facet joint
- Spondylolisthesis
- Endplate sclerosis
- Degenerative subchondral cystic change

Bibliography

1. Kirkaldy-Willis WH, Farfan HF. Instability of the lumbar spine. Clin Orthop Relat Res. 1982;165:110–23.

3 Imaging of the Spine

Samuel E. Smith

Take-Home Message

- X-rays: easy, inexpensive, best to see bony pathology and deformity.
- Risk is radiation.
- CT: detailed bony anatomy, neurologic information improved with myelography.
- Risk is high doses of radiation.
- MRI: useful for anatomic information from bone and neurologic structure and provides some physiologic information.
- Best for tumor, imaging of spinal cord and nerves, imaging of discs.
- Risks not entirely known as yet.
- DEXA: essential to define bone density, osteoporosis is a huge health problem now and into the future.
- Nuclear medicine is useful but not as specific, and radiation dose is high; indium labeling may be useful with infection.
- Understand the need to relate the imaging findings with the patient's history and physical assessment; large number of patients with degenerative changes and no symptoms.

Bibliography

1. Boden SD, Wiesel SW. Lumbar spine imaging: role in clinical decision making. J Am Acad Orthop Surg. 1996;4(5):238–48.

4 Spine Infection

Samuel E. Smith

Take-Home Message
- Requires high index of suspicion.
- Post-op infection rate varies in the literature, depends on length and complexity of the procedure and patient comorbidities.
- Obesity and diabetes increase risk of surgical site infection.
- Spondylodiscitis – mostly treated with antibiotics.
- Epidural abscess with neurologic deficit requires surgery, but remember these occur often in patients who are immunocompromised.

Definition

- SSI or surgical site infection – infection within 30 days of surgery, can be superficial or deep and can be hard to distinguish.
- Spondylodiscitis/osteomyelitis is a hematogenous infection – often associated with IV drug abuse and in immunocompromised patients.

Etiology

- SSI: contamination at surgery.
- Obesity increases risk.
- Poor diabetic control increases risk.
- Longer operating times.
- Hematogenous seeding.

Pathophysiology

- SSI: bacteria contaminate with local wound immune compromise due to hematoma and dead space
- Hematogenous spread from other sources, i.e., poor oral health, open sore

Radiographs

- X-ray: not often useful for SSI; spondylodiscitis may show endplate erosions and disc collapse.
- CT: can show bony destruction and soft tissue swelling or fluid collection
- MRI: bright signal in disc, endplate erosion, may show epidural abscess or epidural phlegmon, may need contrast to see rim enhancement

Classification

- SSI: superficial or deep

Treatment

- SSI

Nonoperative

- Antibiotics alone for cellulitis
- Antibiotics and bracing for spondylodiscitis
- Antibiotics alone for some cases of epidural abscess without neurologic deficit

Operative

- SSI: surgical debridement for deep infections of all necrotic debris, need to remove bone graft that is not adherent to soft tissue, save hardware if stable, remove if loose
- Spondylodiscitis for cases of instability or deformity
- Epidural abscess with neurologic changes; most favor surgery, but studies are mixed.

Complications

- Death from sepsis and multiorgan failure
- Neurologic injury
- Failure to clear infection

Special Situations

- Granulomatous disease – will likely need anterior/posterior surgery for kyphosis or neurologic deficit
- Antibiotic important for TB especially and may need control of disease before surgery
- Stage surgery when possible
- Pediatric discitis – mostly antibiotic and surgery only for refractory cases

Bibliography

1. Arko 4th L, Quach E, Nguyen V, Chang D, Sukul V, Kim BS. Medical and surgical management of spinal epidural abscess: a systematic review. Neurosurg Focus. 2014;37(2):E4. doi:10.3171/2014.6.FOCUS14127.
2. Hsieh PC, Wienecke RJ, O'Shaughnessy BA, Koski TR, Ondra SL. Surgical strategies for vertebral osteomyelitis and epidural abscess. Neurosurg Focus. 2004;17(6):E4.

5 Spine Tumors

Samuel E. Smith

Take-Home Message
- Need to define spinal stability and risk of deformity.
- Need to determine neurologic status.
- Pain caused by tumor and above factors.
- Metastatic disease most common.

Definition

- Tumor is present in the bone and surrounding tissues of the spine, causing destruction and potentially making the spine unstable or prone to neurologic injury.

Etiology

- Metastatic disease:
  - Breast, lung, thyroid, prostate, renal
- Multiple myeloma is the most common primary tumor, often presents as osteoporotic compression fracture.
- Other primary bone tumors are very rare:
  - Osteoid osteoma (most often posterior elements), osteoblastoma, osteosarcoma, chondrosarcoma, GCT, ABC

Pathophysiology

- Neoplastic growth
- Causes osteoclasts to resorb bone

Radiographs

- X-rays: bony destruction, deformity, and fracture; look for destruction of the pedicle on AP view of the lumbar spine.
- CT: bony definition of the spine and canal.
- MRI: neurologic compromise, bone and soft tissue involvement.
- Bone scan: screen for bony metastases throughout skeleton.
- PET scan.

Classification

- Depends on tumor staging classifications

Treatment

- Work up tumor and get tissue type.

Nonoperative

- Radiation.
- Chemotherapy.
- Try to avoid bracing for palliative measures.

Operative

- Stabilize.
- Decompress.
- If metastatic disease, try to operate prior to radiation.
- En bloc resection for curable primary tumors.
- With short life expectancy, try to make spine immediately stable.
- Renal cell carcinoma is vascular and may benefit from preop embolization.

Complications

- Failure of fixation
- Infection
- Local recurrence
- Neurologic injury
- DVT/PE – malignancy increases hypercoagulability
- Bleeding

Bibliography

1. Perrin RG, Laxton AW. Metastatic spine disease: epidemiology, pathophysiology, and evaluation of patients. Neurosurg Clin N Am. 2004;15:365–73.
2. White AP, Kwon BK, Lindskog DM, Friedlaender GE, Grauer JN. Metastatic disease of the spine. J Am Acad Orthop Surg. 2006;14(11):587–98.

Inflammatory Disorders

Samuel E. Smith

1 Ankylosing Spondylitis

Samuel E. Smith

> **Take-Home Message**
> - Inflammatory enthesopathy, facet inflammation
> - Related to HLA-B27 antigen, males more often than females
> - Causes bamboo spine appearance
> - Involves SI joints
> - Osteoarthritis of the hips

Definition

- Enthesis – where the tendon, muscle, or ligament attaches to bone.
- Ankylosing spondylitis is an inflammatory disorder where the anterior longitudinal ligament attaches to bone.

Etiology

- Autoimmune phenomenon
- Associated with HLA-B27 antigen

S.E. Smith, MD
Department of Orthopaedics, Denver Health Medical Center,
777 Bannock Street, Denver 80204, CO, USA
e-mail: samuel.smith@dhha.org

C. Mauffrey, D.J. Hak (eds.), *Passport for the Orthopedic Boards and FRCS Examination*, DOI 10.1007/978-2-8178-0475-0_14

Pathophysiology

- Enthesitis of discs and facets.
- Syndesmophytes are marginal.
- SI joints involved.
- Other organ systems involved.
- Causes kyphosis especially the cervicothoracic junction.
- Fractures can occur with little trauma.

Radiographs

- X-rays: Marginal syndesmophytes
- CT: Bony definition in case of fracture
- MRI: Can identify occult fracture
- Nuclear medicine to look for occult fracture and SI inflammation

Classification None

Treatment

Nonoperative

- NSAIDs.
- DMARDs: TNF-alpha-blockers.
- Postural and flexibility exercises.
- Treat bone density.

Operative

- Fractures may need posterior and anterior fixation.
- Epidural hematoma may need draining.
- Chin on chest deformity: Cervicothoracic osteotomy.
- May need corrective osteotomies anywhere in the thoracic or lumbar spine areas.

Complications

- Failure of fixation
- Neurologic injury very high risk
- Death
- Failure around long lever arm

Bibliography

1. de Peretti F, Hovorka I, Aboulker C, Bonneau G, Argenson C. Fracture of the spine, spinal epidural haematoma and spondylitis. Report of one case and review of the literature. Eur Spine J. 1993;1(4):244–8.
2. Masiero S, Bonaldo L, Pigatto M, Lo Nigro A, Ramonda R, Punzi L. Rehabilitation treatment in patients with ankylosing spondylitis stabilized with tumor necrosis factor inhibitor therapy: a randomized controlled trial. J Rheumatol. 2011;38(7):1335–42. doi:10.3899/jrheum.100987. Epub 2011 Apr 1.

2 Rheumatoid Spondylitis

Samuel E. Smith

Take-Home Message

- Cranial settling because C1 can settle on C2 as distinct from basilar invagination which may occur with osteoporosis of the skull base
- C1/C2 instability fundamental, erosion of transverse ligament of the atlas
- Subaxial subluxations
- Pain and myelopathy

Definition

- Rheumatoid arthritis is a synovial proliferative disease.

Etiology

- Viral, autoimmune causing synovial proliferation

Pathophysiology

- Anterior arch of C1, synovial joint exists between odontoid and tranverse ligament of the atlas, facet and synovial joints are relatively large compared to the overall motion segment in the cervical spine, thoracic and lumbar spines are spared
- Rheumatoid pannus possible behind the odontoid, instability possible between C1/C2 and occiput C2

Radiographs

- X-ray: C1/C2 instability, check flexion/extension films, ADI greater than 3 mm
- Review Ranawat, McGregor, Chamberlin, etc. lines, define the relationship of the odontoid to foramen magnum
- MRI: C1/C2 relationship and pannus formation, spinal cord compression and cord signal, cervicomedullary angle should be less than 135°, can be compressed by the odontoid in the foramen magnum
- Myelography/CT when MRI not possible or when bony anatomy needs definition for operative therapy

Classification

- Know classification schemes for myelopathy, Nurick, Ranawat, Japanese Orthopedic Association.

Treatment

Nonoperative

- DMARDs
- Steroids
- Observation

Operative

- Occipitocervical fusion, C1/C2 fusion, C1 posterior arch resection or enlargement of the foramen magnum with fusion, transoral odontoid and pannus removal, multilevel fusion which may span from the occiput to cervical spine depending upon pathology

Complications

- Death with or without operative therapy
- Neurologic injury
- Pseudarthrosis
- Vertebral artery injury and posterior or cerebellar stroke
- CSF leak
- Sagittal sinus injury from occipital fixation
- Continued progression of myelopathy in spite of adequate decompression
- DVT/PE

Bibliography

1. Shen FH, Samartzis D, Jenis LG, An HS. Rheumatoid arthritis: evaluation and surgical management of the cervical spine. Spine J. 2004;4(6):689–700.

Trauma

Samuel E. Smith

1 Spinal Cord Injury

Samuel E. Smith

Take-Home Message

- Know the different cord syndromes, anterior, posterior (rare), central, and Brown-Sequard (hemisection).
- Use of steroids for spinal cord injury is controversial, may cause root sparing, and complication rate is high in some series.
- Know how to define level of injury.

Definition

- Damage to tissue of the spinal cord altering its function and causing varying degrees of paralysis
- Level of spinal cord injury defined by lowest level of normal sensory and motor function bilaterally

Etiology

- Blunt trauma
- Penetrating trauma – this is where hemisection is more likely.

S.E. Smith, MD
Department of Orthopaedics, Denver Health Medical Center,
777 Bannock Street, Denver 80204, CO, USA
e-mail: samuel.smith@dhha.org

C. Mauffrey, D.J. Hak (eds.), *Passport for the Orthopedic Boards and FRCS Examination*, DOI 10.1007/978-2-8178-0475-0_15

Pathophysiology

- Direct trauma
- Edema
- Vascular insult
- Free radicals

Radiographs

- Needs myelogram/CT or MRI to look at the cord
- MRI – only way to see substance of the cord

Classification

- ASIA (American Spinal Injury Association)
- A – complete, B – sensory preservation distally, C – sensory and motor activity less than Grade 3, D – sensory and motor activity greater than Grade 3, E – normal

Treatment

- Steroids are controversial.
- Stabilize the spine injury from the field to the ER.
- Decompress the spinal canal when appropriate and operatively stabilize the spine.
- DVT prophylaxis – rate of DVT and PE high
- Gunshot wound – leave alone unless intrathecal or causing progressive neurologic deficit

Complications

- DVT
- Pressure sores
- Urinary tract infection
- Autonomic dysfunction – bradycardia, hypotension, autonomic dysreflexia from visceral distention especially the bladder

Bibliography

1. Eidelberg E. The pathophysiology of spinal cord injury. Radiol Clin North Am. 1977;15(2):241–6.

2 Cervical Spine Injury

Samuel E. Smith

Take-Home Message

- Look for other injuries – head, chest.
- Look for noncontiguous spine fractures, vertebral artery injury.
- Protect the spinal cord.
- Know protocol or have one in place at your institution for collar removal.

Definition

- Injury to the bone and ligamentous structure of the cervical spine from the occiput to C7

Etiology

- Trauma:
  - Fall, MVC, penetrating trauma
- Beware of spine injury associated with ankylosing spondylitis, diffuse idiopathic skeletal hyperostosis, ossification of the posterior longitudinal ligament, osteoporosis, and cervical spondylosis (risk of central cord syndrome even without fracture).
- Risk by mechanism: high-speed MVC, fall greater than 10 ft, head injuries.

Pathophysiology

- Fracture
- Ligament injury
- Cord injury
- Edema
- Bleeding
- Vertebral artery injury

Radiographs

- Clearance protocols
- CT scans for intoxicated patients, distracting injuries, i.e., other fractures, midline tenderness
- CT-angiogram for high risk of vertebral artery injury (C1/C2 or transverse foramen injuries)

Classification

- Depends on specific injury

Treatment

- Depends on specific injury

Complications

- Airway compromise
- Respiratory failure
- Neurologic injury

Bleeding into the canal or cord

- DVT/PE
- Pressure sores

Pediatric Cervical Spine Trauma

- Occiput/C1 injuries more common.
- X-rays interpreted differently due to immature skeleton.
- More physiologic motion can be confused with instability.
- Soft tissues anterior to the cervical spine wider than in the adult, i.e., 6 mm at C2 and 22 mm at C6.
- ADI in kids 5 mm compared to 3 mm in adults.
- Account for the size of the child's head compared to the thorax when stabilizing the cervical spine, relatively large head causes flexion on a flat surface.
- Beware that atlantoaxial instability can occur with pharyngitis.

Bibliography

1. Lebl DR, Bono CM, Velmahos G, Metkar U, Nguyen J, Harris MB. Vertebral artery injury associated with blunt cervical spine trauma: a multivariate regression analysis. Spine (Phila Pa 1976). 2013;38(16):1352–61. doi:10.1097/BRS.0b013e318294bacb.
2. McCall T, Fassett D, Brockmeyer D. Cervical McCall T, Fassett D, Brockmeyer D. Cervical spine trauma in children: a review. Neurosurg Focus. 2006;20(2):E5.

3 Occiput/C1 Injuries

Samuel E. Smith

Take-Home Message
- Rarely survive but survival more common with improved resuscitation of patients at the scene
- By definition occiput/C1 dissociation unstable
- Always needs surgery

Definition

- Disruption of ligamentous connection between occiput, C1, and C2

Etiology

- High-energy trauma:
  - Children more susceptible due to relatively large size of the head compared to the trunk

Pathophysiology

- Disruption of occiput/C1 joint capsule
- Disruption of paired alar ligaments of the dens

Radiographs

- Difficult to see, review Power's ratio – establishes anterior/posterior relationship of occiput to C1
- CT – essential to see bony relationships
- MRI to look for soft tissue and spinal cord injuries

Classification

- Anterior
- Posterior
- Distractive

Treatment

- Operative always as it is grossly unstable:
  - Occiput to C1 or more commonly C2 fusion, wiring or screw, occipital plate and rods

Complications

- Neurologic injury pentaplegia
- CSF leak from occipital screws
- Injury to transverse sagittal sinus with potential for death
- DVT/PE
- Infection

Bibliography

1. Gire JD, Roberto RF, Bobinski M, Klineberg EO, Durbin-Johnson B. The utility and accuracy of computed tomography in the diagnosis of occipitocervical dissociation. Spine J. 2013;13(5):510–9. doi:10.1016/j.spinee.2013.01.023. Epub 2013 Feb 22.
2. Lador R, Ben-Galim PJ, Weiner BK, Hipp JA. The association of occipitocervical dissociation and death as a result of blunt trauma. Spine J. 2010;10(12):1128–32. doi:10.1016/j.spinee.2010.09.025.

4 Fractures of the Atlas

Samuel E. Smith

Take-Home Message

- 7 mm of lateral mass displacement combined defines rupture of the transverse ligament of the atlas.
- Otherwise atlas fractures mostly stable.
- The canal of the occiput to C2 is wide and accounts in part for reduced risk of neurologic injury with these fractures.
- Beware of high rate of contiguous and noncontiguous spine fractures and head injury.

Definition

- Fracture of one or both arches of C1 with or without displacement of the lateral masses

Etiology

- Usually axial trauma

Pathophysiology

- Trauma with axial load to the lateral masses causing a disruption of the C1 ring typically involving the arches

Radiographs

- X-ray: open mouth, shows widening between dens and lateral masses and overhang of C1 lateral masses on C2 superior facets
- CT: shows best and defines fracture complexity
- MRI sometimes to show rupture of TAL from bone

Classification

- Type I: anterior arch fracture
- Type II: bilateral arch fractures from bursting injury to C1
- Type III: unilateral mass displacement

Treatment

Nonoperative

- Typically bracing with semirigid collar for 6–8 weeks

Operative

- If transverse ligament of the atlas is ruptured, C1/C2 fusion with instrumentation needed
- C1 lateral mass and C2 pedicle screws or Magerl's transarticular technique
- Preop CT needed to make sure that screws can be passed safely without entering the foramen transversarium

Complications

- Neurologic injury: rare
- Infection
- DVT/PE
- Greater occipital nerve injury
- Vertebral artery injury
- Dural tear or leak

Bibliography

1. Jackson RS, Banit DM, Rhyne 3rd AL, Darden 2nd BV. Upper cervical spine injuries. J Am Acad Orthop Surg. 2002;10(4):271–80. Review.
2. Vergara P, Bal JS, Hickman Casey AT, Crockard HA, Choi D. C1-C2 posterior fixation: are 4 screws better than 2? Neurosurgery. 2012;71(1 Suppl Operative): 86–95. doi:10.1227/NEU.0b013e318243180a.

5 Hangman's Fracture

Samuel E. Smith

Take-Home Message

- Classic presentation of C2 pars fractures with separation of the vertebral body from posterior elements. but there are many variations where fractures involve lateral masses.
- High association with fractures at other levels of the spine.
- Because of the wide canal at this level, patients mostly present neurologically normal.
- Most fracture types are stable and do not require operative treatment.
- Avoid traction in IIA fractures as they have a distraction component and traction therefore dangerous.

Definition

- C2 fracture separating posterior elements from the anterior elements, sometimes with subluxation of C2 on C3

Etiology

- Hyperextension, fracturing the pars with subsequent flexion which may cause C2/C3 subluxation
- Motor vehicle accidents

Pathophysiology

- Most fractures caused by initial hyperextension followed by flexion.
- IIA fractures include flexion/distraction component and require different treatment.

Radiographs

- X-rays define basic injury.
- CT best for details of the bony injury.
- CTA to detect vertebral artery injury.
- MRI to look at the cord if needed, also may help define flexion/distraction component.

Classification

- Type I – may have up to 3 mm anterior displacement but no angulation
- Type II – have displacement up to 3 mm and angulation of C2/C3
- Type IIA – very important distinction, have no displacement but are angulated and represent a flexion/distraction injury, do not use traction
- Type III – same as Type I but with dislocated facets at C2/C3

Treatment

Nonoperative

- Type I fractures can be treated in rigid orthosis – autofusion of C2/C3 facets likely.
- Type II fractures can be treated with traction and halo.
- Type IIA fractures should not be treated in traction, and rather they are placed in extension and then compressed in a halo.

Operative

- Type III fractures are treated operatively.
- Anterior C2/C3 discectomy, fusion with plate fixation.
- Posterior C1 to C3 fusion.
- Repair of pars fractures by direct screw fixation.
- Some Type II fractures with 5 mm or more of displacement may need surgery.

Complications

- Neurologic injury
- Vertebral artery injury
- Nonunion

- Malunion usually well tolerated
- Infection
- DVT/PE
- Decubiti from being in one position for traction

Bibliography

1. Effendi B, Roy D, Cornish B, Dussault RG, Laurin CA. Fractures of the ring of the axis. A classification based on the analysis of 131 cases. J Bone Joint Surg Br. 1981;63-B(3):319–27.
2. Levine AM, Edwards CC. The management of traumatic spondylolisthesis of the axis. J Bone Joint Surg Am. 1985;67(2):217–26.
3. Vaccaro AR, Madigan L, Bauerle WB, Blescia A, Cotler JM. Early halo immobilization of displaced traumatic spondylolisthesis of the axis. Spine (Phila Pa 1976). 2002;27(20):2229–33.

6 Rotatory Atlantoaxial Instability

Samuel E. Smith

Take-Home Message

- Mostly nontraumatic but rather associated with inflammation or ligamentous laxity

Definition

- Rotation of C1 on C2 with subluxation or dislocation of C1/C2 lateral mass joints, can also be associated with translational change if there is disruption of the transverse ligament of the atlas

Etiology

- Pharyngeal inflammation: Grisel's syndrome
- Joint laxity as in Down's syndrome or juvenile arthritis

Pathophysiology

- Inflammatory changes weakening the ligamentous structures of C1/C2 or underlying ligamentous laxity

Radiographs

- Open-mouth X-ray: can look for asymmetry of odontoid lateral mass relationship but sometimes hard to see

- CT with dynamic views: best study
- MRI: may be hard to interpret but best way to see the cord and its relationship to the canal

Classification

- Type I: rotational subluxation of C1 on C2 with the odontoid being the axis of rotation
- Type II: rotation about one of the facet joints as the axis with potential injury to transverse ligament of the atlas
- Type III: both C1 lateral masses translated anteriorly in addition to rotation and defines disruption of the transverse ligament of the atlas
- Type IV: posterior displacement and rotation and very rare

Treatment

- For the first week can be observation, perhaps ibuprofen, and wait for spontaneous location
- Skull traction over 1–3 days to try and relocate
- Manipulation with tongs
- May require halo placement
- May in rare circumstance require C1/C2 fusion

Complications

- Mostly a problem in children and complications rare
- Infection
- Malrotation and fixed deformity

Bibliography

1. Pang D. Atlantoaxial rotatory fixation. Neurosurgery. 2010;66(3 Supp):161–83. doi:10.1227/01.NEU.0000365800.94865.D4.

7 Odontoid Fracture

Samuel E. Smith

Take-Home Message

- Nonunion higher risk with Type II fractures with any of the following:
  - 5 mm displacement
  - Comminution
  - Angulation more than 10°
  - Age greater than 50
- Normal atlanto-dens interval on X-ray 3 mm for adult and 5 mm for children

Definition

- Fractures of the odontoid process

Etiology

- Both flexion and extension mechanisms
- Type I fractures may be associate with occipitocervical injuries

Pathophysiology

- Disrupts the relationship between C1 and C2 with respect to stability.
- Type I injuries include alar ligament avulsions which attach to C1 and to the occiput.

Radiographs

- X-rays: check lateral and open-mouth views
- CT: ADI of greater than 10 mm or SAC (space available for the cord) less than 17 mm highly associated with neurologic deficit
- CT/angiography to look for vertebral artery injury
- MRI: looks at the spinal cord and signal changes

Classification

- Anderson and D'Alonzo
  - Type I: apical avulsion-type fractures
  - Type II: waist fractures at the level of the transverse ligament of the atlas
  - Type III: involving the vertebral body

Treatment

Nonoperative

- Halo for young people with Type II odontoid
- Rigid collar for elderly people, more complication with halo party due to osteoporosis

Operative

- Odontoid screw fixation to preserve rotation about the odontoid
- C1/C2 posterior fixation and fusion with wires, screws, and rods and bone grafting, eliminates rotation between C1 and C2 which is at least 50 % of the total cervical rotation but not all odontoid fractures can be fixed with a screw

Complications

- DVT/PE especially with spinal cord injury
- Infection
- Nonunion and malunion
- Neurologic
- Blindness
- Positional neuropathies

Bibliography

1. Anderson LD, D'Alonzo RT. Fractures of the odontoid process of the axis. J Bone Joint Surg Am. 1974;56(8):1663–74.
2. Konieczny MR, Gstrein A, Müller EJ. Treatment algorithm for dens fractures: non-halo immobilization, anterior screw fixation, or posterior transarticular C1-C2 fixation. J Bone Joint Surg Am. 2012;94(19):e144(1–6). doi:10.2106/JBJS.K.01616.

8 Subaxial Cervical Spine Trauma

Samuel E. Smith

Take-Home Message
- Know the SLIC
- Combination of bone, ligament, and neurologic deficit to define stability of injury and, therefore, operative vs. nonoperative treatment
- Requires bony and soft tissue imaging in conjunction with physical findings to accurately define stability

Definition

- Trauma to the bone, ligament, and nerve structures of the cervical spine

Etiology

- Different mechanism of force applied to the spine from motor vehicle, trauma, falls, penetrating trauma, violence, etc.
- Flexion, flexion/distraction, axial load, hyperextension, sheer, lateral bending, and rotational forces
- For example, hyperextension injuries in the face of preexisting pathology, like DISH

Pathophysiology

- Post-injury inflammatory change of bone, ligament and neurologic tissue
- Sometimes leads to neurologic deficit
- Fracture pattern depends on force direction

Radiographs

- X-ray: defines bony injury and overall spinal alignment.
- CT: gives accurate 3-D image of bony injury and facet joint location.
- MRI defines neurologic and soft tissue injuries.

Classification

- SLIC classification-point system – 4 points is in between, less than four nonoperative, and more than four definitely operative
- Morphology

Compression fracture	1
Burst fracture	2
Distraction (can be disc hyperextension or facet perch)	3
Translation/rotation	4

- Neurologic involvement

Root injury	1
Complete cord	2
Incomplete cord	3
Continued compression in the face of neurologic deficit	

- Posterior ligamentous complex

Intact	0
Injury suspected/indeterminate	2
Definitely Injured	3

Treatment

Nonoperative

- Nonoperative can be observation or bracing, may require halo

Operative

- Depends on pathology, comminution of any burst component and the need to decompress any neurologic injury.
- Can be anterior, posterior, or combined and possibly staged.
- Goal is to decompress, stabilize the spine, and mobilize the patient.

Complications

- DVT/PE especially with spinal cord injury
- Infection
- Neurologic
- Blindness
- Positional neuropathies
- Decubiti

Bibliography

1. Kwon BK, Vaccaro AR, Grauer JN, Fisher CG, Dvorak MF. Subaxial cervical spine trauma. J Am Acad Orthop Surg. 2006;14(2):78–89.

2. Patel AA, Hurlbert RJ, Bono CM, Bessey JT, Yang N, Vaccaro AR. Classification and surgical decision making in acute subaxial cervical spine trauma. Spine (Phila Pa 1976). 2010;35(21 Suppl):S228–34. doi:10.1097/BRS.0b013e3181f330ae.
3. Whang PG, Goldberg G, Lawrence JP, Hong J, Harrop JS, Anderson DG, Albert TJ, Vaccaro AR. The management of spinal injuries in patients with ankylosing spondylitis or diffuse idiopathic skeletal hyperostosis: a comparison of treatment methods and clinical outcomes. J Spinal Disord Tech. 2009;22(2):77–85. doi:10.1097/BSD.0b013e3181679bcb.

9 Thoracolumbar Spine Trauma

Samuel E. Smith

Take-Home Message

- Know the TLICS.
- Combination of bone, ligament, and neurologic deficit to define stability of injury and, therefore, operative vs. nonoperative treatment.
- Requires bony and soft tissue imaging in conjunction with physical findings to accurately define stability.

Definition

- Trauma to the bone, ligament, and nerve structures of the spine

Etiology

- Different mechanism of force applied to the spine from motor vehicle, trauma, falls, penetrating trauma, violence, etc.
- Flexion, flexion/distraction, axial load, hyperextension, sheer, lateral bending, and rotational forces

Pathophysiology

- As per the definition above
- Post-injury inflammatory change of bone, ligament, and neurologic tissue
- Sometimes leads to neurologic deficit

Radiographs

- X-ray: defines bony injury and overall spinal alignment.
- CT: gives accurate 3-D image of bony injury and facet joint location.
- MRI defines neurologic and soft tissue injuries.

Classification

- TLICS classification-point system – 4 points is in between, less than four nonoperative, and more than four definitely operative
- Morphology

Compression fracture	1
Burst fracture	2
Translation/rotation	3
Distraction	4

- Neurologic involvement

Incomplete	3
Complete	2
Cauda equina	3

- Posterior ligamentous complex

Intact	0
Injury suspect/indeterminate	2
Injured	3

Treatment

- Nonoperative can be observation or bracing, historically burst fractures treated aggressively but many can be treated closed, from the University of Iowa study

Operative

- Depends on pathology, comminution of any burst component, and the need to decompress any neurologic injury.
- Can be anterior, posterior, or combined and possibly staged.
- Goal is to decompress, stabilize the spine, and mobilize the patient.

Complications

- DVT/PE especially with spinal cord injury
- Infection
- Neurologic
- Blindness
- Positional neuropathies
- Decubiti
- Death

Bibliography

1. Cao Y, Krause JS, DiPiro N. Risk factors for mortality after spinal cord injury in the USA. Spinal Cord. 2013;51(5):413–8. doi:10.1038/sc.2013.2. Epub 2013 Feb 5.
2. Patel AA, Vaccaro AR. Thoracolumbar spine trauma classification. J Am Acad Orthop Surg. 2010;18(2):63–71.
3. Weinstein JN, Collalto P, Lehmann TR. Thoracolumbar "burst" fractures treated conservatively: a long-term follow-up. Spine (Phila Pa 1976). 1988;13(1):33–8.

10 Osteoporotic Vertebral Fractures

Samuel E. Smith

Take-Home Message
- Most common fragility fracture.
- Multiple fractures are likely.
- No history of trauma always.
- Can affect life expectancy due to pulmonary function deficits.

Definition

- Fracture due to insufficient strength of the vertebral body caused by loss of bone density, i.e., osteoid and mineral loss

Etiology

- Vertebral bodies largely cancellous bone and are therefore more susceptible to bone loss.
- Osteoporosis with or without trauma can lead to fracture.

Pathophysiology

- Osteoporosis leading to decrease strength in bone and fracture
- Also changes in structure of bone leading to weakness in the bone

Radiographs

- X-rays may show "codfish" vertebra or simple wedging.
- Vertebral bodies may appear with vertical striations.

- CT defines bony anatomy of the fracture, whether or not there is burst component.
- MRI defines the canal and may show fatty replacement of the marrow.
- DEXA – dual energy X-ray absorptiometry

Classification

- WHO definition of osteoporosis is greater than 2.5 deviations below the mean peak bone mass of young adults based on DEXA.

Treatment

- Many patients are asymptomatic.

Nonoperative

- Observation
- Bracing

Operative

- Vertebroplasty – AAOS makes strong recommendation against vertebroplasty because of cement extravasation in the neurologically intact patient.
- Kyphoplasty.
- Decompression and stabilization, hardware, may need cement supplementation.

Complications

- Infection
- DVT/PE
- Neurologic injury
- Chronic pain
- Adjacent segment fractures

Bibliography

1. Link TM. Osteoporosis imaging: state of the art and advanced imaging. Radiology. 2012;263(1):3–17. doi:10.1148/radiol.12110462.
2. McGuire R. AAOS clinical practice guideline: the treatment of symptomatic osteoporotic spinal compression fractures. J Am Acad Orthop Surg. 2011;19(3):183–4.
3. Patil S, Rawall S, Singh D, Mohan K, Nagad P, Shial B, Pawar U, Nene A. Surgical patterns in osteoporotic vertebral compression fractures. Eur Spine J. 2013;22(4):883–91. doi:10.1007/s00586-012-2508-4. Epub 2012 Sep 28.

11 Fractures of the Sacrum

Samuel E. Smith

Take-Home Message

- This section is for sacral fractures as distinct from fractures of the pelvic ring.
- U-shaped fractures of the sacrum represent a dissociation of the spine from the pelvis.
- Transverse sacral fractures differ in terms of whether or not they are high or low.
- Neurologic involvement common.

Definition

- U-shaped fractures of the sacrum are where proximal sacral segments are no longer connected by bony or soft tissue to the distal ala, lower sacrum, and pelvis; spinopelvic dissociation.
- Transverse fractures of the sacrum may involve a sacral kyphosis, and stabilization of the SI joints may be needed as well as sacral laminectomy to decompress canal.

Etiology

- Motor vehicle trauma
- Falls
- Insufficiency fractures

Pathophysiology

- Axial forces from falls often cause this
- Osteoporosis leading to sacral insufficiency fracture

Radiographs

- Often missed on X-ray, needs high index of suspicion with pelvic pain and perianal sensation changes.
- CT is the best study.
- MRI to look at cauda equina.

Classification

- Know the Denis classification, covered elsewhere.
- Transverse fractures subdivided but this does not direct treatment.

Treatment

Nonoperative

- Simple observation and symptomatic treatment – controversial

Operative

- Lumbopelvic fixation, triangular osteosynthesis
- Percutaneous fixation with SI screws of appropriate length or bilateral fixation, at least two screws to prevent further kyphosis
- Sacral laminectomy
- Bilateral lateral sacral fixation for some transverse sacral fractures

Complications

- Infection
- Neurologic deficit
- DVT/PE
- Wound dehiscence
- Chronic pain

Bibliography

1. Fountain SS, Hamilton RD, Jameson RM. Transverse fractures of the sacrum. A report of six cases. J Bone Joint Surg Am. 1977;59(4):486–9.
2. König MA, Jehan S, Boszczyk AA, Boszczyk BM. Surgical management of U-shaped sacral fractures: a systematic review of current treatment strategies. Eur Spine J. 2012;21(5):829–36. doi:10.1007/s00586-011-2125-7. Epub 2011 Dec 23.
3. Nork SE, Jones CB, Harding SP, Mirza SK, Routt Jr ML. Percutaneous stabilization of U-shaped sacral fractures using iliosacral screws: technique and early results. J Orthop Trauma. 2001;15(4):238–46.
4. Roy-Camille R, Saillant G, Gagna G, Mazel C. Transverse fracture of the upper sacrum. Suicidal jumper's fracture. Spine (Phila Pa 1976). 1985;10(9):838–45.

Deformity

Samuel E. Smith

1 Pediatric-Adolescent Idiopathic Scoliosis

Samuel E. Smith

Take-Home Message
- Right thoracic curve common, can be progressive
- Left thoracic curve needs MRI
- Large curves can cause cardiopulmonary compromise
- More common in females

Definition

- Lateral curvature of the spine in the coronal plane of unknown cause

Etiology

- Unknown
  - Family history of first-degree relatives important
- Inner ear problem, proprioceptive cord problem, hormonal

Pathophysiology

- Unknown
- Lateral curvature causes rotational deformity and lends to progression

S.E. Smith, MD
Department of Orthopedics, Front Range Orthopedic Center,
1551 Professional Ln Suite 200, Longmont, CO 80501, USA
e-mail: samuel.smith@dhha.org

C. Mauffrey, D.J. Hak (eds.), *Passport for the Orthopedic Boards and FRCS Examination*, DOI 10.1007/978-2-8178-0475-0_16

Radiographs

- X-rays: Full-length standing films, first film AP and lateral as there can be sagittal plane imbalances as well, protect reproductive organs
- Document Cobb angle and spinal balance, spinal rotation, apical vertebrae, stable vertebra, check clavicle angle (important for determining whether or not to include upper thoracic curve)
- Use flexibility x-rays to further define curve behavior when deciding on operative treatment
- Check pelvis for Risser grade (0–4)
- MRI for left-sided curves and then look at whole spinal axis

Classification

- King classification – older and less often used at meetings
- Lenke classification – more complex but better able to use for treatment and especially for level selection, takes into account sagittal plane abnormalities in deciding structural nature of the curve

Treatment

Nonoperative

- Observation for small curves and to document progression
- Bracing for curves 25–45°
- Type of brace determined by apex of curve, above T7 need Milwaukee-type brace, otherwise can use underarm orthosis
- Brace wear should be full time, i.e., 23 h out of 24, but there are studies showing that less than full-time wear okay
- Trying to halt progression, duration of brace wear at least 1 year and otherwise until skeletal maturity defined by multiple factors

Operative

- Posterior fusion and fixation
- Anterior fusion and fixation especially lumbar and thoracolumbar curves
- Combined approaches for more severe or inflexible curves

Complications

- Loss of correction
- Adding on of the curve
- Crankshaft phenomenon in pediatric patients
- Pseudarthrosis
- Infection
- Neurologic injury
- SMA syndrome can cause postop ileus

Special Situations

Infantile idiopathic scoliosis

- Boys are more commonly affected
- Left thoracic curve more common
- Other congenital defects more common
- Curves less than 30° can be observed
- Look at study by Mehta, Cobb greater than 20°, RVA greater than 20°, and a phase 2 relationship define progression
- Treatment casting, dual growing rods, or VEPTR

Bibliography

1. Lenke LG. Lenke classification system of adolescent idiopathic scoliosis: treatment recommendations. Instr Course Lect. 2005;54:537–42.
2. Mehta MH. The rib-vertebra angle in the early diagnosis between resolving and progressive infantile scoliosis. J Bone Joint Surg Br. 1972;54(2):230–43.
3. Ward WT, Rihn JA, Solic J, Lee JY. A comparison of the lenke and king classification systems in the surgical treatment of idiopathic thoracic scoliosis. Spine (Phila Pa 1976). 2008;33(1):52–60. doi:10.1097/BRS.0b013e31815e392a.

2 Adult Spine Deformity

Samuel E. Smith

Take-Home Message
- High complication rate treated operatively
- Nonoperative treatment successful often
- Severe pain and dysfunction attributable to positive sagittal balance
- Difficult decision sometimes as to when or when not to fuse to the pelvis

Definition

- Scoliosis especially of the lumbar spine caused by asymmetric development of lumbar spondylosis
- May occur in preexisting adolescent idiopathic curve

Etiology

- Degenerative cascade describe by Kirkaldy-Willis which is asymmetric

Pathophysiology

- Degenerative cascade leads to disc and facet degeneration, and when this occurs, asymmetrically curve or deformity ensues
- Frequently associated and exacerbated by osteoporosis and associate fractures
- Can occur in preexisting AIS
- When advanced can lead to flattening of lordosis beyond the ability of the pelvis to retrovert, normal lumbar lordosis roughly equal to pelvic incidence
- Olisthesis, lateral, anterior, or retro often associated

Radiographs

- X-rays: signs of spondylosis, Cobb angle, sagittal plane deformity, olisthesis
- Must get full-length films to evaluate global balance
- CT: defines bony anatomy and stenosis, more informative if done with myelographic contrast
- MRI useful to evaluate for stenosis both centrally and in the foramen, radicular symptoms commonly in the concavity of the curve

Classification

- Schwab classification: thoracic, TL/L, double curve, along with a description of the mismatch between the pelvic incidence and the lumbar lordosis as well as the SVA, i.e., the number of centimeters the C7 vertebra is in front of S1

Treatment

Nonoperative

- Exercises, PT
- Manipulative therapy
- NSAIDs
- Avoid opioids

Operative

- Anterior release and reconstruction
- Posterior release and reconstruction
- Have to decide when and when not to fuse to the pelvis
- Osteotomies sometimes employed, Ponte, PSO, VCR
- Combined approaches

Complications

- Infection
- Loss of fixation, often bone density is poor
- Pseudarthrosis especially L4/L5 and L5/S1
- Smoking increases risk of failure of treatment both with respect to pain relief and fusion success
- Neurologic injury

Bibliography

1. Bess S, Schwab F, Lafage V, Shaffrey CI, Ames CP. Classifications for adult spinal deformity and use of the Scoliosis Research Society-Schwab Adult Spinal Deformity Classification. Neurosurg Clin N Am. 2013;24(2):185–93. doi:10.1016/j.nec.2012.12.008.
2. Kotwal S, Pumberger M, Hughes A, Girardi F. Degenerative scoliosis: a review. HSS J. 2011;7(3):257–64. Epub 2011 Jun 11.

3 Adult Thoracic Kyphosis

Samuel E. Smith

Take-Home Message
- Normal kyphosis T2 to T12 20–40°, 45° max
- Normal sagittal balance defined by sagittal vertical axis 0–4 cm
- Most of the time will respond to conservative measures
- Patients in positive sagittal balance more at risk for pain and disability

Definition

- Abnormal kyphosis caused by degenerative disease or prior Scheuermann's kyphosis

Etiology

- Prior Scheuermann's
- Osteoporosis and compression fractures
- Thoracic spondylosis
- Tumor
- Infection

Pathophysiology

- Above issues cause loss of anterior spinal column height
- Gibbus acute kyphosis over short distance from fracture, tumor, or infection

Radiographs

- X-rays: vertebral body wedging caused by trauma or bone destruction from tumor or infection, old Scheuermann's kyphosis
- Cobb angle: need upright scoliosis films to measure sagittal balance parameters, define bone density
- DEXA scan to measure bone density

- CT: sometimes need this to define bony anatomy
- MRI: prior to surgery to define soft tissues and look at the cord and its relationship to the kyphosis, MRI will look at tumor and infection well

Classification

None

Treatment

Nonoperative

- NSAIDs
- Hyperextension exercises to strengthen paraspinous muscles
- Modification of activity

Operative

- Anterior/posterior
- Posterior alone with osteotomies
- Combined approaches
- Depends on diagnosis and rigidity of the curve and the degree of sagittal imbalance

Complications

- Complication rate high
- Loss of correction
- Neurologic injury including paralysis
- Proximal junctional kyphosis above the construct
- DVT/PE
- Pseudoarthrosis
- Donor site complications
- Bone graft substitutes and their complications

Bibliography

1. Bae JS, Jang JS, Lee SH, Kim JU. Radiological analysis of lumbar degenerative kyphosis in relation to pelvic incidence. Spine J. 2012;12(11):1045–51. doi:10.1016/j.spinee.2012.10.011. Epub 2012 Nov 14.

4 Other Scolioses

Samuel E. Smith

Take-Home Message
- Congenital: hemivertebra and unsegmented bars
- Neuromuscular: CP, myelomeningocele, spinal muscular atrophy, Duchenne's muscular dystrophy, myelomeningocele

Definition

- Congenital: vertebral segmentation abnormalities during gestation
- Neuromuscular: spinal muscular imbalance during growth secondary to neurologic abnormality

Etiology

- Congenital: maternal diabetes, Etoh abuse during pregnancy, genetic
- Neuromuscular: variable etiologies

Pathophysiology

- Congenital: hemivertebrae and unsegmented bars
  - Other systems involved: genitourinary, cardiac
- Neuromuscular: spine deformity alters sitting or positioning imbalances leading to difficult care, pressure sores

Radiographs

- X-rays

  Congenital: look for hemivertebra
  - Neuromuscular: follow curve progression
- CT: define bony anatomy, diastomatomyelia
- MRI: tethered cord, intradural lipoma, Arnold-Chiari malformations

Classification

- None

Treatment

Nonoperative

- Observation
- Do not brace congenital curves
- Can brace neuromuscular curves until surgery appropriate

Operative

- Congenital scoliosis: fit operation to pathology, most likely to progress with hemivertebra and unsegmented contralateral bar, posterior, anterior/posterior, hemivertebra resection, growing rods, VEPTR
- Neuromuscular: often fuse to the pelvis to control pelvic obliquity

Complications

- Crankshaft phenomenon
- Short stature from fusion in childhood
- Neurologic injury
- Infection

Bibliography

1. Bowen RE, Abel MF, Arlet V, Brown D, Burton DC, D'Ambra P, Gill L, Hoekstra DV, Karlin LI, Raso J, Sanders JO, Schwab FJ. Outcome assessment in neuromuscular spinal deformity. J Pediatr Orthop. 2012;32(8):792–8. doi:10.1097/BPO.0b013e318273ab5a.
2. Hedequist D, Emans J. Congenital scoliosis: a review and update. J Pediatr Orthop. 2007;27(1):106–16.

5 Scheuermann's Kyphosis

Samuel E. Smith

Take-Home Message
- Wedging of three consecutive vertebrae
- Schmorl's nodes
- Growth abnormality of ring apophysis
- Males more commonly affected

Definition

- Kyphosis of the thoracic spine caused by wedging of multiple vertebrae, defined radiographically by 5° of wedging over three adjacent vertebrae

Etiology

- Unknown and probably multifactorial
  - May be autosomal dominant

Pathophysiology

- There are abnormalities of the growth plate of the anterior vertebrae represented by the disruption of the ring apophysis, may be a secondary effect to the ring apophysis rather than an intrinsic abnormality

Radiographs

- X-rays: normal thoracic kyphosis 20–40°
- Greater than 45° of thoracic kyphosis is abnormal
- Severe kyphosis greater than 75°
- MRI: sometimes need to identify herniated thoracic disc

Classification

- Need to distinguish from postural kyphosis which will be flexible and will correct with improved posture
- No classification but you must be able to define Cobb angle and establish flexibility of the curve

Treatment

Nonoperative

- Observation for progression, like scoliosis progresses with growth
- Bracing can be effective in growing child to prevent further deformity; at one time, it was felt that bracing can improve deformity but no longer believed to be the case

Operative

- Posterior surgery with or without osteotomies, posterior shortening
- Anterior surgery with rods, open or VATS, to release anterior structures
- Anterior/posterior surgery
- Fuse to first lordotic disc

Complications

- MRI preop
- Cord can be draped over kyphosis, beware of anterior lengthening causing neurologic deficit
- Infection
- DVT/PE
- Proximal junctional kyphosis

Bibliography

1. Bradford DS, Moe JH. Scheuermann's juvenile kyphosis. A histologic study. Clin Orthop Relat Res. 1975;110:45–53.
2. Miladi L. Round and angular kyphosis in paediatric patients. Orthop Traumatol Surg Res. 2013;99(1 Suppl):S140–9. doi: 10.1016/j.otsr.2012.12.004. Epub 2013 Jan 1.

6 Adult and Pediatric Spondylolisthesis

Samuel E. Smith

Take-Home Message

- Know Wiltse classification
- Know Meyerding grades
- Dysplastic forms have more risk of neurologic sequelae

Definition

- Anterior slippage of typically L5 on S1 caused by instability of the motion segment

Etiology

- Multifactorial
- Isthmic defect most common
- Traumatic pedicle fractures
- Dysplastic facets with stretching or fracture of the pars, posterior elements sometimes come forward too

Pathophysiology

- Instability of the motion segment
- Stenosis, central and neuroforaminal depending on type of slip
- Problems with sagittal balance
- Sometimes hyperlordotic lumbar spine in patient with high pelvic incidence
- Sometimes lumbosacral kyphosis with higher slip grades

Radiographs

- X-rays: pars defects, slip, dysplastic changes of facet and remodeling changes of dome of sacrum and trapezoidal shape at L5
- Degenerative slip rarely greater than grade 2, has associated spondylotic change, facet degeneration and subluxation seen
- Review pelvic incidence, pelvic tilt, and sacral slope, and understand pelvic incidence is a fixed number and that sacral slope plus the pelvic tilt equals the pelvic incidence
- CT: better defines pars defects, bony stenosis, facet joints
- MRI to look at soft tissue associated with pars defects, neurologic visualization especially foramina

Classification

- Wiltse classification: type I – congenital; type II – isthmic; type III – degenerative; type IV – traumatic, acute, usually pedicles are fractured; type V – pathologic
- Meyerding classification based on percentage of slip of L5 on S1, hard to define with dysplastic and remodeling changes

Treatment

Nonoperative

- Most of the time nonoperative therapy is successful
- PT and exercises
- NSAIDs
- Activity modification

Operative

- Depends on pathology
- Dysplastic and remodeling changes may require dome osteotomy and reduction of lumbosacral kyphosis
- Degenerative slip can be approached anterior or lateral alone, front and back or posterior alone with or without cages, may need decompression
- Isthmic slip can also be approached variably depending upon pathology and surgeon preference
- Spondyloptosis: L5 in front of the pelvis may need anterior/posterior surgery with complete L5 removal and reduction and fusion of L4 to the sacrum with fixation to the ilium

Complications

- L5 root palsies
- Infection
- DVT/PE
- Pseudarthrosis
- Repeat surgery

Bibliography

1. Alfieri A, Gazzeri R, Prell J, Röllinghoff M. The current management of lumbar spondylolisthesis. J Neurosurg Sci. 2013;57(2):103–13.
2. Labelle H, Roussouly P, Berthonnaud E, Dimnet J, O'Brien M. The importance of spino-pelvic balance in L5-s1 developmental spondylolisthesis: a review of pertinent radiologic measurements. Spine (Phila Pa 1976). 2005;30(6 Suppl):S27–34.
3. Wiltse LL, Newman PH, Macnab I. Classification of spondylolysis and spondylolisthesis. Clin Orthop Relat Res. 1976;117:23–9.

Degenerative Disorders

Samuel E. Smith

1 Cervical Spondylosis

Samuel E. Smith

Take-Home Message
- Degenerative Cascade
- Degenerative disc changes and facet arthrosis
- Can lead to stenosis
- Changes of aging vs. pathologic change

Definition

- Disc degeneration and facet arthropathy leading to a variety of changes which can cause axial and radicular pain can cause neurologic changes

Etiology

- Age related
- Motion and wear and tear over time
- Injuries
- Smoking
- Occupation
- Genetic

S.E. Smith, MD
Department of Orthopedics,
Front Range Orthopedic Center,
1551 Professional Ln Suite 200, Longmont,
CO 80501, USA
e-mail: samuel.smith@dhha.org

C. Mauffrey, D.J. Hak (eds.), *Passport for the Orthopedic Boards and FRCS Examination*, DOI 10.1007/978-2-8178-0475-0_17

Pathophysiology

- Degenerative cascade
- DDD with instability, micro or macro
- Annular tearing
- Facet degeneration leading to stenosis

Radiographs

- X-rays: Disc narrowing, endplate sclerosis, marginal osteophytes, uncal hypertrophy, and foraminal narrowing seen on obliques, subluxation
- CT: Defines bony anatomy but not good at seeing stenosis unless done with myelography
- MRI: Disc desiccation, foraminal stenosis, central stenosis, disc herniation
- Discography controversial

Classification

- Subjective
- Mild, moderate, severe

Treatment

- Natural history favorable

Nonoperative

- Physical therapy
- Chiropractic care
- Massage
- NSAIDs
- Relative rest

Operative – depends on pathoanatomy

- Decompression
- Fusion
- Instrumentation

Complications

- DVT: PE
- Infection
- Neurologic injury
- Covered in other sections

Bibliography

1. Kelly JC, Groarke PJ, Butler JS, Poynton AR, O'Byrne JM. The natural history and clinical syndromes of degenerative cervical spondylosis. Adv Orthop. 2012;2012:393642.

2 Cervical Disc Herniation

Samuel E. Smith

Take-Home Message

- Typically causes radiculopathy with nerve compression in the foramen, i.e., C6 nerve root in the C5/C6 foramen
- Central herniations can cause spinal cord compression and myelopathy
- Herniations with axial pain only do not do well with surgery

Definition

- Disruption of the annulus fibrosis of the intervertebral disc leading to displacement of the nucleus pulposus away from the center of the disc

Etiology

- Degenerative cascade
- Microtrauma leading to annular tearing
- Genetic predisposition

Pathophysiology

- Annular tearing as a repetitive phenomenon
- Tears coalesce into a larger annular fissure
- Nucleus displaces from the center of the disc into the canal or foramen or both
- Most commonly cause radiculopathy but can cause myelopathy

Radiographs

- Sometimes normal
- Degenerative disc space narrowing sometimes seen
- CT does not show herniation in the cervical spine well
- MRI "gold standard" for diagnosis
- Myelogram/CT for when MRI not possible

Classification

- No accepted classification

Treatment

- Natural history of cervical radiculopathy is favorable

Nonoperative

- Bracing
- Traction: Controversial as to whether it helps or not

- Manipulation
- Medication
- PT
- Spinal injections

Operative

- Anterior cervical discectomy with or without fusion. Most favor fusion to prevent collapse of disc into kyphosis
- Fixation vs. stand-alone graft
- Plates or interlocking cages
- Disc arthroplasty
- Posterior foraminotomy avoids fusion and results can be comparable to ACD/ACF and is amenable to less invasive approach

Complications

- Dysphagia
- Aspiration
- Esophageal injury
- Injury to recurrent laryngeal nerve-latest information suggests equal risk from right or left sided approach, review the anatomy as it relates to the aortic arch for the RLN
- Dural tear
- Infection
- DVT/PE

Bibliography

1. Lees F, Turner JW. Natural history and prognosis of cervical spondylosis. Br Med J. 1963;2(5373):1607–10.
2. Rhee JM, Yoon T, Riew KD. Cervical radiculopathy. J Am Acad Orthop Surg. 2007;15(8):486–94.

3 Cervical Spinal Stenosis

Samuel E. Smith

Take-Home Message

- Can be congenital, developmental with degenerative disease, or associated with OPLL
- Most common source degenerative osteophytes from margins of disc, facet hypertrophy, and degenerative hypertrophy of the uncovertebral "joint"
- Vertebral subluxation a potential factor
- Can cause radiculopathy, myelopathy, or both

Definition

- Decreased space for the spinal cord and exiting nerve roots of the cervical spine from a variety of causes
- Congenital stenosis defined by Torg ratio or a sagittal diameter of less than 10 mm
- Not everyone with stenosis has symptoms

Etiology

- Degenerative marginal osteophytes and hypertrophy of the abovementioned structures decrease the space available for the cord and nerve roots
  - Congenital stenosis can have superimposed degenerative stenosis
- Familial tendency
- Smoking
- Occupational factors
- OPLL ethnic and genetic factors

Pathophysiology

- Degenerative cascade of Kirkaldy-Willis
- OPLL dealt with separately
- Can lead to spinal cord compromise and signs of myelopathy (Hoffman's, clonus, poor tandem walking, hyperactive reflexes, incoordination)
- Radiculopathy (Spurling's)

Radiographs

- X-rays: May show osteophytes, deformity, subluxation, and congenital stenosis
- MRI good with canal dimensions and direct visualization of cord and nerve roots
- Detects signal change in cord
- Defines operative anatomy, limited diagnostically but very useful if used with myelography

Treatment

Nonoperative

- Physical therapy
- Chiropractic care
- NSAIDs
- Opioid therapy for only brief periods

Operative

- Approach depends on specific pathoanatomic problems
- Anterior
- Posterior
- Anterior/posterior
- With or without fusion

- ACD/ACF most common procedure and can be single or multiple levels
- Laminoplasty for myelopathy in some cases
- You must correlate symptoms and physical findings to imaging studies, i.e., does the patient have deformity, myelopathy, or radiculopathy? Does the patient need pain relief or prevention of further neurologic deterioration?

Complications

- Paralysis
- Nerve root injury either directly or indirectly. Traction palsies possible and usually resolve with time
- Esophageal injury with anterior approach
- Recurrent laryngeal nerve injury with anterior approach
- Horner's syndrome
- Infection
- DVT/PE
- Pseudarthrosis
- If use BMP anteriorly, risk of airway compromise from seroma

Bibliography

1. Emery SE. Cervical spondylotic myelopathy: diagnosis and treatment. J Am Acad Orthop Surg. 2001;9(6):376–88.
2. Fountas KN, Kapsalaki EZ, Nikolakakos LG, Smisson HF, Johnston KW, Grigorian AA, Lee GP, Robinson Jr JS. Anterior cervical discectomy and fusion associated complications. Spine (Phila Pa 1976). 2007;32(21):2310–7.

4 Thoracic Herniated Disc

Samuel E. Smith

Take-Home Message
- Very rare
- Often calcified and may only see that on CT, this may indicate adherence of the herniation to the dura
- More common at the lower thoracic levels where there is more spinal mobility

Definition

- Migration of nucleus pulposus through weakened annulus through microtears of the annulus

Etiology

- Degenerative cascade

Pathophysiology

- As per lumbar herniated disc

Radiographs

- X-rays: Thoracic spondylosis, Schmorl's nodes
- CT: Calcification of the herniation
- MRI: Shows exact nature of herniation and looks at thoracic roots and the spinal cord

Classification

- Central vs. foraminal
- Myelopathy vs. radiculopathy or combination

Treatment

Nonoperative

- Natural history favorable
- NSAIDs
- Exercise and PT
- Manipulation
- Massage

Operative

- Discectomy: Anterior, costotransversectomy or lateral approach, may need fusion
- VATS

Complications

- Spinal cord injury
- Dural tear
- Infection, DVT/PE
- Recurrent surgery
- Pneumothorax
- Vascular injury

Bibliography

1. Vanichkachorn JS, Vaccaro AR. Thoracic disk disease: diagnosis and treatment. J Am Acad Orthop Surg. 2000;8(3):159–69.

5 Lumbar Spondylosis

Samuel E. Smith

Take-Home Message
- Degenerative cascade of Kirkaldy-Willis
- Disc degeneration and facet arthropathy
- Can lead to deformity, stenosis, subluxation
- Not always a cause of symptoms and therefore must correlate history and physical with imaging findings

Definition

- Degenerative disc disease and facet arthropathy which can cause axial and referred pain, or disc herniation or stenosis with radiculopathy or neurogenic claudication

Etiology

- Changes of aging vs. pathologic change
- Smoking
- Genetic
- Occupation

Pathophysiology

- Disc degeneration
- Facet arthropathy
- Stenosis
- Deformity
- Causes in some case positive sagittal balance, covered in adult deformity and kyphosis sections

Radiographs

- X-rays: Disc narrowing, endplate sclerosis, subluxation, Schmorl's nodes, marginal osteophytes, facet hypertrophy/arthropathy, and stenosis

- MRI: Disc dessication, disc herniation, stenosis either central, lateral recess, or foramen or combination
- CT alone can be useful when MRI cannot be done or when bony definition important for surgery
- Myelography with CT better at defining stenosis
- Discography – controversial

Classification

- Subjective
- Mild, moderate, severe

Treatment

- Natural history favorable

Nonoperative

- Physical therapy
- Manipulation
- Massage
- NSAIDs
- Short-term periods of rest
- Short-term opioid therapy

Operative

- Depends on pathoanatomy and its relationship to history and physical exam
- Ranges from decompression to fusion and from single-level procedure to multilevel procedure

Complications

- Neurologic injury
- Infection
- Blood loss
- Dural leak
- Blindness
- Plexopathy-brachial, lumbar
- Major vessel, visceral injury

Bibliography

1. Torgerson WR, Dotter WE. Comparative roentgenographic study of the asymptomatic and symptomatic lumbar spine. J Bone Joint Surg Am. 1976;58(6):850–3.

6 Lumbar Discogenic Back Pain

Samuel E. Smith

Take-Home Message

- Operative treatment controversial
- Confirming disc as real source of pain difficult
- Discography controversial
- Success related to psychosocial issues

Definition

- Pain caused by disc degeneration

Etiology

- Degenerative cascade – discussed elsewhere

Pathophysiology

- Chondrocyte degeneration
- Disc desiccation
- Instability
- Inflammatory cytokines

Radiographs

- X-ray: Marginal osteophytes, disc narrowing, endplate sclerosis, and cyst formation
- Discography: Subjective test and controversial in terms of interpreting disc as source of pain, requires control, and disc injection can induce degenerative change
- CT: Facet degeneration and possible facet source of pain, important if disc arthroplasty is a consideration

Classification

- Modic changes I, II, and III worth knowing but type of changes not definitively known to relate to pain and instability

Treatment

- Conservative treatment emphasized

Nonoperative

- NSAIDs
- PT
- Massage
- Manipulation

Operative

- Disc arthroplasty, one level typically, two levels can be done, done to reduce adjacent segment degeneration and further surgery
- Arthrodesis, front alone, back alone, front and back
- Cage placement vs. posterior fusion alone
- Avoid operating on multilevel disease as results are not good
- Consider psychosocial screening in these patients
- Results not as good in workers' compensation cases

Complications

- Infection
- Chronic regional pain
- Repeat surgery and adjacent segment degeneration
- DVT, PE

Bibliography

1. Dickerman RD, Zigler J. Re: Carragee EJ, Lincoln T, Parmar VS, et al. A gold standard evaluation of the 'discogenic pain' diagnosis as determined by provocative discography. Spine 2006;31:2115–23. Spine (Phila Pa 1976). 2007;32(2): 287–8; author reply 288–9.
2. Maghout Juratli S, Franklin GM, Mirza SK, Wickizer TM, Fulton-Kehoe D. Lumbar fusion outcomes in Washington State workers' compensation. Spine (Phila Pa 1976). 2006;31(23):2715–23.

7 Lumbar Herniated Disc

Samuel E. Smith

Take-Home Message

- Know traversing vs. exiting nerve root
- Typical posterolateral HNP affects traversing root, e.g., L4/L5 HNP causes L5 symptoms and signs
- Foraminal HNP affects exiting root, e.g., L4/L5 HNP causes L4 root compression
- Natural history of lumbar HNP is favorable
- Large numbers of people have asymptomatic HNP, must correlate symptoms and signs

Definition

- Migration of nucleus pulposus through weakened annulus through microtears of the annulus

Etiology

- Part of the degenerative cascade
- Genetics
- Smoking
- Working or driving in an environment where patient is exposed to vibration, controversial
- Repetitive labor

Pathophysiology

- Microtears of the annulus
- Torsional strain
- Disc desiccation

Radiographs

- X-rays: May be normal or show signs of lumbar spondylosis
- CT: May show displacement of disc but does not define type of herniation
- CT/myelography: More definitive in showing nerve root or thecal sac displacement
- MRI: Disc desiccation, defines protrusion vs. extrusion vs. sequestration, shows cauda equina well

Classification

- Disc protrusion with displaced disc material and canal or foraminal encroachment but with intact annulus, disc edge distance less than the base distance
- Disc extrusion through annulus and disc edge distance is more than the base distance
- Disc sequestration is when displaced nucleus has separated from the main disc

Treatment

- Natural history favorable within 6 weeks to 3 months from the onset of symptoms
- NSAIDS, PT, massage, manipulation
- Discectomy: Open vs. minimally invasive, operating microscope
- Fusion not necessary in vast majority of cases, true even with the first recurrence
- Cauda equina with central HNP, may consider fusion, not always necessary to treat cauda equina as emergency but this is controversial

Complications

- Dural tear
- Discitis which is not always infectious
- Nerve root injury
- Recurrent HNP
- Chronic regional pain
- Vascular and visceral injury from violating annulus anteriorly

Bibliography

1. Kostuik JP, Harrington I, Alexander D, Rand W, Evans D. Cauda equina syndrome and lumbar disc herniation. J Bone Joint Surg Am. 1986;68(3):386–91.
2. Lee JK, Amorosa L, Cho SK, Weidenbaum M, Kim Y. Recurrent lumbar disk herniation. J Am Acad Orthop Surg. 2010;18(6):327–37.
3. Weinstein JN, Lurie JD, Tosteson TD, Tosteson AN, Blood EA, Abdu WA, Herkowitz H, Hilibrand A, Albert T, Fischgrund J. Surgical versus nonoperative treatment for lumbar disc herniation: four-year results for the Spine Patient Outcomes Research Trial (SPORT). Spine (Phila Pa 1976). 2008;33(25):2789–800. doi:10.1097/BRS.0b013e31818ed8f4.

8 Lumbar Spinal Stenosis

Samuel E. Smith

Take-Home Message
- Verbiest – the first clinical description
- End result of the degenerative cascade
- Know sites for stenosis
- Can cause neurogenic claudication as distinct from vascular claudication

Definition

- Reduced dimension of the spinal canal by bony and ligamentous degenerative hypertrophy
- Stenosis can be central, lateral recess, or neuroforamen

Etiology

- Degenerative cascade causing bony and ligamentous hypertrophy secondary to instability

Pathophysiology

- Cartilage degeneration leading to loss of disc height, facet instability, and reactive hypertrophic change in nature's response to instability
- Canal dimensions decrease in size and volume

Radiographs

- X-rays show signs of spondylosis discussed elsewhere
- May show olisthesis, deformity or both
- CT shows bony canal and is enhanced by myelography
- MRI: Shows canal best, T1 to look at epidural fat and neuroforamina, T2 gives myelogram effect

Classification

- Subjective: Mild, moderate, severe

Treatment

Nonoperative

- Observation
- NSAIDs
- Physical therapy and flexion exercises
- Manipulation
- Epidural steroid injections – mostly temporary relief
- Opioids for short-term pain control

Operative

- Lumbar decompressive laminectomy is mainstay
- Open or less invasive
- May have to do fusion with instability or deformity, covered elsewhere

Complications

- Infection
- DVT/PE
- Failure of pain relief
- Adjacent segment degeneration
- Blood loss
- Dural leak
- Neurologic injury
- Instability or progression of deformity

Bibliography

1. Verbiest H. A radicular syndrome from developmental narrowing of the lumbar vertebral canal. J Bone Joint Surg Br. 1954;36-B(2):230–7.
2. Weinstein JN, Tosteson TD, Lurie JD, Tosteson A, Blood E, Herkowitz H, Cammisa F, Albert T, Boden SD, Hilibrand A, Goldberg H, Berven S, An H. Surgical versus nonoperative treatment for lumbar spinal stenosis four-year results of the Spine Patient Outcomes Research Trial. Spine (Phila Pa 1976). 2010;35(14):1329–38. doi:10.1097/BRS.0b013e3181e0f04d.

Miscellaneous

Samuel E. Smith

1 Diastematomyelia

Samuel E. Smith

> **Take-Home Message**
> • Strong association with congenital scoliosis

Definition

- Longitudinal cleft of the spinal cord

Etiology

- Abnormality of congenital fetal development

Pathophysiology

- Longitudinal cleft that can fix the cord as the spine grows causing neurologic deficit, similar to a tethered cord

Radiographs

- Ultrasound – in utero.
- X-rays may show widening of the pedicles.
- CT/myelography can best detect bony diastema.
- MRI defines neurologic anatomy.

S.E. Smith, MD
Department of Orthopedics, Front Range Orthopedic Center,
1551 Professional Ln Suite 200, Longmont, CO 80501, USA
e-mail: Samuel.smith@dhha.org

C. Mauffrey, D.J. Hak (eds.), *Passport for the Orthopedic Boards and FRCS Examination*, DOI 10.1007/978-2-8178-0475-0_18

Treatment

Nonoperative

- Observation

Operative

- Surgery to resect and repair
- Must deal with diastema operatively if also doing deformity correction

Complications

- Dural leak
- Retethering of neurologic structures

Bibliography

1. Cheng B, Li FT, Lin L. Diastematomyelia: a retrospective review of 138 patients. J Bone Joint Surg Br. 2012;94(3):365–72. doi:10.1302/0301-620X.94B3.27897.

2 Myelomeningocele

Samuel E. Smith

Take-Home Message
- Higher neurologic levels more likely to cause scoliosis
- Pressure ulceration from sitting imbalance
- Can have neurologic progression from tethered cord
- Urosepsis common

Definition

- Failure of the tissue closure causing midline defect

Etiology

- Multifactorial
  - Diabetes
  - Folate deficiency during pregnancy

Pathophysiology

- Midline defect that is sometimes just the bone, sometimes the bone and meninges, and sometimes the bone, meninges, and neural elements

Radiographs

- X-rays: Monitor her spinal deformity especially.
- MRI: If there is a change in neurologic status with respect to myelopathy, consider tethered cord.
- CT scan: Better definition of bony anatomy for spine surgery.

Classification

- Spina bifida occulta
- Meningocele: Sac does not include neural elements.
- Myelomeningocele: Sac includes neural elements.
- Try to determine neurologic level for prognostic and treatment purposes.

Treatment

- Bracing is not effective but observation can be appropriate.
- When spine surgery is indicated it often requires anterior/posterior approach because posterior arthrodesis is very difficult due to deficient posterior elements.
- As with other neuromuscular deformities, fusion to the pelvis is indicated.

Complications

- Infection risk with surgery high
- Pressure sores
- Failure fixation, failure of fusion
- Urosepsis
- DVT/PE

Bibliography

1. Keessen W, van Ooy A, Pavlov P, Pruijs JE, Scheers MM, Slot G, Verbout A, Wijers HM. Treatment of spinal deformity in myelomeningocele: a retrospective study in four hospitals. Eur J Pediatr Surg. 1992;2 Suppl 1:18–22.

3 Diffuse Idiopathic Skeletal Hyperostosis

Samuel E. Smith

Take-Home Message

- Clinical implications similar to ankylosing spondylitis but it is not inflammatory
- Causes non-marginal syndesmophytes
- Does not involve facets unlike AS

Definition

- Non-marginal syndesmophyte formation over three or more motion segments

Etiology

- Unknown

Pathophysiology

- Ankylosis at the disc
- Pain, stiffness
- Associated at times with stenosis
- Risk of unstable fracture

Radiographs

- X-rays: Syndesmophytes have flowing appearance.
- Superimposed upon signs of lumbar spondylosis.
- CT: Bony anatomy in cases of suspected fracture.
- MRI and nuclear medicine to check for occult fracture.
- MRI to evaluate associated stenosis.

Classification

None

Treatment

Often associated with poor bone density

Nonoperative

- NSAIDs
- Brace wear
- PT
- Bisphosphonates

Operative

- Stenosis: May need decompression
- Fractures are intrinsically unstable and require surgery most of the time
- May need posterior stabilization alone or combined approach
- Mortality with cervical fractures is high and operative therapy preferred

Complications

- Neurologic injury
- Death
- Risk of heterotopic ossification anywhere in the body

Bibliography

1. Belanger TA, Rowe DE. Diffuse idiopathic skeletal hyperostosis: musculoskeletal manifestations. J Am Acad Orthop Surg. 2001;9(4):258–67.

4 Ossification of the Posterior Longitudinal Ligament

Samuel E. Smith

Take-Home Message
- More common is East Asian populations.
- Can be adherent to dura.

Definition

- Ossification of the posterior longitudinal ligament of the cervical spine

Etiology

- Genetics
- East Asian more common

Pathophysiology

- Fibroblastic infiltration, followed by vascular invasion and ultimately ossification
- Encroaches on the canal and can adhere to dura
- Can cause myelopathy

Radiographs

- Films show degenerative change which is sometimes hard to see and therefore need CT.
- CT defines problem and identifies morphologic type.
- K-line defines the size of mass and canal encroachment relative to cervical lordosis.
- MRI shows cord compression and signal.
- PLL very dark on MRI.

Classification

- Single segment
- Multisegmental
- Continuous
- Mixed

Treatment

Nonoperative

- Observation if no neurologic symptoms and canal encroachment minimal

Operative

- If canal encroachment more than 60 % or crosses K-line than myelopathy likely
- Anterior

- Posterior – laminoplasty or laminectomy and fusion
- Combined approaches

Complications

- Dural tear
- Paralysis
- Continued progression of myelopathy
- Stiffness even after laminoplasty
- RLN injury
- Esophageal injury
- Nerve root traction injury usually C5
- Postop hematoma

Bibliography

1. An HS, Al-Shihabi L, Kurd M. Surgical treatment for ossification of the posterior longitudinal ligament in the cervical spine. J Am Acad Orthop Surg. 2014;22(7):420–9. doi:10.5435/JAAOS-22-07-420.

5 Spondylolysis

Samuel E. Smith

Take-Home Message
- Isthmic pars fracture without slip
- Can be biologically active or inert
- Does not always cause pain

Definition

- Stress fracture without displacement of the pars interarticularis

Etiology

- Genetic predisposition
- Six percent of the population
- Increased risk in gymnastics and football lineman, i.e., whenever hyperextension is emphasized

Pathophysiology

- Pars interarticularis is an area of high stress especially with extension.
- Occurs in 25 % of first-degree relatives.

Radiographs

- May be difficult to see on plane films
- Oblique films to look for scotty dog sign
- Bone scan to look for signs of bone turnover – lots of radiation, however
- CT scan may be needed – lots of radiation, however
- MRI to look for bone edema

Treatment

- Depends on activity of defect, i.e. is there potential for healing?

Nonoperative

- Activity modification
- PT with modalities
- Bracing or casting
- NSAIDs

Operative

- Pars repair – ideally in biologically active lesion with no or minimal displacement
- Fusion

Complications

- Failure of healing of pars repair, fusion is the salvage
- Nonunion
- Infection
- DVT:PE
- Nerve injury

Bibliography

1. Menga EN, Kebaish KM, Jain A, Carrino JA, Sponseller PD. Clinical results and functional outcomes after direct intralaminar screw repair of spondylolysis. Spine(PhilaPa1976).2014;39(1):104–10.doi:10.1097/BRS.0000000000000043.
2. Sakai T, Sairyo K, Suzue N, Kosaka H, Yasui N. Incidence and etiology of lumbar spondylolysis: review of the literature. J Orthop Sci. 2010;15(3):281–8. doi:10.1007/s00776-010-1454-4. Epub 2010 Jun 18.

Part V
Paediatric Orthopaedics

Ashok Johari and Ratna Maheshwari

Juvenile Arthritis

Ashok Johari, Ratna Maheshwari, and Shalin Maheshwari

> **Take-Home Message**
> - Age of onset <16 years, with symptoms >6 weeks.
> - Can be associated with uveitis.
> - Can present with limb-length discrepancy.
> - Positive rheumatoid factor and antinuclear antibody (ANA) may indicate a more aggressive course.

Definition Juvenile Idiopathic arthritis is an autoimmune inflammatory arthritis of joints in children lasting more than 6 weeks.

The American College of Rheumatology has established five criteria for the diagnosis of JRA.

- Age at onset younger than 16 years
- Arthritis of one or more joints
- Symptom duration of at least 6 weeks
- An onset type, after 6 months' observation, of the polyarthritic form (five or more affected joints), the oligoarthritic form (fewer than five joints affected), or the systemic form with arthritis and characteristic fever
- Exclusion of other forms of arthritis

Positive rheumatoid factor and antinuclear antibody (ANA) may indicate a more aggressive course.

A. Johari, MD (✉) • R. Maheshwari, MD • S. Maheshwari, MD
Childrens' Orthopedic Centre,
2nd Floor, Bobby Apartments, 143 L. J. Road, Mahim (W), Mumbai 400016, India
e-mail: drashokjohari@hotmail.com

C. Mauffrey, D.J. Hak (eds.), *Passport for the Orthopedic Boards and FRCS Examination*, DOI 10.1007/978-2-8178-0475-0_19

Etiology

- Remains unknown, but the predominant common factors involve the immune system. Children with JRA have altered immune systems.
- Heredity factors may play a role.
- Infection – *Mycoplasma fermentans*, rubella virus, and *Bartonella henselae* may play a role in the etiology of systemic-onset JRA. Perinatal infection with influenza virus with expression of the disease many years later has also been proposed as an etiology.

Pathoanatomy

- T-lymphocyte abnormalities have been reported frequently, but their exact role in pathogenesis has yet to be determined.
- Human leukocyte antigen (HLA) product, T-cell receptor, and an antigen, together called a *trimolecular complex,* play a critical role in JRA pathogenesis.
- As in adult RA, autoimmune erosion of cartilage occurs.

Radiology and Evaluation

- Ultrasonography and MRI are useful in the early stages of disease to identify joint effusion and synovial hypertrophy.
- The earliest changes seen on plain films include periarticular soft tissue swelling; osteopenia, especially around the joint; and widening of the joint space. As the disease progresses, the radiographic joint space narrows owing to destruction of articular cartilage.

Classification

- Systemic JIA/JRA (Still disease)
  - Rash, high fever, multiple inflamed joints, and acute presentation are typical.
  - Anemia and/or a high white blood cell (WBC) count may occur.
  - Serositis, hepatosplenomegaly, lymphadenopathy, and pericarditis may be present.
  - Usually presents at age 5–10 years; girls and boys affected equally.
  - Poorest long-term prognosis.
  - Least common type of JIA (accounts for 20 %).
  - Remission occurs in approximately 29–50 % of children within 10 years of diagnosis.
- Oligoarticular JIA
  - Most common type of JIA (accounts for 30–40 %).
  - Four or fewer joints are involved; usually large joints, commonly knees and ankles, are affected.
  - Peak age 2–3 years; four times as common in girls as in boys.
  - A limp that improves during the day is typical.
  - 20 % have uveitis. Ophthalmology evaluation needed every 4 months if ANA positive, every 6 months if ANA negative.

  - Limb-length discrepancy with the affected side often longer is another sequela.
  - Best prognosis for long-term remission (70 %).

- Polyarticular JIA/polyarticular JRA
  - Five or more joints are involved; often, small joints (hand/wrist) are affected.
  - Uveitis sometimes present, but less common than in oligoarticular JIA.
  - More common in girls.
  - Prognosis is good (60 % remission).

Treatment

- Medical management with NSAIDs or DMARDs by a rheumatologist is usual. Low-dose methotrexate and other cytotoxic drugs may have a rapid effect on resistant disease.
- Physical and occupational therapy must be initiated to maintain joint range of motion.
- An arthrocentesis or synovial biopsy may be needed for diagnosis. Steroid injections and synovectomy may help if medical management fails.
- The development of flexion contractures of the hip and knee results in the loss of walking efficiency, with both increased loading on the knee and increased pain. Surgical releases of the hip and knee may result in long-term improvement in range of motion and function.
- Growth disturbances are most often seen at the knee. When a valgus deformity is present, either growth modulation or percutaneous partial epiphysiodesis will correct the deformity without major surgical trauma.
- Limb-length discrepancy may require epiphysiodesis; arthroplasty may be needed in adulthood for destroyed joints.

Bibliography

1. Chantler JK, Tingle AJ, Petty RE. Persistent rubella virus infection associated with chronic arthritis in children. N Engl J Med. 1985;313:1117.
2. Grom AA, Giannini EH, Glass DN. Juvenile rheumatoid arthritis and the trimolecular complex (HLA, T cell receptor, and antigen): differences from rheumatoid arthritis. Arthritis Rheum. 1994;37:601.
3. Sherry DD. What's new in the diagnosis and treatment of juvenile rheumatoid arthritis. J Pediatr Orthop. 2000;20:419.
4. Tsukahara M, Tsuneoka H, Tateishi H, et al. Bartonella infection associated with systemic juvenile rheumatoid arthritis. Clin Infect Dis. 2001;32:E22.
5. Williams MH. Recovery of mycoplasma from rheumatoid synovial fluid. In: Duthie JJR, Alexander WRM, editors. Rheumatic diseases. Baltimore: Williams & Williams; 1968. p. 172.

Birth Injuries

Ashok Johari, Ratna Maheshwari, and Shalin Maheshwari

1 Brachial Plexus Birth Palsy

Ashok Johari, Ratna Maheshwari, and Shalin Maheshwari

Take-Home Message

- Failure of antigravity biceps recovery by 3–6 months is an indication for microsurgery in BPBP

Definition

- Brachial plexus birth palsy (BPBP) is a traction or compression injury sustained to the brachial plexus during birth.
- Incidence reported to be 0.1–0.4 % of live births.

Etiology

- Risk factors include macrosomia, shoulder dystocia/difficult delivery, prior BPBP. Vacuum- or forceps-assisted deliveries are also at risk.
- Vertex presentation accounts for most of the cases (94–97 %), breech presentations account for 1–2 % of cases, and caesarean deliveries account for 1 % of cases.

A. Johari, MD (✉) • R. Maheshwari, MD • S. Maheshwari, MD
Pediatric Orthopedics, Childrens' Orthopedic Centre, Mumbai, India
e-mail: drashokjohari@hotmail.com

C. Mauffrey, D.J. Hak (eds.), *Passport for the Orthopedic Boards and FRCS Examination*, DOI 10.1007/978-2-8178-0475-0_20

Pathophysiology

- The mechanism of injury is forceful separation of the head from the shoulder by lateral flexion of the cervical spine and depression of the shoulder.

Classification

-
  - Anatomic: Upper trunk, lower trunk, total plexus.
  - Neurologic: *Neurapraxia* is paralysis in the absence of peripheral degeneration; the delay to recovery may be long, but recovery will be complete. *Axonotmesis* is damage to nerve fiber with complete peripheral degeneration but with intact external tissues to provide support for accurate spontaneous regeneration. Good recovery is anticipated, and no intervention can improve the outcome. In *neurotmesis* all essential structures, both neural and supporting tissues, have been disrupted. This category includes neuroma in continuity, division of nerve, and anatomic disruption.
- Narakas Classification
  - Group I: The classic Erb (C5–C6) palsy with initial absence of shoulder abduction and external rotation, elbow flexion, and forearm supination. Wrist and digital flexion and extension are intact. Successful spontaneous recovery as high as 90 %.
  - Group II: Includes involvement of C7 along with C5 and C6 impairment.
  - Group III: Flail extremity but without a Horner's syndrome.
  - Group IV: The most severe involvement is a flail extremity and Horner's syndrome. Preganglionic lesions are avulsions from the cord that will not spontaneously recover motor function. Preganglionic lesion is suggested by the presence of a Horner's syndrome, elevated hemidiaphragm, winged scapula, and the absence of rhomboid, rotator cuff, and latissimus dorsi function.
- Functional status – Toronto test score (see Table 1).

Table 1 Toronto test score

Elbow flexion	0–2
Elbow extension	0–2
Wrist extension	0–2
Digital extension	0–2
Thumb extension	0–2
Total score	0–10

A score of 0 denotes no function and score of 2 denotes full or normal function

- Modified Mallet Classification is used to assess residual deformity at shoulder. It is scored on the following parameters: global abduction; global external rotation; ability to take hand to neck, hand to spine, and hand to mouth; and internal rotation.

Evaluation

- EMG and NCV may help differentiate neuropraxia from axonal degeneration.
- CT myelography and MRI can identify preganglionic nerve root injuries if they are associated with traumatic pseudomeningoceles.
- X-ray changes may be seen in late presentation like retroversion of the glenoid, posterior subluxation, and medial flattening of the humeral head.

Management

- Initial phase involves giving rest to the extremity up to 3 weeks followed by gradual mobilization at the end of 3 weeks.
- If antigravity biceps function recovers by 2 months, full recovery is anticipated. If biceps function recovers at or after 5 months, incomplete recovery is likely. The presence of Horner's syndrome is associated with worse prognosis.
- Indications for surgery: When no clinical recovery of deltoid and biceps at 3 months supported by EMG and total palsy at birth with Horner's syndrome. Current recommendations for the timing of microsurgical repair range between the ages of 3 and 9 months.

  If biceps function is absent at 3 months, one may consider microsurgery or observe for a further 3 months

  Later, children with residual shoulder problems may be treated with appropriate musculotendinous lengthening, tendon transfer, or osteotomies.

- In patient with a total brachial plexus palsy, the classic priorities of repair include elbow flexion by biceps/brachialis muscle reinnervation, shoulder stabilization – abduction – external rotation by suprascapular nerve reinnervation, brachiothoracic pinch by reinnervation of the pectoralis major, sensation below the elbow in C6–C7 area by reinnervation of the lateral cord, wrist extension, and finger flexion by reinnervation of the lateral and posterior cord.
- Microsurgical treatment includes nerve transfers/neurotizations in avulsion injuries. In nerve ruptures, consider excision of neuroma and nerve grafting.
- Secondary procedures
  - Tendon transfers: Latissimus dorsi and teres major tendon transfers to rotator cuff (Sever-L'Episcopo procedure), often combined with releases of the pectoralis major, subscapularis, and coracobrachialis muscles, to improve shoulder abduction and external rotation
  - Humeral osteotomy: External rotation osteotomy of the distal humeral segment; recommended in setting of advanced glenohumeral joint dysplasia
  - Biceps rerouting will help improve forearm pronation.

Bibliography

1. Gilbert A. Long- term evaluation of brachial plexus surgery in obstetrical palsy. Hand Clin. 1995;11:583–94.
2. Waters PM. Obstetric brachial plexus injuries: evaluation and management. J Am Acad Orthop Surg. 1997;5:205–14.
3. Waters PM. Update on management of pediatric brachial plexus palsy. J Pediatr Orthop. 2005;25:116–26.

2 Torticollis

Ashok Johari, Ratna Maheshwari, and Shalin Maheshwari

Take-Home Message

- It is important to assess sternomastoid muscle spasm or contracture. Absence of the same must alert one to ocular, neurogenic, or psychogenic causes.
- Investigate to rule out atlantoaxial instability in case of recent onset torticollis with pain.
- Aim of management is to correct the deformity and restore range of motion of cervical spine.
- Stretching measures are usually unsuccessful after 1 year of age in congenital muscular torticollis.

Definition Torticollis is a combined deformity of the neck with tilt of the head to one side and rotation of the chin to the opposite side. It could be a symptom of cervical spine abnormality. For its differential diagnosis, see Table 2.

Table 2 Differential diagnosis of torticollis

Congenital-nonpainful	Acquired-painful	Acquired painful/nonpainful
Congenital muscular	Traumatic	Paroxysmal torticollis of infancy
	Atlantoaxial rotatory displacement	
	Os odontoideum	
Vertebral anomalies	Inflammatory	Tumors of posterior fossa, cervical cord
Failure of segmentation or formation	Grisel's syndrome	
	Juvenile rheumatoid arthritis	
	Diskitis	
	Tumors	Syringomyelia
	Eosinophilic granuloma	
	Osteoid osteoma	
		Oculogyric crisis
		Associated with ligamentous laxity, e.g., Down's

Etiology

- Acute wryneck: It is a condition seen after minimal trauma or associated with an upper respiratory tract infection with muscle spasm
- Osseous causes: Occipitocervical synostosis, basilar impression, odontoid anomalies. The most common cause of acquired, painful torticollis is atlantoaxial rotatory subluxation.
- Nonosseous causes:
  - Ocular: Weakness of the superior oblique muscle, Duane syndrome
  - Neurogenic: Posterior fossa tumor or tumor of the lower cranial nerves, Chiari malformation, syringomyelia. Intermittent torticollis is a feature of cervical dystonia.
  - Psychogenic
  - Muscular torticollis: It is the most common form of torticollis in infants and children. Primiparous, breech, or a difficult delivery causing birth trauma resulting into muscle trauma has been postulated as a cause.

Pathophysiology of Muscular Torticollis

- Mesenchymal cells remain in the sternocleidomastoid from fetal embryogenesis.
- Anoxia is the cause of fibrosis: The extent of fibrosis can vary from a relatively short segment to fibrosis of the entire length of the muscle.
- More recently, the fibrosis as a sequel of compartment syndrome due to intrauterine position has been suggested.
- Injury to the spinal accessory nerve and secondary fibrosis.
- Osseous-type lesion arises from a malformation of mesenchymal anlages at the occipitovertebral junction.

Evaluation

- Important points from history are age of onset, presence of precipitating factors, painful or painless, and constant or intermittent
- Examination
  - Contraction of sternocleidomastoid
  - Facial asymmetry
  - Short neck/low hairline/webbed neck
  - Eye movements and vision
  - Hip adduction contracture, foot deformities as part of packaging disorder
  - Gait and balance

Radiology

- In case of osseous torticollis, lateral radiograph of skull and upper cervical spine is used to assess basilar impression. Common lines used are Chamberlain's, McRae's, and McGregor's.
- X-ray beam directed 90° perpendicular to the skull gives a satisfactory view of occipitocervical junction. Standard radiographs are difficult to decipher.
- Further studies like CT scan can delineate the anomaly.

Classification

Cheng's Clinical Groups

- Sternocleidomastoid tumor group: Clinically palpable sternocleidomastoid tumor
- Muscular group: Clinical thickening and tightness of sternocleidomastoid muscle
- Postural torticollis: No tightness or tumor of sternocleidomastoid muscle

Treatment After ruling out other causes of torticollis, muscular torticollis must be addressed in the following way:

- Congenital muscular torticollis usually disappears within a year.
- Manual stretching and active positioning: Recommended in infancy.
- Recalcitrant cases: Use of botulinum toxin type A gives satisfactory results. However, it has little effect on established contracture.
- Stretching measures are usually unsuccessful after 1 year of age in congenital muscular torticollis. Surgery may be unipolar or bipolar release. Undertaken if deformity is not corrected by 1 year. Postoperative stretching with orthotic support for 3 months is usually sufficient.

Complications

- Structures that can be injured during surgery are the spinal accessory nerve, anterior and external jugular veins, carotid vessels and sheath, and facial nerve.

Bibliography

1. Canale ST, Griffin DW, Hubbard CN. Congenital muscular torticollis: a long term follow up. J Bone Joint Surg Am. 1982;64:810.
2. Cheng JC, Tang SP. Outcome of surgical treatment of congenital muscular torticollis. Clin Orthop Relat Res. 1999;362:190–200.
3. Cheng JC, Tang SP, Chen TM, Wong MW, Wong EM. The clinical presentation and outcome of treatment of congenital muscular torticollis in infants – a study of 1,086 cases. J Pediatr Surg. 2000;35:1091–6.
4. Cheng JCY, Wong MWN, Tang SP, et al. Clinical determinants of the outcome of manual stretching in the treatment of congenital muscular torticollis in infants. J Bone Joint Surg Am. 2001;83:679–8.
5. Davids JR, Wenger DR, Mubarak SJ. Congenital muscular torticollis: sequela of intrauterine or perinatal compartment syndrome. J Pediatr Orthop. 1993;13: 141–7.
6. Joyce MB, de Chalain TM. Treatment of recalcitrant idiopathic muscular torticollis in infants with botulinum toxin type a. J Craniofac Surg. 2005;16:321–7.

Cerebral Palsy

Ashok Johari, Ratna Maheshwari, and Shalin Maheshwari

Take-Home Message

- The CNS lesion in cerebral palsy is static, but the peripheral manifestations of CP often change over time.
- Botulinum toxin blocks the presynaptic release of acetylcholine and generally relaxes the muscles into which it is injected for 3–6 months.
- Scoliosis occurs in >50 % of patients with quadriplegia.
- Varus foot deformities are due to overactivity of the anterior tibialis, posterior tibialis, or both. Dynamic electromyography (EMG) is helpful in distinguishing the etiology.
- Soft tissue transfers alone will not suffice to correct a rigid foot deformity. Bone surgery will be needed in such cases as well.
- The most common causes of intoeing in children with CP are femoral anteversion and internal tibial torsion. Varus foot deformities commonly cause intoeing in patients with hemiplegia but not in patients with diplegia or quadriplegia.

Definition Cerebral palsy is a disorder of movement and posture that appears during infancy or early childhood. It is caused by nonprogressive damage to the brain before, during, or shortly after birth. CP is not a single disease but a name given to a wide variety of static neuromotor impairment syndromes occurring secondary to a lesion in the developing brain. The damage to the brain is permanent and cannot be cured, but the consequences can be minimized. Progressive musculoskeletal pathology occurs in most affected children.

A. Johari, MD (✉) • R. Maheshwari, MD • S. Maheshwari, MD
Pediatric Orthopedics, Childrens' Orthopedic Centre, Mumbai, India
e-mail: drashokjohari@hotmail.com

C. Mauffrey, D.J. Hak (eds.), *Passport for the Orthopedic Boards and FRCS Examination*, DOI 10.1007/978-2-8178-0475-0_21

Table 1 Risk factors for cerebral palsy

Prenatal	Perinatal	Postnatal (0–2 years)
Prematurity (gestational age less than 36 weeks)	Prolonged and difficult labor	CNS infection (encephalitis, meningitis)
Low birth weight (less than 2,500 g)	Premature rupture of membranes	Hypoxia
Maternal epilepsy	Presentation anomalies	Seizures
Hyperthyroidism	Vaginal bleeding at the time of admission for labor	Coagulopathies
Infections (TORCH)	Bradycardia	Neonatal hyperbilirubinemia
Bleeding in the third trimester	Hypoxia	
Incompetent cervix		
Severe toxemia, eclampsia		
Hyperthyroidism		
Drug abuse		
Trauma		
Multiple pregnancies		
Placental insufficiency		

Etiology The incidence of CP among babies who have one or more risk factors is higher than among the normal population. See Table 1.

Classification

- *Clinical classification*

Tonus	Lesion site
Spastic	Cortex
Dyskinetic	Basal ganglia – extrapyramidal system
Hypotonic/ataxic	Cerebellum
Mixed	Diffuse

The importance of the classification is that, in general, surgical results are more reliable in patients with spasticity compared with patients with dystonia.

- *Anatomical classification*

Location	Description
Hemiplegia	Upper and lower extremity on one side of the body
Diplegia	Four extremities, legs more affected than the arms
Quadriplegia	Four extremities plus the trunk, neck, and face
Triplegia	Both lower extremities and one upper extremity
Monoplegia	One extremity (rare)
Double hemiplegia	Four extremities, arms more affected than the legs

- *Functional classification – gross motor function classification system*
  - Walks independently and speed, balance, and coordination reduced
  - Walks without assistive devices but limitations in community
  - Walks with assistive devices
  - Transported or uses powered mobility
  - Severely limited, dependent on wheelchair

Investigations and Clinical Assessment

- Obtain baseline hip and spine radiographs. It is necessary to monitor hip instability. Reimer's index which is the percentage of femoral head coverage by the acetabulum (Fig. 1).

In a normal hip, the entire femoral head is located medial to the lateral margin of the acetabulum. In a spastic hip, the lateral migration is measured as AC/ AB ×100.

- Cranial magnetic resonance imaging (MRI) – useful for diagnosing lesions in the white matter.
- Electroencephalogram – useful for diagnosis and follow-up of seizure disorders.
- The typical clinical picture is established towards the age of 1 year. Primitive reflexes persist, and advanced postural reactions do not appear in the child with CP.
- Musculoskeletal examination includes evaluation of joint range of motion (ROM), deformities, contractures balance, posture, sitting, and gait.

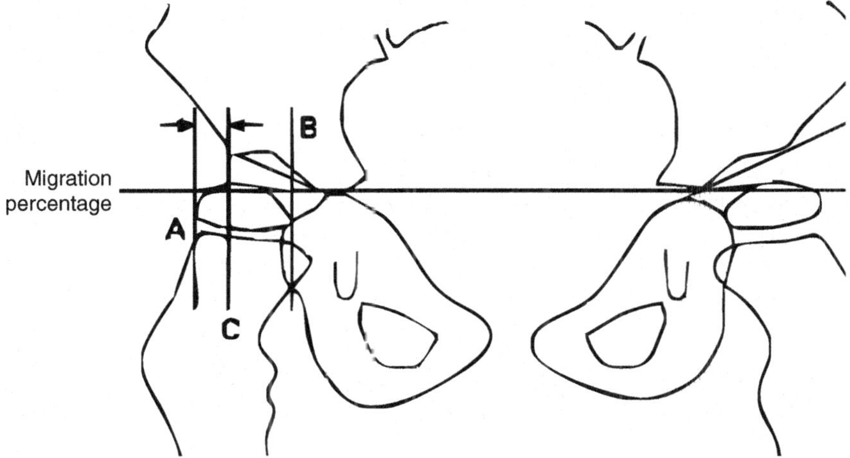

Fig. 1 Reimer's migration index

Assessing Lower Extremities

- Thomas test for hip flexion contracture.
- Range of abduction with hip in flexion and extension. If abduction is limited when the hips are extended but better when they are flexed, then adduction contracture is caused by gracilis and medial hamstring spasticity.
- *The Ely test* shows rectus femoris tightness.
- Test hip rotation in prone position with the knee in flexion. Excessive internal rotation suggests persistent femoral anteversion.
- Measure the popliteal angle to test for hamstring contracture.
- Use the Silfverskiöld test to assess triceps surae tightness.
- Examine tibial torsion with the patient in the prone position. Evaluate the thigh-foot angle with the knee flexed to 90°.
- A spastic posterior tibialis muscle causes hindfoot varus.
- A spastic peroneus or gastrocnemius muscle may cause a valgus deformity.

Assessing Upper Extremities

- Most commonly these patients possess internal rotation contractures at the shoulder, flexion contractures about the elbow, pronation contractures of the forearm, flexion contractures at the wrist, and thumb-in-palm deformity.
- A higher level of use and recognition of the affected upper extremity or extremities leads to more reliable surgical outcomes.
- Commonly used assessment tools include the Manual Ability Classification System, the House functional classification system of upper extremity use (see Table 2), the Zancolli classification system of voluntary grasp and release patterns of the upper extremity (Table 3), and modified House classification for thumb deformities (Table 4).

Table 2 House functional classification for cerebral palsy

Grade	Designation	Activity level
0	Does not use	Does not use
1	Poor passive assist	Uses as stabilizing weight only
2	Fair passive assist	Can hold on to object placed in hand
3	Good passive assist	Can hold on to object and stabilize it for use by the other hand
4	Poor active assist	Can actively grasp object and hold it weakly
5	Fair active assist	Can actively grasp object and stabilize it well
6	Good active assist	Can actively grasp an object and then manipulate it against other hand
7	Spontaneous use, partial	Can perform bimanual activities easily and occasionally uses the hand spontaneously
8	Spontaneous use, complete	Uses hand completely independently without reference to the other hand

Table 3 Zancolli classification of active finger and wrist extension

Level	Designation	Description
1	Minimal flexion spasticity	Can completely extend the fingers with a neutral position of the wrist or with <20° of flexion
2	Moderate flexion spasticity	Fingers can be actively extended but only with >20° of flexion
2A		Can actively extend, partially or totally, the wrist with the fingers flexed
2B		Cannot actively extend the wrist with the fingers flexed because of flaccid paralysis of the wrist extensor muscles
3	Severe flexion spasticity	Cannot extend the fingers even with maximal flexion of the wrist

Table 4 Modified house classification of thumb deformity

Type	Deforming force	Thumb position
1 Intrinsic	Adductor pollicis	Metacarpal adduction
	First dorsal interosseous	MCP joint flexion
	Flexor pollicis brevis	IP joint extension
2 Extrinsic	Flexor pollicis longus	MCP joint flexion
		IP joint flexion
		Metacarpal adduction less marked
3 Combined	Adductor pollicis	Metacarpal adduction
	First dorsal interosseous	MCP joint flexion
	Flexor pollicis brevis	IP joint flexion
	Flexor pollicis longus	(True "thumb-in-palm" deformity)

Management

Principles

- Physical therapy (PT) addresses development of gait and functional mobility with gait trainers, walkers or crutches, and prevention of contracture. Bracing is used part time in most children. The ground reaction ankle foot orthosis prevents excessive ankle dorsiflexion and crouch gait. Knee orthosis is generally used as resting splints. Neurofacilitation techniques use sensory input to the CNS that produces reflex motor output.
- Occupational therapy (OT) addresses fine motor function, activities of daily living (ADLs), self-feeding, self-dressing, and communication through speech or adaptive equipment.
- Speech therapy is often requisite, particularly in children with significant bulbar involvement.
- Antispasticity medicines like baclofen – oral administration is common, but dosage needs to be adjusted if relaxation is accompanied by an unacceptable amount of sedation.

- Botulinum toxin affects the neuromuscular junction by irreversibly binding synaptic proteins to block the presynaptic release of acetylcholine. It results in 3–6 months of relaxation in spastic muscles. It is useful for dynamic spasticity only, not for fixed contractures. Botulinum toxin may be considered a temporizing measure to delay surgery.
- The aim of orthopedic surgery is to obtain plantigrade stable feet, stable hips, good hip, and knee extension in the ambulatory child. Factors to consider in surgical selection include selective motor control, balance, cognitive function, visual impairment, apraxia, sensation, and neurological involvement level.
- Surgical intervention is generally undertaken when a patient has reached a plateau or worsened in regard to function and/or deformity despite nonsurgical interventions.

Spine Problems Specific to CP

- *Scoliosis* – the incidence and severity are related to the severity of CP. Scoliosis progression is common after skeletal maturity in patients with quadriplegia.

  Treatment

  - Bracing may not be an effective treatment of neuromuscular scoliosis in children with CP, but it may be effective in the treatment of idiopathic curves in children with mild involvement.
  - Surgery, typically fusion that is performed from the upper thoracic spine to the pelvis in nonambulatory patients, may be indicated for large curves that cause pain and/or interfere with sitting.

- *Lumbar hyperlordosis*

  - Lumbar hyperlordosis can occur.
  - It is almost always secondary to hip flexion contractures.

Hip Problems Specific to CP

- Subluxation

  Epidemiology/overview

  - Subluxation is uncommon in the ambulatory patient, but it is very common in the nonambulatory patient.
  - Subluxation (usually posterosuperior) is due to adductor and iliopsoas spasticity and non-weight-bearing status.
  - If abduction of either hip drops below 45° or the MI is >25 %, the hips are at risk and an anteroposterior pelvic radiograph should be obtained at each examination.
  - Hip subluxation will develop in 50 % of quadriplegic CP patients.
  - 50–75 % of dislocated hips will become painful. Hips with migration index (MI) >50 % do not reduce spontaneously; approximately one third will progress to dislocation.

Treatment

- Goals are to prevent hip subluxation and dislocation, maintain comfortable seating, and facilitate care and hygiene.
- Treatment is based on radiologic assessment with the Reimer migration percentage.
- Nonsurgical treatment consists first of PT and range of motion (ROM), hip abduction orthosis, with consideration of botulinum toxin injections to adductors.
- Soft tissue releases include adductor longus, aponeurotic psoas, and partial adductor brevis myotomy. Obturator neurectomy can lead to overcorrection.
- Soft tissue releases work in 50 % of patients, much less in quadriplegics. Over age 5 or once subluxation is over 50 %, soft tissue surgery is not likely to be sufficient. At this point bony anatomy and balance needs to be restored.
- This includes proximal femoral osteotomy (varus derotational osteotomy – VDRO) and possible pelvic osteotomy (Dega or Albee type). Older children with closed triradiate cartilage or those with recurrent subluxation may benefit from a Schanz or Chiari pelvis osteotomy. Children with failed hip reconstruction or older children with arthritis, even without previous surgery, may require resection arthroplasty (Castle procedure) for pain relief.
  - Pitfalls – the Castle procedure requires careful interposition of the hip capsule and muscle in the joint space, and the recovery time is often prolonged (6 months or more).
- Scissoring
  - Scissoring (due to adductor tightness) at the hip joint can interfere with gait and hygiene and is treated with proximal adductor release.
  - Obturator neurectomy should not be performed.
- Hip flexion contracture is treated with intramuscular iliopsoas lengthening.

Lever Arm Dysfunction Associated with CP

- Lever arm dysfunction results in posterior displacement of the ground reaction force relative to the knee and often results in crouch and power abnormalities in gait.
- Intoeing from femoral anteversion can be treated with femoral rotational osteotomies.
- Intoeing from internal tibial torsion can be treated with supramalleolar tibial osteotomies (concurrent fibular osteotomy is not needed).

Knee Problems Specific to CP

- Crouched gait
  - Causes – the most common cause is tight hamstrings, although crouch may be secondary to excessive ankle dorsiflexion or ankle equinus.
  - Treatment

- Nonsurgical treatment includes PT, bracing (such as knee immobilizers at night), and botulinum toxin injection.
- Surgical treatment is medial hamstring lengthening. Lengthening medial and lateral hamstrings in an ambulatory patient carries an increased risk of recurvatum.

- Stiff-knee gait
  - Stiff-knee gait causes difficulties with foot clearance in swing phase and tripping.
  - The cause is often overactivity of the rectus femoris (RF) in swing phase.
  - Treatment is with distal RF transfer. Indications for surgery are decreased magnitude and/or delayed timing of peak knee flexion in swing phase in conjunction with overactivity of the RF in swing phase.
- Knee contracture – in a nonambulatory patient, hamstring release may be useful to maintain leg position in a standing program.

Foot and Ankle Abnormal position or ROM at the foot and ankle causes gait abnormalities and decreases push-off power. Goals of treatment include a painless, plantigrade (stable) foot.

- Equinus deformity results from gastrocnemius-soleus muscle complex spasticity. It can create toe-walking or a back-knee (genu recurvatum) gait.
  - Nonsurgical treatment includes stretching, PT for ROM, AFO use, and botulinum toxin injection.
  - Surgical treatment should be considered only in patients with fixed contractures.
    - Testing under anesthesia helps determine whether a gastrocnemius recession or Achilles tendon lengthening is appropriate. If the ankle is in equinus with the knee flexed and extended, then the soleus is also tight, and an Achilles tendon lengthening should be performed. If the ankle comes above neutral with the knee flexed (gastrocnemius relaxed), then a gastrocnemius recession should be performed.
    - Overlengthening the heel cord may cause crouched gait, calcaneus foot position, and poor push-off power. This is less of a problem with a gastrocnemius recession than with an Achilles tendon lengthening.
- Equinovarus foot deformity can cause painful weight bearing over the lateral border of the foot and instability in stance phase.
  - The anterior tibialis and/or the posterior tibialis (the invertors) overpowers the peroneals (the evertors), whereas a tight gastrocnemius-soleus muscle causes equinus.
  - Dynamic EMG is useful in distinguishing whether the anterior tibialis and/or the posterior tibialis is causing the varus.
  - Clinically, the tibialis anterior can be checked using the confusion test. The patient sits on the edge of the examining table and flexes the hip

actively. The tibialis anterior will fire. If the forefoot supinates as it dorsiflexes, the varus is at least partially due to the tibialis anterior. If the forefoot just dorsiflexes, the varus is likely not due to the tibialis anterior.

- Clinically, the posterior tibialis is assessed by tightness as the hindfoot is positioned in valgus.
- Generally, isolated forefoot supination comes from the tibialis anterior, while hindfoot varus comes from the posterior tibialis.
- Anterior tibialis and/or posterior tibialis split tendon transfers are recommended rather than full tendon transfers because whole tendon transfers may lead to overcorrection.
- Tibialis posterior lengthenings are helpful in less severe deformities that are caused by the posterior tibialis.
- Pitfalls
  - Rigidity of the varus must be assessed preoperatively to determine the need for calcaneal ostectomy.
  - A soft tissue procedure will not be sufficient if the hindfoot deformity is rigid.
  - In rigid feet, soft tissue and bone procedures are both needed.

- Pes planus (pes valgus)
  - Pes planus is common in patients with diplegia and quadriplegia.
  - The foot is externally rotated due to spastic gastrocnemius, soleus, and peroneal muscles, with weak tibialis posterior function.
  - Patients bear weight on the medial border of the foot, on the talar head. The foot is unstable in push-off.
  - Weight-bearing AP radiographs of the ankles must be obtained because ankle valgus may also contribute to deformity.

  Treatment

  - Mild planovalgus feet can be treated with SMOs or AFOs.
  - Moderate to severe deformities can be treated with a calcaneal osteotomy. Calcaneal lengthening osteotomy (best undertaken after age of 6 years) is able to restore normal anatomy and is combined with peroneus brevis lengthening and tightening of the medial talonavicular joint capsule and/or posterior tibial tendon. Avoid peroneus longus lengthening because this can cause increased first ray dorsiflexion. Calcaneal (medial) sliding osteotomy brings the calcaneus in line with the weight-bearing axis of the tibia.
  - Severe deformities can be treated with subtalar fusion, although this is usually only needed in very large children and/or those with extreme laxity. (Triple arthrodesis is almost never required.)
  - Compensatory midfoot supination can be treated with first ray plantar flexion osteotomy, often with a peroneus brevis lengthening.

- Hallux valgus
  - Occurs frequently with pes valgus, equinovalgus, and equinovarus feet.
  - Toe straps added to AFOs or nighttime hallux valgus splinting may be helpful.
  - Severe hallux valgus should be treated with a fusion of the first metatarsophalangeal (MTP) joint.
  - Pes valgus must be simultaneously corrected to avoid recurrence.
  - Pitfalls – at the time of hallux valgus correction, consider that the patient will often also have valgus interphalangeus, which should be treated with a proximal phalanx (Akin) osteotomy.

- Dorsal bunion
  - Overview/Etiology
    - Dorsal bunion is a deformity in which the great toe is flexed in relation to an elevated metatarsal, causing a prominence over the uncovered metatarsal head, which can be painful with shoe wear.
    - Dorsal bunion may be iatrogenic, occurring after surgery to balance the foot.
    - The deformation may either be caused by an overpowering tibialis anterior or an overpowering flexor hallucis longus (FHL).
  - Treatment
    - Nonsurgical treatment is with shoes with soft, deep toe boxes.
    - Surgical treatment is needed in recalcitrant cases. Flexible deformities are treated with lengthening or split transfer of the anterior tibialis and transfer of the FHL to the plantar aspect of the first metatarsal head. Osteotomies of the medial column are rarely needed. Rigid deformities require fusion of the first MTP joint and lengthening or split transfer of the anterior tibialis. Osteotomies are rarely needed.

Upper Extremity Problems Specific to CP

- Nonsurgical treatment
  - OT is useful in early childhood for ADL, stretching, and splinting.
  - Botulinum toxin is useful for dynamic deformities.
  - Constraint-induced therapy (splinting of the uninvolved upper extremity to encourage use of the involved arm) in patients with hemiplegia is gaining popularity but does not have a long track record.

- Surgical treatment
  - Surgical treatment is undertaken primarily for functional concerns, hygiene, and sometimes for appearance.
  - If shoulder adduction and internal rotation contractures are interfering with hand function, they may be treated with subscapularis release and pectoralis major lengthening. A proximal humeral derotational osteotomy is rarely necessary.

- Elbow flexion contractures may be treated with lacertus fibrosis resection, biceps and brachialis lengthening, and brachioradialis origin release.
- Elbow pronation contractures should be treated with pronator teres release or rerouting.
- Radial head dislocation is uncommon and, if symptomatic, may be treated with radial head excision when the patient reaches maturity.
- The goal of surgical procedures on the wrist and fingers is to allow the fingers to open with wrist flexion for release and to close with wrist extension for grasp. Wrist deformities usually include flexion contracture with ulnar deviation and are associated with weak wrist extension and a pronated forearm.
  - If finger extension is good and there is little wrist flexion spasticity, the flexor carpi ulnaris (FCU) or flexor carpi radialis (FCR) should be lengthened.
  - Releasing the wrist and finger flexors and the pronator teres from the medial epicondyle of the humerus weakens wrist and finger flexion but is nonselective.
  - In severe spasticity, an FCU transfer is recommended. If grasp is good, release is weak, and the FCU is active in release; it should be transferred to the extensor digitorum communis (EDC). If grasp is weak with the wrist flexed, release is good, and the FCU is active in grasp; it should be transferred to the extensor carpi radialis brevis (ECRB). A concurrent FCR release should not be performed, to avoid overweakening the wrist flexion.
  - Some believe that the extensor carpi ulnaris is often overactive as an ulnar deviator but remains in phase as an extensor and is the preferred tendon to transfer into the extensor carpi radialis brevis. This transfer has less of a supinatory torque than the Green procedure does (transfer of the flexor carpi ulnaris to the extensor carpi radialis brevis).

Hand Deformities

- Thumb in palm – caused by metacarpal adduction contracture with metacarpophalangeal (MCP) flexion or extension contracture, sometimes with interphalangeal (IP) joint flexion contracture. The approach to the thumb-in-palm deformity is to release contracted soft tissue and then augment weak extensors and abductors often by EPL translocation.
- Clawing of the fingers, with wrist flexion and MCP hyperextension, can be treated with FCR or FCU transfer to the ECRB.
- Finger flexion contracture is treated with flexor digitorum sublimis (FDS) and flexor digitorum longus (FDL) lengthening or tenotomies.
- Swan neck deformities of the fingers are a result of intrinsic tightness and extrinsic overpull. These deformities are sometimes caused by wrist flexion or weak wrist extensors and can sometimes be helped by correcting the wrist flexion deformity.

Bibliography

1. Crankshaft effect after posterior spinal fusion and unit rod instrumentation in children with cerebral palsy. J Pediatr Orthop. 2001;21:108–12.
2. Dabney KW, Miller F. Cerebral palsy. In Abel MF editor. Orthopaedic knowledge update: pediatrics 3. Rosemont: American Academy of Orthopaedic Surgeons; 2006. p 93–109.
3. Flynn JM, Miller F. Management of hip disorders in patients with cerebral palsy. J Am Acad Orthop Surg. 2002;198–209.
4. House JH, Gwathmey FW, Fidler MO. A dynamic approach to the thumb-in palm deformity in cerebral palsy. J Bone Joint Surg Am. 1981;63:216–25.
5. Kerr Graham H, Selber P. Musculoskeletal aspects of cerebral palsy. J Bone Joint Surg Br. 2003;85:157–66.
6. Zancolli EA, Zancolli ER Jr. Surgical management of the hemiplegic spastic hand in cerebral palsy. Surg Clin North Am. 1981;61:395–406.

Deformities

Ashok Johari, Ratna Maheshwari, and Shalin Maheshwari

1 Amelia/Phocomelia/Ectromelia

Ashok Johari, Ratna Maheshwari, and Shalin Maheshwari

Overview/Definition

- Congenital limb defects are rare foetal anomalies with a birth prevalence of 0.55 per 1,000.
- Amelia: Rare birth defect with complete absence of the skeletal parts of a limb is generally thought to be a sporadic anomaly. It is a terminal transverse deficiency.
- Ectromelia: Total or partial absence of one or more long bones or limbs.
- Phocomelia: Absence of the arm and forearm in the upper limb or the thigh and leg in the lower limb (i.e. the hands or feet sprout directly from the trunk); the deficiency may be proximal (arms or thighs missing) or distal (forearms or legs missing). This is an intercalary transverse deficiency.

Aetiology

- Amelia can be isolated defect or with associated malformations, particularly abdominal wall and renal anomalies.
- Teratogens such as thalidomide, alcohol, vascular compromise by amniotic bands or other causes and maternal diabetes have been reported to cause this severe limb deficiency.
- Amelia may be attributed to the early stages of health complications during pregnancy, including infection, failed abortion or even the complications associated with removal of an IUD after pregnancy.

A. Johari, MD (✉) • R. Maheshwari, MD • S. Maheshwari, MD
Pediatric Orthopedics, Childrens' Orthopedic Centre, Mumbai, India
e-mail: drashokjohari@hotmail.com

C. Mauffrey, D.J. Hak (eds.), *Passport for the Orthopedic Boards and FRCS Examination*, DOI 10.1007/978-2-8178-0475-0_22

- Different modes of inheritance have been involved in the aetiology of amelia including autosomal recessive, X-linked dominant and autosomal mode of inheritance which indicate the genetic heterogeneity of this condition. Tetra-amelia syndrome appears to have autosomal recessive pattern of inheritance.

Pathoanatomy

- By 7 weeks of embryonic life, the formation of all parts of the upper and lower limbs is essentially complete.
- Most limb deficiencies occur early in the period of limb morphogenesis, when there is rapid proliferation and differentiation of cells and tissues. This "sensitive period" of limb formation peaks during the fifth and sixth weeks after fertilisation.
- The subclavian artery disruption sequence has been proposed as a common pathway, but this remains speculative.
- The presence of ectoderm-derived tissues (skin, nails, distal phalangeal tufts) supports the concept of failure of normal mesodermal proliferation.

Evaluation

- Prenatal diagnosis including detailed ultrasound and amniocentesis plays a major role in counselling parents with foetal anomalies.
- Children with phocomelia can have abnormalities in the face, ears, nose and vessels in addition to limbs. Infants will have a petite head with sparse hair that may appear "silvery blonde". Haemangioma can develop around facial area at birth with hypertelorism.

Treatment

- Advances in prosthetic limbs with the use of new materials have increased greatly. Myoelectric prosthetic limbs can detect electrical signals from the nervous system and muscles.
- Infants as early as 6 months are fitted with prosthetic mitten, enabling them to get used to the prosthesis.

Bibliography

1. Baron E, Clarke S, Solomon C. The two stage myoelectric hand for children and young adults. Orthot Prosthet. 1983;37:11.
2. Bavinck JN, Weaver DD. Subclavian artery supply disruption sequence: hypothesis of a vascular etiology for Poland, Klippel-Feil, and Mobius anomalies. Am J Med Genet. 1986;23:903.
3. Froster-Iskenius UG, Baird PA. Amelia: incidence and associated defects in a large population. Teratology. 1990;41(1):23–31. doi:10.1002/tera.

2 Radioulnar Synostosis

Ashok Johari, Ratna Maheshwari, and Shalin Maheshwari

Take-Home Message

- Majority of children with radioulnar synostosis have forearm fixed in pronation.
- The magnitude of functional limitations must be considered while planning therapy.
- Any corrective surgery if considered necessary should be undertaken before the child adapts to the current position of the forearm.
- There are no good long-term reports for resection of synostosis as a procedure.
- Rotation osteotomy can be considered in bilateral cases, with severe pronation deformity, with significant disability in activities of daily living. However, this procedure is associated with a high complication rate.

Definition

- This condition represents a failure of differentiation in the proximal forearm.
- It is an isolated anomaly in one-third of cases, and bilateral involvement is seen in 60 % of affected children.

Aetiology

- The exact event that causes failure of separation is unknown.
- Syndromes such as Poland syndrome, Apert syndrome, arthrogryposis, Klinefelter syndrome and many others are associated with congenital radioulnar synostosis.

Pathophysiology

- Congenital radioulnar synostosis represents a failure of differentiation in the primitive mesenchymal condensations that occur in the proximal forearm at approximately 5 weeks of gestation.
- The humerus, radius and ulna all arise from a shared mesenchymal anlage that later condenses into cartilage and separates into individual bones. Failure of this process to properly occur can result in radioulnar synostosis.
- The process of separation occurs at the time the foetal forearm is in a position of pronation; this explains why in the majority of children with congenital radioulnar synostosis, the forearm is fixed in pronation.

Radiology and Classification

- Type I involves a smooth fusion of the radius and ulna proximally for a variable distance, typically 2–6 cm.
- Type II is a fusion just distal to the proximal radial epiphysis associated with a congenital dislocation of the radial head. There may be compromised elbow extension in this type.

Treatment

- Nonoperative
  - The magnitude of functional limitations must be considered while planning therapy.
  - Pronation is a good position for writing and keyboard tasks when they become adults. Increased compensatory rotation at the carpus, wrist and shoulder is usually adequate for most activities.
  - In rare bilateral cases with marked pronation deformities, the child may have difficulties in daily functional activities.

- Operative: The surgical decision should be based on the difficulties in forearm functioning affecting the quality of life, rather than just the degree of pronation.
  - Resection

    The procedure of resection of synostosis is technically demanding, and results are often unsatisfactory. One reason for failure is the reformation of synostosis. Interposition of various materials in the resection gap has been tried, and of these, vascularised fat graft seems to be the most promising. However, there are no good long-term reports of this method, and so most surgeons do not choose this procedure.
  - Rotational osteotomy

    This is the favoured procedure when functional limitations are severe enough to require repositioning of the forearm. Surgically increasing supination can improve forearm function, and the loss of pronation can be easily compensated by the shoulder. The site of osteotomy can be either through the synostosis or in the diaphyses of both bones. It is recommended that in bilateral cases, the dominant hand should be left in 20° of pronation and the nondominant hand in neutral.
  - Fixation can be by cast, intramedullary nail and cross-pin fixation. In older children, low-profile plates can be used.
  - Ideally, any corrective surgery should be undertaken before the child adapts to the current position of the forearm.

Complications Rotational osteotomies can cause nerve palsies, vascular compromise, compartment syndrome and malunion.

Bibliography

1. Green WT, Mital MA. Congenital radio-ulnar synostosis: surgical treatment. J Bone Joint Surg Am. 1979;61:738–43.
2. Kanaya F, Ibaraki K. Mobilization of a congenital proximal radio-ulnar synostosis with use of free vascularized fascio-fat graft. J Bone Joint Surg Am. 1998;80:1186–92.
3. Shingade VU, Shingade RV, Ughade SN. Results of single- staged rotational osteotomy in a child with congenital proximal radioulnar synostosis: subjective and objective evaluation. J Pediatr Orthop. 2014;34:63–9.
4. Simmons BP, Southmayd WW, Riseborough EJ. Congenital radioulnar synostosis. J Hand Surg [Am]. 1983;8:829–38.

3 Madelung Deformity

Ashok Johari, Ratna Maheshwari, and Shalin Maheshwari

Take-Home Message

- Volar and ulnar aspect of distal radial physis slows or stops growth prematurely. Continued normal growth of both ulnar physis and remaining dorsal, radial aspect of radial physis, results in ulnar overgrowth, carpal subluxation and radial articular deformity.
- The treatment principle of physiolysis involves resection of abnormal volar, ulnar physeal region of radius and fat interposition.
- Aberrant tethering anatomic structures are excised.
- Patient presenting late with marked deformity and symptoms is addressed with corrective osteotomy. Ulnar overgrowth is treated with an ulnar shortening procedure.

Definition

- Madelung deformity is described as a growth deformity of the distal radius. The deformity in classical Madelung deformity is an ulnar and volar deviation of the wrist with prominence of the lower end of the ulna.
- The deformity is more frequently seen in girls, usually appearing at around 12 years of age, during time of adolescent growth spurt, and gradually progressing until skeletal maturity.

Aetiology

- Generally sporadic in nature.
- Can be associated with Léri-Weill syndrome, a dyschondrosteosis form of mesomelic dwarfism.
- It has also been associated with Hurler mucopolysaccharidosis, Turner syndrome, osteochondromatosis, achondroplasia and Ollier disease.

Pathoanatomy

- The arrest of volar, radial aspect of distal radial physis causes subsequent deformity of radiocarpal, radioulnar and ulnocarpal joints.
- Vickers et al. have described abnormal tethering of soft tissues from distal radius to carpus and ulna.
- The soft tissue tether is usually a strong abnormal ligament and pronator quadratus muscle insertions that links the proximal pole of the lunate to the palmar and ulnar cortex of the distal radius.

Radiology

- Increased tilt of radial articular surface from dorsal radial corner of styloid to the volar, ulnar aspect of depleted lunate fossa.
- The ulnar variance is more positive, with carpal overload and dorsal subluxation.
- The carpus migrates more proximal into the increasing diastasis between radius and ulna on anteroposterior radiograph.

Treatment

- Physiolysis
  - Early physiolysis has been recommended by Vickers and Nielsen, who have shown that the procedure can arrest progression of the deformity and restore normal growth of the radius quite effectively.
  - The operation entails resection of a sliver of bone from the ulnar aspect of the distal radius, identifying the growth plate, ensuring that any bone bridge is removed and placing fat graft astride the growth plate to prevent a bridge from reforming.
- Resection of the soft tissue tether.
  - Should be done whenever physiolysis is undertaken. The wrist joint has to be opened as the abnormal ligament is attached to the lunate. When done in conjunction with physiolysis, the entire ligament can be followed to its proximal attachment to the radius and excised.
- Corrective osteotomy of the distal radius.
  - An established deformity in a long-standing case can be improved by an osteotomy of the distal radius. In classical Madelung deformity, a dorsal- and lateral-based wedge of bone is excised from the distal radius close to the articular surface.
  - Excision of the distal ulna can remove the unsightly prominence in the older patient with established deformity. This may be combined with the osteotomy of the distal radius.

Bibliography

1. Nielsen JB. Madelung's deformity: a follow- up study of 26 cases and a review of literature. Acta Orthop Scand. 1977;48:379.
2. Ranawat CS, DeFieore J, Straub LR. Madelung's deformity: an end- result study of surgical treatment. J Bone Joint Surg Am. 1975;57:772.
3. Vickers DW. Madelung deformity. In: Gupta A, Kay SPJ, Scheker LR, editors. The growing hand. London: Harcourt; 2000. p. 791–8.
4. Vickers D, Nielsen G. Madelung's deformity: treatment of osteotomy of the radius and Lauenstein procedure. J Hand Surg Am. 1987;12:202.

4 Radial Club Hand

Ashok Johari, Ratna Maheshwari, and Shalin Maheshwari

Take-Home Message
- RLD is commonly associated with other congenital anomalies, including TAR, Fanconi anaemia, Holt-Oram syndrome and VACTERL association.
- Elbow stiffness precludes surgery.

Definition Radial club hand is a complex congenital anomaly involving failure of formation of structure on the preaxial border of the upper limb. The deficiency involves the skeleton, muscles and tendons, nerves and vessels and other soft tissues of the entire upper limb to a greater or lesser extent.

Aetiology Radial club hand may be an isolated anomaly or may be associated with one of a host of complex syndromes. Unilateral radial club hand is often an isolated anomaly, while the bilateral form is more frequently associated with syndromes.

RLD is associated with several congenital conditions and syndromes:

- Thrombocytopenia-absent radius (TAR)—Low platelet count that normalises over time
- Fanconi anaemia—Platelet and blood cell counts normal at birth but decrease dramatically during first few years of life; diagnosed with mitomycin-C chromosomal challenge test; treated with bone marrow transplantation
- Holt-Oram syndrome—RLD with congenital heart disease, typically atrial or ventricular septal defects
- VACTERL—Constellation of anomalies including *v*ertebral, *a*nal, *c*ardiac, *t*racheal, *e*sophageal, *r*enal, and *l*imb

Pathophysiology In addition to skeletal deficiencies, there are similar deficiencies of soft tissue structures (e.g. radial artery, median nerve, flexor carpi radialis).

Radiology and Classification

Bayne classification

- Delayed appearance of distal epiphysis, slightly shortened radius
- Deficient growth proximal and distal, considerably shortened radius
- Partial absence of the radius (distal and middle thirds most common)
- Completely absent radius (most common)

Evaluation

Look for the following:

- Elbow flexion contracture
- Shortened and/or bowed forearm
- Radial deviation of the wrist
- Aplasia or hypoplasia of the thumb

Treatment No intervention is the preferred option if either the function of the hand is so near normal that surgery is unlikely to make a difference or when surgery may actually jeopardise existing function.

Elbow stiffness also precludes surgery.

Surgery should also be avoided if the child has adjusted to his deformity.

- In type I, radial club hand with mild radial deviation of the wrist and stability of wrist joint serial manipulation and casting in early infancy is effective in correcting the deformity. In cases of wrist instability, radial lengthening may be an effective option.
- For severe degrees of types II, III and IV radial club hand, centralisation or more recently radialisation is a popular surgery.
- Corrective osteotomy of the bowed ulna may be performed in conjunction with either an operation to stabilise the wrist (radialisation or centralisation) or at the time of ulnar lengthening.

Bibliography

1. Bayne LG, Klug MS. Long-term review of the surgical treatment of radial deficiencies. J Hand Surg [Am]. 1987;12:169–79.
2. D'Arcangelo M, Gupta A, Scheker LR. Radial club hand. In: Gupta A, Kay SPJ, Scheker LR, editors. The growing hand. London: Harcourt Publishers Limited; 2000. p. 147–70.
3. Dobyns JH, Wood VE, Bayne LG. Congenital hand deformities. In: Green DP, editor. Operative Hand Surgery, vol. 1. 3rd ed. New York: Churchill Livingstone; 1993. p. 288–303.

5 Ulnar Haemimelia

Ashok Johari, Ratna Maheshwari, and Shalin Maheshwari

Take-Home Message
- Typically, the wrist is stable, but elbow function is compromised.
- The main problems that can arise in an ulnar club hand include progressive bowing of radius, proximal migration of dislocated radial head, hand anomalies and loss of elbow motion.

Definition Ulnar club hand is a longitudinal deficiency of the postaxial border of the upper limb with abnormalities of the elbow, forearm, wrist and hand.

Aetiology

- Ulnar club hand is frequently associated with other anomalies or syndromes. Can be associated with rare inheritable syndromes, such as ulnar mammary syndrome, Klippel-Feil syndrome and other nongenetic syndromes such as Cornelia de Lange syndrome.
- Usually sporadic with rare autosomal dominant inheritance patterns.
- Contralateral upper extremity deficiencies of phocomelia, transverse arrest, radial deficiency and aphalangia occur commonly.

Pathophysiology

- Progressive bowing of the radius attributed to the presence of a fibrous tether between the cartilaginous anlage and the ulnar side of the distal radial epiphysis.
- The elbow may be in severe flexion in children with a cubital pterygium syndrome, or it may be stiff in extension in children with synostosis.

Radiology and Classification

Dobyns classification (see Table 1)

A significant proportion of children with ulnar club hand have thumb anomalies. Thumb anomalies include deficiency, duplication, syndactyly of the first web and adduction deformity.

Table 1 Classification of ulnar club hand

Type	Ulna	Elbow	Radial head	Radius	Wrist and hand
I. Hypoplasia	Short but both proximal and distal ulnar epiphyses are present	Well formed	Dislocation+/– no proximal migration	Mild bowing present but does not increase	Wrist not deviated. Hand anomalies frequent and may be severe
II. Partial aplasia	Small ossified segment + Cartilage anlage in distal third	Humeroulnar articulation formed	Dislocation+ Proximal migration occurs	Short	Wrist deviated. Sloping distal radial epiphysis. Hand anomalies frequent and may be severe
				Bowing present which may progress	
III. Total aplasia	Absent	Fixed flexion deformity	No proximal radioulnar joint as ulna is totally absent	+/– Bowing	Hand anomalies severe
	No cartilage remnant	May be associated with cubital pterygium syndrome			
IV. Synostosis	Small remnant present	Radiohumeral fusion or ulnohumeral fusion	No proximal radioulnar joint	+/– Bowing	Variable

Treatment

Aim of management

- To tackle the main problems that can arise in an ulnar club hand which include progressive bowing of radius, proximal migration of dislocated radial head, hand anomalies and loss of elbow motion
- Attempt must be made to prevent the radius from bowing.

Treatment options

- Specific hand anomalies can be corrected like syndactyly release, first web space release and surgery on the hypoplastic thumb. Separation of thumb and index finger by 6 months of age and of central syndactyly by 18 months of age.
- Forearm splintage in the infant and young child may help to minimise severity of radial bowing.
- In cases with significant proximal migration of radial head, function can be improved by radial head excision and creation of synostosis of radius and ulna (type 2).
- Exclusion of cartilaginous anlage of distal ulna may reduce the severity of radial bowing.
- Internal rotation deformity of humerus may also require surgical intervention.
- If there is no useful elbow function and no potential improving hand function, with cubital pterygium syndrome, consideration can be given to above elbow amputation.

Bibliography

1. Cole PJ, Manske PR. Classification of ulnar deficiency according to the thumb and first web space. J Hand Surg (Am). 1997;22:479–88.
2. Dobyns JH, Wood VE, Bayne LG. Congenital hand deformities. In: Green DP, editor. Operative hand surgery, vol. 1. New York: Churchill Livingstone; 1993. p. 251–548.
3. Lloyd- Roberts GC. Treatment of defects of the ulna in children by establishing cross union with the radius. J Bone Joint Surg Br. 1973;55:327–30.
4. Mulligan PJ. The elbow in ulnar club hand. In: Gupta A, Kay SPJ, Scheker LR, editors. The growing hand. London: Harcourt Publishers Limited; 2000. p. 197–202.

6 Typical and Atypical Cleft Hand

Ashok Johari, Ratna Maheshwari, and Shalin Maheshwari

Take-Home Message

- A typical cleft hand has the following: bilaterality, positive inheritance, foot involvement, V-shaped cleft and syndactyly.
- The atypical cleft refers to a unilateral anomaly that is nonfamilial, U-shaped cleft with no foot involvement.
- Cleft closure and thumb reconstruction are the goals of surgical management.

Definition

- Typical cleft hand represents a partial or complete longitudinal deficiency in the central portion of hand. The elbow, forearm and wrist are usually normal.
- Atypical cleft hand has now been classified as part of symbrachydactyly. Symbrachydactyly is defined by unilateral central digital deficiencies and simple syndactylies.

Aetiology

- Typical cleft hand has an autosomal dominant inheritance pattern, with variable penetrance.
- Can be associated with other syndromes and malformations, such as cleft lip/palate, other craniofacial syndromes, Cornelia de Lange syndrome, congenital heart disease, ocular malformations and imperforate anus.
- Symbrachydactyly is a sporadic event, with no associated anomalies.

Evaluation

- A typical cleft hand has the following: bilaterality, positive inheritance, foot involvement, V-shaped cleft and syndactyly.
- The atypical cleft refers to a unilateral anomaly that is nonfamilial, U-shaped cleft with no foot involvement.
- The severity of the cleft ranges from a cleft between middle and ring fingers to oligodactylous radial digits and syndactylous ulnar digits.
- Clefting can occur without absence of digit; however, most cases have absence of one or more digits and may have varying degrees of polydactyly and syndactyly.
- Often the middle finger alone is missing and the defect may extend to produce a deep V-shaped cleft with absence of the metacarpal.

Treatment

- Cleft closure and thumb reconstruction are the goals.
- Syndactyly when present should be released early, because it may affect the growth potential of two neighbouring digits.
- Thumb reconstruction may require anywhere between web space deepening to tendon transfers to rotation osteotomies to toe to hand transfer.
- Web deepening should always follow cleft closure; otherwise, difficulty may be encountered in raising flaps for cleft closure.

Bibliography

1. Buss PW. Cleft hand/foot: clinical and developmental aspects. J Med Genet. 1994;31:726.
2. Kay SPJ. Congenital hand deformities: cleft hand. In: Green DP, Hotchkiss RN, Pederson WC, editors. Green's operative hand surgery. 4th ed. New York: Churchill Livingstone; 1999. p. 402.

7 Syndactyly

Ashok Johari, Ratna Maheshwari, and Shalin Maheshwari

Take-Home Message
- When performing syndactyly release, only one side of an affected digit should be operated on at a time to avoid vascular embarrassment.

Definition

- Failure of separation of digits occurs in utero.
- Most common congenital hand condition, occurring in 1 per 2,000–2,500 live births
- Males affected more commonly than females; whites affected more commonly than blacks

Aetiology

- Autosomal dominant inheritance with variable penetrance
- Associated conditions
  - Poland syndrome: congenital absence of the sternocostal head of the pectoralis major, limb hypoplasia and symbrachydactyly
  - Apert syndrome (also known as acrocephalosyndactyly): mental retardation; premature fusion of cranial sutures resulting in high, broad forehead, occipital flattening, and bulging low-set eyes; and acrosyndactyly (spadelike hand)
  - Carpenter syndrome: acrocephalopolysyndactyly

Pathoanatomy

- Normal differentiation of digits occurs during the fifth to 8 weeks of gestation.
- Failure of normal programmed cell death results in syndactyly.

Radiology

- May reveal osseous union and marked joint and bony malalignment.
- In infancy, areas of chondral abnormalities will not be visible on radiographs.

Classification

- Simple syndactyly defined by web formed by soft tissue only.
- Complex syndactyly denotes fusion of adjacent phalanges.
- Complicated syndactyly refers to interposition of accessory phalanges or abnormal bones.
- Complete syndactyly refers to webbing that extends to the tips of the involved digits.

- Incomplete syndactyly does not extend to the digital tips.
- Acrosyndactyly involves webbing of tip of all fingers.
- The third web is most commonly affected, followed by the fourth, second and first web spaces.

Management

- If the syndactyly does not extend beyond the PIP joint, this will not limit function.
- Surgery is generally performed at around 12 months of age.
- Release digits of differing sizes first to avoid growth disturbance.
- Do not operate on both sides of the digit at the same time to avoid vascular embarrassment.
- Use local skin flaps to reconstitute the web commissure to avoid scar contracture and "web creep".
- Use zigzag lateral flaps to avoid longitudinal scar contracture.
- Use full-thickness skin grafts to cover bare areas.

Complications

- The most worrisome complication of an avascular digit is avoidable, by not operating on both sides of the digit.
- Flap necrosis and scar contractures are common. Flaps should be secured without tension, and vascularity should be checked.
- Web space creep is common with growth, but often does not require reoperation.

Bibliography

1. Light TR. Congenital anomalies: syndactyly, polydactyly and cleft hands. In: Peimer CA, editor. Surgery of hand and upper extremity. New York: McGraw-Hill; 1996. p. 2111.
2. Percival NJ, Skyes PJ. Syndactyly: a review of the factors which influence surgical treatment. J Hand Surg Br. 1989;14:196.

8 Preaxial and Postaxial Polydactyly

Ashok Johari, Ratna Maheshwari, and Shalin Maheshwari

Take-Home Message

- Surgical management of preaxial polydactyly involves ablation of the bony elements of the more underdeveloped (usually radial) thumb and reconstruction of the (radial) collateral ligament and, in Wassel type IV thumbs, transfer of the thenar muscles from the ablated proximal phalanx to the preserved (ulnar) proximal phalanx.

- Late deformity following surgery of preaxial polydactyly occurs due to failure to recognise a pollex abductus, inadequate correction of the longitudinal thumb alignment, inadequate reconstruction of the collateral ligament and failure to centralise the extensor and/or flexor tendons.

Definition

- Thumb duplication may be a misnomer because it implies that there are two normal thumbs, whereas in fact, both thumbs are hypoplastic.

Aetiology

- Preaxial polydactyly is usually unilateral and sporadic.
- Not associated with syndromes except type VII. Type VII associations include Fanconi anaemia, Holt-Oram syndrome, Diamond-Blackfan syndrome, hypoplastic anaemia, imperforate anus, cleft palate and tibial defects.
- Postaxial polydactyly is commonly inherited (autosomal dominant) and is more common in African-American than white children. In black children, it is usually an isolated condition, but in whites, nearly 30 % have an internal organ disorder associated with it.

Pathoanatomy

- The pathoanatomy is dependent on the type of polydactyly. The nails, bones, joints, ligaments, muscles, tendons, nerves and blood vessels are split among the two digits.
- There can be hypoplasia or aplasia of any of the normal anatomic elements of a thumb.
- Both the radial and ulnar components have structures that must be preserved and reconstructed to provide a stable, mobile and functional thumb.
- In Wassel type II, the radial digit has the radial collateral ligament insertion, and the ulnar digit has the ulnar collateral ligament insertion of the interphalangeal (IP) joint.
- In Wassel type IV, the thenar muscles insert on the more radial digit, and the adductor pollicis inserts on the more ulnar digit.
- Pollex abductus is an abnormal connection between the extensor pollicis longus (EPL) and flexor pollicis longus (FPL) tendons, seen in approximately 20 % of hypoplastic and duplicated thumbs; presence of a pollex abductus is suggested by abduction of the affected digit and absence of IP joint creases.

Classification

Wassel classification of preaxial polydactyly (see Fig. 1)

Type I: bifid distal phalanx
Type II: at the interphalangeal joint
Type III: bifid proximal phalanx
Type IV: at the metacarpophalangeal joint (most common)
Type V: at the thumb metacarpal level

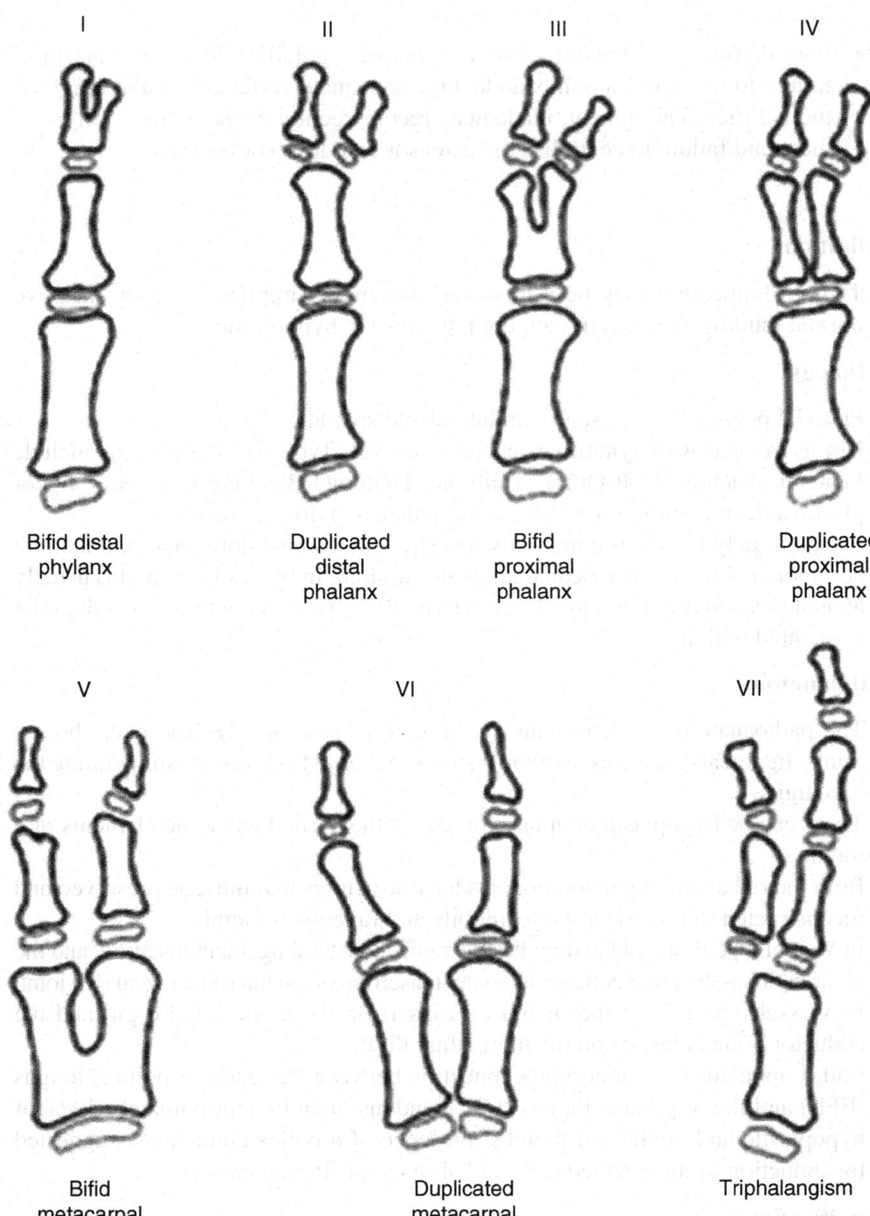

Fig. 1 The Wassel classification of preaxial polydactyly

Type VI: the CMC joint level
Type VII: triphalangeal thumb (two types, first one with an extra wedge-shaped ossicle called delta phalanx, other with a normal-sized additional phalanx)

- Stelling and Turek classification of postaxial polydactyly

  Type 1: duplication of soft parts only
  Type 2: partial duplication of the digit, including the osseous structures
  Type 3: complete duplication of the ray, including the metacarpal

Management

Goal of surgical correction in preaxial polydactyly is to construct a thumb that is at least 80 % the size of contralateral thumb size.

- Types I and II: Bilhaut-Cloquet procedure. This involves removing the central composite tissue segments from each thumb and combining the two into one. However, the Bilhaut-Cloquet procedure is technically difficult and often results in an aesthetically unpleasing thumb with physeal mismatch and articular incongruity.
- Another combination procedure is preferred involving ablation of the bony elements of the more underdeveloped (usually radial) thumb and reconstruction of the (radial) collateral ligament and, in Wassel type IV thumbs, transfer of the thenar muscles from the ablated proximal phalanx to the preserved (ulnar) proximal phalanx.
- Chondroplasty of the metacarpal head and/or corrective osteotomy of an abnormally shaped phalanx or metacarpal may need to be performed to restore the longitudinal alignment of the thumb.
- Adduction contracture of the first web space should be treated with Z-plasty to deepen the web space.
- Wassel types V and VI are rare and complex duplications requiring reattachment of the abductor tendons and reconstruction of the basal joint of the thumb.

  Treatment options for postaxial polydactyly include the following:

- Type 1, suture ligation of the pedicle is done. The digit will eventually become gangrenous and fall off. When performed in a newborn nursery, complications like infection, bleeding and incomplete removal have been noted, hence best avoided in such environment.
- Types II and III require formal reconstruction with reorganisation of any important collateral ligaments or muscles that attach to the ablated digit.

Complications

- Approximately 15–20 % of patients develop late deformity following surgery of preaxial polydactyly. Causes include failure to recognise a pollex abductus, inadequate correction of the longitudinal thumb alignment, inadequate reconstruction of the collateral ligament and failure to centralise the extensor and/or flexor tendons.

Bibliography

1. Light TR. Treatment of preaxial polydactyly. Hand Clin. 1992;8:161–75.
2. Marks T, Bayne L. Polydactyly of the thumb: abnormal anatomy and treatment. J Hand Surg Am. 1978;3:107.
3. Wassel H. The results of surgery for polydactyly of the thumb. Clin Orthop. 1969;64:175.

9 Macrodactyly

Ashok Johari, Ratna Maheshwari, and Shalin Maheshwari

- "Overgrowth" according to IFSSH classification
- Typically unilateral, involving radial digits
- Usually isolated, but may occur in the setting of neurofibromatosis, proteus syndrome, or Klippel-Trenaunay-Weber syndrome
- May be static or progressive, with asymmetric digital nerve involvement, and may result in radioulnar or flexion deformity
- Classification
  - Type I: macrodactyly and lipofibromatosis; most common type, associated with fibrofatty proliferation in the distribution of a digital or peripheral nerve, which is typically enlarged and tortuous
  - Type II: macrodactyly and neurofibromatosis
  - Type III: macrodactyly and hyperostosis
  - Type IV: macrodactyly and hemihypertrophy
- Surgical options
  - Include soft tissue debulking, epiphysiodesis of affected phalanges, bony and soft tissue reduction procedures and amputation
  - Individualised according to the anatomic distribution, degree of deformity and skeletal growth remaining

9.1 Brachydactyly

- Shortening of the metacarpal or fingers is often inherited as an autosomal trait or may be associated with a variety of conditions such as Poland, Holt-Oram, Cornelia de Lange or Silver syndromes. Rarely finger lengthening procedures are appropriate.
- *Finger lengthening* of up to 10 mm in single stage and 30 mm by gradual distraction may be achieved. Metacarpal lengthening improves pinch function in children with either transverse deficiency or constriction band syndromes. Finger lengthening improves appearance in children with brachydactyly. These lengthening procedures are rarely indicated.

Bibliography

1. Gallant GG, Bora FW. Congenital deformities of the upper extremity. JAAOS. 1994;4:162
2. Guidera KJ et al. Overgrowth management in Klippel-Trenaunay-Weber and Proteus syndromes. JPO. 1993;13:459.
3. Ogino T et al. Digital lengthening in congenital hand deformities. J Hand Surg. 1994;19B:120

10 Hypoplastic Thumb

Ashok Johari, Ratna Maheshwari, and Shalin Maheshwari

Take-Home Message

- The finding of a thumb deficiency in a neonate should prompt a thorough multiple-system examination for other malformations.
- Thumb hypoplasia includes a contracted first web space, unstable MCP joint, thenar weakness and interphalangeal joint stiffness or instability.
- Types 2 through 3A consider surgical reconstruction—first web deepening, MCP stabilisation and opponensplasty.
- Types 3B through 5 consider index pollicisation with or without ablation of thumb.

Aetiology

- Often bilateral; males and females equally affected.
- Universally seen in radial dysplasia.
- Associated conditions include Holt-Oram, TAR, Fanconi anaemia and VACTERL.

Pathoanatomy

In general, thumb hypoplasia includes the following pathologies:

- Contracted first web space
- Unstable MCP joint
- Thenar weakness
- Interphalangeal joint instability or weakness

Classification

Buck-Gramcko modification of Blauth classification

- Type 1: minor hypoplasia, thumb looks smaller than normal.
- Type 2: narrow first web space, laxity of the ulnar collateral ligament of the metacarpophalangeal joint and thenar muscle hypoplasia.

- Type 3: global thenar weakness and metacarpophalangeal joint collateral ligament instability, partial aplasia of the first metacarpal and extrinsic weakness.
  3A: as in the previous category, with proximal metacarpal and carpometacarpal joints present.
  3B: absent proximal metacarpal, with deficient carpometacarpal joint.
- Type 4: *pouce flottant* (floating thumb); no bony support.
- Type 5: total absence of thumb.

Management

Aims of treatment: Provide a thumb that can oppose and ensure that the thumb has stable, cosmetically acceptable appearance

- Type 1 deficiency—function is normal. No intervention is required.
- Types 2 to 3A deficiency—active opposition is absent. Abductor digiti minimi transfer or opponensplasty with flexor digitorum superficialis of the ring finger. Palmaris longus can be transferred as free graft. Ulnar collateral ligament has to be reconstructed. First web space deepening.
- Type 3B/4/5 deficiency—pollicisation of index finger is recommended for non-functional thumb. If normal index finger is not available for transfer, then microvascular toe transfer can be done. Pollicisation is generally performed between 6 and 18 months of age.
- Principles of pollicisation
  - Use of local skin flaps to reconstitute first web space
  - Bony reduction to recreate metacarpal and phalanges of pollex in appropriate position (120–140° pronation, 15° extension, 40° palmar abduction)
  - Transfer of index finger on neurovascular pedicles to new position
  - Tendon transfers (extensor digitorum communis [EDC] to abductor pollicis longus [APL], extensor indicis proprius [EIP] to EPL, first dorsal interosseous [DIO] to abductor pollicis brevis [APB], first volar interosseous [VIO] to adductor pollicis [AdP])

Complication

- The quality of the pollicised digit is dependent on the quality of the original index finger, in terms of tendon function and joint motion.
- Patients with thumb aplasia and radial dysplasia generally do more poorly, because the involved index finger has deficient musculature and camptodactyly.

Bibliography

1. Buck-Gramcko D. Pollicization of the index finger. Method and results in aplasia and hypoplasia of the thumb. J Bone Joint Surg Am. 1971;53(8):1605.
2. Manske PR, McCaroll Jr HR. Index finger pollicization for a congenitally absent or nonfunctioning thumb. J Hand Surg [Am]. 1985;10(5):606.
3. Tay SC, Moran SL, Shin AY, Cooney WP. The hypoplastic thumb. J Am Acad Orthop Surg. 2006;14:354–66.

11 Trigger Thumb

Ashok Johari, Ratna Maheshwari, and Shalin Maheshwari

Take-Home Message

- Abnormality of tendon sheath at A1 pulley, with constriction of flexor pollicis longus.
- Surgical release of constricting A1 pulley and flexor tendon sheath is the treatment of choice. This is indicated in infants without spontaneous resolution by 1 year of age and in older child presenting with a locked trigger thumb.

Definition Trigger thumb represents an abnormality of the flexor pollicis longus and its tendon sheath at the A1 pulley. There is a palpable mass, representing the flexor pollicis longus constriction at A1 pulley.

Aetiology

- Though initially defined as congenital, this condition is acquired in the first 2 years of life.
- Unlike adult trigger digits, this does not appear to be an inflammatory component.
- Trigger digits are seen with neurologic syndromes like trisomy 18 and mucopolysaccharidoses.
- There is no familial inheritance pattern.

Pathoanatomy

- The cause appears to be a size mismatch between flexor pollicis longus and A1 pulley leading to progressive constriction.
- If the trigger is long-standing, compensatory hyperextension of MCP joint develops to effectively bring the thumb out of the palm.
- Trigger digits are more often multiple and can be associated with central nervous system disorders and syndromes. The pathology appears to predominate at the decussation of flexor tendons under the A2 pulley, not A1 pulley alone. Triggering occurs when the flexor digitorum profundus passes through the chiasm of flexor digitorum superficialis.

Management

- In infants younger than 9 months of age, 30 % of trigger thumbs may resolve spontaneously. In infants older than 1 year of age, less than 10 % of trigger thumb resolves spontaneously.
- Benefit of splinting is limited.

- Surgical release of constricting A1 pulley and flexor tendon sheath is the treatment of choice. This is indicated in infants without spontaneous resolution by 1 year of age and in older child presenting with a locked trigger thumb.

Complication

- Care must be taken to avoid iatrogenic injury to the superficial digital neurovascular bundles.
- Oblique pulley needs to be preserved to prevent flexor tendon bowstringing.

Bibliography

1. Buchman M, Gibson T, McCallum D, et al. Transmission electron microscopic pathoanatomy of congenital trigger thumbs. J Pediatr Orthop. 1999;19:411.
2. Dinham JM, Meggit DF. Trigger thumbs in children. J Bone Joint Surg Br. 1974;56:153.
3. Rodgers WB, Waters PM. Incidence of trigger digits in newborns. J Hand Surg Am. 1994;19:35.
4. Slakey JB, Hennrikus WL. Acquired thumb flexion contracture in children. J Bone Joint Surg Br. 1996;78:481.
5. Tsuyuguchi Y, Toda K, Kawaii H. Splint therapy for trigger fingers in children. Arch Phys Med Rehabil. 1983;64:75.
6. Van Heest AE, House J, Krivit W, et al. Surgical treatment of carpal tunnel and trigger digits in children with mucopolysaccharide storage disorders. J Hand Surg Am. 1998;23:236.

12 Constriction Band

Ashok Johari, Ratna Maheshwari, and Shalin Maheshwari

Take-Home Message

- Amniotic band syndrome usually occurs distal to the wrist and typically involves the central digits.
- The anatomy is normal proximal to the constriction ring.

Definition

- Congenital constriction band syndrome, otherwise known as amniotic band syndrome, is a common cause of terminal congenital malformation of the limbs.
- The three main manifestations include acrosyndactyly, superficial or deep constriction bands involving a digit or extremity and intrauterine amputation.

Aetiology

- It is proposed to be sporadic, not hereditary.
- Commonly associated with other anomalies (e.g. clubfoot, cleft lip/palate, craniofacial defects).

Pathophysiology The theory behind the formation of constriction bands is that amniotic disruption releases strands of membrane that circumferentially wrap around the developing upper limb.

Evaluation

- The bands lie perpendicular to longitudinal axis of the affected digit/limb.
- More than 90 % occur distal to wrist. Central digits are more commonly affected with varying depths of constriction.
- If no amputation, secondary syndactyly or bony fusions may occur with proximal epithelialised sinus tracts.

Classification

Patterson 1961

- Simple constriction ring
- Deformity distal to ring (lymphedema)
- Fusion of distal parts
- Amputation

Treatment

- Type I: observation versus excision/release of constriction ring.
- Type II: excision of constriction ring with local flaps (Z-plasty).
- Type III: syndactyly release.
- Type IV: Function may be improved with reconstructive procedures, including bony lengthenings, web deepenings, "on top" plasties, nonvascularised toe phalanx transfers or free vascularised toe transfers.
- Clubfeet in neonates with constriction band can be treated with serial manipulation and casting, if there is no significant foot oedema or evidence of neurovascular compromise.

Complications

- The compressed neurovascular structures can be difficult to distinguish and may be inadvertently damaged.

Bibliography

1. Allington NJ, Jay Kumar S, Guille IT. Clubfeet associated with congenital constriction bands of ipsilateral lower extremity. J Pediatr Orthop. 1995;15:599.
2. Patterson TJS. Congenital ring constrictions. Br J Plast Surg. 1961;14:1.

13 Sprengel Shoulder and Klippel-Feil Anomaly

Ashok Johari, Ratna Maheshwari, and Shalin Maheshwari

Take-Home Message

- Beware of midline cutaneous defects such as hairy patch, sinus or haemangioma that may be harbingers of intraspinal anomalies such as diastematomyelia or diplomyelia.
- Surgery after 8 years in Sprengel shoulder is associated with highest risk of nerve impairment.
- Feil's triad in Klippel-Feil syndrome includes short neck, low posterior hairline and limited range of motion of neck.

Definition Congenital deformity of the scapula with inadequate descent of this bone from the cervical to the thoracic area during the third month of pregnancy is seen in Sprengel shoulder.

Aetiology

- The condition usually occurs sporadically, although a familial occurrence has been observed.
- The deformity is associated with other malformations in 75 % of cases, e.g. presence of cervical ribs, malformations of ribs, Klippel-Feil syndrome, scoliosis, intraspinal anomalies and some renal or pulmonary diseases.

Pathophysiology

- In 50 % of patients, a fibrous band, cartilaginous bar or omovertebral bone extends from the vertebral border of the superior scapular angle to posterior element of C4 to C7.
- Malrotation of scapula positions the acromion process as a fixed anatomic block to glenohumeral motion, especially abduction.
- Dysplasia of muscles about the shoulder girdle, especially the levator scapulae, rhomboideus major and minor and trapezius, may contribute to limited shoulder motion.
- Klippel-Feil anomaly is caused due to failure of segmentation of mesoderms of vertebrae during the 3rd–8th weeks of intrauterine life.

Radiography

- Elevated and rotated scapula.
- The omovertebral bone can be identified on axial views of the scapula.

- An associated Klippel-Feil syndrome will show osseous fusions of cervical spine at craniocervical junction and/ or subaxial level. Intervertebral disc spaces are narrowed or obliterated, with flattened or widened vertebral bodies.

Classification

Cavendish grading for Sprengel shoulder

- Grade 1: Very mild, the deformity is unobservable when patient is dressed, shoulder joint at same level.
- Grade 2: Mild with shoulder joints slightly unaligned. Prominence in the neck when patient is dressed.
- Grade 3: Moderate deformity with shoulder joint at higher level (2–5 cm) compared to opposite side.
- Grade 4: Severe with superior angle of scapula near the occiput and webbing may be present.

Feil classification (in Klippel-Feil anomaly)

Type 1: block fusion of all cervical and upper thoracic vertebrae
Type 2: fusion of one or two pairs of cervical vertebra
Type 3: cervical fusion in combination with lower thoracic or lumbar fusion

Treatment

- No treatment is necessary if deformity is mild.
- Generally surgery is done between the ages of 3 and 8 years. Clavicular osteotomy is recommended in older children to lessen the risk of brachial plexus impingement with scapular descent.
- Role of surgical treatment in Klippel-Feil anomaly is not clearly defined. In the presence of neurologic symptoms, decompression and fusion becomes mandatory.
- Surgical options for Sprengel shoulder include the following:
  - Green's procedure—involves extraperiosteal detachment of scapular insertion.
  - Woodward procedure—scapula is moved distally by detachment and reattachment of parascapular muscles at their origins on the spinous process.
  - The modified Woodward procedure includes resection of superior pole of scapula
  - Wilkinson and Campbell's vertical scapular osteotomy is reserved for older children.

Complications

- Surgery after 8 years is associated with highest risk of nerve impairment.

Bibliography

1. Carson WG, Lovell WW, Whitesides Jr TE. Congenital elevation of scapula. Surgical correction by the woodward procedure. J Bone Joint Surg Am. 1981;63:1199.
2. Greitemann B, Rondhuis JJ, Karbowski A. Treatment of congenital elevation of the scapula. 10 (2–18) year follow-up of 37 cases of Sprengel's deformity. Acta Orthop Scand. 1993;64(3):365–8.
3. Grogan DP, Stanley EA, Bobechko WP. The congenital undescended scapula. Surgical correction by the woodward procedure. J Bone Joint Surg Br. 1983;65:598.
4. Wilkinson JA, Campbell D. Scapular osteotomy for Sprengel's shoulder. J Bone Joint Surg Br. 1980;62-B:486.

Limb-Length Discrepancy

Ashok Johari, Ratna Maheshwari, and Shalin Maheshwari

Take-Home Message

- Limb equalization procedures must take into account the final projected LLD, not the LLD present at the time of surgery.
- Scanogram provides reliable measurements with minimal magnification; however, a full-length standing AP computed radiograph (teleoroentgenogram) is a more comprehensive assessment technique, with similar costs at less radiation exposure.
- A proximal fibular epiphysiodesis should be included with proximal tibial epiphysiodesis if more than 2–3 years of growth remain.
- Undercorrection of an LLD associated with paralysis facilitates the foot clearing the floor during the swing phase of gait and is especially important if the patient walks with a brace in which the knee is locked in extension.

Overview

- Differences between the lengths of the upper and/or lower arms and the upper and/or lower legs are called limb-length discrepancies (LLDs).
- Small (up to 2 cm) limb-length discrepancies (LLDs) are common, occurring in up to two thirds of the general population.

Secondary Problems from LLD

- *Gait problems*, such as limping, toe-walking, or rotation of the leg. A knee that is chronically hyperextended on the short side and flexed on the long side.

A. Johari, MD (✉) • R. Maheshwari, MD • S. Maheshwari, MD
Pediatric Orthopedics, Childrens' Orthopedic Centre, Mumbai, India
e-mail: drashokjohari@hotmail.com

C. Mauffrey, D.J. Hak (eds.), *Passport for the Orthopedic Boards and FRCS Examination*, DOI 10.1007/978-2-8178-0475-0_23

- The prevalence of back pain may be higher with large discrepancies (>2 cm), but the evidence is limited.
- During double-limb stance, the hip on the long side is relatively less covered by the acetabulum. Osteoarthritis is seen more commonly (84 % of the time) on the long-leg side.
- LLD increases the incidence of structural scoliosis to the short side. In up to one third of cases, the scoliosis is in a noncompensatory direction.

Etiology

- An injury, such as in a *fracture* that damages the cells responsible for growth of the bone, while the corresponding bone on the other leg grows normally. Some fractures can also lead to overgrowth of the bone during the healing process.
- Diseases of the bone, such as *osteomyelitis*, can injure the growth plate, so that a discrepancy occurs gradually over time.
- Congenital conditions
- Bone tumors and treatments designed to eradicate them.
- Functional leg-length discrepancy can also result from congenital problems that alter alignment of the hips, such as coxa vara and *developmental dislocation of the hip*.
- Neuromuscular problems, such as *cerebral palsy*, which causes problems with alignment and posture, can also lead to a functional discrepancy.

Evaluation

- Discrepancy can be measured by placing blocks under the short leg to level the pelvis.
- Clinical methods such as the use of a tape measure and standing blocks were noted as useful screening tools, but not as accurate as imaging modalities.
- Hip, knee, and ankle contractures will affect the apparent limb length and must be ruled out. A hip adduction contracture causes an apparent shortening of the adducted side.
- Orthoroentgenogram utilizes three radiographic exposures centered over the hip, knee, and ankle joints in order to reduce magnification error. A single large cassette is used.
- Scanogam utilizes three radiographic exposures over the hip, knee, and ankle. Standard length cassette is moved over three exposures.
- A teleoroentgenogram consists of single long cassette placed behind patient, while x-ray beam is centered over the knee joint. This is subjected to magnification error but has less radiation exposure and opportunity to comprehensively assess the entire extremity for underlying etiology and deformity analysis.
- Scanogram provides reliable measurements with minimal magnification; however, a full-length standing AP computed radiograph (teleoroentgenogram) is a more comprehensive assessment technique, with similar costs at less radiation exposure.
- Up to 6 % of patients with LLD from hemihypertrophy develop embryonal cancers (e.g., Wilms tumor). Routine abdominal ultrasounds are recommended until age 6 years.

Prediction Methods

- Rule of thumb method
  - Assumes growth ends at age 14 years for girls and 16 years for boys
  - Estimates the annual contribution to leg length of each physis near skeletal maturity (during the last 4 years of growth)
    - Proximal femoral physis—4 mm
    - Distal femoral physis—10 mm
    - Proximal tibial physis—6 mm
    - Distal tibial physis—5 mm
- Growth remaining method—LLD prediction based on Green and Anderson tables of extremity length for a given age.
- Moseley straight line graph method
  - This method improves the accuracy of Green and Anderson prediction by reformatting the data in graph form.
  - It accounts for differences between skeletal age and chronologic age.
  - It minimizes errors of arithmetic or interpretation by averaging serial measurements.
- Multiplier method
  - This method predicts final limb length by multiplying the current discrepancy by a sex- and age-specific factor. It is most accurate for discrepancies that are constantly proportional (e.g., congenital).

Classification

- In congenital conditions, the absolute discrepancy increases, but the relative percentage remains constant (e.g., a short limb that is 70 % of the long side at birth will be 70 % of the long side at maturity).
- Children with paralysis usually have shortening of the more severely affected side.
- Static discrepancies (e.g., a malunion of the femur in a shortened position) must be differentiated from progressive discrepancies (e.g., physeal growth arrest).

Treatment It is sometimes advisable to correct coexisting deformities before correcting leg-length discrepancy, because the correction of some deformities changes the treatment goal

- Physeal bar excision
  - Physeal bars following trauma tend to be more discrete (and more amenable to excision) than are bars resulting from infection or ischemia.
  - Bridge resection is indicated if the bony bridge involves <50 % of the physis in patients with at least 2 years of growth remaining.

- Discrepancy correction
  - General guidelines expressed in terms of the magnitude of the predicted discrepancy can be used to choose from among the major treatment categories:

    0–2 cm: No treatment
    2–6 cm: Shoe lift, epiphysiodesis, shortening
    6–20 cm: Lengthening, which may or may not be combined with other procedures
    >20 cm: Prosthetic fitting

  - Nonsurgical—Any size discrepancy can be corrected with a shoe lift, but shoe lifts >5 cm are poorly tolerated because they are heavy and may result in subtalar and ankle inversion injuries.
  - Surgical
    - General principles
      - The surgical correction must address the anticipated final LLD, not just the current discrepancy.
      - In paralytic conditions (such as myelodysplasia, cerebral palsy, or polio), it is often best to leave the LLD undercorrected to facilitate foot clearance of the weak leg. This is especially important if the patient walks with a brace that locks the knee in extension.
    - Shortening techniques
      - Epiphysiodesis is the treatment of choice for discrepancies of 2–5 cm because of the very low complication rate. If proximal tibial epiphysiodesis is performed, concomitant proximal fibular epiphysiodesis should also be performed if more than 2–3 years of growth remain (to prevent proximal fibular overgrowth and prominence).
      - Acute osseous shortening is typically used for discrepancies of 2–5 cm after skeletal maturity.
    - Lengthening techniques
      - Methods
        - Uniplanar or multiplanar external fixation
        - External fixation with intramedullary nail
        - Intramedullary distraction
      - Pearls
        - Lengthen at metaphyseal level whenever possible.
        - Ilizarov recommended corticotomy, a technique in which the cortex is cut but care is taken that the medullary contents are not disturbed.
        - Delay the onset of distraction by 5–7 days after the corticotomy is performed.

- Lengthen at a rate of 1 mm/day (0.25 mm four times/day).
- Limit the lengthening goal to <20 % of the individual bone length per lengthening period.

Complications

- Incomplete arrest or angular deformity can result from either open or percutaneous epiphysiodesis techniques.
- Common complications of lengthening include pin-site infection, pin or wire failure, regenerate deformity or fracture, delayed union, premature cessation of lengthening, and joint subluxation/dislocation.

Bibliography

1. Anderson M, Green W, Messner M. Growth and predictions of growth in the lower extremities. J Bone Joint Surg. 1963;45-A:1.
2. Paley D, Bhave A, Herzenberg J, et al. Multiplier method for predicting limb-length discrepancies. J Bone Joint Surg. 2000;59A:1432–46.
3. Sabharwal S, Kumar A. Methods for assessing leg length discrepancy. Clin Orthop Relat Res. 2008;466(12):2910–22.

Paediatric Hip Conditions

Ashok Johari, Ratna Maheshwari, and Shalin Maheshwari

1 Developmental Dysplasia of the Hip

Ashok Johari, Ratna Maheshwari, and Shalin Maheshwari

Take-Home Message

- Ultrasound is a better test than plain radiographs in the first 4–6 months of life.
- Routine ultrasound screening should be performed for infants with risk factors for the condition. Because of the poor specificity of ultrasonography in children younger than 1 month, hip ultrasonography should be deferred until after 1 month of life.
- Pavlik harness treatment should be discontinued if the dislocated hip does not relocate within 3–4 weeks, to avoid Pavlik harness disease.
- Excessive hip flexion in the Pavlik harness results in an increased risk of femoral nerve palsy. Excessive hip abduction in the Pavlik harness results in an increased risk of osteonecrosis of the femoral head.
- Hip abduction does not become limited in DDH until approximately 6 months of age.

Definition

- Developmental dysplasia of the hip (DDH) refers to the complete spectrum of pathologic conditions involving the developing hip, ranging from acetabular dysplasia to hip subluxation to irreducible hip dislocation.

A. Johari, MD (✉) • R. Maheshwari, MD • S. Maheshwari, MD
Pediatric Orthopedics, Childrens' Orthopedic Centre, Mumbai, India
e-mail: drashokjohari@hotmail.com

C. Mauffrey, D.J. Hak (eds.), *Passport for the Orthopedic Boards and FRCS Examination*, DOI 10.1007/978-2-8178-0475-0_24

- Teratologic dislocation of the hip occurs in utero and is irreducible on neonatal examination. This condition always accompanies other congenital anomalies or neuromuscular conditions, most frequently arthrogryposis and myelomeningocele.

Aetiology

- Multifactorial—genetic, hormonal and mechanical. Maternal hormone like relaxin may play a role.
- It is more common in females with the left hip more commonly involved than the right hip.
- There is an increased incidence in breech deliveries. It is associated with oligohydramnios, torticollis, talipes calcaneovalgus and metatarsus adductus (intrauterine packaging disorder).
- Primary acetabular dysplasia may run in families.

Pathoanatomy

- The femoral head and neck are anteverted. The head is pulled proximally and laterally by abductors.
- Hip joint fills by fibrofatty tissue (pulvinar).
- Acetabular labrum becomes inverted and enlarged. Limbus blocks reduction of the femoral head.
- Acetabulum becomes dysplastic.
- Ligamentum teres becomes lengthened and redundant. Transverse acetabular ligament is pulled superiorly.
- Capsule becomes expanded.
- Muscles crossing the hip joint—hamstring, hip adductors and psoas—become shortened and contracted and block reduction.

Evaluation

- Clinical presentation—The clinical presentation varies with age.
  - In the neonatal period, instability of the hip is the key clinical finding.
  - Hip clicks are nonspecific physical findings.
  - Because asymmetric skin folds are common in children with normal hips, children with such asymmetry have a high rate of false positives.
  - In infants older than 6 months, limitation of motion and apparent limb shortening are common findings.
  - In toddlers, in addition to restricted motion and limb-length inequalities, a limp or waddling gait may be appreciated.
  - In adolescents, all the above findings may be present in addition to fatigue and pain in the hip, thigh or knee.

- Physical examination—Accuracy of the physical examination requires that the child be relaxed.
  - The Galeazzi (or Allis) test is positive only in unilateral severe subluxations or dislocations. In the Galeazzi test, the hips are flexed to 90°; the test is positive if one knee (the involved side) is lower than the other.

Table 1 Graf classification

Types	Alpha angle	Beta angle	Description	Treatment
1	>60	<55	Normal	None
2	43–59	55–77	Physiological in child <3 months, delayed ossification in child >3 months	?
3	<43	>77	Lateralization	Pavlik harness
4	Unmeasurable		Dislocated and labrum interposing between the head and acetabulum	Pavlik harness/closed or open reduction

- The Barlow test is performed by applying a posterolateral force to the extremity with the hip in a flexed and adducted position. The test is positive if the hip subluxates or even dislocates.
- The Ortolani test is performed by abducting and lifting the proximal femur anteriorly. The test is positive if the dislocated hip is reducible.
- Range of motion (ROM) testing of the hip is important, with decrease in abduction as the most sensitive test for DDH. ROM however will be normal in children younger than 6 months because contractures will not yet have developed.

• Diagnostic tests

- Ultrasonography—In the first 4 months of life, plain radiographic evaluation is unreliable because the femoral epiphysis has not yet ossified. Ultrasonography of the infant hip (before the appearance of the proximal femoral ossific centre) is useful in confirming a diagnosis of DDH and also in documenting reducibility and stability of the hip in an infant undergoing treatment with a Pavlik harness or brace.

  Graf classification (Table 1)—after taking a midcoronal section, alpha angle is measured between the line of the ilium and bony acetabulum. The beta angle is the angle between the line of the ilium and cartilaginous acetabular roof.
- Radiology

  Radiographic lines in DDH (Fig. 1)

  • The Hilgenreiner line is a line drawn horizontally through each triradiate cartilage of the pelvis.
  • The Perkin line is drawn perpendicular to the Hilgenreiner line at the lateral edge of the acetabulum.
  • The Shenton line is a continuous arch drawn along the medial border of the femoral neck and superior border of the obturator foramen.
  • The acetabular index is the angle formed by an oblique line (through the outer edge of the acetabulum and triradiate cartilage) and the Hilgenreiner line.

    - In the newborn, a normal value averages 27.5°.
    - By 24 months of age, the acetabular index decreases to 21°.

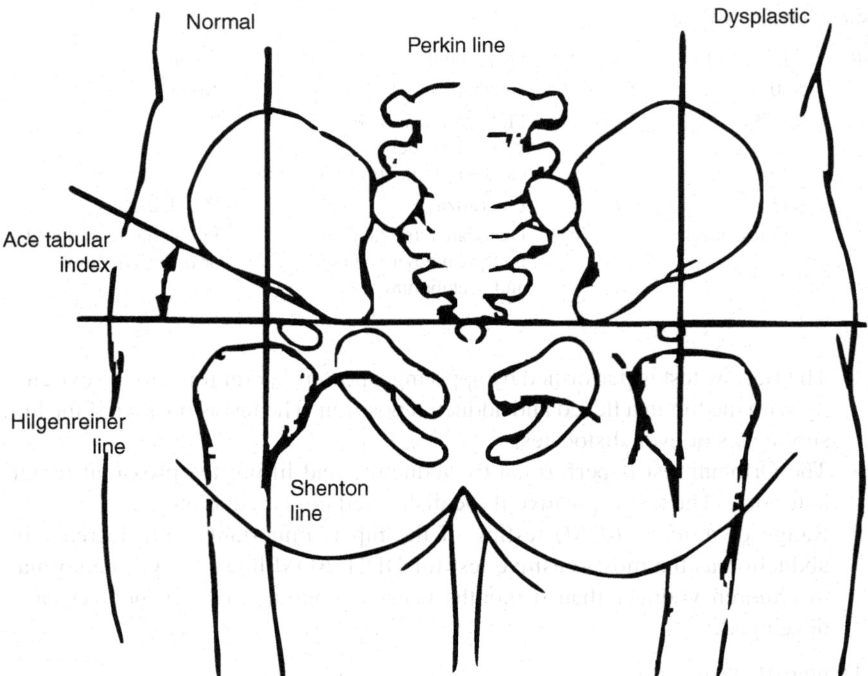

Fig. 1 Radiographic lines in DDH. Hilgenreiner line is drawn through the triradiate cartilages. The Perkin line is drawn perpendicular to the Hilgenreiner line at the margin of the bony acetabulum. The Shenton line curves along the femoral metaphysis and connects smoothly to the inner margin of the pubis. The acetabular index is the angle between a line drawn along the margin of the acetabulum and the Hilgenreiner line. It averages 27.5° in normal newborn and decreases with age

- The centre–edge angle of Wiberg is the angle formed by a vertical line through the centre of the femoral head and perpendicular to the Hilgenreiner line and an oblique line through the outer edge of the acetabulum and centre of the femoral head. The centre–edge angle is reliable only in patients older than 5 years. A centre–edge angle <20° is considered abnormal.

– Arthrography of the hip—Useful in confirming the acceptability of a closed reduction and in diagnosing the blocks to reduction, such as capsular narrowing and labral hypertrophy.
– CT—The standard for confirming acceptable reduction for a patient in a spica cast following closed or open procedures.
– Magnetic resonance imaging:
  - MRI can also be used to confirm acceptable reduction of the hip following closed or open procedures.
  - MRI can also be useful in an older patient with suspected labral pathology.

Management

Based on the age of the child, stability of the hip (unstable versus dislocated hip) and severity of acetabular dysplasia. The aim of management is to obtain concentric, congruent and stable hips.

- Dysplastic hip in neonate through 6 months of age
  - In a child with an abnormal α angle on ultrasound or with an unstable hip (subluxatable hip on examination), initial treatment usually includes a Pavlik harness.
    - Proper positioning of the Pavlik harness is critical.
      - The hips should be flexed to 100° with mild abduction (two to three finger breadths between knees when knees are flexed and adducted).
      - Excessive flexion should be avoided to lower the risk of femoral nerve palsy.
      - Excessive abduction should be avoided to lower the risk of osteonecrosis; osteonecrosis can occur in both the normal and dysplastic hip.
    - The child can be weaned from the Pavlik harness over a 3- to 4-week period when ultrasound parameters become normal.
    - Success rates for Pavlik harness treatment in this setting have been reported at >90 %.
    - The recurrence rate is 10 %; therefore, follow-up evaluation until maturity is necessary.
  - In a relatively large child or in a child older than age 6 months with a dysplastic hip or with hip subluxation, a fixed abduction orthosis or spica casting is an option. Pavlik harness treatment is ineffective in this setting because the child generally "overpowers" the brace.
- Dislocated hip in neonate through 6 months of age
  - If the hip is Ortolani positive, Pavlik harness treatment is initiated.
    - Frequent (every 1–2 weeks) re-examination (clinical plus ultrasound) is necessary to ensure that the hip is reduced.
    - Once the hip becomes stable, treatment is the same as the protocol described above for treatment of dysplastic hip.
    - Success rate (i.e. the hip becomes reduced) is reported to be 85 %.
    - The risk of osteonecrosis is low (<5 %), especially if treatment is initiated early (i.e. in the first 3 months of life).
  - If the hip is Ortolani negative, initial treatment still includes a Pavlik harness. If reduction is not achieved by 3–4 weeks (confirmed by ultrasound), however, Pavlik harness treatment is abandoned, and closed reduction is necessary.
    - Pavlik harness treatment should be discontinued if the dislocated hip does not relocate within 3–4 weeks, to avoid Pavlik harness disease.

    - In Pavlik harness disease, the femoral head sits up against the edge of the acetabulum and worsens the acetabular dysplasia, particularly the postero-lateral rim.

- Dislocated hip in children 6–18 months of age
  - Closed reduction is the preferred method of treatment in children age 18 months or younger.
  - Secondary femoral or acetabular procedures are rarely necessary in this age group.
  - The evidence for preliminary traction is equivocal. Given this and the possible complications of skin slough and leg ischaemia, most centres have abandoned preliminary traction.
  - Closed reduction is performed under general anaesthesia.
    - Adductor tenotomy frequently is necessary.
    - Hip arthrography is used intraoperatively to confirm adequacy of reduction.
    - There should be <5 mm of medial contrast pooling between the femoral head and acetabulum.
    - The safe and stable zones for abduction/adduction, flexion/extension and internal/external rotation should be established.
    - A spica cast is applied with the hip maintained in the "human position" (hip flexion of 90–100° and abduction). Hip abduction should be <60° to minimize the risk of osteonecrosis.
    - The reduction of the hip in the cast must be confirmed.
      - Presently, CT is the standard.
      - MRI is used in some centres to confirm adequacy of reduction of the hip.
    - Cast immobilization is continued for 3–4 months.
      - Cast change is sometimes necessary.
      - Removable abduction brace is used afterwards until the acetabulum normalizes.

- Dislocated hip in children >18 months of age
  - Open reduction is the preferred treatment.
    - Unilateral dislocation: Surgical treatment is generally indicated in children up to 8 years of age with a unilateral dislocation. After 8 years of age, the risks of surgery are felt to outweigh the benefits.
    - Bilateral dislocation: The upper age limit for surgical treatment in these children is typically 5–6 years.
  - Femoral shortening is indicated in children with significantly high-riding dislocations.
    - This is necessary in most, but not all, children ≥2 years of age.
    - Pelvic osteotomy is needed for significant acetabular dysplasia (typical in children >18–24 months old). If a pelvic osteotomy is performed in this

age group at the time of initial surgery, the rate of reoperation is reduced significantly.

- Open reduction
  - Open reduction is indicated if concentric closed reduction cannot be achieved or when excessive abduction (>60°) is required to maintain reduction.
  - The goal of open reduction is to remove the obstacles to reduction and/or safely increase its stability.
    - Impediments to congruent reduction are the iliopsoas, hip adductors, capsule, ligamentum teres, pulvinar and transverse acetabular ligament. An infolded labrum may be an impediment in some cases.
    The most commonly used approaches are anterior, anteromedial and medial.
- Secondary procedures
  - Secondary femoral and/or pelvic procedures are frequently necessary in children older than 2 years of age to achieve and maintain concentric reduction and minimize the risk of osteonecrosis.
  - Femoral osteotomy
    - Femoral osteotomy provides shortening (to decrease pressure on the femoral head, thereby minimizing the risk of osteonecrosis), derotation (external rotation to address the abnormally high femoral anteversion in DDH) and varus.
    - Avoid excessive varus, because the greater trochanter can impinge against the acetabulum and prevent concentric reduction.
  - Pelvic osteotomy
    - Indications for pelvic osteotomy include persistent acetabular dysplasia and hip instability.
    - There is considerable variability in clinical practice with regard to pelvic osteotomy in children >2 years of age.
    - The two general types of pelvic osteotomy are reconstructive and salvage:
      - Reconstructive osteotomies redirect or reshape the roof of the acetabulum with its normal hyaline cartilage into a more appropriate weight-bearing position. A prerequisite to a reconstructive pelvic osteotomy is a hip that can be reduced concentrically and congruently. The hip must also have near-normal ROM. Redirectional osteotomies include single innominate (Salter), triple innominate (Steel) and peri-acetabular (Ganz). Redirectional osteotomies involve complete cuts through various pelvic bones, and those that cut all three pelvic bones provide the ability to obtain greater coverage. Reshaping osteotomies involve incomplete cuts, and hinge on different aspects of triradiate cartilage can decrease volume. It must be done in patients with open triradiate cartilage. These include Dega and Pemberton osteotomies.

– Salvage procedures are typically indicated in adolescents with severe dysplasia in whom acetabular deficiency precludes the use of a redirectional osteotomy. In salvage procedures, weight-bearing coverage is increased by using the joint capsule as an interposition between the femoral head and bone above it. The intent of these osteotomies is to reduce point loading at the edge of the acetabulum. These osteotomies rely on fibrocartilaginous metaplasia of the interposed joint capsule to provide an increased articulating surface. Salvage osteotomies include Chiari and shelf osteotomies.

Complications

- Pavlik harness treatment should be discontinued if the dislocated hip does not relocate within 3–4 weeks, to avoid Pavlik harness disease.
- Excessive hip flexion in the Pavlik harness results in an increased risk of femoral nerve palsy. Excessive hip abduction in the Pavlik harness results in an increased risk of osteonecrosis of the femoral head.

Bibliography

1. Gillingham BL, Sanchez AA, Wenger DR. Pelvic osteotomies for the treatment of hip dysplasia in children and young adults. J Am Acad Orthop Surg. 1999;7:325–37.
2. Staheli LT. Surgical management of acetabular dysplasia. Clin Orthop Relat Res. 1991;264:111–21.
3. Vitale MG, Skaggs DL. Developmental dysplasia of the hip from six months to four years of age. J Am Acad Orthop Surg. 2001;9:401–11.
4. Weinstein SL, Mubarak SJ, Wenger DR. Developmental hip dysplasia and dislocation: Part I. J Bone Joint Surg Am. 2003a;85:1824–32.
5. Weinstein SL, Mubarak SJ, Wenger DR. Developmental hip dysplasia and dislocation: Part II. J Bone Joint Surg Am. 2003b;85:2024–35.
6. Wientroub S, Grill F. Ultrasonography in developmental dysplasia of the hip. J Bone Joint Surg Am. 2000;82:1004–18.

2 Perthes Disease

Ashok Johari, Ratna Maheshwari, and Shalin Maheshwari

Take-Home Message

- The disease more commonly affects boys than girls (4:1–5:1).
- The hips are involved bilaterally in 10–12 % of cases.
- The Herring classification is the most reliable classification scheme and is related to prognosis.
- The older the child, the poorer is the prognosis.
- The most important factor that influences the outcome in Perthes' disease is extrusion of the epiphysis.

Definition
Perthes' disease is a self-limiting form of osteochondrosis of the capital femoral epiphysis of unknown aetiology that develops in children commonly between the ages of 5 and 12 years.

Aetiology

The exact aetiology of LCPD is unknown.
Risk factors: Family history is positive in 1.6–20 % of cases.
LCPD is associated with attention-deficit/hyperactivity disorder (33 %).
Patients are commonly skeletally immature, with bone age delayed in 89 % of cases.

Pathophysiology

- Current theories propose that a disruption of the vascularity of the capital femoral epiphysis occurs, resulting in necrosis and subsequent revascularization.
  - Deficient vascularity may be due to interruption of the blood supply to the femoral head.
  - The vascularity of the capital femoral epiphysis may also be threatened by thrombophilia and/or various coagulopathies (protein C and S deficiency, activated protein C resistance).
    - Thrombophilia has been reported to be a possible causative factor in 50 % of children with LCPD.
    - As many as 75 % of patients with LCPD will have a coagulopathy.
    - The capital epiphysis and physis are abnormal histologically, with disorganized cartilaginous areas of hypercellularity and fibrillation.

Evaluation
Onset is insidious, and children with LCPD will commonly have a limp and pain in the groin, hip, thigh or knee regions.

- Examination of the child with LCPD may reveal an abnormal gait (antalgic and/or Trendelenburg).
- ROM testing will often reveal decreased abduction and internal rotation. Hip flexion contractures are seen rarely.

Radiology

- Standard AP and frog-leg lateral views of the pelvis are critical in making the initial diagnosis and assessing the subsequent clinical course.
- LCPD typically proceeds through four radiographic stages.
  - Initial stage—Early radiographic findings are a sclerotic, smaller proximal femoral ossific nucleus (due to failure of the epiphysis to increase in size) and widened medial clear space (distance between the teardrop and femoral head).
  - Fragmentation stage—Segmental collapse (resorption) of the capital femoral epiphysis follows, with increased density of the epiphysis.
  - Reossification or reparative stage—Necrotic bone is resorbed with subsequent reossification of the capital femoral epiphysis.
  - Remodeling stage—Remodeling begins when the capital femoral epiphysis is completely reossified.

Classification

These stages are those of avascularity (stage I), fragmentation (stage II), regeneration (stage III) and complete healing (stage IV). The first three stages of the disease can be further subdivided into early (substage a) and late (substage b) parts of each respective stage:

- The Herring (lateral pillar) (Fig. 2) classification is based on the height of the lateral pillar of the capital epiphysis on AP view of the pelvis:
  - Group A—No involvement of the lateral pillar, with no density changes and no loss of height of the lateral pillar.
  - Group B—More than 50 % of the lateral pillar height is maintained.
  - Group C—Less than 50 % of the lateral pillar height is maintained.
  - B/C border group—This group has been added more recently to increase the consistency of readings and to increase prognostic accuracy of the lateral pillar classification. In this group, the lateral pillar is narrow (2–3 mm wide) or poorly ossified, or exactly 50 % of lateral pillar height is maintained.
  - The Herring classification is the most reliable classification scheme and is related to prognosis. Its limitation is that the final classification cannot be determined at the time of initial presentation.
- The Catterall classification is based on the amount of epiphyseal involvement. Although commonly used in the past, it has more recently been criticized for its poor interobserver reliability.
  - Group I—Involvement is limited to the anterior part of the capital epiphysis.
  - Group II—The anterior and central parts of the capital epiphysis are involved.
  - Group III—Most of the capital epiphysis is involved, with sparing of the medial and lateral parts of the epiphysis.
  - Group IV—The entire epiphysis is involved.
  - Catterall also described four at-risk signs, which indicate a more severe disease course.
    - Gage sign (radiolucency in the shape of a V in the lateral portion of the epiphysis)
    - Calcification lateral to the epiphysis
    - Lateral subluxation of the femoral head
    - A horizontal physis

Treatment

The older the child, the poorer is the prognosis. Irreversible deformation of the femoral head occurs either by the late fragmentation stage (stage IIb) or in the early stage of regeneration (stage IIIa), and containment should be achieved before the disease progresses to this stage. The most important factor that influences the outcome in Perthes' disease is extrusion of the epiphysis. Extrusion occurs almost invariably in children who are over the age of 7 years at the onset of the disease. Containment is indicated in children younger than 7 years in stage 1 or 2 of disease only if epiphyseal extrusion is present. Extrusion of the epiphysis will occur sooner or later in these older children, and since the results of surgery early in the

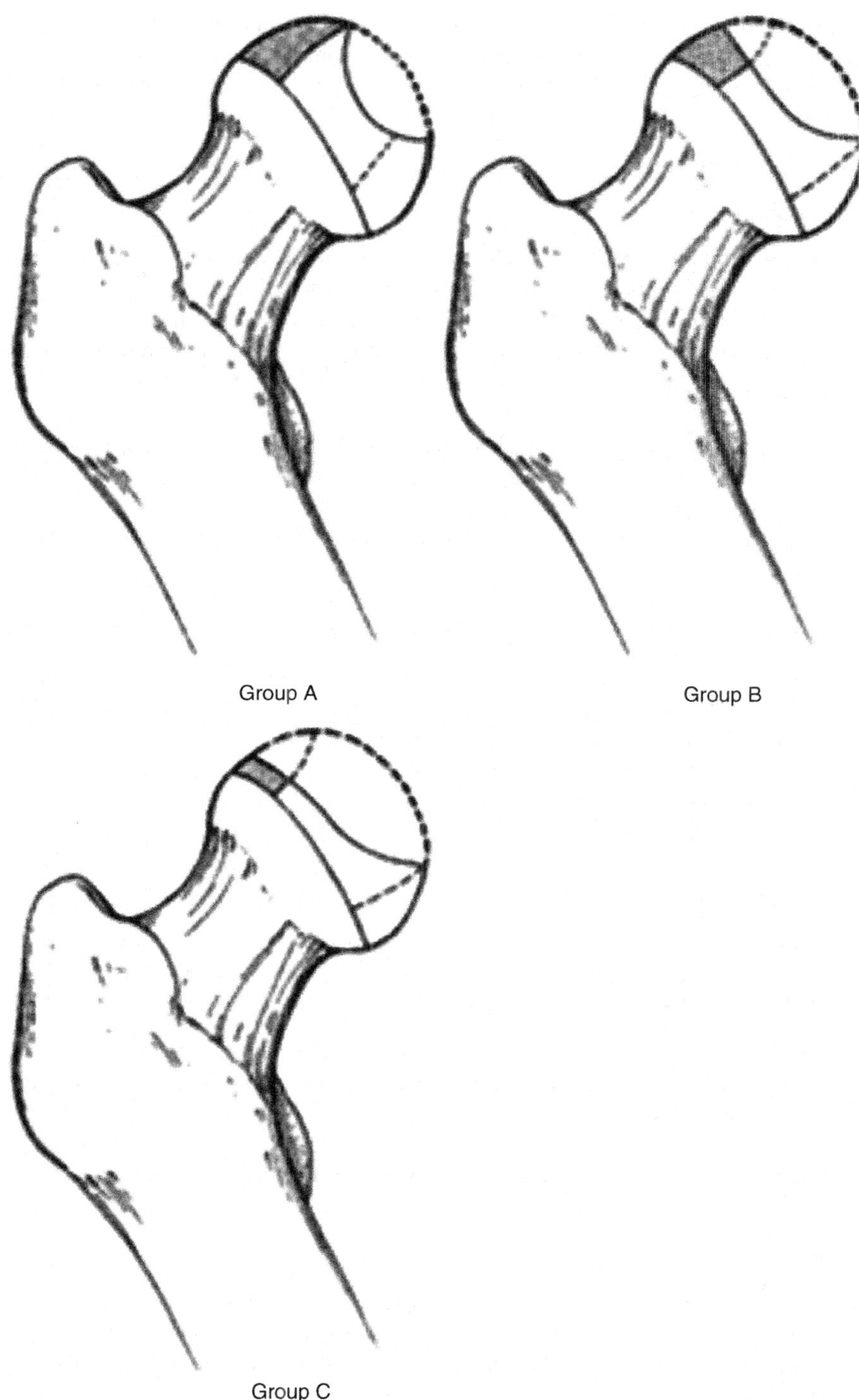

Fig. 2 Herring classification

course of the disease (in stages Ia, Ib or IIa) are distinctly superior to the results of surgery later in the disease, containment is recommended even before there is any demonstrable extrusion in children over the age of 7 years at the onset of symptoms.

- Containment treatment
  - Nonsurgical
    - Containment may be achieved by nonsurgical means, specifically by casting or bracing in an abducted and internally rotated position.
    - Petrie casts and a variety of abduction orthoses have been used.
    - The long-term benefit of casting and bracing has been called into question.
  - Surgical
    - Several surgical methods (described below) have been recommended to preserve containment. The results of these methods are comparable.
    - For these methods to be effective, the hips must be "containable", i.e. relatively full ROM with congruency between the femoral head and acetabulum.
    - Surgical containment may be approached from the femoral side, the acetabular side or both sides of the hip joint, according to surgeon's preference.
      - On the femoral side, a proximal femoral varus osteotomy is an option.
      - On the acetabular side, a pelvic osteotomy (Salter, triple innominate, Dega or Pemberton) may be performed.
      - A shelf arthroplasty can also be performed to prevent subluxation and lateral overgrowth of the capital epiphysis.
      - An arthrodiastasis (hip distraction) for 4–5 months has also been advocated in some centres, although this is more complicated and cumbersome for the patient.
- Once the hip is no longer containable, or for patients presenting late with deformity, treatment strategy focuses on salvage procedures, and the goals of treatment are relief of symptoms and restoration of stability.
  - These patients are at risk for hinge abduction, i.e. lateral extrusion of the femoral head resulting in the femoral head impinging on the edge of the acetabulum with abduction.
  - An abduction–extension proximal femoral osteotomy should be considered.
  - Pelvic osteotomy procedures such as a Chiari osteotomy and shelf arthroplasty may be beneficial.

Complications

- The wide range of complications includes femoral head deformity, premature physeal arrest patterns, osteochondritis dissecans, labral injury and late arthritis.
- The most important prognostic factors are the shape of the femoral head and its congruency at skeletal maturity and patient age at onset of disease. Stulberg correlated worse long-term outcomes to greater deformities in the femoral head at maturity.

- Long-term follow-up studies indicate that most patients with LCPD do well until the fifth or sixth decade of life, at which time degenerative changes in the hip joint are common.

Bibliography

1. Joseph B, Nair NS, Rao NLK, Mulpuri K, Varghese G. Optimal timing for containment surgery for Perthes' disease. J Pediatr Orthop. 2003;23:601–6.
2. Joseph B, Varghese G, Mulpuri K, Rao NLK, Nair NS. The natural evolution of Perthes' disease: a study of 610 children under 12 years of age at disease onset. J Pediatr Orthop. 2003;23:590–600.
3. Muirhead-Allwood W, Catterall A. The treatment of Perthes' disease: the results of a trial of management. J Bone Joint Surg Br. 1982;64:282–5.
4. Stulberg SD, Cooperman DR, Wallensten R. The natural history of Legg-Calve-Perthes' disease. J Bone Joint Surg Am. 1981;63:1095–108.

3 Slipped Capital Femoral Epiphysis

Ashok Johari, Ratna Maheshwari, and Shalin Maheshwari

Take-Home Message
- ROM testing may reveal obligate external rotation, i.e. external rotation of the hip as the hip is brought into flexion.
- Forceful manipulation is never indicated because it is associated with an increased risk of complications, including osteonecrosis.
- In situ fixation involves placement of a single-cannulated screw in the centre of the epiphysis and gives excellent results in stopping SCFE progression with minimal risk of chondrolysis.

Definition

The term SCFE is a misnomer because the epiphysis is held in the acetabulum by the ligamentum teres. The slippage results in a 3-dimensional deformity with the metaphysis displaced on the epiphysis in varus in the coronal plane, in extension in the sagittal plane and in external rotation in the axial plane.

Aetiology

- The precise aetiology is unknown. It can occur without any obvious underlying aetiology (idiopathic).
- It is slightly more common in boys than girls and tends to occur in children who are obese (>95th percentile weight for age, or BMI >25 kg/m^2).
- Conditions that weaken the physis include endocrinopathies such as hypothyroidism, panhypopituitarism, growth hormone abnormalities, hypogonadism and

hyper- or hypoparathyroidism; systemic diseases such as renal osteodystrophy; and a history of previous radiation therapy to the femoral head region.

- Decreased femoral anteversion and decreased femoral neck–shaft angle are also associated with SCFE.

Pathophysiology

- The physis is abnormally widened with irregular organization. The slip occurs through the proliferative and hypertropic zones of the physis.
- In general, SCFE is thought to be the result of mechanical insufficiency of the proximal femoral physis to resist load. This can occur because of either physiologic loads across an abnormally weak physis or abnormally high loads across a normal physis.
- The natural history is one of gradual increase in the SCFE as time passes and, as the severity of the SCFE increases, so does the incidence of degenerative hip disease later in life.

Radiology

- Plain radiographs—standard AP and frog-leg lateral views of the pelvis are recommended.

  - The Klein line, a line tangential to the superior border of the femoral neck on the AP view, intersects the proximal femoral epiphysis in a normal hip. The Klein line may fail to intersect the proximal femoral epiphysis in a hip involved with SCFE or will be asymmetric in the two hips.
  - The metaphyseal blanch sign—superimposition of the posteriorly displaced epiphysis on the femoral neck (seen on AP view).

Classification

- The Loder classification is the most widely used classification and is based on SCFE stability. The value of the Loder classification is its superior ability to predict osteonecrosis.

  - The SCFE is stable if the patient is able to weight bear on the involved extremity (with or without crutches).
  - The SCFE is unstable if the patient is unable to weight bear on the involved extremity.

- The traditional classification is temporal and based on duration of symptoms but has largely been replaced by the Loder classification because of the superior prognostic value of the latter.

  - The SCFE is chronic when symptoms have been present for >3 weeks.
  - The SCFE is acute when symptoms have been present for <3 weeks.
  - The SCFE is acute on chronic when there is an acute exacerbation of symptoms following a prodrome of at least 3 weeks.

- Radiographic classifications
  - Depending on the amount of slip (percentage of epiphyseal displacement relative to metaphyseal width of the femoral neck [on AP or lateral radiographs]), the SCFE is mild (0–33 %), moderate (33–50 %) or severe (>50 %).
  - Depending on the difference in Southwick angle between the involved and uninvolved sides, the SCFE is mild (<30° difference), moderate (30–50°) or severe (>50°). The Southwick angle, or the head–shaft angle, is the angle formed by the proximal femoral physis and femoral shaft on lateral radiographs.

Treatment

Aim of treatment is to prevent progression of slip and reduce the chances of avascular necrosis, chondrolysis and late degenerative arthritis.

Surgical Procedures

- In situ fixation involves placement of a single-cannulated screw in the centre of the epiphysis and gives excellent results in stopping SCFE progression with minimal risk of chondrolysis.
  - Forceful manipulation is never indicated because it is associated with an increased risk of complications, including osteonecrosis.
  - An anterior starting point allows the screw to be targeted to the centre position of the femoral head and perpendicular to the physis on both AP and lateral views.
  - It is important to detect problematic impingement before the occurrence of irreversible intra-articular hip joint pathology that can occur in association with residual slip deformity.
  - Subsequently, early surgical correction of residual deformity should be considered in attempting to minimize the occurrence of degenerative pathology. Options include intertrochanteric proximal femoral osteotomy, or osteochondroplasty or modified Dunn procedure through safe surgical hip dislocation for residual deformity.
  - For residual deformities, intracapsular osteotomies, such as cuneiform osteotomy through the growth plate, correct the deformity at the apex, but they are associated with increased risk of avascular necrosis and chondrolysis. In contrast, extracapsular osteotomies, such as intertrochanteric osteotomy, have low risk of avascular necrosis, but are limited by the severity of the deformity that can be corrected because the deformity is addressed indirectly.
- Bone peg epiphysiodesis—a bone graft is placed across the physis which acts as both an internal fixation device and also incites a rapid physeal closure, thus preventing the SCFE from progressing.

- For severe deformities, in SCFE a proximal femoral osteotomy at the subcapital, femoral neck, intertrochanteric or subtrochanteric level can be performed as the primary procedure. Osteotomy at the subcapital and femoral neck levels can provide the most correction but in general requires technical expertise because the complication rates are the highest among all osteotomies.
- Priorities in the treatment of an unstable slip include avoidance of avascular necrosis, avoidance of chondrolysis, prevention of further slip and correction of the deformity to prevent secondary femoroacetabular impingement (FAI) and coxarthrosis.
  - Emergent treatment and decompression either with capsulotomy or aspiration are currently recommended in all unstable SCFE to optimize blood flow to the femoral head.
  - In situ pinning remains the gold standard for management of unstable slips.
  - The more severe the residual deformity, the greater likelihood of developing labral tears.
  - Surgical hip dislocation is a promising technique in the management of unstable SCFE with moderate to severe slippage with initial reported rates of osteonecrosis ranging from 0 to 6.7 % in all series.
- Indications for prophylactic fixation of the contralateral hip include age younger than 10 years and associated at-risk conditions such as endocrinopathies, renal osteodystrophy and a previous history of radiation therapy.

Complications

- Risk of AVN—unstable SCFE inherently has a high risk of AVN. Attempts at forceful reduction can increase this risk.
- Risk of chondrolysis—it is more frequent in severe SCFEs and is increased if there is permanent penetration of the joint with internal fixation devices.
- Late degenerative arthritis of the hip.

Bibliography

1. Aronson DD, Carlson WE. Slipped capital femoral epiphysis: a prospective study of fixation with a single screw. J Bone Joint Surg Am. 1992;74:810–9.
2. Carney BT, Weinstein SW, Noble J. Long-term follow-up of slipped capital femoral epiphysis. J Bone Joint Surg Am. 1991;73:667–74.
3. Crawford AH. Role of osteotomy in the treatment of slipped capital femoral epiphysis. J Pediatr Orthop B. 1996;5:102–9.
4. Loder RT, Richards BS, Shapiro PS, Reznick LR, Aronson DD. Acute slipped capital femoral epiphysis: the importance of physeal stability. J Bone Joint Surg Am. 1993;75:1134–40.
5. Lykissas MG, McCarthy JJ. Should all unstable slipped capital femoral epiphysis be treated open? J Pediatr Orthop. 2013;33:S92–8.

4 Coxa Vara

Ashok Johari, Ratna Maheshwari, and Shalin Maheshwari

Take-Home Message

- The Hilgenreiner–epiphyseal angle is prognostic and critical in treatment decision-making. Surgery is indicated for an angle >60° and observation for an angle <45°. Those with angles between 45° and 59° require observation for potential progression.
- It is necessary to determine the aetiology of coxa vara. Coxa vara caused by trauma will often spontaneously improve, bypassing the need for an osteotomy. Developmental and dysplastic coxa vara often progress and will either need surgery at presentation or later.

Definition

Coxa vara is a deformity of the proximal femur that results in a reduction of the normal neck–shaft angle, and it includes a wide spectrum of types with varying pathologies and differing sites of deformity.

Aetiology and Classification

The exact cause remains unknown; however, there appears to be a genetic predisposition.

- Congenital coxa vara
  Congenital coxa vara is the type associated with a congenital short femur and proximal femoral focal deficiency. It is characterized by a primary cartilaginous defect in the femoral neck.
- Developmental coxa vara
  This occurs in early childhood, when the child begins to ambulate with a Trendelenburg limp. Developmental coxa vara is bilateral in up to one half of cases.
- Dysplastic coxa vara
  Dysplastic coxa vara is due to an underlying bony abnormality such as fibrous dysplasia, vitamin D-resistant rickets, osteopetrosis and various generalized skeletal dysplasias.
- Acquired coxa vara
  This can develop following trauma or iatrogenically following surgery. It can also be the result of septic processes.

Pathophysiology

- The deformity in the proximal femur is most widely attributed to a primary defect in endochondral ossification in the medial part of the femoral neck.
- Large amounts of fibrous tissue rather than the cancellous bone has been found in the medial part of metaphysic of the femoral neck. This dystrophic tissue fatigues with weight bearing.
- Also the vertical orientation of physis converts the compressive forces into shear forces.

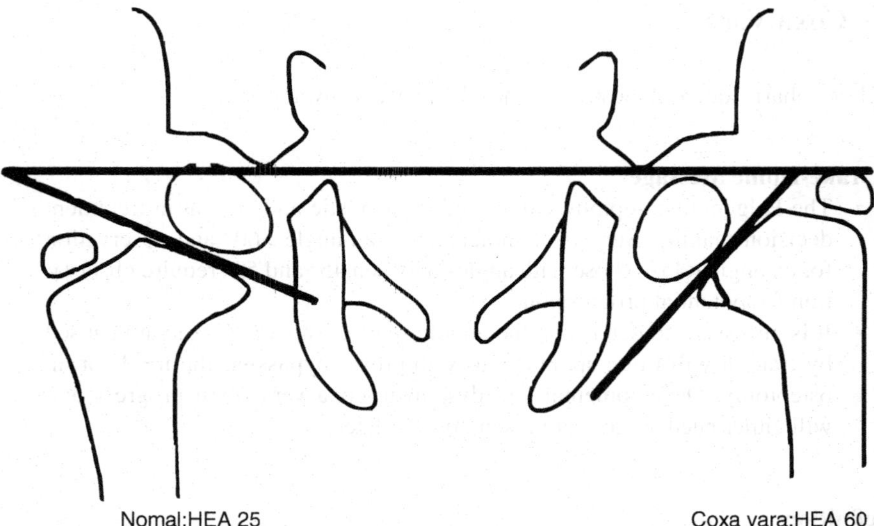

Fig. 3 Quantification of the extent of radiographic deformity of the proximal femur in developmental coxa vara. The Hilgenreiner–epiphyseal angle is the angle between the Hilgenreiner line and a line drawn parallel to the capital femoral physis

Radiography

- A decrease in the femoral neck–shaft angle
- The pathognomonic radiographic sign is the inferior and posterior bony metaphyseal fragment in the femoral neck—the inverted Y sign.
- Vertical orientation of physis with a short femoral neck.
- Associated femoral retroversion, acetabular dysplasia.
- Varus can be quantified by measuring the neck–shaft angle, the head–shaft angle or the Hilgenreiner–epiphyseal (H–E) angle· The H–E angle has prognostic value (see Fig. 3).

Treatment

- If the deformity is due to an underlying metabolic condition, then appropriate medical management is needed first. Surgical recommendations are based on the H–E angle.
  - If the HEA is >60°, all will progress, those between 45 and 60° may or may not progress and <45° often correct spontaneously.
  - Correction of the HEA to <30° is suggested to minimize the risk of recurrence in those with developmental coxa vara.
- Procedures
  - The standard procedure is a proximal femoral valgus derotational osteotomy.

- The osteotomy can occur at the intertrochanteric or subtrochanteric level as described by Langenskiöld (intertrochanteric), Pauwel (Y-shaped intertrochanteric) and Borden (subtrochanteric).
- Osteotomy at the femoral neck level should be avoided because higher morbidity rates and poorer clinical results have been reported.

- Timing of surgery—As soon as the bony development of the child is deemed adequate by the treating surgeon to allow secure fixation of the surgeon's preference.

Complications

- Recurrence of varus deformity
- Premature closure of the proximal femoral physis can occur leading to limb-length inequality and/or trochanteric overgrowth.

Bibliography

1. Beals RK. Coxa vara in childhood: evaluation and management. J Am Acad Orthop Surg. 1998;6:93–9.
2. Desai SS, Johnson LO. Long-term results of valgus osteotomy for congenital coxa vara. J Pediatr Orthop. 1993;294:204–10.
3. Gillespie R. Classification of congenital abnormalities of the femur. In: Herring JA, Birch JG, editors. The child with a limb deficiency. Rosemont: American Academy of Orthopaedic Surgeons; 1998. p. 63–72.
4. Weinstein JN, Kuo KN, Millar EA. Congenital coxa vara: a retrospective review. J Pediatr Orthop. 1984;4:70–7.

5 Angular and Rotational Deformities

Ashok Johari, Ratna Johari, and Shalin Maheshwari

Take-Home Message

Tibia Vara (Blount's Disease)

- Beware of internal tibial torsion with tibia vara. The patella should be pointed directly anterior on all weight-bearing lower extremity radiographs.
- To avoid undercorrection, fix the distal fragment in slight valgus, lateral translation and external rotation.
- The risk of postoperative compartment syndrome is decreased if an anterior compartment fasciotomy is performed at the time of surgery.
- Confirm the new mechanical alignment on the surgical table with bovie cord. A cord held directly over the centre of the femoral head and ankle should pass over the lateral tibial plateau.

- One or two pins and a cast are all the fixation necessary for infantile cases. Plate or external fixation is necessary for fixation in adolescent Blount's disease.
- Recurrence is less when the osteotomy is done before age 4 years.

Tibial Bowing

- Anterolateral bowing is typical of congenital pseudarthrosis of the tibia and is often associated with neurofibromatosis.
- Posterolateral bowing is often associated with development of a limb-length discrepancy.

Genu Valgum

- Unilateral genu valgum following a Cozen fracture almost always resolves spontaneously.
- Physeal tethers must be placed extraperiosteally to avoid unintended arrest.
- Physeal tethers (staples or eight-plate systems) must be placed in the mid-coronal plane to prevent recurvatum or procurvatum deformities.
- Nomograms are available to appropriately time a permanent hemiepiphysiodesis (or predict the duration necessary for correction with a temporary physeal tethering).
- If an isolated distal tibial osteotomy is performed, rotation of >30° generally results in translation of the distal fragment. This is of no clinical consequence and will remodel rapidly in growing children.

Rotational Deformities

- Brace-dependent ambulators (e.g. patients with cerebral palsy or myelodysplasia) tolerate less tibial torsion because the compensatory mechanisms (knee and subtalar joint motion) are unavailable.
- Lever-arm dysfunction in children with neuromuscular disorders is the reason osteotomies are frequently indicated in such children.
- Estimate anteversion clinically by measuring the degree of internal rotation of the hip necessary to make the greater trochanter maximally prominent laterally (trochanteric prominence angle test).
- Amount of rotation to correct excess anteversion = (prone internal rotation – prone external rotation)/2.

5.1 *Physiological Bowing and Blount's Disease*

Introduction

- Normal physiologic knee alignment includes periods of "knock knees" and "bowed legs". Symmetric genu varum before 2 years of age is rarely pathological. After which there is some degree of genu valgum is seen after which adult tibiofemoral angle of 6° is reached at 6–7 years of age (Fig. 4).

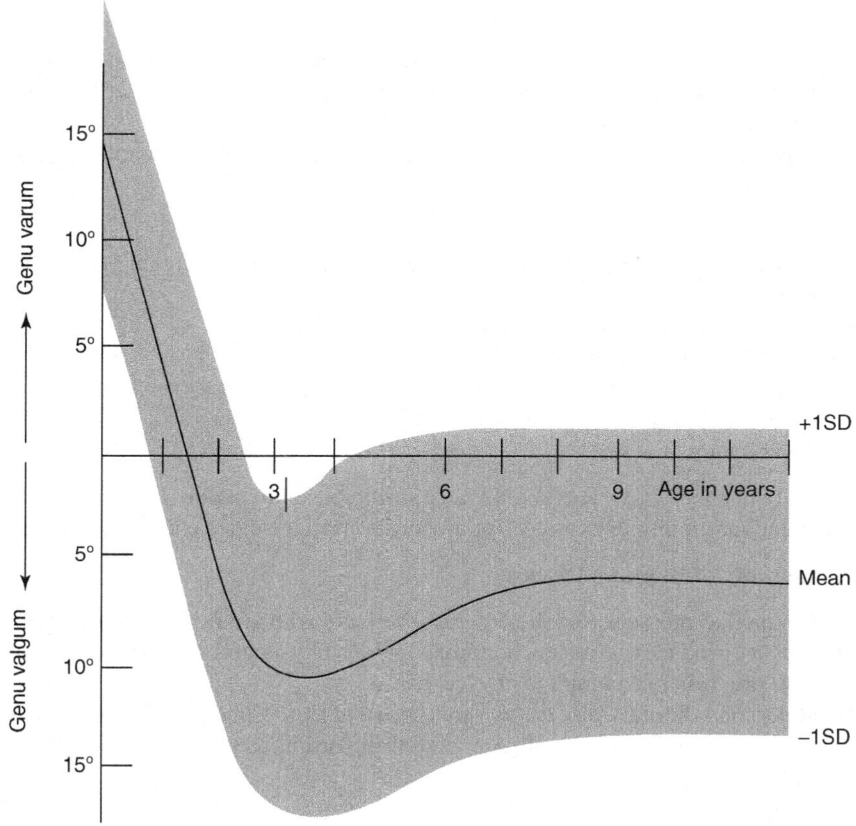

Fig. 4 Normal development of tibiofemoral angle during growth (after Salenius). Symmetric genu varum is often present before 2 years of age, which gradually progresses to genu valgum, after which adult tibiofemoral angle of 6° is reached at around 6 years of age

- Genu varum is more likely to be pathological if it is:
  - Present after 2 years of age
  - Unilateral
  - Associated with shortening (of the limb or of stature)
  - Severe
  - In a child with obesity
- Blount's disease, or tibia vara, is a progressive varus deformity occurring at the medial part of the proximal tibial physis. There are two main types: infantile Blount's which begins during the early childhood years, and late-onset or adolescent Blount's which begins in late childhood and the early teen years.

Aetiology

- Infantile Blount's disease is usually bilateral. Physiologic bowing is a continuum with Blount's disease. They share the common aetiological factor of early weight bearing by a child who may or may not be overweight.
- Variable increase in physeal shear stress and eventual disruption in medial physeal and bony growth
- Aetiological causes of pathological genu varum include:
  - Trauma or infection (including meningococcal) producing a bony bar at the proximal tibial physis
  - Rickets (including the vitamin D-resistant variety)
  - Blount's disease (tibia vara)
  - Generalized or focal osteochondrodysplasias, e.g. hereditary multiple exostoses, achondroplasia and focal fibrocartilaginous dysplasia
  - Tibial hemimelia
- A family history of bow legs should raise suspicions of hypophosphataemic rickets, hereditary multiple exostoses or a bone or cartilage dysplasia.

Pathoanatomy of Blount's Disease

- Excess medial pressure (e.g. heavy, early walkers who are in physiologic varus alignment) produces an osteochondrosis of the physis and adjacent epiphysis that can progress to a complete physeal bar.
- In adolescent Blount's disease, a varus moment at the knee during the stance phase of gait inhibits medial physeal growth according to the Heuter–Volkmann principle.

Evaluation

- Clinical findings suggestive of pathologic bowing:
  - Proximal tibial location of bowing
  - Sharply angular deformity
  - Asymmetric bowing of the two legs
  - Progressive deformity on serial examinations
  - Lateral thrust during gait
  - Very severe deformity
- Features to differentiate between infantile and adolescent Blount's disease (see Table 2)
- Infantile Blount's involves definite radiographic changes in both the proximal tibial physis and metaphysis that are progressive. These changes have been classified into six stages by Langenskiöld (see Fig. 5).
  Depression of the articular surface of the medial tibial plateau is evident in stages IV, V and VI, and premature physeal arrest is seen in stage VI.

Table 2 Infantile versus adolescent Blount's disease

Feature	Infantile Blount's	Adolescent Blount's
Physeal changes	Progressive and often severe	Mild
Physeal bar formation	Frequent	Does not occur
Metaphyseal changes	Progressive changes	No changes seen
Joint deformity	Common	Rare
Internal tibial torsion	Common	Rare
Recurrence	Often seen	Seldom seen

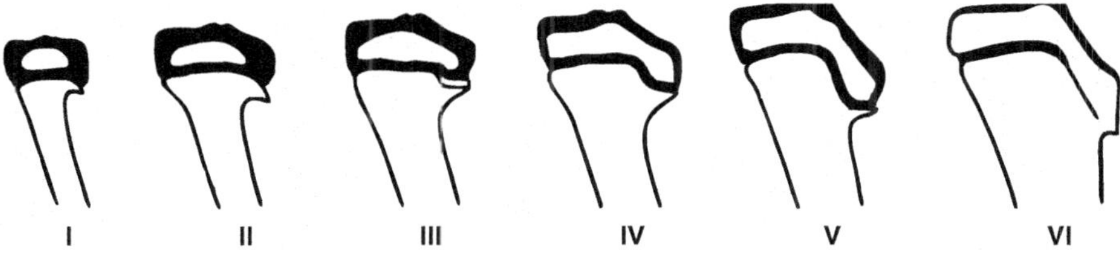

Fig. 5 Langenskiöld classification of infantile tibia vara in six progressive stages with increasing age. The prognostic implications suggested by Langenskiöld are that simple osteotomy can be effective up to stage IV (Redrawn from Langenskiöld A. Tibia vara; a survey of 23 cases. Acta Chir Scand. 1952;103:9)

- Radiographic distinction between physiologic bowing and Blount's disease may not be initially obvious, because Langenskiöld changes diagnostic of Blount's disease typically are not distinctive until 2–3 years of age.
- When the metaphyseal–diaphyseal (MD) angle (Fig. 6) is <10°, there is 95 % chance the bowing will resolve. If the MD angle is >16°, there is 95 % chance of progression. For MD angles between 11° and 16°, there is considerable overlap between physiologic genu varum and Blount's disease.

Treatment

Aims of Treatment

- Restore normal alignment of the tibia
  Restoring the normal alignment of the tibia and restoring the normal mechanical axis of the limb is the foremost important goal.
- Correct joint deformity
  If the tibial articular surface is depressed, it needs to be corrected. In severe cases, elevation of the medial tibial epiphyseal depression should be considered along with proximal tibial osteotomy.
- Equalize limb length
- Maintain correction and prevent recurrence
  In infantile disease, recurrence is commonly encountered.
  The best chance of preventing recurrence is to correct the deformity in the very early stages of the disease

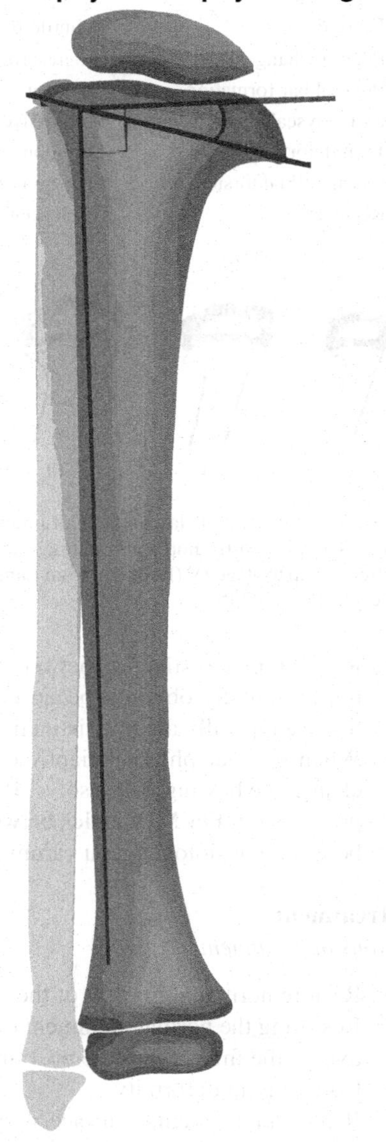

Fig. 6 Metaphyseal–diaphyseal angle. It is the angle created by the intersection of a line connecting the most prominent medial portion of the proximal tibial metaphysis (the "beak") and the most prominent lateral point of the metaphysis with a line drawn perpendicular to the long axis of the tibial diaphysis. Radiographic Blount's subsequently develop in patients with MDA > 11°

- Prevent neurovascular complications
  - Nonsurgical
    - Bracing efficacy is controversial.
    - Bracing is indicated only in patients 2–3 years of age with mild disease (stage 1–2).
    - Poor results are associated with obesity and bilaterality.

    - Improvement should occur within 1 year.
    - Bracing must be continued until the bony changes resolve, which usually takes 1.5–2 years.
- Surgical
    - If the child has not achieved complete correction by the age of 4 years or has progressed to Langenskiöld stage III disease, then immediate tibial osteotomy is indicated.
- General surgical principles
    - To avoid undercorrection, the distal fragment is fixed in slight valgus, lateral translation and external rotation.
    - Performing an anterior compartment fasciotomy at the time of surgery decreases the postoperative risk of compartment syndrome.
    - The mechanical axis can be confirmed intraoperatively by holding the bovie cord directly over the centre of the femoral head and ankle. The cord should pass over the lateral tibial plateau.
- Infantile Blount's disease
    - Patients older than 3 years require proximal tibial valgus and rotational osteotomy. One or two pins and a cast provide fixation. Fibular osteotomy is needed to allow for sufficient correction. The risk of recurrence is much less if the surgery is performed before age 4 years.
    - If a bony bar is present, a bar resection with interposition of methyl methacrylate (epiphysiolysis) is performed concomitantly.
    - If significant depression of the medial tibial plateau exists, a medial tibial plateau elevation and realignment osteotomy may be necessary.
- Adolescent Blount's disease
    - Temporary or permanent epiphysiodesis prevents deformity progression and may allow some correction in adolescents with mild to moderate Blount's in whom at least 15–18 months of growth remain.
    - Severe deformities require proximal tibial osteotomy and occasionally a femoral osteotomy (if distal femoral varus exceeds 7–10°).
    - Fixation is generally with a plate or external fixation.

Bibliography

1. Greene WB. Infantile tibia vara. J Bone Joint Surg Am. 1993;75:130–43.
2. Henderson RC, Kemp GJ Jr, Greene WB. Adolescent tibia vara: alternatives for operative treatment. J Bone Joint Surg Am. 1992;74:342–50.
3. Loder RT, Johnston II CE. Infantile tibia vara. J Pediatr Orthop. 1987;7:639–46.
4. Schoenecker PL, Meade WC, Pierron RL, Sheridan JJ, Capelli AM. Blount's disease: a retrospective review and recommendations for treatment. J Pediatr Orthop. 1985;5:181–6.

5. Slawski DP, Schoenecker PL, Rich MM. Peroneal nerve injury as a complication of pediatric tibial osteotomies: a review of 255 osteotomies. J Pediatr Orthop. 1994;14:166–72.

5.2 *Torsional Deformities*

5.2.1 Femoral Anteversion

Definition

The normal average femoral anteversion is around 40° at birth, and as the child matures into adulthood, it decreases to around 10–15°. Femoral anteversion is around 5° higher in females than in males.

Aetiology

Increased femoral anteversion can be idiopathic, or associated with other conditions such as developmental hip dysplasia and cerebral palsy.

Pathoanatomy

- Rotation variations have not been directly correlated to degenerative changes of the hip or knee.
- Patellofemoral pain can arise with increasing femoral anteversion, but a pathologic threshold has not been identified.
  - Brace-dependent ambulators (such as those with cerebral palsy or myelodysplasia) tolerate less tibial torsion because the compensatory gait mechanisms (knee and subtalar motion) are unavailable.
  - Lever-arm dysfunction in children with neuromuscular disorders is the reason osteotomies are frequently indicated in such children.

Evaluation

- In-toeing gait with medially rotated patellae is indicative of femoral anteversion.
- In-toeing from femoral anteversion is most evident between 3 and 6 years of age.
- The torsional profile consists of four components: gait progression, hip rotation, thigh–foot angle and foot border profiles.
  - The gait progression angle simply describes the deviation of the child's gait from a straight-ahead pattern; a negative angle indicates an in-toeing gait, and a positive angle indicates an out-toeing gait relative to a completely straight-ahead gait.
  - Passive hip rotation assessment involves measurement of both internal and external rotation; as femoral anteversion increases, internal rotation increases at the expense of external rotation. The passive ranges of hip rotation measured with the hips in extension and also in flexion can be recorded on a grid for documenting change in the movement as the child grows.

  - The thigh–foot angle indicates the amount of tibial torsion; an external thigh–foot angle indicates relative external tibial torsion, while an internal thigh–foot angle indicates relative internal tibial torsion. This is extremely important when the physician is considering the possibility of a miserable malalignment syndrome.
  - The foot borders indicate whether there is a torsional component from the foot itself. A concave medial border indicates the likelihood of metatarsus adductus; a concave lateral border indicates the likelihood of a significant pes valgus.
- CT or MRI can quantify anteversion most accurately, but they are unnecessary in most cases.

Management

Aims of Management

- Improve cosmesis of gait
  If the gait is so unsightly as to cause concern to the child, correction of the anteversion may be considered.
- Relieve anterior knee pain in the miserable malalignment syndrome
  To relieve the child's anterior knee pain by improving the normal anatomic relationship between the femur and tibia with respect to torsion.
- Improve stability of the unstable hip
  In situations where the increased femoral anteversion is contributing to hip instability, the stability needs to be improved by correcting the anteversion.

Treatment

- Shoes, orthoses, and braces are ineffective.
- Observation of the in-toeing gait is the most widely selected option. Since the natural history is one of gradual resolution, the aim of observing the child over time is to simply document this natural improvement
- For able-bodied children after age 10 years with unacceptable awkward gait or pain and <10° external hip rotation, a derotation osteotomy is indicated. The amount of rotation needed to correct excessive anteversion = (prone internal rotation – prone external rotation)/2.
- The osteotomy can be performed at the intertrochanteric level with blade-plate fixation, at the mid-diaphysis with intramedullary nail fixation or at the distal metaphyseal level with dynamic compression plate fixation.
- If there are significant patellofemoral malalignment issues, and if they can be corrected by a more distal osteotomy, then the procedure should occur at that level.
- In the presence of the miserable malalignment syndrome, tibial rotational osteotomy should also be performed.

Complications

- Infection, avascular necrosis, loss of fixation, nonunion, malunion and nerve palsies

5.2.2 Tibial Torsion

Definition
Tibial torsion is the angular difference between the bimalleolar axis at the ankle and the bicondylar axis of the knee (normal is 20° of external rotation).

Evaluation
Most evident between the ages 1 and 2 years and usually resolves by age 6 years.

Management

- Parent education is the primary treatment.
- Special shoes and braces do not change the natural history.
- Derotation osteotomy is rarely needed in able-bodied children.
- If an isolated distal tibial rotational osteotomy is performed, rotation >30° generally results in translation of the distal fragment. This is not clinically significant and will remodel quickly in growing children.

5.3 Tibial Bowing

5.3.1 Anterolateral Bowing of the Tibia

Definition
Congenital anterolateral bowing of the tibia is a potentially troublesome deformity, particularly when it is associated with either neurofibromatosis or fibrous dysplasia. The bowed tibia may fracture, and the fracture may fail to unite, progressing on to a frank pseudarthrosis. The fracture usually develops once the child begins to walk although it can occur in infancy.

Epidemiology

- 50 % of patients with anterolateral bowing have neurofibromatosis.
- 10 % of patients with neurofibromatosis have anterolateral bowing.

Evaluation and Classification

- The presence of sclerosis, cysts, fibular dysplasia and narrowing are the basis of the Boyd and Crawford classifications. Neither is predictive of prognosis.
  - Type I is characterized by anterior lateral bowing with increased cortical density and a narrow but normal medullary canal.
  - Type IIA, by anterior lateral bowing with failure of tubularization and a widened medullary canal.
  - Type IIB, by anterior lateral bowing with a cystic lesion before fracture or canal enlargement from a previous fracture.

  - Type IIC, by frank pseudarthrosis and bone atrophy with "sucked candy" narrowing of the ends of the two fragments.

- There are other growth abnormalities of the tibia, fibula and the ipsilateral femur that may need to be taken into consideration while planning treatment. These include abnormal inclination of the proximal tibial physis, posterior bowing of the proximal third of the tibial diaphysis, proximal migration of the lateral malleolus, fibular hypoplasia, fibular pseudarthrosis, ankle valgus and calcaneus deformity.

Natural History

- Spontaneous resolution is unusual. Good prognostic signs include:
  - Duplicated hallux
  - Delta-shaped osseous segment in the concavity of the bow

Management

- Aims of treatment:
  - The primary goal of treatment is prevention of pseudarthrosis.
  - Achieve union
  - Prevent refracture
  - Correct limb-length inequality
  - Correct associated growth abnormalities
  - Prevent ankle deformity and arthritis
- Treatment
  - A clam-shell total contact brace is used.
  - Osteotomies to correct bowing are contraindicated because of the risk of pseudarthrosis of the osteotomy site.
  - Fracture risk decreases at skeletal maturity.

Pseudarthrosis

- Excision of the pseudarthrosis involves excising the tapered ends of the bone until fresh bleeding is encountered. The thick periosteum surrounding the entire area of the pseudarthrosis is excised.
- All treatment options have limited success (Table 3).
  - Intramedullary rod and bone grafting.
  - Circular fixator with bone transport: the chances of obtaining union following the Ilizarov procedure are low in children under 3 or 4 years of age.
  - Vascularized fibular graft: it is technically difficult to perform a microvascular-free fibular transfer in a very young child.
- Amputation is indicated for persistent pseudarthrosis (usually after two or three failed surgeries.

Table 3 Factors to be taken into consideration while choosing the primary procedure

Factors to be considered	Microvascular free fibular transfer	Ilizarov technique	Intramedullary rodding and bone grafting
Reported union rate	>70 %	>70 %	>70 %
Success in children less than 3 years	Poor	Poor	Good
Ability to reduce risk of refracture	Does not	Does not	Reduces risk
Simultaneous correction of limb-length inequality	Not possible	Possible	Not possible
Simultaneous correction of all deformities	Not possible	Possible	Not possible
Prevention of late ankle valgus	Not possible	Not possible	Possible

5.3.2 Posteromedial Bowing of the Tibia

Definition

Congenital posteromedial bowing of the tibia and fibula is an isolated, congenital lower limb malformation. The malformation occurs in fetal period most probably as a result of the pressure on the plantar surface of the foot, which comes to the position of maximum dorsal bowing pressing the tibia and fibula.

Aetiology

The malformation has no connection with neurofibromatosis, pathologic fractures, and congenital pseudoarthrosis of the tibia and fibula.

Natural History

- Posteromedial bowing tends to resolve, to a great extent, spontaneously as the child grows. Unlike anterolateral bowing, in children with posteromedial bowing, there is no risk of the tibia fracturing and a pseudarthrosis developing.
- It is corrected gradually and spontaneously following the child's growth. After the growth is complete, only the leg must be shortened—on average by 13 % of the normal length of the tibia and fibula.

Evaluation

- After the child is born, the most distinctive feature is a talipes calcaneovalgus. The foot adheres to the front lateral surface of the tibia and fibula with its dorsal surface.
- This is accompanied by posteromedial bowing of the tibia.
- However, leg shortening is often missed, and directly after birth, it is minor. LLDs at maturity are usually in the 3–8 cm range.

Management

- No intervention is necessary if adequate resolution of the deformity of the foot and the tibia has occurred and if the limb-length inequality is less than 2 cm at skeletal maturity.

- If the anticipated shortening at skeletal maturity is likely to exceed 2 cm, limb-length equalization is needed.
- If complete or near-complete resolution of the tibial deformity occurs, no active intervention is needed in this regard. However, if the residual deformity is clinically visible, correction may be justified.

Bibliography

1. Grill F, Bollini G, Dungl P, et al. Treatment approaches for congenital pseudarthrosis of tibia: results of the EPOS multicenter study. European Paediatric Orthopaedic Society (EPOS). J Pediatr Orthop. 2000;9:75–89.
2. Hofmann A, Wenger DR. Posteromedial bowing of the tibia. Progression of discrepancy in leg lengths. J Bone Joint Surg Am. 1981;63:384–8.
3. Hubbard DD, Staheli LT, Chew DE, Mosca VS. Medial femoral torsion and osteoarthritis. J Pediatr Orthop. 1988;8:540–2.
4. Shands AR Jr, Steele MK. Torsion of the femur. A follow-up report on the use of the Dunlap method for its determination. J Bone Joint Surg Am. 1958;40: 803–16.
5. Staheli LT, Lippert F, Denotter P. Femoral anteversion and physical performance in adolescent and adult life. Clin Orthop Relat Res. 1977;129:213–6.
6. Svenningsen S, Apalset K, Terjesen T, Anda S. Regression of femoral anteversion. A prospective study of intoeing children. Acta Orthop Scand. 1989;60:170–3.
7. Wientroub S, Grill F. Congenital pseudarthrosis of the tibia: Part 1. European Pediatric Orthopaedic Society multicenter study of congenital pseudoarthrosis. J Pediatr Orthop B. 2000;9:1–2.

Paediatric Feet Conditions

Ashok Johari, Ratna Johari, and Shalin Maheshwari

1 Club Feet

Ashok Johari, Ratna Johari, and Shalin Maheshwari

Take-Home Message

- The most common cause of a late failure after initial club foot correction with Ponseti casts is poor compliance with the Denis Browne brace.
- Most club feet treated with the Ponseti method (up to 90 %) require percutaneous Achilles tenotomy at the time the final cast is applied.
- Anterior tibial tendon transfer (split or whole transfer) is needed in one third to one half of club feet treated with the Ponseti method.

Definition

Club foot is a congenital foot deformity consisting of hindfoot equinus and varus as well as midfoot and forefoot adduction and cavus. It is more common in males and is the most common birth defect (1 in 750 live births).

Aetiology

Considered to be multifactorial

- Mechanical block by extrinsic pressure in utero
- Primary germ plasm defect in the talus
- Retracting fibrosis—myofibroblast contraction
- Neurogenic theory—increased type 1 muscle fibres in the calf muscle
- Myogenic theory—atrophy of leg muscles

A. Johari, MD (✉) • R. Johari, MD • S. Maheshwari, MD
Pediatric Orthopedics, Childrens' Orthopedic Centre, Mumbai, India
e-mail: drashokjohari@hotmail.com; drratnajohari@gmail.com

C. Mauffrey, D.J. Hak (eds.), *Passport for the Orthopedic Boards and FRCS Examination*, DOI 10.1007/978-2-8178-0475-0_25

- Hypotrophic anterior tibial artery
- Genetic factors

Pathoanatomy

- The talus is smaller, and there is short talar neck. There is medial and plantar deviation of the anterior end of the talus. Talar neck body axis is reduced to less than 90°.
- The axes of the anterior and middle facet of the calcaneus create a more acute angle than a normal foot, with the anterior facet oriented inward. Calcaneus is medially rotated and pronated.
- There is talonavicular subluxation. The navicular is displaced medially over the head of the talus. The forefoot deformity is the result of medial displacement of the navicular.
- Although the entire foot is supinated, the forefoot pronation relative to the hindfoot causes the cavus.
- Among the various structures that may be abnormal and contribute to the deformity are the gastrocnemius–soleus and the tibialis posterior. These muscles may be contracted.
- Other soft-tissue contractures, including the joint capsules, develop subsequently. In longstanding cases, adaptive bony changes ensue.

Evaluation

- Common clinical findings are a small foot, small calf and slightly shortened tibia, and the skin creases medially and posteriorly.
- Nonidiopathic club feet must be identified. Club feet associated with arthrogryposis, myelodysplasia, diastrophic dysplasia and amniotic band syndrome are resistant to casting treatment.
- Radiography: Minimal ossification of the foot in the newborn limits the utility of radiographs. In both the AP and lateral views of a club foot, the talus and calcaneus are less divergent and more parallel (smaller talocalcaneal angle) than normal.

Classification

- Dimeglio Classification
  Each major components of club foot (equinus, heel varus, medial rotation of carpopedal block, forefoot adduction) are given points accordingly.

  –20° and 0°: 1 point
  0–20°: 2 points
  20–45°: 3 points
  45–90°: 4 points

  Additional 1 point each are added for the following:

  - Deep posterior crease
  - Medial crease
  - Cavus
  - Poor muscle condition

Grade I: if score less than 5
Grade II: if score is 5–9
Grade III: if score is 10–14
Grade IV: if score is more than 15

- Pirani Scoring
  Each component may score 0, 0.5 or 1. This includes the following:
  Hindfoot contracture score

  - Posterior crease
  - Empty heel
  - Rigid equinus

  Midfoot contracture score

  - Medial crease
  - Curvature of lateral border
  - Position of the head of the talus

Treatment

- Nonsurgical—the Ponseti serial casting.
  - Outcome is much better than with historical casting techniques (80–90 % success versus 10–50 %).
  - Sequence of deformity correction is *c*avus, *a*dductus, *v*arus and finally *e*quinus (CAVE).
  - Important Ponseti casting concepts:
    - Forefoot is supinated, not pronated.
    - Lateral pressure is applied to the neck of the talus only.
    - Long-leg casts.
    - Weekly cast changes.
    - Percutaneous Achilles tenotomy is frequently done before final cast application to address residual equinus (up to 90 % of feet).
  - The most common cause of failure after initial correction with the Ponseti casting is poor compliance with the Denis Browne brace. Recommended use is 23 h/day for 3 months after casting and then at night for 2–3 years.
  - Anterior tibial tendon transfer (split or whole transfer) is needed in one third to one half of club feet treated with the Ponseti method.

- Surgical
  Complete posteromedial release indications: persistent deformity after casting, syndrome-associated club foot and delayed presentation (older than 1–2 years of age). Secondary or residual deformities may require surgical intervention.
  - Hindfoot varus

    <2–3 years: Modified McKay procedure
    3–10 years: Isolated heel varus—Lateral closing wedge osteotomy of the calcaneus. Short medial column: Dillwyn Evan's procedure—this consists

of medial and posterior release with calcaneocuboid fusion. Long lateral column: Lichtblau procedure—consists of resection of the lateral end of the os calcis.

10–12 years: Triple arthrodesis

Equinus: Mild to moderate deformity—tendo-Achilles lengthening and post-capsulotomy of the ankle and subtalar joints. Severe deformity—Lambrinudi procedure

Complications

- Vascular compromise—immediate placement of cast in neutral position predisposes to this complication.
- Injury to infant's tarsal bone—transaction of the head of the talus and sustentaculum tali can occur during capsulotomies.
- Injury to posterior tibial physis, distal fibular physis or first metatarsal physis.

Bibliography

1. Bensahel H, Guillaume A, Czukonyi Z, et al. Results of physical therapy for idiopathic clubfoot: a long-term follow-up study. J Pediatr Orthop. 1990;10:189–92.
2. Carroll NC. Pathoanatomy and surgical treatment of resistant clubfoot. Instr Course Lect. 1988;37:93–106.
3. Dimeglio A, Bensahel H, Souchet P, et al. Classification of clubfoot. J Pediatr Orthop B. 1995;4:129–36.
4. Ippolito E, Ponseti IV. Congenital clubfoot in the human fetus. A histological study. J Bone Joint Surg Am. 1980;62:8–22.
5. Ponseti IV. Congenital clubfoot: fundamentals of treatment. Oxford: Oxford University Press; 1996.

2 Metatarsus Adductus

Ashok Johari, Ratna Maheshwari, and Shalin Maheshwari

Take-Home Message

- Metatarsus adductus is a medial deviation of the forefoot with normal alignment of the hindfoot.
- Avoid treating a deformity which spontaneously improves.
- Most cases of metatarsus adductus improve; those that improve need no active treatment.
- Correction of the deformity should be considered for cases that do not resolve, particularly if the deformity is severe.

Definition

In children born with this foot deformity, the forefoot is deviated inward relative to the hindfoot. Some authors distinguish between metatarsus adductus and metatarsus varus by the degree of rigidity of the deformity, the latter being the stiffer type.

Aetiology

- Intrauterine compression has been long presumed as the cause.
- Abnormal insertion of tibialis posterior on first cuneiform, or peroneal weakness with overactive tibialis anterior.
- May be associated with torticollis and developmental dysplasia of the hip.

Pathophysiology

- Shape of medial cuneiform found to be altered, with medial deviation of articular surface
- Adduction of metaphysis of the second through fifth metatarsal

Radiography

Medial deviation of metatarsals at the tarsometatarsal level (see Fig. 1)

Classification

Bleck Classification

Mild: Forefoot can be clinically abducted to the midline of the foot and beyond.
Moderate: Flexibility to allow abduction of forefoot to the midline, and not beyond.
Rigid: The forefoot cannot be abducted at all.

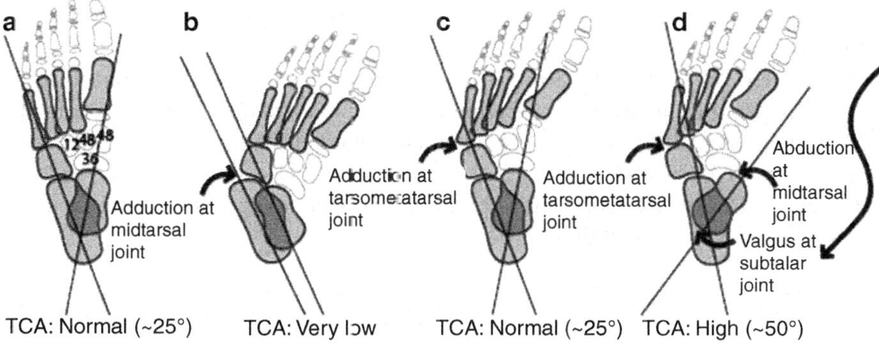

Fig. 1 Talocalcaneal angle in various foot deformities. (**a**) In the normal foot—the T–C angle is around 25°. (**b**) In a club foot—The T–C angle is very low. (**c**) In metatarsus adductus—the T–C angle is normal; however, there is adduction at tarsometatarsal joints. (**d**) In skewfoot—the T–C angle is very high, with adduction at tarsometatarsal joints

Treatment

- Nonsurgical
  - Spontaneous resolution of metatarsus adductus occurs in 90 % of children by age 4 years.
  - Passive stretching is recommended for mild deformity but does not improve final outcome.
  - Serial casting is useful in children between 6 and 12 months of age with moderate deformity. Unlike cast treatment for club feet, the fulcrum for applying an external rotation torque when moulding the cast is located over the cuboid.
- Surgical
  - Surgery is indicated only in children with severe deformities uncorrected by conservative measures or when there are problems with shoe wear and pain or objectionable appearance.
  - 2–4 years: Tarsometatarsal capsulotomies and/or abductor hallucis release.
  - >4 years: A medial column lengthening (opening wedge osteotomy of cuneiform) and lateral column shortening (closing wedge of the cuboid) produce good results with fewer complications.
  - If the child has a skewfoot (hindfoot valgus in addition to the metatarsus adductus), then hindfoot osteotomy is required in addition to the midfoot osteotomy.

Complications

- Recurrence is the most common complication.

Bibliography

1. Asirvatham R, Stevens P. Idiopathic forefoot-adduction deformity: medial capsulotomy and abductor hallucis lengthening for resistant and severe deformities. J Pediatr Orthop. 1997;17:496–500.
2. Heyman CH, Herndon CH, Strong JM. Mobilization of the tarsometatarsal and intermetatarsal joints for the correction of resistant adduction of the fore part of the foot in congenital club-foot or congenital metatarsus varus. J Bone Joint Surg Am. 1958;40:299–309.
3. Ponseti IV, Becker JR. Congenital metatarsus adductus: the results of treatment. J Bone Joint Surg Am. 1966;48:702–11.

3 Congenital Vertical Talus

Ashok Johari, Ratna Maheshwari, and Shalin Maheshwari

Take-Home Message

- The diagnosis of the vertical talus should prompt the orthopaedic surgeon to look for neural tube defects or arthrogryposis.
- Early use of nonoperative treatment (usually manipulation and serial casts) in combination with limited surgery appears to be an evolving general principle in the management.
- One must be able to distinguish subtler forms of congenital vertical talus from flexible flatfoot or the oblique talus. A lateral radiograph of foot in plantar flexion helps to distinguish the same.

Definition

Congenital vertical talus is an irreducible dorsal dislocation of the navicular on the talus, with the navicular displaced dorsally and the head of the talus pointing plantarward. Occasionally, the dislocation affects the calcaneocuboid joint. The heel is in equinus and valgus, the forefoot dorsiflexed and abducted producing in severe cases a rocker-bottom foot.

Aetiology

Some cases of isolated deformity are transmitted as an autosomal dominant trait with incomplete penetrance.

Rare condition (1 in 150,000 births) is commonly (~50 %) associated with neuromuscular disease (myelodysplasia, arthrogryposis, diastematomyelia) or chromosomal abnormalities such as trisomy 18.

Pathophysiology

- The navicular is dislocated dorsolaterally.
- The deformity also includes eversion of the calcaneus, contracture of the dorsolateral muscles and Achilles tendon and attenuation of the spring ligament. The dorsal capsule of talonavicular joint is thickened and contracted. The hindfoot is in a fixed equinovalgus position.
- The midfoot is dorsiflexed and abducted on the hindfoot and cannot be plantar flexed.

Evaluation

- Clinically, the foot has a rigid convex plantar surface with a prominent talar head (rocker-bottom).
- Unlike flexible flatfoot, the arch will not reconstitute upon standing on the toes or hyperextending the great toe.
- An awkward, calcaneal-type gait pattern results from limited push-off power, limited (if any) forefoot contact and excessive heel contact.
- Radiographs

- The radiographic view that is diagnostic for a vertical talus is a lateral view in forced plantar flexion (Fig. 2). The talus, calcaneus and metatarsals are ossified at birth, and the cuboid generally ossifies within the first month of life. The navicular remains dorsally dislocated in this view. This differs from oblique talus, in which the navicular reduces on this view.
- Prior to ossification of the navicular (age 3 years), the first metatarsal is used as a proxy for the dorsal alignment of the navicular on the lateral view.

Treatment

- Nonsurgical
  - Initial treatment begins with casting.
  - Casting is usually insufficient to correct a vertical talus but may help stretch the tight dorsolateral soft tissues. The foot is stretched into plantar flexion and inversion.
  - The talonavicular joint is reduced by the serial casts or, if incomplete, openly reduced (through a small medial incision) and held with a Kirschner wire.

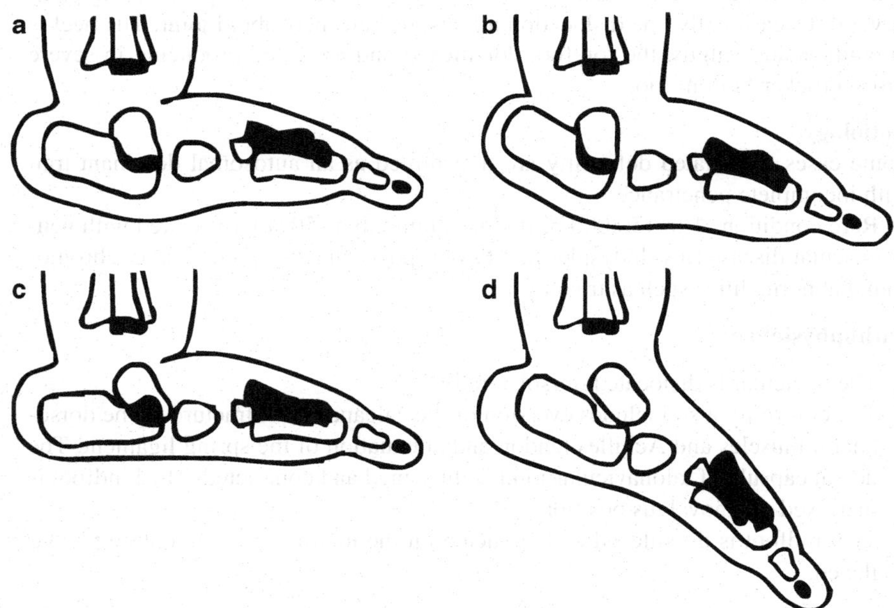

Fig. 2 Radiographic features differentiating CVT and flexible flatfoot. (**a**) Vertical talus: (*top figure left*) the talus plantar flexed. Grossly elevated talocalcaneal angle. Long axis of the first metatarsal not in line with the long axis of the talus. (**b**) On attempting plantar flexion: (*top figure right*) forefoot cannot be plantar flexed. Normal tarsal relationships are not restored. (**c**) Flexible flatfoot: (*bottom figure left*) the talus plantar flexed. Grossly elevated talocalcaneal angle. Long axis of the first metatarsal not in line with the long axis of the talus. (**d**) On plantar flexion: forefoot can be plantar flexed, and normal tarsal relationships are restored

- Surgical
  - Surgery is usually performed between 12 and 18 months of age.
  - Surgical treatment includes extensive talar release with lengthening of the Achilles, toe extensors and peroneal tendons and pinning of the talonavicular joint. The split tibialis anterior tendon is generally transferred to the talar neck, to maintain reduction by preventing the talus from plantar flexing.
  - Outcome of reconstruction after age 3 years is less predictable. Triple arthrodesis is rarely needed as a salvage procedure.
  - Aftercare following the removal of casts and wires includes stretching exercises performed by the child's parents and the use of a night-time brace consisting of two shoes held parallel by a connecting metal bar until the child has learnt to walk. Thereafter, a solid ankle–foot orthoses moulded in 15° plantar flexion and 15° adduction are used until the age of 2.

Complications

- Avascular necrosis of the talus can be a potential complication of extensive talar release.
- Complete transfer of the tibialis anterior can lead to progressive cavus deformity.

Bibliography

1. Dodge L, Ashley R, Gilbert R. Treatment of the congenital vertical talus: a retrospective review of 36 feet with long- term follow up. Foot Ankle. 1987;7:326.
2. Drennan J, Sharrard W. The pathological anatomy of convex pes valgus. J Bone Joint Surg Br. 1971;53:445.
3. Hamanishi C. Congenital vertical talus: classification with 69 cases and new measurement system. J Pediatr Orthop. 1984;4:318.
4. Jacobsen S, Crawford A. Congenital vertical talus. J Pediatr Orthop. 1983;3:306.
5. Lamy L, Weissman L. Congenital convex pes planus. J Bone Joint Surg. 1939;21:79.

4 Cavus Foot

Ashok Johari, Ratna Maheshwari, and Shalin Maheshwari

Take-Home Message

- Percutaneous plantar fascia release is insufficient to correct a cavus foot.
- Simultaneous plantar fascia release should be avoided with an Achilles tendon lengthening. An intact Achilles tendon provides the resistance necessary to stretch the divided plantar tissues.
- A key to surgical decision-making is the flexibility of the hindfoot.

Definition

- Cavus refers to a fixed equinus deformity of the forefoot in relation to the hindfoot (anterior cavus), or less frequently from excessive calcaneal dorsiflexion (posterior cavus), resulting in an abnormally high arch.
- The heel may be in a neutral, varus, valgus, calcaneus or equinus position.
- There may be an accompanying clawing of toes.

Aetiology

- Cavus is a manifestation of a neuromuscular disorder with muscle imbalance, until proven otherwise.
- Two thirds of patients with a cavus foot have a neurologic problem (most commonly Charcot–Marie–Tooth disease).
- Calcaneocavus is seen exclusively in children with myelomeningocele and poliomyelitis.

Pathoanatomy

- The primary structural problem is forefoot plantar flexion, particularly of the first ray.
- For the lateral half of the foot to be in contact with the ground, the hindfoot must deviate into varus.
- First-ray plantar flexion may result from a weak tibialis anterior relative to the peroneus longus, but it is more commonly due to intrinsic weakness and contracture.
- Over time, the plantar fascia contracts, and the hindfoot varus deformity becomes more rigid.

Evaluation

- Instability of gait and frequent falling, a feeling of ankle "giving out".
- A neurologic examination and family history are essential.
  - Unilateral involvement suggests a focal diagnosis (e.g. spinal cord anomaly or nerve injury).
  - Bilateral involvement and a positive family history are common with Charcot–Marie–Tooth disease.
- Hindfoot flexibility is assessed by placing a block under the lateral border of the foot (Coleman block test).
- Standing AP and lateral radiographs of the foot are indicated on initial evaluation. There is normally a straight line relationship between the axis of the talus and that of the first metatarsal on lateral view. An apex dorsal angulation indicates a cavus deformity.
- Other possible investigations include DNA blood tests for Charcot–Marie–Tooth disease, electromyography with nerve conduction studies and muscle biopsy.
- MRI of the spine is indicated for unilateral involvement.

Management

- Shoe modifications may be used to ameliorate symptoms during the time it takes to diagnose and if possible treat the underlying cause.
- There is little role for nonoperative treatment as most are progressive and of advanced degree of severity at the time of diagnosis.
- Indications for surgery are progressive deformity, calluses beneath the metatarsal heads or base of the fifth metatarsal or ankle instability.
- Surgical treatment of pes cavus can be divided into soft-tissue surgery, osteotomies and triple arthrodesis. Soft-tissue surgery is always part of the surgical reconstruction of a cavus foot. Because the deformity is driven by muscular imbalance, contractures must be released and the forces exerted by the tendons rebalanced.
- In young patients with flexible deformities, soft-tissue surgery is adequate to address the deformity. Percutaneous plantar fascia release is insufficient to correct a cavus foot. At minimum, an open release and soft-tissue rebalancing are needed.
- In older patients, flexibility is lost as adaptive bony changes occur, and an osteotomy will be necessary to restore a plantigrade foot. Joint-sparing procedures are preferred whenever possible.
- A key to surgical decision-making is the flexibility of the hindfoot.
- In patients who have flexible hindfoot varus on the Coleman block test, plantar flexion of the medial part of the forefoot may be correctable by first metatarsal osteotomy.
- In global equinus of the forefoot, with the medial and lateral aspects of the forefoot equally plantar flexed, multiple metatarsal osteotomies have been performed to elevate the forefoot and correct the cavus.
- Calcaneal osteotomy is indicated in children with inflexible hindfoot varus on the Coleman block test.
- Several osteotomies of the midfoot have been proposed for surgical reconstruction of a cavus foot. These osteotomies all involve removing a dorsally based V-shaped wedge of the bone from the midfoot at or just proximal to the apex of the cavus deformity.

Complications

- Simultaneous plantar fascia release should be avoided with an Achilles tendon lengthening. An intact Achilles tendon provides the resistance necessary to stretch the divided plantar tissues.

Bibliography

1. Brewerton D, Sandifer P, Sweetnam D. "Idiopathic" pes cavus: an investigation into its aetiology. Br Med J. 1963;2:659.
2. Mosca VS. The cavus foot. J Pediatr Orthop. 2001;21:423.
3. Paulos L, Coleman S, Samuelson K. Pes cavovarus: review of a surgical approach using selective soft-tissue procedures. J Bone Joint Surg Am. 1980;62:942.
4. Watanabe RS. Metatarsal osteotomy for the cavus foot. Clin Orthop Relat Res. 1990;252:217.

5 Flexible Flatfoot

Ashok Johari, Ratna Maheshwari, and Shalin Maheshwari

Take-Home Message

- It is rarely symptomatic, is common in childhood and resolves spontaneously in most cases.
- It is an anatomic variant, and not a potentially disabling deformity.
- The differential of flatfoot includes tarsal coalition, congenital vertical talus and accessory navicular.
- Surgery is reserved for rare cases in which pain is recalcitrant to nonsurgical treatment.

Definition

- Flexible flatfoot is a physiologic variation of normal. It is defined by a decreased longitudinal arch and a valgus hindfoot during weight bearing. Flexibility refers to the mobility of the subtalar joint and longitudinal arch and ability of both to reverse their malalignment.
- Flexible flatfoot is present in 20–25 % of adults.

Aetiology

- It is an anatomic variant, and not a potentially disabling deformity.

Pathoanatomy

- Generalised ligamentous laxity is common.
- Subclinical muscle weakness is a theory supported by many.
- The role of intrinsic muscles and extrinsic factors like shoe wear have been investigated.
- Approximately one fourth of flexible flatfeet have a contracture of the gastrocnemius–soleus complex. Only these cases are associated with disability.

Evaluation

- An arch should be evident when toe-standing, dorsiflexing the hallux or not weight bearing.
- Subtalar motion should be full and painless.
- On a lateral radiograph, the talus is plantar flexed relative to the first metatarsal (Meary angle has a plantar apex). Also there is plantar flexion of the calcaneus, measured by the calcaneal pitch.
- Dorsiflexion of the navicular on the head of the plantar-flexed talus creates a midfoot sag. It can also be used to assess the accessory navicular bone.
- Apparent hindfoot valgus may actually be due to ankle valgus (particularly in children with myelodysplasia). If there is any suspicion of ankle valgus, ankle radiographs should be obtained.

Classification Flatfoot should be categorised into three groups:

- Flexible flatfoot without tight heel cord
- Flexible flatfoot with tight heel cord
- Rigid flatfoot

The differential of flatfoot includes tarsal coalition, congenital vertical talus and accessory navicular.

Management

- No treatment is indicated for asymptomatic patients.
- Nonsurgical
  - Shoes or orthoses do not promote arch development.
  - Use of athletic shoes with arch and heel support can help relieve pain.
  - The University of California Biomechanics Lab (UCBL) orthosis is a rigid orthotic insert designed to support the arch and control the hindfoot. The rigid material may be poorly tolerated. A soft moulded insert is an alternative but may be inadequate to control hindfoot valgus.
  - In the presence of the contracted Achilles tendon, it may prevent normal dorsiflexion of the ankle joint and shifts the stress to the subtalar joint. An aggressive stretching programme for the Achilles tendon, performed with subtalar inversion, may relieve symptoms.
- Surgical
  - Surgery is reserved for rare cases in which pain is recalcitrant to nonsurgical treatment.
  - Procedures that rely entirely on soft-tissue plications and tendon transfers fail in short term.
  - A calcaneal neck lengthening with soft-tissue balancing is the treatment of choice. It corrects deformity while preserving motion and growth. Arthrodesis and arthroereisis are rarely, if ever, indicated.

Bibliography

1. Harris RJ, Beath T. Army foot survey: an investigation of foot ailments in Canadian soldiers. Ottawa: National Research Council of Canada; 1947.
2. Koutsogiannis E. Treatment of mobile flatfoot by displacement osteotomy of the calcaneus. J Bone Joint Surg Br. 1971;53:96.
3. Meary R. On the measurement of the angle between the talus and the first metatarsal. Symposium: Le Pied Creux Essential. Rev Chir Orthop. 1967;53:389.
4. Mosca VS. Flexible flatfoot and skewfoot. In: Drennan JC, editor. The child's foot and ankle. New York: Raven; 1992. p. 355.
5. Rao U, Joseph B. The influence of footwear on the prevalence of flatfoot: a survey of 2300 children. J Bone Joint Surg Br. 1992;64:525.
6. Steel MI, Johnson K, DeWitz M, et al. Radiographic measurements of normal adult foot. Foot Ankle. 1980;1:151.

6 Skewfoot

Ashok Johari, Ratna Maheshwari, and Shalin Maheshwari

Take-Home Message
- This deformity combines adduction deformity of forefoot with valgus deformity of the hindfoot.
- Can be idiopathic or occur due to improper cast treatment of metatarsus adductus and club foot.
- Surgery is indicated when nonoperative management fails to relieve pain or callosities.

Definition
- It is a poorly defined foot shape that combines adduction deformity of forefoot with valgus deformity of hindfoot.
- Disability caused by this condition is most often related to hindfoot deformity.

Aetiology
- Idiopathic
- Can occur due to improper cast treatment of metatarsus adductus and club foot

Pathogenesis
- Can be created in a foot with metatarsus adductus by applying abduction pressure to the forefoot without stabilising the hindfoot.
- Idiopathic cases—the medial cuneiform is trapezoid shaped. A thickened portion of tibialis anterior courses along an oblique dorsal-to-plantar groove on the concave medial border of the medial cuneiform.

Evaluation
- It is challenging to differentiate metatarsus adductus from skewfoot in an infant. In some infant feet with forefoot adductus, the subtalar joint is sufficiently everted so that the head of the talus can be visualised and palpated medially.
- Valgus deformity of the hindfoot, with adduction of the forefoot, can be better appreciated in older children.
- The skew deformity is present in both the frontal and sagittal planes in the radiographs.

Management
The prevalence of long-term disability attributable to residual deformity, which does not undergo resolution, is unknown. But children can have pain, callosities and difficulty wearing shoes, as early as the first decade of life.

- In infancy, it is reasonable to treat all feet with partly flexible and inflexible adductus with serial long-leg casting. It may take longer to correct a skewfoot. Valgus stress must be avoided.

- Older children having pain under the prominent head of plantar-flexed talus have contracture of the Achilles tendon. Attempts can be made to stretch the tendon by means of exercises and cast.
- Surgery is indicated when nonoperative management fails to relieve pain or callosities. Correction of symptomatic skewfoot can be done for the individual deformities of the forefoot and hindfoot. Calcaneal lengthening osteotomy, medial cuneiform opening wedge osteotomy and lengthening of the Achilles tendon can be combined for a satisfactory result.

Complications

- Painful callus can develop under the head of the talus.
- Shoe may wear unevenly in untreated cases.

Bibliography

1. Berg E. A reappraisal of metatarsus adductus and skewfoot. J Bone Joint Surg Am. 1986;68:1185.
2. McCormick DW, Blount WP. Metatarsus adductovarus: "skewfoot". JAMA. 1949;141:449.
3. Mosca VS. Skewfoot deformity in children: correction by calcaneal neck lengthening and medial cuneiform opening wedge osteotomies. J Pediatr Orthop. 1993;13:807.
4. Mosca VS. Flexible flatfoot and skewfoot. Instr Course Lect. 1996;45:347.
5. Peterson H. Skewfoot (forefoot adduction with heel valgus). J Pediatr Orthop. 1986;6:24.

7 Tarsal Coalition

Ashok Johari, Ratna Maheshwari, and Shalin Maheshwari

Take-Home Message

- Preoperative CT assessment is helpful before tarsal coalition excision because multiple coalitions are present in 10–20 % of feet with tarsal coalition.
- The most common solitary coalitions are talocalcaneal (usually involving the middle or anterior facets of the subtalar joint) and calcaneonavicular.
- Tarsal coalitions most commonly present as rigid pes planovalgus foot. However, equinovarus deformity or forefoot inversion may occur in some forms of massive and multiple tarsal coalitions.
- Apparent hindfoot valgus may actually be the result of ankle valgus. If there is any suspicion of ankle valgus, radiographic views of the ankle should be obtained.

- Harris axial radiographs have a high false-positive rate for tarsal coalition. If the view is slightly oblique to the posterior or middle facet, it will appear as if a coalition is present when it is not.
- Tarsal coalitions are bilateral in 50–60 % of cases.

Definition

Tarsal coalition is a failure of segmentation of mesenchymal tissue in the hind- and midfoot with secondary failure of formation of the normal hindfoot or midfoot joints. It can be osseous, cartilaginous or fibrous connection between the bones.

Classification with Aetiology

- Solitary coalitions: They involve part of two adjacent tarsal bones. The most common solitary coalitions include talocalcaneal and calcaneonavicular.
- Massive coalitions: Associated with other limb anomalies, in particular, fibular hemimelia, proximal focal femoral deficiency and Apert syndrome.
- Multiple tarsal coalitions are seen in genetic syndromes such as multiple synostosis syndromes where coalitions of carpal bones, symphalangism and congenital fusion of the elbow may also be present.

Pathophysiology

- The lack of segmentation of the cartilaginous anlage occurs, and it is possible that a fibrous connection between bones undergoes metaplasia to cartilage (syndesmosis to synchondrosis) and finally to synostosis.
- The onset of symptoms usually coincides with the transition of a cartilaginous coalition to the bone during late childhood and early adolescence, causing restriction of subtalar motion. Pain can be associated with stress fracture at the time of progressive ossification or limited and altered mobility of joints.

Evaluation

Clinical Presentation

Child presents with rigid planovalgus foot. Failure to reconstitute a medial longitudinal arch when the child attempts to go into a weight-bearing equinus position is seen. Restriction of subtalar and/or midtarsal joints may occur.

Radiology

- Standing anteroposterior, lateral radiographs and a non-weight-bearing oblique radiograph should be done.
- The calcaneonavicular bar is visualised on the oblique radiograph; on the lateral radiograph, the "anteater" sign is often seen. This represents the ossified bar as it extends from the calcaneus to the navicular.

- Talocalcaneal bars are difficult to visualise on the lateral radiograph, and all that is seen is a valgus foot, a C sign and, perhaps, talar beaking.
- Secondary degenerative arthritis may develop in subtalar and midtarsal joints over a period of time if they are left untreated.

Other Investigations

Since radiographs may often be negative for talocalcaneal coalitions, fine cut CT scan is a must in the child with "peroneal spastic foot". Also since only solitary coalitions are resected, it is important that the surgeon confirm the same with a CT scan. It is also useful to quantitate the area of the joint involved. Patients having less than a third of the joint surface involved have a high likelihood of success with resection.

Treatment

Nonoperative: Those who present with minimal pain need only simple shoe modifications. These may include heel cups, medial longitudinal arch supports or other orthotics. Trial of immobilisation in short-leg cast may be of help if patients are more symptomatic.

Operative: This should be considered in children where nonoperative interventions have failed to relieve symptoms. Resection of coalitions can be considered if they are solitary, with no degenerative changes in the joints.

Calcaneonavicular coalitions: The mainstay procedure is resection of the cartilaginous or osseous bar with interposition of the extensor digitorum brevis muscle belly.

The talocalcaneal coalition: The bar, which involves the anterior and middle facet of the subtalar joint, is identified from a medial approach and excised from a superior direction, leaving the sustentaculum tali untouched. After bar resection, bone wax is first placed onto the raw surfaces, followed by a fat graft.

Subtalar or triple arthrodesis: This procedure is reserved for failed resections or coalitions associated with degenerative changes.

Bibliography

1. Comfort TK, Johnson LO. Resection for symptomatic talocalcaneal coalition. J Pediatr Orthop. 1998;18:283–8.
2. Harris R, Beath T. Etiology of peroneal spastic flatfoot. J Bone Joint Surg Br. 1948;30:624.
3. Rebello G, Joseph B. The foot in multiple synostoses syndromes. J Foot Ankle Surg. 2003;9:19–24.
4. Wilde PH, Torode IP, Dickens DR, Cole WG. Resection for symptomatic talocalcaneal coalition. J Bone Joint Surg Br. 1994;76:797–801.

Neuromuscular Conditions

Ashok Johari, Ratna Maheshwari, and Shalin Maheshwari

1 Myelodysplasia

Ashok Johari, Ratna Maheshwari, and Shalin Maheshwari

Take-Home Message

- Supplementation with folic acid decreases the risk of myelodysplasia, but only if taken in the first weeks following conception.
- Serial neurologic examinations are critical. Changes in strength and/or spasticity are early signs of a tethered cord.
- Prior to kyphectomy surgery, ventriculoperitoneal (VP) shunt function must be checked. It must be patent and functioning or the patient must be shunt independent.
- Hip dislocations in children with myelodysplasia rarely require treatment.
- Fusions should be avoided during foot surgery to decrease the risk of pressure sores.
- Prenatal diagnosis via maternal serum α-fetoprotein is 60–95 % accurate.
- L4 level or lower (active quadriceps) is considered necessary for community ambulation.

A. Johari, MD (✉) • R. Maheshwari, MD • S. Maheshwari, MD
Pediatric Orthopedics, Childrens' Orthopedic Centre, Mumbai, India
e-mail: drashokjohari@hotmail.com

C. Mauffrey, D.J. Hak (eds.), *Passport for the Orthopedic Boards and FRCS Examination*, DOI 10.1007/978-2-8178-0475-0_26

Definition
Myelodysplasia is part of a spectrum of deformities resulting from failure of closure of the neural tube late in the first month following conception.

Etiology

- Multifactorial pattern of inheritance.
- Environmental factors include genetic, geography, and drugs (valproic acid and carbamazepine).
- History of previously affected pregnancy, low folic acid intake, pregestational maternal diabetes, high maternal alcohol intake.

Pathoanatomy

- Lesions can occur at any level along the spinal column but predominate in the lumbosacral area. The next most common site is the cervical spine.
- The basic deformity of myelomeningocele is an open neural placode, which represents the embryologic form of the caudal end of the spinal cord. A narrow groove passes down the placode in the midline. This represents the primitive neural groove and is directly continuous with the central canal of the closed spinal cord above (and occasionally below) the neural placode.

Classification
Spina bifida may be subdivided into:

- Spina bifida cystica, where there is a visible cyst present
- Spina bifida occulta, where the defect is hidden but may be suspected because of the presence of a dimple, a patch of hair, pigmentation, or a lipoma
- Types of spina bifida cystic
- Myeloschisis – The vertebral arches are deficient with neural plate material spread out in the surface, commonly over a cystic swelling of the meninges.
- Myelomeningocele – This is a cystic swelling lined by dura and arachnoid, protruding through a defect in the vertebral arches. The spinal cord and nerve roots are carried into the fundus of the sac.
- Meningocele – It is a cystic swelling of dura and arachnoid, protruding through a defect in the vertebral arches under the skin. The cord is confined within the vertebral arches.

Evaluation
Antenatal diagnosis:

- Maternal serum alpha-fetoprotein is usually tested routinely as a screening test between the 16th and 20th week of pregnancy.
- Ultrasound at 16–18 weeks identifies virtually all anencephalics and over 80 % of spina bifidas.

Assessment of neurosegmental levels: (Table 1)

Treatment

- Walking ability is related to level of paralysis, knee flexion deformity, mental status, family compliance, and gait training. It is not related to hip reduction status.

Table 1 Motor level and functional status for myelomeningocele

Lesion level	Muscle involvement	Function
Thoracic	No active movement of limbs	Sitter
L1	Iliopsoas grade 2 or better	Wheelchair dependant
L2	Iliopsoas, sartorius, and adductors grade 3 or better	Possible household ambulators with RGO
L3	Quadriceps grade 3 or better	Household/community ambulator with KAFO or AFO
L4	Medial hamstring or tibialis anterior grade 3 or better	Significant difference between L3 and L4 level, medial hamstring needed for community ambulation
L5	Lateral hamstrings grade 3 or better + criteria for L4	Community ambulators as adults, wheelchair for long distances
	Gluteus medius grade 2 or better	
	Peroneus tertius grade 4 or better	
	Tibialis posterior grade 3 or better	
Sacral	Quadriceps and gluteus medius function	Community ambulator with AFO, UCBL, or none
High sacral	No gastrosoleus strength	Community ambulator with AFO, UCBL, or none. May have gluteus lurch and excessive pelvic obliquity and rotation during gait
Low sacral	Good gastrocnemius-soleus strength, normal gluteus medius, maximus	Walk without AFO, gait close to normal

RGO reciprocating gait orthosis, *UCBL* University of California/Berkeley Lab (orthosis), *KAFO* knee-ankle-foot orthosis, *AFO* ankle-foot orthosis, *HKAFO* hip-knee-ankle-foot orthosis

- The long-term medical and skeletal issues associated with myelodysplasia are often best addressed by multidisciplinary teams.
  - Nonsurgical treatment
    - Frequent skin checks for pressure sores.
    - Well-fitting braces and wheelchairs are important because these patients often have significant sensory deficits.
    - Rehabilitation efforts should include early mobilisation, PT, bracing, and functional wheelchair fitting.
    - Bracing – Hip-knee-ankle-foot orthoses (HKAFOs), knee-ankle-foot orthoses (KAFOs), or AFOs are frequently used to support stance and/or to prevent contracture.
  - Surgical
    - Spine – Neurosurgeons perform closure of myelomeningocele within 48 h with a shunt for hydrocephalus. Later issues can develop with the shunt, a tethered cord, or syrinx, so diligent neurologic examinations need to be repeated and documented.

  - Tethered cord can cause progressive scoliosis, change functional levels, or cause spasticity.
  - Syrinx, shunt problems, or new hydrocephalus can cause new upper extremity symptoms such as weakness or increasing spasticity.
  - Arnold-Chiari malformation is often addressed with shunting in infancy but may require later decompression.
  - Scoliosis and kyphosis may be progressive. Ninety per cent of patients with thoracic myelodysplasia may require kyphectomy and posterior fusion. Prior to kyphectomy, it is important to check shunt function, because shunt failure can result in acute hydrocephalus and death when the spinal cord is tied off during the kyphectomy.
  - Scoliosis may cause suprapelvic obliquity increasing the risk of decubitus ulcer formation, sitting problems, and impaired hand function. Severe or progressive deformity must be corrected and the pelvis must be levelled to distribute skin loading evenly under the pelvis.
  - Poor soft-tissue coverage, contractures, impaired sensation, fragile bone, and deficient posterior elements complicate treatment. Pseudoarthrosis rates are decreased with combined anterior-posterior fusions and rigid segmental instrumentation.

- Hip
  - Flexion contractures are common but are often not severe. If the contracture is >40° in patients with lower lumbar level involvement, they may require flexor release.
  - Hip dysplasia and/or dislocation – Currently, the trend in treatment is not to reduce a dislocated hip in any child with myelodysplasia, as the recurrence rate is high.
  - Operative indications include painful dysplasia in the ambulatory patient and fixed pelvic obliquity, which makes sitting difficult or skin care unmanageable.

- Knee
  - Flexion contracture >20° should be treated with hamstring lengthening, capsular release, and/or distal femoral extension osteotomy. There is, however, a significant rate of recurrence after extension osteotomy in growing children.
  - Extension contracture can be treated with serial casting or V-Y quadriceps lengthening.
  - Knee valgus, often with associated external tibial torsion and femoral anteversion, is common in patients with midlumbar level involvement because they lack functional hip abductors and have a significant trunk shift when walking with AFOs. This can be addressed by the use of KAFOs or crutches with AFOs.
  - External tibial torsion can be addressed with a distal tibial derotational osteotomy.

– Foot

  - About 30 % of children with myelodysplasia have a rigid clubfoot. This deformity in myelomeningocele patients is truly teratologic, in that the deformity is nearly always rigid, with less propensity to respond to conservative treatment; requires extensive surgery to correct; and is likely to recur. It can be initially managed with serial casting. It may need extensive posteromedial release, in addition to bony procedures or salvage procedures like talectomy.
  - With surgical treatment, a portion of the tendons (e.g. Achilles, posterior tibialis, FHL, flexor digitorum communis [FDC]) may be resected rather than lengthened to decrease the risk of recurrence.
  - Calcaneus foot position can occur with unopposed tibialis anterior (L3–L4 level). Manage with an orthotic, anterior tibialis and ankle release, tenodesis of the tendoachilles, or transfer of the anterior tibialis to the Achilles tendon.
  - Equinovarus, equinus, and calcaneal foot deformities often are best treated with simple tenotomy rather than tendon transfer, achieving a flail but braceable foot.
  - Valgus foot deformities are common in L4–L5 level patients. If surgery is necessary to achieve a plantigrade foot, fusion should be avoided to maintain foot flexibility and to decrease the risk of pressure sores.
  - Planovalgus foot is best managed by calcaneal lengthening, which provides correction and maintains foot mobility.
  - Vertical talus deformities require operative correction during the first year. Correct with a single-stage procedure.
  - Cavus deformity often causes skin breakdown and significant disability. Manage in two stages. First perform a plantar medial release. Follow with osteotomies and tendon transfers to maintain correction.
  - Toe deformities include dorsal bunion, clawing, or simple flexion deformities. Manage by releases and osteotomies to preserve function. Avoid fusions when possible.
  - Ankle valgus is secondary to a triangular distal tibial epiphysis. Manage by placing a medial malleolar screw that restricts medial physeal growth to correct the valgus. A valgus deformity at the end of growth may require a distal tibial osteotomy for correction.

Complications

- Pathologic fractures may follow minimal trauma, manipulative treatments, or operative procedures. Pathologic fractures may be confused with osteomyelitis.
- Cord tethering is suggested by loss of function, increasing deformity, or pain.
- Skin breakdown includes sacral decubitus and foot ulcers. Reduce risk by correcting rigid foot deformities and severe pelvic obliquity.
- Latex allergy occurs in about 5 % of patients.

Bibliography

1. Beaty JH, Canale ST. Orthopaedic aspects of myelomeningocele. J Bone Joint Surg Am. 1990;72:626–30.
2. Frischhut B, et al. Foot deformities in adolescents and young adults with spina bifida. J Pediatr Orthop B. 2000;9:161.
3. Gabrieli AP, Vankoski SJ, Dias LS, Milani C, Lourenco A, Filho JL, Novak R. Gait analysis in low lumbar myelomeningocele patients with unilateral hip dislocation or subluxation. J Pediatr Orthop. 2003;23:330–6.
4. Rodgers WB, Frim DM, Emans JB. Surgery of the spine in myelodysplasia. An overview. Clin Orthop Relat Res. 1997;338:19.
5. Snela S, Parsch K. Follow-up study after treatment of knee flexion contractures in spina bifida patients. J Pediatr Orthop B. 2000;9:154.
6. Thompson JD. Myelomeningocele. In: Abel MF, editor. Orthopaedic knowledge update: pediatrics 3. Rosemont: American Academy of Orthopaedic Surgeons; 2006. p. 111–22.

2 Hereditary Motor Sensory Neuropathy

Ashok Johari, Ratna Maheshwari, and Shalin Maheshwari

Take-Home Message

- The most common cause of bilateral cavus feet is Charcot-Marie-Tooth disease.
- If foot surgery is required, soft-tissue balancing and avoidance of fusions are important.
- Scoliosis is very common and often does not respond to brace treatment.

Definition

- These are a group of variously inherited chronic progressive peripheral neuropathies.

Pathoanatomy/Classification

- HMSN I (myelinopathy Charcot-Marie-Tooth disease)
  - HMSN I is the most common HMSN (1 in 2,500 children). The age at onset is the first to second decade of life.
  - Peripheral myelin degeneration occurs with decreased motor nerve conduction. Peroneal muscle weakness, absent deep tendon reflexes. EMG is slow (<38 mm/s).

  - HMSN I is commonly caused by a mutation in 17p11 (*PMP-22*) or X-linked connexin 32.
  - Autosomal dominant inheritance is most common but can also be autosomal recessive, X-linked, or sporadic.
- HMSN II (neuropathy Charcot-Marie-Tooth disease)
  - The myelin sheath is intact, but Wallerian axonal degeneration occurs. The age at onset is the second decade of life or later
  - Characterised by persistently normal reflexes, sensory and motor nerve conduction times are only mildly abnormal.
  - Autosomal dominant inheritance is most common, but it can also be autosomal recessive, X-linked, or sporadic.
- HMSN III (Dejerine-Sottas disease)
  - HMSN III is characterised by peripheral nerve demyelination with severely decreased motor nerve conduction.
  - Autosomal recessive inheritance is common, with the mutation in the *MPZ* gene.
  - HMSN III presents in infancy.
  - It is characterised by enlarged peripheral nerves, ataxia, and nystagmus. The patient stops walking by maturity.

Evaluation

- Diagnosis is made by conduction testing and genetic studies.
- Biopsy of muscle and nerve can confirm the same.

Management

- The major orthopaedic problems include pes cavovarus, hip dysplasia, spinal deformity, and hand and upper extremity dysfunction.
- HMSN commonly presents as distal weakness, affecting intrinsic and extrinsic muscles.
- Cavus foot
  - It develops from contracted plantar fascia, weak tibialis anterior, weak peroneals, and tight foot intrinsic muscles with normal FDL and FHL. The peroneus longus is generally somewhat stronger than the peroneus brevis and anterior tibialis. As the first metatarsal becomes increasingly plantarflexed, there is increasing hindfoot varus.
  - Surgery typically involves plantar release and posterior tibial tendon transfer to the dorsum or split posterior tibial tendon transfer.
  - Forefoot equinus should be corrected with plantar release and possibly midfoot osteotomies.
  - Achilles tendon lengthening is occasionally needed, but only if there is true hindfoot equinus.

- Osteotomies to correct bony deformities in adolescence include a calcaneal osteotomy (Dwyer) for fixed hindfoot varus (determined by Coleman block test).
- Fusions should be avoided as far as possible to maintain flexibility.

• Hip dysplasia

- Typical findings include acetabular dysplasia, coxa valga, and subluxation.
- Soft-tissue releases can be used to correct contractures and restore muscle balance.
- Pelvic or proximal femoral varus derotation osteotomies may be needed to stabilise and adequately realign the hip.

• Spinal deformity

- Scoliosis or kyphoscoliosis is seen in 15–37 % of children with HMSN and up to 50 % of patients with HMSN who are skeletally mature – more commonly in HMSN I and girls
- Orthotic management can be effective in arresting deformity in a minority of cases.
- If progression reaches 45–50°, a posterior spinal fusion and segmental spinal instrumentation can effectively stabilise the deformity.
- Intraoperative somatosensory cortical-evoked potentials may show no signal transmission because of the underlying disease.

• Claw toes may become rigid and require treatment, such as IP fusion, often in conjunction with Jones transfers of the extensor tendons to the metatarsal heads.
• Hand intrinsics, thenar, and hypothenar muscles may also show wasting, creating clawing of the thenar and hypothenar eminences, limiting thumb abduction, and compromising pinch power. Surgically, sometimes transfer of the FDS, nerve decompression, contracture releases, and joint arthrodesis may be helpful.

Bibliography

1. Daher YH, Lonstein JE, Winter RB, Bradford DS. Spinal deformities in patients with Charcot-Marie-tooth disease. A review of 12 patients. Clin Orthop. 1986;202:219.
2. Pailthorpe CA, Benson MKD'A. Hip dysplasia in hereditary motor and sensory neuropathies. J Bone Joint Surg Br. 1992;74:538.
3. Paulos L, Coleman SS, Samuelson KM. Pes cavovarus. Review of a surgical approach using selective soft-tissue procedures. J Bone Joint Surg Am. 1980;62:942.
4. Shapiro F, Bresnan MJ. Current concepts review. Orthopaedic management of childhood neuromuscular disease. Part 2: peripheral neuropathies, Friedreich's ataxia and arthrogryposis multiplex congenital. J Bone Joint Surg Am. 1982;64:949.
5. Walker JL, Nelson KR, Stevens DB, et al. Spinal deformity in Charcot-Marie – tooth disease. Spine. 1994;19:1044.

3 Friedreich Ataxia

Ashok Johari, Ratna Maheshwari, and Shalin Maheshwari

Take-Home Message

- Friedrich ataxia (FA) is the most common form of the uncommon spino-cerebellar degenerative diseases. It occurs in 1 in 50,000 births.
- Clinical triad of ataxia, areflexia of knees and ankles, and a positive plantar response. Onset is before age of 25 years.
- The age of onset of the disease is related to the number of GAA repeats.
- Common orthopaedic problems include pes cavovarus and scoliosis.

Definition

It is the most common form of spinocerebellar degenerative disease, characterised by slow and progressive spinocerebellar degeneration.

Etiology and Pathophysiology

- Autosomal recessive
- Defect on chromosome 9q13
- Trinucleotide repeat of GAA, results in loss of expression of frataxin protein

Evaluation

- Clinical triad of ataxia, areflexia of knees and ankles, and a positive plantar response. Onset is before age of 25 years. High incidence of scoliosis is present.
- Most individuals are wheelchair bound by second or third decade.
- Muscle weakness is usually symmetric, initially proximal, and more severe in lower extremities. The first muscle to be involved is the gluteus maximus.
- Death is usually due to progressive hypertrophic cardiomyopathy, pneumonia, or aspiration.
- Nerve conduction studies show decreased or absent sensory action potentials in the digital and sural nerves.
- EMG shows loss of motor units and increase in polyphasic potentials.

Treatment

The major orthopaedic problems are pes cavovarus, spinal deformity, and painful muscle spasms.

- Pes cavovarus
  - Orthotics is usually ineffective.
  - Surgical procedures can be used in ambulatory patients to improve balance and walking ability. Tendoachilles lengthening and tibialis posterior

tenotomy, lengthening, and anterior transfer to dorsum of foot are all shown to be effective procedures.
  - In fixed and rigid deformities, triple arthrodesis may be necessary to achieve a plantigrade foot.

- Spinal deformity
  - Scoliosis essentially occurs in all patients with Friedrich ataxia.
  - If disease onset is before 10 years of age and scoliosis is before 15 years of age, most patient curves usually progress to greater than 60°.
  - Pattern of scoliosis are similar to adolescent idiopathic scoliosis. About two-thirds of patients develop an associated kyphosis.
- A TLSO may be tried in ambulatory patients having 25–40° curves. In progressive curves greater than 60°, especially in older adolescents, a single-stage posterior spinal fusion stabilises the curve.
  - Fusion to sacrum is usually unnecessary except in C-shaped thoracolumbar curves with associated pelvic obliquity.
  - Anterior surgery, with or without instrumentation, usually followed by a posterior spinal fusion and instrumentation is limited to rigid curves greater than 60° associated with poor sitting balance.

- Painful muscle spasms
  - Hip adductors and knee extensors are commonly involved. If conservative measures like heat or muscle relaxants fail, then patients may benefit by tenotomies.

Complications

- Thorough evaluation is a must before surgical intervention to avoid cardiopulmonary problems.

Bibliography

1. Chamberlain S, Shaw J, Rowland A, et al. Mapping of mutation causing Friedreich's ataxia to human chromosome 9. Nature. 1998;334:248.
2. Labelle H, Tohme S, Duhaime M, et al. Natural history of scoliosis in Friedreich's ataxia. J Bone Joint Surg Am. 1986;68:564.
3. Labelle H, Beauchomp M, LaPierre Duhaime M, Allard P. Pattern of muscle weakness and its relation to loss of ambulatory function in Friedreich's ataxia. J Pediatr Orthop. 1987;7:496.
4. Labelle H, Duhaime M, Allard P. Spinal deformities in Friedreich's ataxia. In: Weinstein SL, editor. The pediatric spine: principles of practise. New York: Raven; 1994. p. 999.
5. Shapiro F, Specht L. Current concepts review. The diagnosis and orthopaedic treatment of childhood spinal muscular atrophy, peripheral neuropathy, Friedreich ataxia and arthrogryposis. J Bone Joint Surg Am. 1993;75: 1699.

4 Poliomyelitis

Ashok Johari, Ratna Maheshwari, and Shalin Maheshwari

Take-Home Message

- The paralysis in poliomyelitis is asymmetric. In the presence of symmetric paralysis of limbs and trunk, a paralytic disease other than poliomyelitis should be considered.
- Fusion of foot in corrected position should be combined with tendon rerouting to restore balance, or else deformity will recur.
- Because triple arthrodesis may exert excessive ligamentous strain on ankle joint, it is imperative to determine the stability of body of talus in ankle mortise.

Definition

Polio is caused by a viral infection localised in the anterior horn cells of the spinal cord and certain brainstem motor nuclei.

Etiology

- The virus a member of enteroviral group has 3 subtypes.
- The route of transmission is from the gastrointestinal and respiratory tract hematogenously to the CNS.

Pathoanatomy

- The lumbar and cervical enlargements of the cord are most commonly affected.
- The anterior horn cells get damaged directly by the viral cytotoxicity and indirectly by ischemia, edema, and hemorrhage in the surrounding tissue.
- Destruction in spinal cord is evident focally following which Wallerian degeneration begins.

Stages

- Acute stage: Lasts up to 10 days. Symptoms range from mild malaise to generalised encephalomyelitis with widespread paralysis.
- Convalescent stage: Begins 2 days after the temperature returns to normal and continues for 2 years. Muscle power improves spontaneously during this stage.
- Chronic stage: Usually begins 24 months after the acute illness.

Treatment

Early recognition, postural care, physiotherapy, corrective plastering, traction, and orthosis are useful.

Treatment of fixed deformities

- Shoulder: If scapular muscles are strong arthrodesis is a good option.
- Elbow and forearm: Transferring the flexor origin more proximally can restore elbow flexion.
- Pronation can be strengthened by transferring the active FCU tendon across the forearm to the radial border.
- Supination can be restored by transferring the ECU across the back of the forearm.
- Wrist deformity: It is treated by arthrodesis.
- Thumb opposition: It is restored by Bunnel's transfer of FDS of ring finger to first metacarpal.
- Hip: There is gradual development of subluxation due to the following:
  - Pelvic obliquity associated with scoliosis
  - Growth abnormality of proximal femur leading to persistent increase in anteversion, coxa valga, and underdevelopment of acetabular socket
    - Correction of scoliosis and reducing pelvic obliquity.
    - Overcoming muscle imbalance by suitable tendon transfers – iliopsoas to lateral aspect of greater trochanter (Mustard) or entire iliacus transferred posteriorly (Sharrad's operation), external oblique abdominis muscle transfer for gluteal paralysis.
    - Proximal femoral osteotomy to correct malalignment.
    - Acetabuloplasty can deepen acetabular sockets.
    - Fixed flexion at hip can be treated with Soutter's operation (release of structures from ASIS).
    - Fixed abduction: Young's operation, division of iliotibial tract and fascia lata.
- Knee
  - Instability due to relative weakness of knee extensors can be compensated by putting finger on the front of thigh and pushing knee into extension.
  - Corrected by usage of calliper or supracondylar extension osteotomy.
  - Fixed flexion deformity: Flexor to extensor transfer.
  - Genu recurvatum: Treated by supracondylar flexion osteotomy.
- Foot
  - Instability controlled by below knee calliper and foot drop by toe raising spring.
  - In the immature and supple foot, transfer of suitable power is undertaken for prevention and correction of deformities.
  - Fusion in corrected position should be combined with tendon rerouting to restore balance, or else deformity will recur.
  - Varus/valgus deformities

- Grice green subtalar arthrodesis
- Triple arthrodesis
- Lambrinudi's modification if associated with foot drop

– Calcaneocavus foot: Elmslie's operation
– Claw toes: Transfer of flexors to extensors

Bibliography

1. Das K, Maitra TK, Acharyya B. Management of post polio residual paralysis of lower limb in present Indian scenario. Indian J Orthop. 2004;38(4):226–32.
2. Yount CC. The role of tensor fasciae femoris in certain deformities of the lower extremities. J Bone Joint Surg Am. 1967;40:1275.

5 Spinal Muscular Atrophy

Ashok Johari, Ratna Maheshwari, and Shalin Maheshwari

Take-Home Message

- Progressive weakness starts proximally and moves distally.
- Major orthopaedic abnormality includes soft-tissue contractures of lower extremities, hip subluxation and dislocation, and spinal deformities.
- The course and prognosis of SMA are directly related to the age at onset.
- Scoliosis progression is not impacted by use of a TLSO.
- Hip dislocation rarely requires treatment.

Definition

This is a group of disorders characterised by degeneration of anterior horn cells of spinal cord and occasionally neurons of lower bulbar motor nuclei, resulting in muscle weakness and atrophy.
Spinal muscle atrophy (SMA) is the most common genetic disease resulting in death during childhood, with an incidence of 1 in 10,000 live births.

Pathoanatomy

- Autosomal recessive disorder
- C5 mutations cause deficient survival motor neuron (SMN) protein resulting in progressive loss of α-motor neurons in the anterior horn cells.
- Large-scale deletions involving genes like SMN and NAIP correspond to a more severe phenotype.

- Soft-tissue contracture is the result of progressive muscle degeneration and replacement with fibrous tissue.

Evaluation

- Symmetric limb and trunk weakness and muscle atrophy that affects the lower extremities more than the upper extremities and proximal muscles more than distal muscles.
- Hypotonia and areflexia are present.
- Sensation and intelligence is normal.
- EMG/ NCV and muscle biopsy are used for initial diagnosis. EMG shows typical neuropathic changes, such as increased amplitude and duration of response. Muscle biopsy shows muscle fibre degeneration and atrophy of fibre groups.
- Recent advent of genetic testing is possible for gene deletions.

Classification

Type 1 – Acute Werdnig-Hoffman disease

- Onset between birth and 6 months of age
- Severe involvement with marked weakness and hypotonia
- Usually die from respiratory failure between 1 and 24 months

Type 2 – Chronic Werdnig-Hoffman disease

- Clinical onset varies between 6 and 24 months.
- Less involved than type1, but never able to walk.
- May live into the fourth or fifth decade.

Type 3 – Kugelberg-Welander disease

- Onset is between 2 years and usually before 10 years.
- Walking is possible up to late childhood.
- Motor capacity decreases with time.
- Gowers' sign may be positive.

Treatment

Major orthopaedic abnormality include soft-tissue contractures of lower extremities, hip subluxation and dislocation and spinal deformities.

- Soft-tissue contractures can be delayed with use of orthosis. Wheelchair-bound child and prolonged sitting enhance hip and knee flexion contractures. Even if released, posture causes recurrence.
- Foot deformities such as equinovarus occur commonly. Rarely, if the patient is ambulatory and retains strength, then gastrocnemius-soleus, posterior tibialis, FDL, and FHL tenotomy may be performed to maintain standing and walking.
- Hip subluxation and dislocation – Management can vary from soft-tissue releases, open reduction and capsulorrhaphy, varus derotation osteotomy, or pelvic procedures depending on the severity of the condition, though it is rarely symptomatic and surgery is rarely indicated.
- Spinal deformity – As the curve progresses there is adverse effect on pulmonary function.

Bracing is ineffective in halting progression. But it can improve sitting balance. TLSO is the most commonly used brace. Curves greater than 40° and an FCV greater than 40 % of normal must be surgically stabilised.
A vertical expandable prosthetic titanium rib (VEPTR) for thoracic insufficiency in young patients with SMA II with curves >50° has had good results.
Flexible curves; often can be fused posteriorly only. Fusion may cause an ambulatory child to lose the ability to walk (and may cause temporary loss of upper extremity function) because of loss of trunk motion.
Fixation to pelvis using Galveston technique is common.

Complications

Excessive blood loss, pulmonary complications, neurologic injury, loss of fixation due to osteopenia, pseudoarthrosis. Aggressive preoperative and postoperative respiratory therapy can decrease complications.

Bibliography

1. Gordon N. The spinal muscular atrophies. Dev Med Child Neurol. 1991;33:930.
2. Lonstein JE. The Galveston technique using Luque or Cotrel-Dubousset rods. Orthop Clin North Am. 1994;25:311–20.
3. Shapiro F, Specht L. Current concepts review. The diagnosis and orthopaedic treatment of childhood spinal muscular atrophy, peripheral neuropathy, Friedreich ataxia and arthrogryposis. J Bone Joint Surg Am. 1993;75:1699.

Neuromuscular Junction Conditions

Ashok Johari, Ratna Maheshwari, and Shalin Maheshwari

1 Myasthenia Gravis

Take-Home Message

- The key feature of myasthenia gravis is a history of muscle weakness precipitated by activity, termed *fatigability*.
- A positive edrophonium chloride (Tensilon) test confirms the diagnosis.
- Patients currently considered appropriate candidates for thymectomy are those whose response to anticholinesterase medications and immunosuppressants is unsatisfactory and those who prefer surgery to long-term immunosuppressant therapy.

Definition

- Myasthenia gravis is a rare autoimmune disease in which antibodies are produced to the nicotinic acetylcholine receptor at the neuromuscular junction. As a result, impulses cannot be transmitted properly across the junction, and the patient experiences muscle weakness or paralysis following repetitive activity.
- Only about 10 % of patients with myasthenia gravis are children.

Etiology

- The exact cause is not fully understood. It is an autoimmune disorder, with antibody production against a protein antigen at the motor end plate.

A. Johari, MD (✉) • R. Maheshwari, MD • S. Maheshwari, MD
Pediatric Orthopedics, Childrens' Orthopedic Centre, Mumbai, India
e-mail: drashokjohari@hotmail.com

C. Mauffrey, D.J. Hak (eds.), *Passport for the Orthopedic Boards and FRCS Examination*, DOI 10.1007/978-2-8178-0475-0_27

- The thymus is considered the site of antibody production. Abnormalities of thymus are frequently found in patients with myasthenia gravis.
- Hormonal influence – postpubertal patients are more likely to be seropositive. In early childhood, there is a nearly equal ratio between females and males (1.3–1), whereas after puberty, the vast majority of patients are female.
- Familial cases have also been reported.

Evaluation

- Three patterns of presentation in children have been described, based on age at onset and clinical features.
  - Neonatal transient myasthenia gravis
    - Generalized muscle weakness, paucity of movement, weak suck, facial weakness, ptosis, and respiratory weakness. Failure to thrive can be a significant problem because of the infant's inability to suck.
    - The symptoms are present at birth and begin to resolve spontaneously within about 4 weeks.
    - The cause of the disease appears to be the passage of maternal antibodies to the acetylcholine receptor through the placenta to the fetus.
    - As the antibodies are destroyed or excreted, the clinical symptoms disappear, usually by 6 weeks of age.
    - The disease can be fatal if untreated, but affected newborns respond to neostigmine therapy. Exchange plasmapheresis is advocated for infants with generalized weakness and high-dose immune globulin therapy has also been used.
  - Congenital myasthenic syndromes
    - Congenital myasthenic syndromes are a group of genetically inherited diseases characterized by an abnormal response to acetylcholine, resulting in myasthenia. In many of these forms, the acetylcholine receptor is abnormal. Congenital myasthenic syndromes are not autoimmune.
    - Most present within the first year of life. Affected infants have poor suck and a weak cry. The spectrum of disease ranges from mild weakness to severe disability with life-threatening respiratory compromise.
    - Patients may present with the typical contractures of arthrogryposis multiplex congenita. Congenital contractures of the extremities may resolve with medical treatment of the myasthenia. Camptodactyly has been reported in these patients. Scoliosis may occur in older children.
  - Juvenile myasthenia gravis
    - The age at onset is 10 years or older.
    - These children most often present with ptosis and ophthalmoparesis or ophthalmoplegia.
    - Weakness of the upper and lower extremities occurs in fewer children, with the weakness more pronounced later in the day.

  - Facial weakness produces a sad expression or flat affect. Weakness in mastication and dysarthria can occur.
  - Respiratory difficulty, which is known as myasthenic crisis, occurs in 40 % of untreated patients and can be fatal.
  - Usually the disease worsens during the first 2 years following onset. However, patients may experience periods of remission lasting months or even years.

- Diagnostic tests
  - A positive edrophonium chloride (Tensilon) test confirms the diagnosis.
  - Electrophysiologic testing can also establish the diagnosis of myasthenia gravis.
  - Assays for anti-acetylcholine receptor antibodies are available.

Management

- Anticholinesterase therapy with neostigmine or pyridostigmine bromide is often used for long-term medical management. Glucocorticosteroids are also commonly used. Plasmapheresis can be helpful in decreasing the amount of antibody to acetylcholine. Intravenous immunoglobulin G has been used to treat rapidly progressive weakness and myasthenic crisis but is of limited benefit as a long-term treatment.
- Surgical treatment consists of removal of the thymus, which is believed to be the primary site of antibody production. Patients currently considered appropriate candidates for thymectomy are those whose response to anticholinesterase medications and immunosuppressants is unsatisfactory and those who prefer surgery to long-term immunosuppressant therapy. Approximately 60 % of children with myasthenia gravis have a good response following thymectomy.

Bibliography

1. Adams C, Theodorescu D, Murphy EG, et al. Thymectomy in juvenile myasthenia gravis. J Child Neurol. 1990;5:215.
2. Bassan H, Muhlbaur B, Tomer A, et al. High-dose intravenous immunoglobulin in transient neonatal myasthenia gravis. Pediatr Neurol. 1998;18:181.
3. Hageman G, Smit LM, Hoogland RA, et al. Muscle weakness and congenital contractures in a case of congenital myasthenia. J Pediatr Orthop. 1986;6:227.
4. Millichap J, Dodge P. Diagnosis and treatment of myasthenia gravis in infancy, childhood, and adolescence: a study of 51 patients. Neurology. 1960;10:1007.

Conditions Affecting Muscle Tissue

Ashok Johari, Ratna Maheshwari, and Shalin Maheshwari

1 Muscular Dystrophies: Duchenne, Beckers, Facioscapulohumeral Dystrophies

Take-Home Message

- Pseudohypertrophy of the calf is classic for DMD, although present in only about 85 % of patients.
- Steroids, when tolerated, slow the progression of DMD. Unfortunately, they are often poorly tolerated because of their significant side effects.
- Early posterior instrumented fusion (curves ≥20°) is recommended in DMD because 95 % of such curves are progressive and because of progressive cardiopulmonary deterioration as children age.
- Malignant hyperthermia is common in children with muscular dystrophy and should be treated with dantrolene.

Definition

Muscular dystrophies are noninflammatory genetically based muscle diseases causing progressive degeneration and weakness of skeletal muscles without apparent cause in peripheral or central nervous system

A. Johari, MD (✉) • R. Maheshwari, MD • S. Maheshwari, MD
Pediatric Orthopedics, Childrens' Orthopedic Centre, Mumbai, India
e-mail: drashokjohari@hotmail.com

C. Mauffrey, D.J. Hak (eds.), *Passport for the Orthopedic Boards and FRCS Examination*, DOI 10.1007/978-2-8178-0475-0_28

Table 1 Gene defect in muscular dystrophy

	Inheritance	Gene defect
Duchenne's	X-linked recessive	Xp21 dystrophin, point deletion, nonsense mutation, no dystrophin protein produced
Becker's	X-linked recessive	Xp21 dystrophin in noncoding region with normal reading frame, lesser amounts of truncated dystrophin produced
Facioscapulohumeral (FSH), adult	AD	4q35
Infantile FSH	AR	Unknown

Etiology and Pathophysiology

- Although genetically based, new mutations are frequent. The common location of gene defect is given below (See Table 1).
- The muscles get degenerated with subsequent loss of fiber, proliferation of connective tissue, and subsequently of adipose tissue.

Classification

- *Sex-linked muscular dystrophy*
  - Duchenne
  - Becker
  - Emery-Dreifuss
- *Autosomal recessive muscular dystrophy*
  - Limb-girdle
  - Infantile facioscapulohumeral
- *Autosomal dominant muscular dystrophy*
  - Facioscapulohumeral
  - Distal
  - Ocular
  - Oculopharyngeal

Evaluation

- Hematologic studies – The serum CPK is markedly elevated in the early stages of Duchenne muscular dystrophy. This may be 200–300 times the normal value but decreases as the disease progresses and muscle mass is reduced.
- Electromyography shows characteristic myopathic changes with reduced amplitude, short duration, and polyphasic motor action potentials.
- Muscle biopsy material is usually examined by routine histology, special histochemical stains, and electron microscopy. Muscles that are involved but functioning are selected.
- More recently, molecular genetic testing has become equally, if not more, important.

1.1 Duchenne Muscular Dystrophy

Overview

- The most common form of muscular dystrophy. The disease is characterized by its occurrence in males.
- Occurs in approximately 1/3,500 live male births.

Evaluation

- Becomes clinically evident when the child is between 3 and 6 years of age. They may demonstrate frequent episodes of falling, with inability to hop and jump normally.
- Progressive weakness in proximal muscle groups which descends symmetrically in both lower extremities, particularly the gluteus maximus, gluteus medius, quadriceps, and tibialis anterior muscles.
- Pseudohypertrophy of calf is common.
- Cardiac involvement is common.
- Patients develop a waddling, wide-based gait with shoulder sway.
- Weakness in the shoulder girdle occurs around 3–5 years later. Tendency for child to slip a truncal grasp has been termed "Meyerson sign."
- Absence of sensory deficits.
- Gower sign: valuable clinical sign – Patient is asked to rise from sitting position on the floor. The patient walks his or her hands up their extremities to compensate for the quadriceps or gluteus weakness.
- Contracture of tendoachilles and IT band are the most consistent deformities.

Management

- Efforts should be made to maintain a daily ambulation program. They progress slowly but continuously. They are usually unable to ambulate effectively by 10 years of age in absence of treatment.
- Orthopedic problems in DMD include decreasing ambulatory ability, soft tissue contractures, and spinal deformity
- Corticosteroid therapy – Prolongs ambulation and slows the deterioration of forced vital capacity (FVC). Treatment carries a high risk of complications.
- Nighttime ventilation significantly prolongs survival.
- Physical therapy and orthosis – Maximum resistance exercises performed several times a day.
- Serial casting may be useful to correct existing deformities; knee flexion contractures of less than 30° may benefit by serial or wedge casting. Orthoses need to be used after casting to maintain correction.

Surgical Intervention

- Surgery is controversial in DMD. It can be done when contractures are painful or interfere with essential daily activities.

- If surgery is performed, the focus should be on early postoperative mobilization and ambulation to prevent deconditioning and deterioration.
- Major contractures include equinus and equinovarus contractures of ankle and foot, knee flexion contractures, and hip flexion and abduction contractures. Contracture releases should be performed when child is still ambulatory.
- Scoliosis develops in 95 % of patients after they transition to a wheelchair (usually around age 12 years). Early posterior instrumented fusion (at 20°) is recommended before loss of FVC occurs due to respiratory muscle weakness and progressively decreasing cardiac output. Stiff curves may require anterior and posterior fusion.

Complications

Malignant hyperthermia is common intraoperatively and is pretreated with dantrolene at surgery.

1.2 Becker's Muscular Dystrophy

Overview

- Less common that DMD. Occurs in 1 in 30,000 live male births.
- It is similar to Duchenne muscular dystrophy in clinical appearance and distribution of weakness but is less severe.

Evaluation

- Onset is generally after 7 years of age; rate of progression is slower. Patients usually remain ambulatory till adolescence or early adult years.
- Pseudohypertrophy of calf is common. Cardiac involvement is frequent.
- Life expectancy is longer.

Treatment

- Treatment is essentially the same as DMD. Incidence of scoliosis is high. Patients require periodic spinal radiographs.

1.3 Facioscapulohumeral Muscular Dystrophy

Overview

- Autosomal dominant disorder manifested by muscular weakness of face, shoulder girdle, and upper arm.
- Onset can occur at any age but is most common in late childhood or early adulthood.
- Can occur in both genders but is more common in females.
- Life expectancy is relatively good.

Evaluation

- Face has a "popeye" appearance. Lack of mobility, incomplete eye closure, pouting lips with a transverse smile, and absence of eye and forehead wrinkles.
- Shoulder and girdle weakness leads to scapular winging.
- Forward-sloping appearance of the shoulders, clavicles assume a horizontal position.
- Decreased scapulothoracic motion, glenohumeral motion is usual preserved.

Treatment

- Winging of scapula and weakness of shoulder flexion and abduction is the major orthopedic problem. Deltoid, supraspinatus, and infraspinatus are usually normal.
- Posterior scapulocostal fusion or stabilization can be beneficial in restoring mechanical advantage of deltoid and rotator cuff. This can result in increased active abduction and forward flexion of shoulder and improved function, as well as cosmesis.

Bibliography

1. Alman BA, Raza SN, Bigger WD. Steroid treatment and the development of scoliosis in males with Duchenne muscular dystrophy. J Bone Joint Surg Am. 2004;86:519–24.
2. Brooke MH, Fenichel GM, Griggs RC, et al. Duchenne muscular dystrophy. Patterns of clinical progression and effects of supportive therapy. Neurology. 1989;39:475.
3. Bunch WH, Siegal IM. Scapulothoracic arthrodesis in fascioscapulohumeral muscular dystrophy. Review of seventeen procedures with three to twenty-one year follow up. J Bone Joint Surg Am. 1993;75:372.
4. Cambridge W, Drennan JC. Scoliosis associated with Duchenne muscular dystrophy. J Pediatr Orthop. 1987;7:436.
5. Dubowitz V. Muscle biopsy. 2nd ed. London: Bailliere Tindall; 1985.
6. Smith SE, Green NE, Cole RJ, et al. Prolongation of ambulation in children with Duchenne muscular dystrophy by subcutaneous lower limb tenotomy. J Pediatr Orthop. 1993;13:331.

2 Larsen Syndrome

Ashok Johari, Ratna Maheshwari, and Shalin Maheshwari

Take-Home Message

- Widely spaced eyes, depressed nasal bridge, and a prominent forehead.
- Unique combination of hypertelorism, multiple joint dislocations, and focal bone deformities.
- Sudden deaths have been reported from exacerbation of cervical compression.

Definition

- Unique combination of hypertelorism, multiple joint dislocations, and focal bone deformities

Etiology

- Autosomal dominant and recessive patterns
- Gene on chromosome 3

Evaluation

- Widely spaced eyes, depressed nasal bridge, and a prominent forehead.
- Cleft palate is common.
- Fingers do not taper distally; thumb has a wide distal phalanx.
- Hypotonia, sudden death from cervical compression can occur.
- Dislocations involve radial heads, hips, and knees.
- Foot deformities involve equinovarus or equinovalgus.
- Spina bifida is common in cervical spine and sometimes in thoracic spine; vertebral bodies may be hypoplastic. Cervical kyphosis is common. Atlantoaxial instability may occur.
- Radiographs may also show accessory calcaneal or carpal ossification centers.

Management

- Cervical kyphosis should be fused posteriorly if it exceeds 35–45°. If kyphosis has progressed to point of myelopathy, anterior corpectomy and fusion will be required.
- Clubfeet are addressed first, with serial casting. Recurrence is common, may need complete subtalar release.
- Hyperextended knees may be treated with casts. Complete dislocations may require open reduction with V-Y quadricepsplasty and anterior capsulotomy.
- Reduction of hip dislocation is controversial. Treatment can be considered of those hips where the dislocation is not too high and acetabulum is not too shallow.

Bibliography

1. Bowen JR, Ortega K, Ray S, et al. Spinal deformities in Larsen's syndrome. Clin Orthop. 1985;197:159.
2. Larsen LJ, Schottstaedt ER, Bost FC. Multiple congenital dislocations associated with characteristic facial abnormality. J Pediatr. 1950;37: 574.
3. Laville JM, Lakermore P, Limouzy F. Larsens's syndrome: review of the literature and analysis of thirty-eight cases. J Pediatr Orthop. 1994; 14:63.

3 Arthrogryposis Multiplex Congenita

Ashok Johari, Ratna Maheshwari, and Shalin Maheshwari

Take-Home Message

- These children are featureless and tubular. Normal skin creases are lacking, but there may be deep dimples over the joints.
- In lower limbs, primary objectives of management are symmetry and stability.
- Most of the rigid deformities require surgical correction.
- Recommendations for surgery include correction of feet at about 4 weeks, knees at 4 months, and hips at 6–8 months.
- The goals of treatment of upper limb are to maximize hand prehension and grasp and to mobilize the shoulder, elbow, and wrist.

Definition

Arthrogryposis, or arthrogryposis multiplex congenita (AMC), is a generic term used to describe the presence of multiple congenital contractures. The word arthrogryposis, *arthro*, joint, *gryp*, curved, literally means curved joint (implying that it is fixed or stuck in the curved position).

Etiology Problems leading to limitation of movement in a fetus:

- Abnormalities of muscle structure or function – myopathic process.
- Abnormalities of nerves that connect to muscles – neuropathic process.
- Abnormalities of connective tissue – tendons, bone, joint, or joint lining develop abnormally as is the case in some forms of distal arthrogryposis.
- Limitation of space within the uterus – e.g., oligohydramnios.
- Maternal illness – e.g., multiple sclerosis, diabetes mellitus, and myasthenia gravis.

Pathophysiology

- Not a problem in formation of joint or limb, but lack of movement is associated with development of extra connective tissue around the joint and plays an important role in formation of contractures.
- Tendons around the joint may not have stretched to their normal length.
- As joint is not used over a period of time, surface of joint begin to assume a flattened contour.

Evaluation

- Accurate history taking in terms of family history, pregnancy history, delivery.
- The most useful tool for prenatal diagnosis is ultrasound. If a mother notices a decrease in fetal movements, a real-time USG may be performed.

- Careful evaluation and description of position of child at rest and joints involved in contractures. Also look for scoliosis, amniotic bands, webbing, abnormal genitalia, malformed nails, eyes, palate, skull, as well as facial features. Document neurological status.
- Radiographs of hip and foot are essential to rule out developmental dysplasia and congenital vertical talus.

Classification

At least 150 specific entities have been recognized that have multiple congenital contractures. Those with mainly limb involvement include

- Amyoplasia- “classic” arthrogryposis
  - Sporadic disorder.
  - Typical symmetric positioning of limbs – severe equinovarus feet, extended elbows, absent muscle tissue with fibrotic replacement, midfacial hemangioma, normal intelligence.
  - Most have all four limbs involved but trunk spared.
  - 10 % have abdominal structural anomalies.
- Distal arthrogryposis
  - Autosomal dominant
  - Characteristic position of hand – medially overlapping fingers, clenched fists, ulnar deviation, foot contractures
  - No associated visceral anomalies
- Contractural arachnodactyly
  - Autosomal dominant
  - Beals syndrome – multiple contractures with long and thin fingers
  - Crumpled ears

Treatment

Principles of Treatment

- Fine motor function is the major objective of upper extremity management. In contrast, in lower limbs, primary objectives are symmetry and stability.
- The primary objective of orthopedic management is to improve function:
- By correcting deformity. Approach treatment with optimism, as most children with amyoplasia have the potential of living a satisfying and productive life. A realistic management plan should be developed.
- Most of the rigid deformities require surgical correction and is undertaken during the infancy phase.
- Nonsurgical methods include cast correction. It is useful for rapid correction of positional deformities, as also to stretch soft tissues prior to surgical correction. Physical and occupational therapy is essential – mobility training, walking, and self-care skills.
- As immobility is an underlying cause of congenital contractures, avoid excessive periods of immobilization.

- Operative treatment should be provided early, briefly, aggressively, and later sparingly and only as absolutely necessary. Correct most lower extremity deformities during the first year. Correct upper extremity deformities in early childhood when deformities that limit function are isolated. Recommendations for surgery include correction of feet at about 4 weeks, knees at 4 months, and hips at 6–8 months.

Lower Extremity

- Hip – Classically hips are flexed, externally rotated, and abducted. Release of contractures is done if they interfere with ambulation. Unilateral dislocations have to be reduced. The appropriateness of reducing bilateral dislocations is controversial. Good results have been reported by medial approach (Ludloff) open reduction if performed during infancy.
- Knee
  Flexion Contactures
  - Arc of motion is not greatly increased by surgery. The objective of surgery is to place the arc of motion in the most functional position.
  - Depending on severity of involvement – Z plasty of skin with lengthening of tendons and capsulotomy may be undertaken. In very severe cases, gradual correction by external fixator or femoral shortening may be undertaken.

  Extension Contractures
  - V-Y quadricepsplasty can be done to reposition the arc of motion.
- Foot
  - Oblique talus does not require treatment.
  - Vertical talus requires surgical correction – Correction of foot deformities is essential regardless of patient's ambulatory status
  - Clubfeet – Cast correction must be started soon after birth and must be discontinued if improvement has plateaued. In such cases soft tissue release is undertaken. Talectomy is a salvage operation. Condition tends to recur.

Upper Extremity
The goals of treatment of upper limb are to maximize hand prehension and grasp and to mobilize the shoulder, elbow, and wrist. Early institution of splinting and range-of-motion treatment is essential.

- Shoulder
  - Limitation of shoulder abduction and external rotation, with muscle weakness.
  - Start passive range of motion early.
  - Primary indication for humeral derotation osteotomy has been to facilitate keyboard use.

- Elbow
- It is often in extension. It is important to consider lower extremity functioning before planning treatment for a stiff elbow. Goal is to obtain flexion to 90°. Posterior elbow release is considered if no improvement with splinting or casting.
  - In case of flexion contractures, functional level is generally high and anterior elbow release is rarely done.
  - Restoration of active elbow flexion by tendon transfer is a consideration, but all transfers come at some cost.
- Wrist
  - They are often flexed and ulnar deviated.
  - Position splints are applied early along with passive range-of-motion exercises.
  - Surgery is rarely performed early, after an adequate trial of splinting. It involves release of volar wrist capsule. Flexor to extensor transfer can be done to maintain the position.
  - Intracarpal extension osteotomy is useful when natural intracarpal fusion exists.
- Hand
  - Primary deformities are the thumb-in-palm and finger flexion contractures. Goals of treatment must be made on individual basis.
  - Early application of corrective splints is done in digital deformities.
  - Surgery can be done for thumb-in-palm deformity if splinting doesn't help. Options include first web skin release, adductor pollicis release, first metacarpal osteotomy, or fusion.

Complications

- The most common complication is the risk of recurrence which continues throughout the period of growth but is more pronounced in infancy.

Bibliography

1. Hall JG, Reed SD, Driscoll EP. Amyoplasia: a common sporadic condition with congenital contractures. Am J Med Genet. 1983;15:571–90.
2. Livingstone IR, Sack Jr GR. Arthrogryposis multiplex congenita occurring with maternal multiple sclerosis. Arch Neurol. 1984;41(11):1216–7.
3. Smit LM, Barth PG. Arthrogryposi multiplex congenita due to congenital myasthenia. Dev Med Child Neurol. 1980;22(3):371–4.
4. Szoke G, Staheli LT, Jaffe K, Hall JG. Medial-approach open reduction of hip dislocation in amyoplasia-type arthrogryplasia. J Pediatr Orthop. 1996;16(1):127–30.
5. Williams P. The management of arthrogryposis. Orthop Clin North Am. 1978;9(1):67–88.

Pediatric Bone and Joint Infections

Ashok Johari, Ratna Maheshwari, and Shalin Maheshwari

1 Acute Osteomyelitis

Ashok Johari, Ratna Maheshwari, and Shalin Maheshwari

Take-Home Message

- A child with bone pain and fever should be assumed to have osteomyelitis until proven otherwise.
- Samples should be sent for culture and histology to rule out neoplasm.
- Acute hematogenous osteomyelitis without abscess can generally be treated medically.
- Most cases of AHO are caused by *S aureus*. In neonates, the most common organism is group B streptococci.
- Because of the prevalence of CA-MRSA, empiric coverage should cover CA-MRSA in most cases.
- Susceptibilities and resistant strains of CA-MRSA vary by community, adding importance to aspiration or biopsy for culture.
- The metaphyseal blood supply crosses the physis to the epiphysis in children younger than 12–18 months, so severe sequelae are more common.
- Preoperative MRI aids surgical planning by delineating the extent of the infection and the location of abscesses.

A. Johari, MD (✉) • R. Maheshwari, MD • S. Maheshwari, MD
Pediatric Orthopedics, Childrens' Orthopedic Centre, Mumbai, India
e-mail: drashokjohari@hotmail.com

C. Mauffrey, D.J. Hak (eds.), *Passport for the Orthopedic Boards and FRCS Examination*, DOI 10.1007/978-2-8178-0475-0_29

Definition

- Osteomyelitis is an inflammation of the bone.
- Two of the following four parameters must be present according to the Peltola and Vahvanen criteria:
  - Pus aspirated from bone
  - Positive bone or blood culture
  - Localized pain, swelling, warmth, and limited ROM of joints
  - Radiographic changes typical of osteomyelitis

Etiology

- Trauma is a common cause of infection.
- *Staphylococcus aureus* still remains the most common organism responsible for acute osteomyelitis; streptococci, *Kingella kingae*, Gram-negative organisms, and salmonella are far less frequently responsible.
- Risk factors for developing acute hematogenous osteomyelitis:
  - Diabetes mellitus
  - Chronic renal disease
  - Hemoglobinopathies
  - Rheumatoid arthritis
  - Concurrent varicella infection
  - Immune compromise

Pathophysiology

- Hematogenous spread—usually involves the metaphysis of the long bones
- Direct inoculation—penetrating injuries and surgical contamination
- From a contiguous focus of infection
  - Slow blood flow in the capillaries of the metaphysis allows bacteria to exit the vessel walls.
  - If a sufficient number of bacteria lodge in the bone to overwhelm the local defenses, an infection occurs.
  - Osteoblast necrosis, activation of osteoclasts, release of inflammatory mediators, recruitment of inflammatory cells, and blood vessel thrombosis cause a purulent exudate.
  - A subperiosteal abscess forms when the exudate penetrates the porous metaphyseal cortex.
  - In bones with an intra-articular metaphysis, the exiting exudate can enter the joint and cause an associated septic arthritis.
  - If pus is not drained and the elevated periosteum remains viable, it will produce new bone over time and involucrum will form.
  - When both medullary and periosteal blood supplies are compromised, large areas of dead bone or sequestra may be formed.

Evaluation

- Clinically acute localized tenderness in the region of the metaphysis of a long bone in the presence of fever should be sufficient grounds to make a tentative diagnosis of acute osteomyelitis. Use of antibiotics may mask the symptoms.

- Laboratory findings
  - Initial blood work should include C-reactive protein (CRP), erythrocyte sedimentation rate (ESR), blood cultures, and white blood cell (WBC) count with differential.
  - Blood cultures may yield an organism 30 % of the time.
  - The WBC is elevated in only 25 % of patients.
- Diagnostic imaging
  - Plain radiographs are of little use in the diagnosis of acute osteomyelitis.
  - In stage I Trueta, there are no plain radiographic changes either in the soft tissue planes or in the bone. In stages II and III, there is loss of definition of soft tissue planes indicative of edema. However, there are still no changes in the bone; bone changes appear 10–14 days after the onset of infection in children.
  - Ultrasound scanning is useful for the diagnosis of a subperiosteal abscess.
  - Technetium Tc 99 m bone scan can help localize the focus and will demonstrate a multifocal infection.
  - MRI detects marrow and soft tissue edema seen early in infection as well as abscesses requiring surgical drainage. It provides good anatomic detail in many planes. In acute osteomyelitis, the low signal intensity in T1 becomes a high signal intensity in T2.

Classification

Trueta divided the clinical stages of acute osteomyelitis into three.

- In stage I, there is severe bone pain and profound local tenderness without any soft tissue inflammation.
- In stage II, the systemic and local signs are more pronounced; this corresponds to the development of a subperiosteal abscess.
- In stage III, there is pus in the soft tissues, and in this stage, it is difficult to distinguish osteomyelitis from cellulitis.

Classification	Description
Anatomic stage	
1	Medullary osteomyelitis
2	Superficial osteomyelitis
3	Localized osteomyelitis
4	Diffuse osteomyelitis
Physiological host status	
A	Normal host
B	Systemic compromise
	Local compromise
	Systemic and local compromise
C	Treatment worse than disease

Stage 1, or medullary, osteomyelitis is confined to the medullary cavity of the bone.

Stage 2, or superficial, osteomyelitis involves only the cortical bone and most often originates from a direct inoculation or a contiguous focus.

Stage 3, or localized, osteomyelitis usually involves both cortical and medullary bones. In this stage, the bone remains stable, and the infectious process does not involve the entire bone diameter.

Stage 4, or diffuse, osteomyelitis involves the entire thickness of the bone, with loss of stability, as in infected nonunion.

Treatment

Identify the organism, select the appropriate antibiotic, deliver the antibiotic to the organism, and stop the tissue destruction are the four principles of treating an infection.

- Aspiration—Aspiration of the suspected area is the first step in management. Aspiration is performed before commencing antibiotics if the clinical condition of the patient allows. A large-bore needle is used. After aspiration, antibiotics may be started according to the guidelines.
- Nonsurgical—If no purulent material is aspirated, the child can be admitted for intravenous antibiotics. Surgery is not indicated if the patient demonstrates clinical improvement within 48 h. Duration of intravenous antibiotics is usually 4–6 weeks.
- Surgical
  - Indications for surgical drainage
    - Aspiration of pus
    - Abscess formation
    - Failure to respond adequately to nonsurgical treatment
  - Procedures
- Surgical drainage requires evacuation of all collections of pus, debridement of devitalized tissue, and drilling the cortex to decompress the bone. The limb should be splinted.
- Samples should be sent for culture and histology to rule out neoplasm.
- With chronic osteomyelitis, a more aggressive débridement may be necessary, at times including excision of the sequestrum.

Complications

- Meningitis
- Chronic osteomyelitis
- Septic arthritis
- Growth disturbance
- Pathologic fracture
- Limb-length discrepancy
- Gait abnormality
- Deep venous thrombosis

Bibliography

1. Howard CB, Einhorn M, Dagan R, Nyska M. Ultrasound in the diagnosis and management of acute haematogenous osteomyelitis in children. J Bone Joint Surg Br. 1993;75:79–82.
2. Kaplan SL. Osteomyelitis in children. Infect Dis Clin North Am. 2005;19: 787–97.
3. McCarthy JJ, Dormans JP, Kozin SH, Pizzutillo PD. Musculoskeletal infections in children: basic treatment principles and recent advances. Instr Course Lect. 2005;54:515–28.
4. Peltola H, Vahvanen V. A comparative study of osteomyelitis and purulent arthritis with special reference to aetiology and recovery. Infection. 1984;12:75.
5. Trueta J. The three types of acute haematogenous osteomyelitis: a clinical and vascular study. J Bone Joint Surg Br. 1959;41:671–80.

2 Subacute Osteomyelitis

Ashok Johari, Ratna Maheshwari, and Shalin Maheshwari

Take-Home Message

- Subacute osteomyelitis may be indistinguishable from tumors on radiographic studies.
- Surgery is required in most cases of subacute osteomyelitis.

Definition

- Subacute osteomyelitis is an uncommon infection characterized by bone pain and radiographic changes without systemic signs. It usually affects lower extremity long bones, but it can occur at other sites. Misdiagnosis and delayed diagnosis are common.

Etiology and Pathoanatomy

- Pathoanatomy is similar to acute osteomyelitis.
- Staphylococcus aureus is responsible in most cases.
- The difference in presentation results from increased host resistance, less virulent organisms, prior antibiotic exposure, or a combination of these factors.

Evaluation

- Intermittent limp or pain is often present. Systemic signs like fever and malaise are absent.
- Point tenderness over involved bone is present.
- Blood test is usually not helpful.

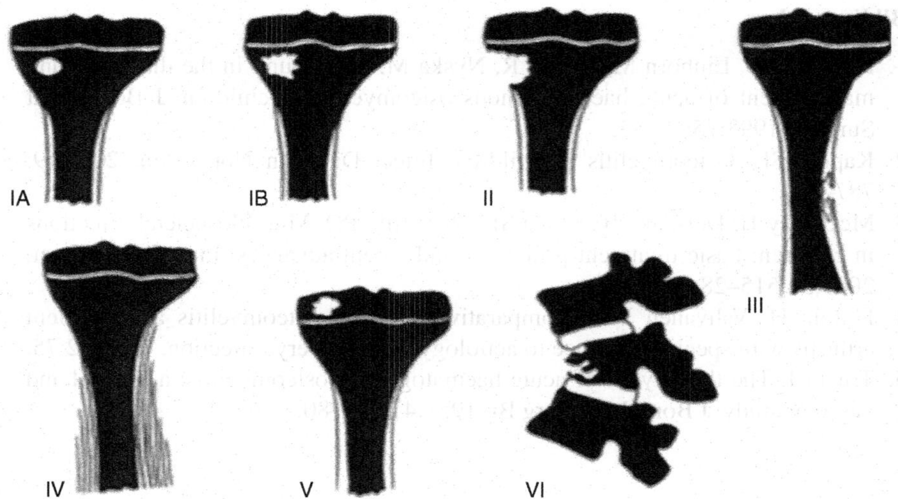

Fig. 1 Radiographic classification of subacute osteomyelitis (Redrawn from Roberts JM, Drummond DS, Breed AL, et al. Subacute hematogenous osteomyelitis in children: A retrospective study. J Pediatr Orthop 1982;2: 249)

- Plain radiographs are positive for changes that range from a well-circumscribed radiolucency in the metaphysis or epiphysis to periosteal new bone formation suggestive of an aggressive malignancy.
- Bone scan is usually positive.
- CT and MRI help characterize the lesion.
- In all cases, the differential diagnosis on x-ray is neoplasm.

Classification

Radiographic classification of subacute osteomyelitis (Fig. 1)

Types IA and IB indicate lucency; type II, metaphyseal involvement with loss of cortical bone; type III, diaphyseal; type IV, onion skinning; type V, epiphyseal; and type VI, spinal involvement.

This classification system is based on the anatomic location, the response of surrounding tissue to infection, and the similarity to benign or malignant tumors

Treatment

- Nonsurgical
  - Lesions without malignant features may respond to antibiotic therapy covering *S. aureus*.
- Surgical
  - Indications
    - Surgical treatment is indicated in all patients with aggressive features on radiographs (types II, III, and IV).
    - A biopsy is required to rule out a malignancy if such radiographic features are present.

– Procedures

  - Once osteomyelitis is confirmed after biopsy and culture, the lesion can be treated with curettage and antibiotics.

Complications

- Growth disturbance (unusual)
- Chronic osteomyelitis

Bibliography

1. Dormans JP, Drummond DS. Pediatric hematogenous osteomyelitis: new trends in presentation, diagnosis, and treatment. J Am Acad Orthop Surg. 1994;2: 333–41.

3 Septic Arthritis

Ashok Johari, Ratna Maheshwari, and Shalin Maheshwari

Take-Home Message
- Septic arthritis more commonly occurs in younger children, with 50 % of cases in children ≤2 years old.
- Septic arthritis is a surgical emergency.
- Children with septic arthritis appear sicker and are in more distress than those with toxic synovitis.
- When managing the hip, err toward drainage in equivocal cases; the morbidity of an arthrotomy is minimal compared to the sequelae of a neglected septic hip.

Overview

- Septic arthritis is more common than osteomyelitis in infancy and childhood. Fifty percent of cases of septic arthritis occur in children younger than 2 years.
- The hip and knee are most frequently involved joints, although other joints may be involved.
- Involvement of multiple joints can occur in about 5 % of children with septic arthritis.

Etiology

- *S. aureus* causes >50 % of cases.
- Other bacteria include group A and group B streptococci. Neonates are more prone to group B streptococcal infection.
- The incidence of *H. influenza* septic arthritis has decreased markedly since the advent of the *H. influenza* vaccine.

Pathoanatomy

- Most cases of septic arthritis result from:
  - Bacteremia seeding the joint
  - Direct inoculation of the joint from trauma or surgery
  - Contiguous spread from adjacent osteomyelitis
- Release of proteolytic enzymes from inflammatory cells, synovial cells, cartilage, and bacteria may cause damage to the articular cartilage within 8 h.
- Increased joint pressure in the hip may cause osteonecrosis of the femoral head if not promptly relieved.
- It can also result into damage to growth plate and joint dislocation.

Evaluation Since cartilage destruction occurs very soon after onset of infection, it becomes exceedingly important to establish a diagnosis as soon as possible and institute treatment.

- On examination
  - Patients have fever and often appear toxic.
  - There is disuse of the extremity and/or refusal to bear weight.
  - Septic joints have an associated effusion, tenderness, and warmth; any motion causes severe pain.
  - The extremity rests in the position that maximizes the volume of the joint; for the hip, this results in hip *f*lexion, *ab*duction, and *e*xternal *r*otation (FABER).
- Laboratory investigations
  - Blood counts, erythrocyte sedimentation rate, and C-reactive protein may help in suggesting that an infective process is going on.
  - The only way the joint infection can be conclusively diagnosed is by demonstrating bacteria in the fluid removed from the joint. However, an organism may be cultured in approximately 60 % of cases of true septic arthritis. Blood cultures should be drawn because these are often positive, even when local cultures are negative.
- Diagnostic imaging
  - Plain radiographs may show joint space widening and are needed to identify any possible bone involvement.
  - Ultrasound confirms the presence of a hip effusion and can be used to guide joint aspiration; ultrasound cannot differentiate between septic and sterile effusions.
  - MRI detects a joint effusion and can assess for adjacent osseous involvement, but it can be difficult to obtain expeditiously.
- Aspiration
  - Joint aspiration is necessary for diagnosis. Fluid samples should be analyzed for cell count with differential, Gram stain, and culture.

Diagnosis and Differential Diagnosis

- Kocher et al. identified clinical and laboratory predictors of septic arthritis. Probability of diagnosis of septic arthritis was 40, 93.1, and 99.6 % if two, three, or four of these predictors, respectively, were present.
  - History of fever
  - Inability to bear weight on the limb
  - ESR > 40 mm/ h
  - WBC count > 12,000/ml
- A CRP >2.0 mg/dL is an independent risk factor for septic arthritis.
- The differential diagnosis includes osteomyelitis, toxic synovitis, viral arthritis, inflammatory bowel disease-associated arthritis, postgastroenteritis arthritis, tuberculosis (TB), Lyme disease, poststreptococcal arthritis, juvenile arthritis, Reiter syndrome, reactive arthritis, villonodular synovitis, leukemia, sickle cell disease, hemophilia, serum sickness, and Henoch-Schönlein purpura.

Treatment

- Treatment starts with joint aspiration, preferably before starting antibiotics empirically.
- Intravenous antibiotics are started after samples are sent for culture and are usually administered for 4 weeks.
- Surgical drainage and irrigation is the standard of care for almost all septic joints, to clear the joint of damaging enzymes. The capsule is not closed following the arthrotomy.
- Rest to the joint either by immobilization in plaster or traction helps to reduce pain.
- Patients may start ROM exercises in the first few days after surgery once the inflammation has reduced.

Complications

- Joint contracture, hip dislocation, growth disturbance, limb-length discrepancy, joint destruction, gait disturbance, and osteonecrosis

Bibliography

1. Frick SL. Evaluation of the child who has hip pain. Orthop Clin North Am. 2006;37:133–40.
2. Jung ST, Rowe SM, Moon ES, et al. Significance of laboratory and radiological findings for differentiating septic arthritis and transient synovitis of the hip. J Pediatr Orthop. 2003;23:368–72.
3. Kim HK, Alman B, Cole WG. A shortened course of parenteral antibiotic therapy in the management of acute septic arthritis of the hip. J Pediatr Orthop. 2000;20:44–7.
4. Kocher MS, Zurakowski D, Kasser JR. Differentiating between septic arthritis and transient synovitis of the hip in children: an evidence-based clinical prediction algorithm. J Bone Joint Surg Am. 1999;81:1662–70.

Other Paediatric Topics

Ashok Johari, Ratna Maheshwari, Ratna Johari, and Shalin Maheshwari

1 Osteogenesis Imperfecta

Ashok Johari, Ratna Maheshwari, and Shalin Maheshwari

Take-Home Message

- Child abuse should not be ruled out in OI patients.
- Bisphosphonates inhibit osteoclasts, yielding increased cortical thickness with decreased fracture rates and pain.
- Olecranon apophyseal avulsion fractures are characteristic in OI patients.

Definition

- It is a heritable disorder of connective tissue, affecting the bone and the soft tissue.
- Most types of osteogenesis imperfecta have been linked to mutations in type 1 collagen.

Aetiology and Pathoanatomy

- Types I through IV are a mutation in the *COL1A1* and *COL1A2* genes that encode type I collagen, the mainstay of the organic bone matrix. The result is bone that has a decreased number of trabeculae and decreased cortical thickness (wormian bone).

A. Johari, MD (✉) • R. Maheshwari, MD • R. Johari, MD • S. Maheshwari, MD
Pediatric Orthopedics, Childrens' Orthopedic Centre, Mumbai, India
e-mail: drashokjohari@hotmail.com; drratnajohari@gmail.com

C. Mauffrey, D.J. Hak (eds.), *Passport for the Orthopedic Boards and FRCS Examination*, DOI 10.1007/978-2-8178-0475-0_30

Classification (Sillence Classification)

- Type 1: Autosomal Dominant

  Bone fragility, blue sclera, onset of fractures after birth
  Type A: Without dentinogenesis imperfecta
  Type B: With dentinogenesis imperfecta

- Type 2: Autosomal Recessive

  Lethal in perinatal period, dark blue sclera, concertina femurs, beaded ribs

- Type 3: Autosomal Recessive

  Fractures at birth, progressive deformity, normal sclera and hearing

- Type 4: Autosomal Dominant

  Bone fragility, normal sclera and normal hearing
  Type A: Without dentinogenesis imperfecta
  Type B: With dentinogenesis imperfecta

Evaluation

- Child abuse should not be ruled out in OI patients; thorough examination is needed.
- Radiographs: Femurs may have a crumpled "concertina" appearance. Long bones appear slender and gracile, with thin cortices and deformities due to multiple fractures. The skull exhibits wormian bones.
- Vertebrae may develop platyspondyly due to multiple fractures and severe scoliosis. Metaphyses may appear cystic. Basilar invagination may occur particularly in types 2 and 3.
- Olecranon apophyseal avulsion fractures are characteristic.

Management

- Type 3 and type 4 represent the greatest challenges.
- Bisphosphonates and growth hormone are used; bisphosphonates inhibit osteoclasts, yielding increased cortical thickness with decreased fracture rates and pain.
- Fractures can be managed with splints/casts.
- For severe bowing of the limbs or recurrent fracture, intramedullary fixation is indicated with or without osteotomy. Telescoping rods allow growth.
- Scoliotic curves tend to advance relentlessly. Fusion can help to stop progress.

Bibliography

1. Acito AJ, Kasra M, Lee JM, et al. Effects of intermittent administration of pamidronate on the mechanical properties of cortical and trabecular bone. J Orthop Res. 1994;12:742.
2. Cole WG. Etiology and pathogenesis of heritable connective tissue diseases. J Pediatr Orthop. 1993;13:392.

3. Lubicky JP. The spine in osteogenesis imperfecta. In: Weinstein SL, editor. The pediatric spine. New York: Raven; 1994. p. 943.
4. Porat S, Heller E, Seidman DS, et al. Functional results of operation in osteogenesis imperfecta: elongating and nonelongating rods. J Pediatr Orthop. 1991;11:200.
5. Sillence DO. Osteogenesis imperfecta: an expanding panorama of variance. Clin Orthop. 1981;159:11.

2 Skeletal Dysplasias

Ashok Johari, Ratna Maheshwari, and Shalin Maheshwari

Take-Home Message

- Lethality and chest circumference: Most critical parameter to determine in the prenatal period.
- Achondroplasia is the most common skeletal dysplasia. It affects the proliferative zone of growth plate.
- The most serious complications of achondroplasia in the infant and toddler are cervical spine and foramen magnum stenosis, which may cause apnoea, weakness and sudden death.
- Cauliflower ears and hitchhiker thumbs are characteristic of diastrophic dysplasia.
- Atlantoaxial instability is common in pseudoachondroplasia, SED, mucopolysaccharidoses, trisomy 21 and McKusick-type metaphyseal dysplasia.
- The mucopolysaccharidoses are all autosomal recessive except for Hunter syndrome, which is X-linked recessive.
- McKusick-type metaphyseal chondrodysplasia: There is an increased risk of malignancy, such as lymphoma, sarcoma and skin cancer. Patients need medical surveillance into adulthood, more than most patients with skeletal dysplasia.

Overview

- Abnormalities of growth, development and maintenance of bones and cartilage give rise to the varied forms of skeletal dysplasia.
- Lethality and chest circumference: Most critical parameter to determine in the prenatal period.
  - Chest circumference to abdominal circumference <0.6.

Evaluation
Clinical Features

- Skeletal dysplasia not recognisable at birth or first year:
  - Storage disorder: Morquio's syndrome
  - Pseudoachondroplasia
  - Multiple epiphyseal dysplasia
  - Metaphyseal dysplasia: McKusick, Schmid
- Anatomical localisation, localisation within the limb:
  - Rhizomelic: Achondroplasia, chondrodysplasia punctata, Larsen's
  - Mesomelic: Ellis–van Creveld syndrome, dyschondrosteosis
  - Acromelic: Pseudohypoparathyroidism, acromesomelic dysplasia, acrodysostosis
- Clinical diagnostic groups:
  - Short limbs/trunk less affected: Achondroplasia, hypochondroplasia
  - Short limbs and short trunk: Kniest dysplasia, diastrophic dysplasia
  - Epiphyseal disorders: Multiple epiphyseal dysplasia, chondrodysplasia punctata
  - Short trunk/limbs less affected: Spondyloepiphyseal dysplasia
  - Metaphyseal dysplasia
  - Abnormal bone density: Increased in osteopetrosis, decreased in hypophosphatasia
- Genetic analysis:
  - FGFR-3 receptor abnormality: Achondroplasia, hypochondroplasia, thanatophoric dysplasia
  - COL2A1 abnormality: Spondyloepiphyseal dysplasia, Kniest dysplasia, Stickler dysplasia
  - Diastrophic dysplasia sulphate transporter defect: Diastrophic dysplasia
  - Cartilage oligomeric matrix protein abnormality: Multiple epiphyseal dysplasia, pseudoachondroplasia
  - TRPV4: Metatropic, SMD (Kozlowski)
  - Storage disorders: MPS
- Features that help to distinguish various dysplasias:
  - Skeletal features:
    - Short trunk vs. short limb
    - Facial features
    - Chest deformity
    - Hand features, e.g. starfish hands in achondroplasia and hitchhikers thumb and symphalangism in diastrophic dysplasia

  - Deformity type: Genu valgum seen in spondyloepiphyseal dysplasia, multiple epiphyseal dysplasias, Morquio's syndrome, Ellis–van Creveld, Kniest syndrome, genu varum and valgum in pseudoachondroplasia
  - Foot and ankle: SED shows ankle valgus, achondroplasia shows ankle varus. Diastrophic dysplasia: Clubfoot and skewfoot

- Extraskeletal features:

  - Hydrocephalus: Achondroplasia
  - Eye: Cataracts in Morquio's, retinal detachment in SEDC and Kniest
  - Ear: Recurrent otitis media in achondroplasia, hearing loss in Kniest
  - Cardiac: Congenital in Ellis–van Creveld syndrome, acquired in Morquio's
  - Respiratory:

- Laryngotracheomalacia in campomelic, diastrophic
- Apnoea: Central± obstructive in achondroplasia
- Restrictive lung disease: Metatropic, thanatophoric, Ellis–van Creveld

  - Immunological: McKusick (metaphyseal chondrodysplasia)

Radiographic Evaluation

- The most powerful single tool for evaluation of dysplasias.
- A complete skeletal survey should be done in children >6 months.
- In newborn and infants <6 months, at least.

  - AP and lateral films of whole spine.
  - AP films of hand.
  - AP of lower extremities.
  - Lateral cervical spine flexion and extension (including skull).

- Some features are pathognomonic.

  - The lumbar spine and pelvis in achondroplasia.
  - Hypoplastic scapulae with non-ossified thoracic pedicles in campomelic dysplasia.

- Several surveys may be required during growth before a specific condition is diagnosed—SED vs. Kniest.
- The survey is evaluated in order to recognise patterns of abnormality.
- Cervical kyphosis is a common feature of diastrophic dysplasia, campomelic dysplasia and Larsen's syndrome.
- Platyspondyly is a common feature of SEDC, pseudoachondroplasia, Morquio's and metatropic dysplasia.
- Coxa vara is a common feature of spondyloepiphyseal dysplasia and its variants, cleidocranial dysplasia and chondrodysplasia punctata.
- Bullet-shaped metacarpals are featured on hand radiographs of Morquio's syndrome.

2.1 Achondroplasia

Definition

This is a form of short-limbed dwarfism with abnormal facies. This is an autosomal dominant, but 90 % are new mutations.

Aetiology

- Mutation affects a single protein in fibroblast growth factor receptor-3 (*FGFR-3*) gene, changing glycine to arginine at position 380, leading to growth retardation of the proliferative zone of the growth plate.

Pathophysiology

- The abnormality seen in the bone of patients with achondroplasia is failure of endochondral ossification. Intramembranous and periosteal ossifications are undisturbed.
- Loss of normal chondrocyte proliferation.
- Because the width of the long bones is a product of intramembranous periosteal ossification, the bones are of normal diameter.

Evaluation

- The growth plates with the most growth (proximal humerus/distal femur) are most affected, resulting in rhizomelic (proximal more than distal) short stature.
- Trunk height tends to be normal, but arm span and standing height are diminished.
- They also have frontal bossing, button nose, trident hands, thoracolumbar kyphosis, lumbar stenosis with lordosis and short pedicles, posterior radial head dislocation, "champagne glass" pelvic outlet and genu varum.
- Radiology: The metaphyses are widened and flared, but the epiphyses are uninvolved. The growth plates are U-shaped or V-shaped. The pelvis characteristically appears broad and flat, with squared iliac wings. The foramen magnum is smaller than normal. There is posterior scalloping of the vertebral bodies and shortened pedicles.
- Prenatal diagnosis of achondroplasia: Ultrasonography does reveal decreased femoral length for gestational age.

Treatment

- Nonsurgical treatment is usual for the thoracolumbar kyphosis present early on. Avoidance of unsupported sitting may help prevent it.
- Genu varum is treated with osteotomies if symptomatic.
- Foramen magnum/upper cervical stenosis may require urgent decompression if cord compression is present; this area does grow bigger in later life.
- The main issue in adult life is lumbar stenosis requiring decompression and/or fusion. A more lateral decompression is often necessary.

- Limb lengthening may be carried out. Adolescence usually is the time when lengthening is undertaken.
- Administration of growth hormone continues on an investigational basis.

2.2 *Hypochondroplasia*

Overview

- Autosomal dominant form due to a cytosine–adenine substitution in FGFR-3 in chromosome 4; but milder form of achondroplasia.
- Rhizomelic shortening of extremities, apparent at 2–3 years.
- Less distinct facial features than achondroplasia.
- Diagnosis is rarely apparent before 2 years.
- Lumbar canal stenosis, genu varum and short stature are seen.
- Treatment is similar to achondroplasia.

2.3 *Diastrophic Dysplasia*

Definition

- Short-limbed and short-trunk dwarfism apparent from birth. Other common findings include cleft palate and hitchhiker thumbs.

Pathoanatomy

- Autosomal recessive
- Mutation in sulphate transport protein that primarily affects cartilage matrix

Evaluation

- Cleft palate is present in 60 %.
- Cauliflower ears are present in 80 % and develop after birth from cystic swellings in the ear cartilage. Compressive wrapping is used for cystic swelling of the ears.
- Cervical kyphosis and thoracolumbar scoliosis are often present.
- Joint contractures (hip flexion, genu valgum with dislocated patellae) and rigid clubfoot or skewfoot are often present.

Treatment

- Surgery is indicated for progressive spinal deformity or cord compromise; note that cervical kyphosis often resolves spontaneously.
- Surgery is also indicated for progressive, symptomatic lower extremity deformity; recurrence is common.

2.4 *Kniest Dysplasia*

Overview

- Autosomal dominant disorder due to mutation in type 2 collagen (COL2A1)
- Short trunk and short limbs

Evaluation

- Features include midface hypoplasia, myopia, retinal detachment and deafness.
- A distinctive feature of Kniest dysplasia is hundreds of small holes in the bone cartilage, making it appear like Swiss cheese on an x-ray. The holes weaken the cartilage, which serves as connective tissue throughout the body and causes joint stiffness and swelling.

Orthopaedic Implication

- Dumbbell-shaped long bones with broad metaphysic and irregular dysplastic epiphysis
- Other features; odontoid hypoplasia, kyphosis, mild scoliosis, joint contractures and limb malalignment, hip dysplasia
- Degenerative arthritis as early as second decade of life

Treatment

- Every child's condition is different, so treatment is determined on a case-by-case basis. Treatment may include nonsurgical options such as bracing and physical therapy or surgical options such as spinal fusion or implanting growing rods to stabilise the child's spine as he continues to grow.

2.5 *Multiple Epiphyseal Dysplasia (MED)*

Overview

- Proportionate dwarfism with multiple epiphyses involved but no spinal involvement (limbs shorter than trunk)
- Often diagnosed in mid childhood

Pathoanatomy

- Autosomal dominant.
- Genes identified causing this phenotype include *COMP*; *COL9A2*, which encodes a chain for type IX collagen (a link protein for type II collagen); and recently a similar gene, *COL9A3*.

Evaluation

- Multiple abnormal and irregular epiphyses.
- Shortened metacarpals and metatarsals are present.
- Valgus knees with a double-layer patella are found.
- May have mild to severe involvement of epiphyses; long-term prognosis ranges from mild joint problems to end-stage OA with severe joint contractures at a young age.
- No spinal involvement.
- For any bilateral Legg–Calvé–Perthes patients, rule out MED.

Treatment

- Progressive genu valgum can be managed by staple hemiepiphysiodesis or osteotomy.
- Painful, stiff joints are managed with therapy and nonsteroidal anti-inflammatory drugs; end-stage OA with joint arthroplasty.

2.6 *Spondyloepiphyseal Dysplasia (SED)*

Overview
Proportionate dwarfism with spinal involvement and a barrel chest

Pathoanatomy

- Most common autosomal dominant form is SED congenital, which is apparent from birth and caused by mutations in *COL2A1*, which encodes type II collagen found in articular cartilage and vitreous humor of the eyes. The proliferative zone of the growth plates is affected with inability of epiphyseal centres to ossify.
- Rarer, X-linked recessive form is SED tarda, which is milder, with later onset from age 8 to 10 years and is thought to involve the *SEDL* gene.

Evaluation

- Hypoplasia of odontoid and atlantoaxial instability is common in both forms.
- Platyspondyly and delayed epiphyseal ossification are present in both, as is premature OA.
- SED congenita: Coxa vara, genu valgum, planovalgus feet, retinal detachment, myopia and hearing loss also present.
- SED tarda: No lower limb bowing, but dislocated hips are sometimes seen.

Treatment

- Cervical instability should be stabilised.
- Progressive, symptomatic lower extremity deformity should be corrected with osteotomies, being careful to assess the whole limb for deformities in joints above and below and recognising that early OA and joint arthroplasty are still likely.

2.7 Metaphyseal Chondrodysplasias

Definition

The metaphyseal chondrodysplasias are actually a group of disorders characterised by metaphyseal irregularity and deformity but with preservation of epiphyseal structure.

The real defect is in the growth plate itself, resulting in failure of uniform ossification of the cartilage columns, with persistence of cartilage islands, underdevelopment and deformity as the sequelae.

The commonest types are McKusick, Schmid and Jansen types, as well as Kozlowski-type spondylometaphyseal dysplasia, which is associated with mild changes in the vertebral bodies.

2.7.1 McKusick-Type Metaphyseal Chondrodysplasia

Overview

- It is also known by the term cartilage–hair hypoplasia.
- The condition is autosomal recessive and maps to chromosome 9. The defect is in the RMRP gene, which encodes a mitochondrial RNA-processing enzyme.

Evaluation

Clinical

- The first thing that distinguishes this group of patients is their fine, light and sometimes sparse hair.
- An alteration in T-cell immunity causes an increased risk of viral infection (especially varicella zoster, which may be more severe in these persons).
- Continued antibiotic prophylaxis in the first 6 months of life has been recommended.
- Anaemia may develop. Haematologic problems have a tendency to become less severe after childhood.
- Hirschsprung disease, intestinal malabsorption and megacolon may also develop. There is an increased risk of malignancy, such as lymphoma, sarcoma and skin cancer. Patients need medical surveillance into adulthood, more than would most patients with skeletal dysplasia.
- Generalised ligamentous laxity is present, but the elbows actually have flexion contractures. There may be mild genu varum. Pectus excavatum or carinatum may be observed.

Radiographic Features

- In the McKusick type of metaphyseal chondrodysplasia, there is more shortening and less varus of the long bones than is seen in the Schmid type.
- The metaphyseal involvement is more evenly distributed, not all on the medial side of the knee.

- Atlantoaxial instability has been reported.
- The sternum is angulated so that the distal end is anterior.

Orthopaedic Implications

- It is prudent to obtain flexion–extension films for atlantoaxial instability. MRI in flexion and extension may be helpful if the plain films seem equivocal diagnostically. Posterior spine fusion should be performed if there is more than 8 mm of translation or if any signs of cord compression are present.
- In congenital hip dislocation, if it is detected early, successful closed reduction may be performed.
- The varus at knee or ankle should be corrected, if severe.

2.7.2 Schmid-Type Metaphyseal Chondrodysplasia

Overview

- The Schmid type is more common than the McKusick type.
- This condition is autosomal dominant with type X collagen mutation in *COL10A1* gene and affects proliferative/hypertrophic zones.

Evaluation

Clinical Features

- Patients with the Schmid dysplasia show rather minimal clinical abnormalities. They are normal at birth. The facial appearance is normal.
- They may present with leg pains, varus knees and ankles, short stature or a waddling gait.
- The adult height is minimally shortened.

Radiographic Features

- The metaphyses of the long bones are widened and flared and may have cysts. The physes are slightly widened.
- There is a varus deformity of the knees. Coxa vara may be present.
- Atlantoaxial instability has been reported but is rare.

Orthopaedic Implications

- The epiphyses are normal, and patients rarely experience degenerative changes.
- Genu varum may need correction.

2.7.3 Jansen Metaphyseal Dysplasia

Overview

- Mutation in parathyroid hormone receptor (affects parathyroid hormone-related protein), which regulates chondrocyte differentiation and affects proliferative/hypertrophic zones; autosomal dominant

Orthopaedic Implications

- Wide eyes, squatting stance, hypercalcemia, bulbous metaphyseal expansion of long bones and extremity malalignment may be present.

2.7.4 Kozlowski-Type (Spondylometaphyseal) Dysplasia

Overview
Clinical Features

- Spondylometaphyseal dysplasia is an uncommon autosomal dominant disorder characterised by spinal as well as metaphyseal changes.
- The disorder is recognised in preschool-aged children by the findings of short stature and mildly increased kyphosis.
- There may be slight limitation of joint movement, a Trendelenburg gait and early osteoarthritis. Adult height reaches approximately 150 cm.

Radiographic Features

- There is mild platyspondyly.
- The bone age of the carpals and tarsals is retarded. The metaphyseal chondrodysplasia is most pronounced in the proximal femur.

2.8 Mucopolysaccharidoses

Overview

- MPS is a type of lysosomal storage disorder where a particular enzyme deficiency leads to accumulation of products in the viscera, joints and brain. This group is characterised by excretion of mucopolysaccharide in urine (Tables 1, subtype II and 2).

Pathoanatomy

- Mucopolysaccharidoses are lysosomal storage diseases that result in the intracellular accumulation of mucopolysaccharides in multiple organs.
- All are autosomal recessive except Hunter syndrome type II, which is X-linked recessive.

Evaluation

- Urine test, using a toluidine blue spot test to see which mucopolysaccharide breakdown products are present
- Testing enzyme activity in skin fibroblast culture
- Chorionic villous sampling

Table 1 Subtypes of mucopolysaccharidoses

Subtype	Cause	Prognosis	Stored substance
Type I H (Hurler syndrome)	Alpha-L-iduronidase deficiency	Death in first decade of life	HS + DS
Type I HS (Hurler–Scheie syndrome)		Death in third decade of life	
Type I S (Scheie syndrome)		Good survival	
Type II (Hunter syndrome)	Sulpho-iduronate-sulphatase deficiency	Death in second decade of life	HS + DS
Type III (Sanfilippo syndrome)	Multiple enzyme deficiency	Death in second decade of life	HS
Type IV (Morquio's syndrome)	Type A (galactosamine-6-sulphate-sulphatase deficiency)	More severe involvement in patients with type IV A than in those with type IV B; survival into adulthood is possible	KS, CS
IV A: Morquio A			
IV B: Morquio B			
IV C: Morquio C			
Type VI (Maroteaux–Lamy syndrome)	Arylsulphatase B deficiency	Poor survival with severe form	DS, CS
Type VII (Sly syndrome)	Beta-glucuronidase deficiency	Poor survival	CS, HS, DS
	Type B (beta-galactosidase deficiency)		

KS keratan sulphate, *HS* heparan sulphate, *CS* chondroitin sulphate, *DS* dermatan sulphate

Clinical Features

- All patients are short statured; additional features vary but often include corneal clouding, enlarged skull, bullet-shaped phalanges, mental retardation, visceromegaly, cervical instability, genu valgum and developmental dysplasia of the hip (DDH) that is later in onset.

Radiological Features

- Vertebra: Platyspondyly (ovoid hypoplastic flat vertebral body usually pointing anteriorly)
- Skull: Abnormal J-shaped sella, thick calvarium
- Chest: Wide oar-shaped ribs, wide clavicles, plump scapula
- Long bones: Foreshortening of long bones with underdevelopment of epiphysis with submetaphyseal overconstriction
- Short tubular bones: Bullet-shaped metacarpals
- Pelvis: Wine glass appearance with shallow acetabulum
- Hip: Coxa valga, fragmented ossification centre of femoral head
- Knee: Genu valgum
- Bone structure: Osteopenic with coarsely laced trabeculae

Table 2 Skeletal dysplasias: genetics and features

Name	Genetics	Features
Achondroplasia	*FGFR-3*; autosomal dominant; 90 % sporadic mutations	Rhizomelic shortening with normal trunk, frontal bossing, trident hands, thoracolumbar kyphosis, lumbar stenosis and lordosis, radial head subluxations, champagne glass pelvic outlet, genu varum
Hypochondroplasia	*FGFR-3* in a different area than achondroplasia; autosomal dominant	Milder than achondroplasia; rhizomelic shortening at 2–3 years, short stature, lumbar stenosis, genu varum. Less distinct facial features
Thanatophoric dysplasia	*FGFR-3*	Rhizomelic shortening, platyspondyly, protuberant abdomen, small thoracic cavity. Death by age 2 years
SED congenital	Type II collagen mutation in *COL2A1* gene; autosomal dominant but usually sporadic mutation	Proportionate dwarfism with spine involvement and barrel chest, abnormal epiphyses including spine (platyspondyly), atlantoaxial instability/odontoid hypoplasia, coxa vara and DDH, genu valgum, premature OA, retinal detachment/ myopia, sensorineural hearing loss
SED tarda	Unidentified mutation likely in type II collagen, X-linked recessive	Late onset (age 8–10 years), premature OA, associated with DDH but not lower extremity bowing
Kniest dysplasia	Type II collagen mutation in *COL2A1* gene, autosomal dominant	Midface hypoplasia, joint contractures, odontoid hypoplasia, kyphosis/scoliosis, dumbbell-shaped femurs, respiratory problems, cleft palate, retinal detachment/myopia, otitis media/ hearing loss, early OA
Cleidocranial dysplasia	Defect in CBFA-1, a transcription factor that activates osteoblast differentiation; autosomal dominant; affects intramembranous ossification	Aplasia/hypoplasia of clavicles, delayed skull suture closure, frontal bossing, coxa vara, delayed ossification pubis, genu valgum
Nail–patella syndrome (osteo-onychodysplasia)	Mutation in LIM homeobox transcription factor 1-β also expressed in eyes/kidneys; autosomal dominant	Aplasia/hypoplasia of the patella and condyles, dysplastic nails, iliac horns, posterior dislocation of the radial head; 30 % will get renal failure and glaucoma as adults
Diastrophic dysplasia	Mutation in sulphate transporter gene affects cartilage matrix. Autosomal dominant	Rhizomelic and truncal shortening, cleft palate, cervical kyphosis, kyphoscoliosis, hitchhiker thumbs, cauliflower ears, rigid clubfeet, skewfoot, severe OA, joint contractures

(continued)

Table 2 (continued)

Name	Genetics	Features
Mucopolysaccharidoses	All defects in enzymes that degrade glycosaminoglycans in lysosomes. The incomplete degradation products accumulate in various organs and cause dysfunction. All autosomal recessive except Hunter syndrome (X-linked recessive)	Visceromegaly, corneal clouding, cardiac disease, deafness, short stature, mental retardation (except Morquio's syndrome, which has normal intelligence). C1–C2 instability is common, as is hip dysplasia and abnormal epiphyses
Metaphyseal dysplasia: Schmid type	Type X collagen mutation in *COL10A1* gene; autosomal dominant; affects proliferative/hypertrophic zones	May appear normal at birth, short stature, coxa vara, genu varum
Metaphyseal dysplasia: Jansen type	Mutation in parathyroid hormone receptor (affects parathyroid hormone-related protein), which regulates chondrocyte differentiation; affects proliferative/hypertrophic zones; autosomal dominant	Wide eyes, squatting stance, hypercalcemia, bulbous metaphyseal expansion of long bones and extremity malalignment
Metaphyseal dysplasia: McKusick type Cartilage–hair hypoplasia	Mutation in *RMRP* gene affects proliferative/hypertrophic zones	C1–C2 instability, hypoplasia of cartilage, small-diameter "fine" hair, intestinal malabsorption and megacolon, increased risk of viral infections and malignancies (immune dysfunction), ligamentous laxity but elbow flexion contractures, pectus abnormalities, genu varum
Pseudoachondroplasia	Mutation in *COMP* on chromosome 19, which is an extracellular matrix glycoprotein in cartilage; autosomal dominant	C1–C2 instability due to odontoid hypoplasia, normal facies, metaphyseal flaring, delayed epiphyses, lower extremity malalignment, DDH, scoliosis, early OA
MED	Mutations in *COMP*, *COL9A2* or *COL9A3* genes (collagen IX, which is a linker for collagen II in cartilage); autosomal dominant	Short stature, epiphyseal dysplasia, genu valgum, hip osteonecrosis and dysplasia, early OA. Spine not involved. Short metacarpals/metatarsals, double-layer patella
Ellis–van Creveld (EVC) syndrome/chondroectodermal dysplasia	Mutation in the *EVC* gene; autosomal recessive	Acromesomelic shortening, postaxial polydactyly, genu valgum, dysplastic nails/teeth, medial iliac spikes, fused capitate/hamate, congenital heart disease
Diaphyseal dysplasia (also known as Camurati–Engelmann syndrome)	Autosomal dominant	Symmetric cortical thickening of long bones most commonly seen in tibia, femur, humerus

Treatment

- Hurler syndrome is now treated with a bone marrow transplant in the first year of life; intelligence is normal in some affected individuals, but short stature and orthopaedic deformities are always present.
- Surgery is indicated for cervical instability (often atlantoaxial—assess with dynamic MRI) and progressive lower extremity deformity.

Bibliography

1. Ain MC, Chaichana KL, Schkrohowsky JG. Retrospective study of cervical arthrodesis in patients with various types of skeletal dysplasia. Spine. 2006;31:E169–74.
2. Mackenzie WG, Ballock RT. Genetic diseases and skeletal dysplasias. In: Vaccaro AR, editor. Orthopaedic knowledge update 8. Rosemont: American Academy of Orthopaedic Surgeons; 2005. p. 663–75.
3. Sponseller PD, Ain MC. The skeletal dysplasias. In: Morrissy RT, Weinstein SL, editors. Lovell and Winter's pediatric orthopaedics. 6th ed. Philadelphia: Lippincott Williams & Wilkins; 2006. p. 205–50.
4. Unger S. A genetic approach to the diagnosis of skeletal dysplasia. Clin Orthop Relat Res. 2002;401:32–8.

3 Neurofibromatosis

Ashok Johari, Ratna Maheshwari, and Shalin Maheshwari

Take-Home Message

- Six or more café-au-lait spots with greatest diameter 5 mm in prepubertal and 15 mm in postpubertal patients are required as a criterion for diagnosing this condition.
- Although 50 % of congenital pseudarthroses of the tibia cases are due to NF, only 10 % of patients with NF have congenital pseudarthrosis of the tibia.
- Scoliosis in patients with NF is often dystrophic (short and sharply angular curve). Surgical success is much higher with combined anterior and posterior fusions.
- 87 % of curves rapidly progress when three or more ribs are pencilled.
- A preoperative MRI scan should be obtained to rule out dural ectasia and intraspinal neurofibromas.

Aetiology

- The two forms of neurofibromatosis (NF) are NF1 and NF2. NF1 is the most common single-gene disorder (1 in 3,000 births). NF1 is autosomal dominant disorder with 100 % penetrance.

Pathophysiology

- The mutation in NF is in the neurofibromin gene located on chromosome 17.
- Neurofibromin regulates cell growth by modulating Ras signalling. This protein acts as a tumour suppressor. Mutation causes disruption of Ras signalling.

Radiology

- Anterolateral bowing of tibia, dystrophic scoliosis (short, four to six levels), with sharp curves, non-union of long bone or overgrowth of part should alert the physician.
- Scalloping of cortex, cystic lesions or permeative bone destruction may also be seen.
- Pelvic radiographs may show coxa valga and protrusio acetabuli.

Diagnostic Criteria and Classification *NF1*

- Von Recklinghausen disease
- Orthopaedic manifestations common

NF 2

- Familial acoustic neuroma.
- Orthopaedic manifestation rare. CNS tumours and rare peripheral manifestations are present.

Diagnostic Criteria for NF 1

Children may exhibit none of the typical findings at birth, but diagnosis can be made as they grow older and develop characteristics necessary to confirm a diagnosis of NF1:

- Six or more café-au-lait spots, with greatest diameter 5 mm in prepubertal and 15 mm in postpubertal patients
- Two or more neurofibromas of any type or one plexiform neurofibroma
- Axillary freckling
- Optic glioma
- Two or more Lisch nodules (iris hamartomas)
- A distinctive osseous lesion
- A first-degree relative with NF1

Treatment

- Anterolateral bowing of the tibia is often treated with prophylactic bracing with total contact orthosis to prevent pseudarthrosis. Fifty per cent of patients with anterolateral bowing have NF, but only 10 % of children with NF have anterolateral bowing:

- Pseudarthrosis may be treated with bone graft and intramedullary rodding and sometimes later will require vascularised bone graft or bone transport by distraction osteogenesis. Amputation is rarely necessary.
- Plexiform neurofibromas (in 40 % of patients with NF1) may cause limb overgrowth. Limb equalisation procedures are indicated for children with projected limb-length discrepancies >2 cm.
- Scoliosis:
  - Scoliosis is common in patients with NF.
  - Nondystrophic scoliosis in NF is treated like adolescent idiopathic scoliosis.
  - Dystrophic scoliosis is short (four to six levels), with sharp curves, and often occurs in children younger than age 6:
    - It is characterised by scalloping end plates, foraminal enlargement and pencilling of ribs.
    - 87 % of curves rapidly progress when three or more ribs are pencilled.
    - The most important risk factors for progression is an early age of onset, a high Cobb angle and an apical vertebra which is severely rotated, scalloped and located in the middle to lower thoracic area.
    - Dystrophic scoliosis in NF is resistant to brace treatment.
    - Dystrophic scoliosis in NF is treated with early anterior and posterior fusion.
    - A preoperative MRI scan should be obtained to rule out dural ectasia and intraspinal neurofibromas.

Complications

- Malignant transformation to neurofibrosarcoma is possible if there is a second mutation in the remaining normal gene.
- Hypertension is a major risk factor for early death, likely to be due to renal artery stenosis or pheochromocytoma.

Bibliography

1. Funasaki H, Winter RB, Lonstein JB, et al. Pathophysiology of spinal deformities in neurofibromatosis. An analysis of 71 patients who had curves associated with dystrophic changes. J Bone Joint Surg Am. 1994;76:692.
2. Joseph KN, Brown JR, MacEwen GD. Unusual orthopaedic manifestations of neurofibromatosis. Clin Orthop Relat Res. 1992;278:17.
3. Morrisy RT. Congenital pseudoarthrosis of tibia. A long term follow up study. Clin Orthop. 1982;166:14.
4. Xu G, O'Connell P, Viskochil D. The neurofibromatosis type 1 gene encodes a protein related to GAP. Cell. 1990;62:608.

4 Upper Limb Paediatric Trauma

Ashok Johari, Ratna Johari, and Shalin Maheshwari

Take-Home Message

- When the diagnosis of child abuse is missed, recurrent injuries occur in about 50 % and it is lethal in 10 % of infants and children.
- Proximal humerus fractures have tremendous remodelling potential, so surgery is rarely needed.
- With fractures of the humeral shaft, primary radial nerve palsies should be observed; however, secondary radial nerve palsies require urgent exploration.
- Ulnar nerve injury with SCH fractures is almost always iatrogenic and is due to medial pin insertion. The risk is greatest if the medial pin is inserted with the elbow in a hyperflexed position.
- The most commonly injured nerve for extension type supracondylar fractures is the AIN and for the flexion type fractures is the ulnar nerve.
- A pulseless, well-perfused hand may be observed following SCH fracture because of the excellent collateral circulation around the elbow.
- The oblique radiograph is the most sensitive for detecting maximal displacement of lateral condyle fractures and must be obtained when contemplating closed treatment.
- During open reduction of lateral condyle fractures, posterior soft-tissue dissection must be avoided to avoid osteonecrosis.
- Elbow dislocations in young children are exceedingly rare, so transphyseal fractures should be suspected in patients with displacement of the proximal radius and ulna relative to the humerus. Elbow arthrography, ultrasonography or MRI may be performed to confirm the diagnosis if the diagnosis is unclear.
- With forearm fractures, bayonet apposition is acceptable in children younger than 10 years of age.
- Isolated radial head dislocations almost never occur in children. These presumed "isolated" injuries are almost always the result of plastic deformation of the ulna with concomitant radial head dislocation (Monteggia fracture).
- With distal forearm physeal fractures, to minimise the risk of iatrogenic physeal injury, no more than one or two reduction attempts should be performed in the emergency department, and rereduction should not be performed more than 5–7 days after injury.
- Single-bone forearm shaft fractures should raise suspicion regarding presence of a Galeazzi- or Monteggia-type injury.

4.1 General Considerations

- A child's bone has growth plate, which facilitates remodelling of residual angulation. However, an injured growth plate can be a cause of deformity.
- The bone has a higher collagen to bone ratio. This reduces the modulus of elasticity of bone. It also has higher cellular and porous content. Bone fails in both tension and compression.
- Periosteum in children is more metabolically active and has more strength. Intact periosteal hinge affects fracture patterns and may aid in reduction.

4.2 Child Abuse

- Because child abuse or nonaccidental trauma is a potentially lethal condition, consider this possibility in every infant or young child with a fracture. When the diagnosis of child abuse is missed, recurrent injuries occur in about 50 % and it is lethal in 10 % of infants and children.
- Suspicion of child abuse increases when the following are present:
  - Any fracture that occurs before walking age
  - Multiple injuries in a child without a witnessed and reasonable explanation
  - Multiple injuries in a child <2 years
  - A child with long-bone injuries and a head injury
- A skeletal survey must be obtained in all children suspected of child abuse to rule out other fractures of differing ages (including examination for skull and rib fractures). A bone scan can show recent injuries if further evaluation is indicated.
- Look for evidence of swelling, pseudoparalysis or soft-tissue trauma. Bruising is more common than fractures.
- Fractures that have a high degree of specificity for abuse are metaphyseal fractures and fractures of the humeral shaft, ribs, scapula, outer end of the clavicle and vertebra. Bilateral fractures, complex skull fractures and those of different ages are suspect.
- Inform social worker. Carefully document findings and evaluation.
- Many fractures are sufficiently healed at the time of presentation to the orthopaedic surgeon that they do not require treatment.

4.3 Evaluation and Resuscitation of a Trauma Patient

- Initial attention and care is directed to the life-threatening injuries:
  - Airway, breathing and circulation (the ABCs) are addressed immediately.
  - Care from a trauma team is requisite to maximise the child's chance of survival.
  - Fluid resuscitation is essential; if venous access is difficult, an intraosseous infusion with a large-bore needle may be necessary.

- Children often remain haemodynamically stable for significant periods of time following significant blood loss:
  - Hypovolaemic shock eventually ensues if fluid resuscitation is inadequate.
  - The “triad of death” (acidosis, hypothermia and coagulopathy) may occur if hypovolaemia persists.
- Because of large head size in young children, a special transport board with an occipital cut-out is necessary when transporting children younger than 6 years to the hospital, to prevent cervical spine flexion and potential iatrogenic cervical spinal cord injury.
- Intracranial pressure (ICP) must be controlled in patients with head injury to minimise ongoing brain damage. ICP can be controlled by elevating the head of the bed, hyperventilation (which lowers pCO_2), limiting intravenous fluids, administration of diuretics and appropriate pain control (including appropriate fracture immobilisation before definitive treatment).

4.3.1 Secondary Evaluation

- Trauma rating systems:
  - Although no single system is optimal for determining prognosis, several trauma rating scores frequently are used, including the Injury Severity Score, the Modified Injury Severity Score (MISS) and the Paediatric Trauma Score.
  - The Glasgow Coma Scale, scored on a scale of 3–15 points, is the tool most commonly used for evaluating head injury:
    - GCS <8 at presentation in verbal children indicates a higher risk of mortality.
    - GCS motor score 72 h postinjury is predictive of permanent disability following traumatic brain injury.
- Abdominal bruising often heralds abdominal visceral injuries and spine fractures.
- Up to 10 % of injuries are initially missed by the treating team because of head injury and/or severe pain in other locations.

4.3.2 Imaging Studies

- Plain radiographs suffice for most extremity fractures.
- CT scans:
  - Only about half of pelvic fractures identified on CT scan appear to be effected by AP pelvic radiographs.
  - CT also helps to delineate fracture patterns in spinal, calcaneal or other intra-articular fractures.
- Intravenous pyelography is used to assess for bladder or urethral injuries, which may occur with anterior pelvic fractures (especially straddle fractures).

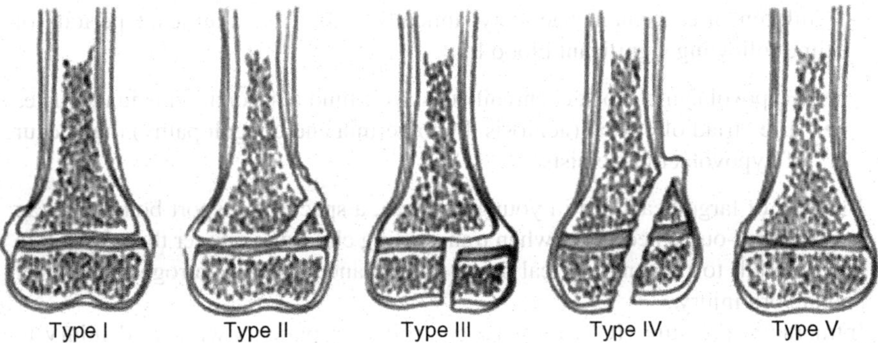

Fig. 1 The Salter–Harris classification: *Type 1* is along the growth plate and can be displaced. *Type 2* is through the metaphysis and along the growth plate. *Type 3* is along the growth plate and through the epiphysis. *Type 4* is through the metaphysis, through growth plate and through the epiphysis. *Type 5* is crush injury to physis

4.4 Physeal Considerations

- Physeal fractures are of great importance, as these injuries can affect subsequent growth and remodelling potential.
- The physis usually fractures through the zone of provisional calcification, sparing the germinal cells so growth is unaffected.
- The most commonly used classification for growth plate fractures is the Salter–Harris classification (Fig. 1).

  – Type I is characterised by a physeal separation.
  – Type II by a fracture that traverses the physis and exits through the metaphysis.
  – Type III by a fracture that traverses the physis before exiting through the epiphysis.
  – Type IV by a fracture that passes through the epiphysis, physis and metaphysis.
  – Type V by a crush injury to the physis.

    - Advantages: Ease of use and prognostic value.
    - One disadvantage of this classification is that Salter–Harris V fractures (which occur rarely) cannot be distinguished from Salter–Harris I fractures at initial presentation; the differentiation often is not made until a growth arrest has occurred.

- Classification of injury type is usually done by radiography. Imaging by CT scans may clarify complex fracture patterns such as those in triplane fractures of the ankle.
- Physeal bridge formation usually follows SH-III, SH-IV, or SH-V injuries. The mechanism is either a crush injury to the germinal layer or a displaced fracture that allows bone to form across the physis.

- Prevention of physeal bridge formation is best achieved by an anatomic reduction of SH-III and SH-IV fractures. Open reduction and internal fixation that does not traverse the physis is best. If fixation is necessary across the growth plate, use small, smooth K wires.

4.5 *Upper Limb Fractures in Children*

- The most common reason for admission to hospital in childhood is for manipulation of an upper limb fracture.
- The majority of upper limb fractures occur as a result of indirect violence, usually a fall on outstretched hand. A minority result from direct violence and are associated with multiple injuries (Table 3).
- The order of appearance of ossification centers is given in Table 3.

4.5.1 Proximal Humerus Fractures

- Salter–Harris type I injury is common in patients under 5 years and Salter–Harris type II is common in children more than 11 years.
- Metaphyseal fractures without epiphyseal fractures predominate in age group 5–11 years.
- 80 % of humeral length is contributed by proximal humeral physis.
- Growth disturbance after proximal humerus fractures is rare.
- Due to the tremendous growth potential, it has tremendous remodelling potential.

Mechanism of Injury

- Fall on outstretched hand

Classification

Neer–Horowitz

- Grade I: 5 mm or less displacement
- Grade II: 1/3 width of shaft displacement
- Grade III: 2/3 width of shaft displacement
- Grade IV: >2/3 width of shaft displacement

Table 3 Order of appearance of ossification centres of the elbow on radiographs

	Age of appearance in girls (years)	Age of appearance in boys (years)
Capitellum	1	1
Radius (proximal)	4–5	5–6
Medial epicondyle	5–6	7–8
Trochlea	8–9	10–11
Olecranon	9	11
Lateral epicondyle	10	11–12

Evaluation

- Since proximal humerus begins to ossify only at 6 months of age, MRI, arthrogram or ultrasound may be necessary for diagnosis.

Management

- Dictated by age, site of injury and degree of displacement.
- Majority are managed by sling, collar and cuff or Velpeau bandage.
- No controversy for treatment of all fractures with Grade I and Grade II displacement: Immobilise (sling and swathe) for approximately 3 weeks, then gradual return to motion and function.
- In children 11 years and younger with Grade III and IV displaced fracture, closed reduction to achieve best possible alignment and immobilise. Even with persistent displacement, remodelling potential leads to good outcome.
- In patients older than 11 years, need for reduction and operative treatment is controversial, with conflicting studies available.
- Consider operative treatment for older adolescents (>11 years) with displaced fractures, Grades III and IV, because of the older age and less remodelling potential. Attempt to reduce to Grade I or II level of displacement, and pin if needed to maintain reduction. Sling and swathe immobilisation.
- If fracture is not able to be reduced closed, interposition of the biceps tendon has been reported. Deltopectoral approach for open reduction and internal fixation is recommended.

4.5.2 Clavicle Shaft Fracture

Mechanism of Injury

- Direct blow (10 %) or fall onto point of the shoulder (85 %)

Epidemiology

- Most commonly fractured bone in children and adults
- 2.5–5 % of all fractures, 10–15 % of fractures in children, 65–90 % midshaft

Other Entities

Birth fracture—seen in neonates with difficult birth
May present with pseudoparalysis of the limb
Heal reliably with abundant callus
Do not confuse with congenital pseudarthrosis of the clavicle
Usually asymptomatic with cartilage cap on histology

Goals of Treatment
Complete healing with resulting minimal pain with activities and full motion, strength and endurance of the shoulder and upper extremity

Nonoperative Treatment

Most clavicle fractures in children are non-displaced or minimally displaced due to thick periosteum and can be treated nonoperatively.
Considered to have excellent remodelling potential in younger children with growth until late teens.
Immobilisation with sling or figure-of-8 brace.

Complications

Non-union (low rate)
Malunion—distal fragment medial, inferior, rotates anteriorly

- Altered shoulder mechanics—thoracic outlet syndrome (extreme cases)
- Pain with overhead activities, decreased strength, endurance
- Improved DASH scores after osteotomy for symptomatic malunion

Operative Treatment

Adults—disability with malunion, randomised trials favour operative treatment if displaced

Indications for acute fixation in kids

Open fractures, floating shoulder, multi-trauma, comminuted (Z) fractures, shortened fractures 15–20 mm (remains controversial—remodelling potential is smaller in adolescents nearing end of growth)

Complications

Non-union, infection, irritating hardware, migration of IM fixation
Refracture after plate removal, incisional numbness (supraclavicular nerve)

Techniques

Anterosuperior plating (tension side, but prominent)
Intramedullary fixation—carefully monitor for migration

4.5.3 Supracondylar Fractures

- Most common elbow fracture in children.
- Young children are prone to this injury because of their physiologic ligamentous laxity.

Mechanism of Injury

- Extension type: Fall on outstretched hand with an extension force.
- Flexion type: Direct trauma or fall on flexed elbow.
- With posteromedial displacement, the periosteum fails laterally. Therefore, forearm pronation can aid in reduction.
- With posterolateral displacement, the periosteum fails medially. Forearm supination usually aids in reduction of these fractures.

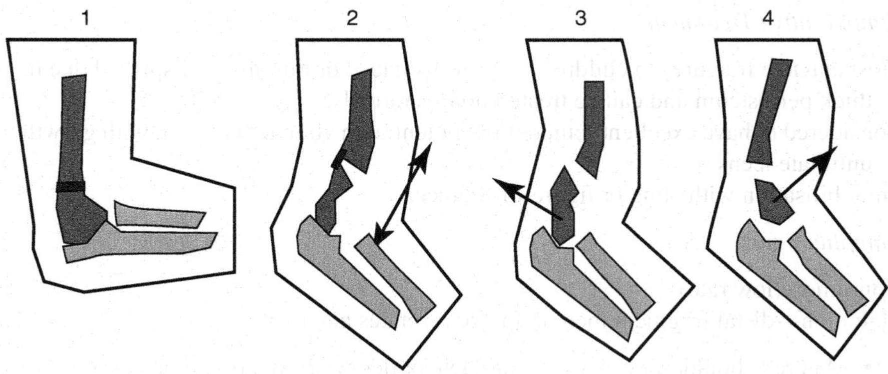

Fig. 2 The Gartland classification. Grade 1, fractures are essentially undisplaced and stable. Grade 2, fractures are partially displaced on the lateral radiographs, but there is some remaining contact. The soft-tissue injury is correspondingly greater. Grade 3, fractures are completely displaced and there is no contact between the proximal and distal fragments on lateral radiographs. Major risks being to brachial artery and median nerve. Grade 4, unstable in flexion and extension

Evaluation

- Baumann angle on AP radiographs. Normal 64–81°, >81° is suggestive of varus.
- Humeral–ulnar angle best reflects the true carrying angle.
- Humerocapitellar angle on lateral radiographs. Normal value is 40°.
- Fat pad sign: Anterior fat pad, posterior fat pad.
- Teardrop of elbow: Oblique orientation of teardrop signifies improper x-ray or fracture.
- Anterior humeral line: Passes through centre of capitellum. This relationship gets altered in fracture.
- Gartland classification (Fig. 2):

  – Type 1: Non-displaced
  – Type 2: Displaced with intact posterior cortex
  – Type 3: Complete displacement, posteromedial or posterolateral

Management

- Type 1: Immobilisation in cast.
- Type 2: Closed reduction and pinning.
- Type 3: Closed reduction and pinning. Two smooth pins from the lateral side are the most commonly used method. If reduction is not obtained, consider open reduction (renewed interest in anterior approach, since it allows for inspection of neurovascular structures and lower incidence of elbow stiffness).
- Closed reduction involves traction to restore length, followed by varus and valgus correction and correction of translation. The elbow is then gradually flexed while applying anterior pressure with thumb over the olecranon.

- Reduction is adequate if the following criteria are fulfilled:
  - The anterior humeral line crosses the capitellum.
  - The Baumann angle is comparative to the opposite side.
  - Oblique views show intact medial and lateral columns.
  - Clinically reduction can be assessed by range of motion and carrying angle.
- The primary indications of an open reduction are interposed tissue in fracture and vascular compromise that does not improve with closed reduction and percutaneous pinning.
- Supracondylar elbow fractures with impaction of the medial condyle: The collapse medially may be subtle and appear insignificant, but if not reduced, the patients developed cubitus varus deformity.

Treatment for Vascular Injuries with Supracondylar Humerus Fractures

- A significant percentage of pulseless patients improve following reduction and fixation.
- Pulse lost after reduction and pinning: Explore brachial artery and treat.
- Pulseless, well-perfused hand: Observe for 24–72 h.
- Pulseless, cool hand: Explore brachial artery and treat.
- Procedures to restore a distal radial pulse have been found to have a high incidence of asymptomatic re-occlusion and re-stenosis of artery in follow-up segmental pressure and MRA studies.
- Pink pulseless hand: Angiography is of little use; colour flow duplex imaging deserves further study.

Complications

- Vascular injury in brachial artery is seen in 1 % of all fractures. The treatment of pink pulseless hand is controversial: Initial observation is recommended, and if there are signs of ischaemia, intervention is necessary.
- Cubitus varus can be associated with higher incidence of lateral condyle fractures, posterolateral rotator instability and ulnar neuropathy.
- 15–20 % are associated with nerve injury. Anterior interosseous component of median nerve is more commonly injured. Usually resolves in 8–12 weeks. Exploration and neurolysis are indicated if no evidence of neural function is present 5 months after injury.
- In case of ulnar nerve palsies after percutaneous cross-pinning, outcomes of studies are controversial with some suggesting that such palsies recover spontaneously and observation is appropriate. Other authors suggest exploration rather than simple pin removal.
- Compartment syndrome: Postsurgical immobilisation should be less than 90° of flexion.

4.5.4 Lateral Condyle Fractures

- 13–18 % of paediatric elbow fractures. Peak age ranges between 6 and 10 years.
- Males >females.
- Most are Salter–Harris type IV fractures.
- They are intra-articular fractures and physeal fractures; hence, anatomic reduction is necessary.

Evaluation

- Oblique x-rays are a must.
- Valgus and varus stress radiograph can provide information about stability of fracture.
- Arthrograms can provide detail about articular congruity but are reserved for intraoperative assessment.

Management

- Non-displaced fractures can be treated with cast but needs weekly x-rays for 3 weeks.
- For minimally displaced fractures, percutaneous pins can be used.
- For displacement greater than 1–2 mm, open reduction with a lateral approach can be used. For anterior joint visualisation, extensor muscles can be peeled off. Dissection posteriorly must be minimal. Pins must be kept for 4 weeks. But fracture may have to be immobilised for a few more weeks.

Complications

- Post-operative stiffness.
- Delayed union can occur even in non-displaced fractures and may be due to poor metaphyseal circulation, bathing of fracture in synovial fluid or tension on the condylar fragment by attached muscles.
- Non-union: It is best to fix in situ with pins or screws and bone graft the site if the non-union has been there for a while.
- Lateral condyle fractures associated with lateral physeal arrest can result in valgus deformity and tardy ulnar nerve palsy.
- Lateral condyle fractures associated with central physeal arrest can result in a "fishtail" deformity.

4.5.5 Radial Neck Fractures

- 7 % of elbow fractures
- Tends to occur between ages of 9–13 years

Mechanism of Injury

- Fall on outstretched hand with a valgus compressive force

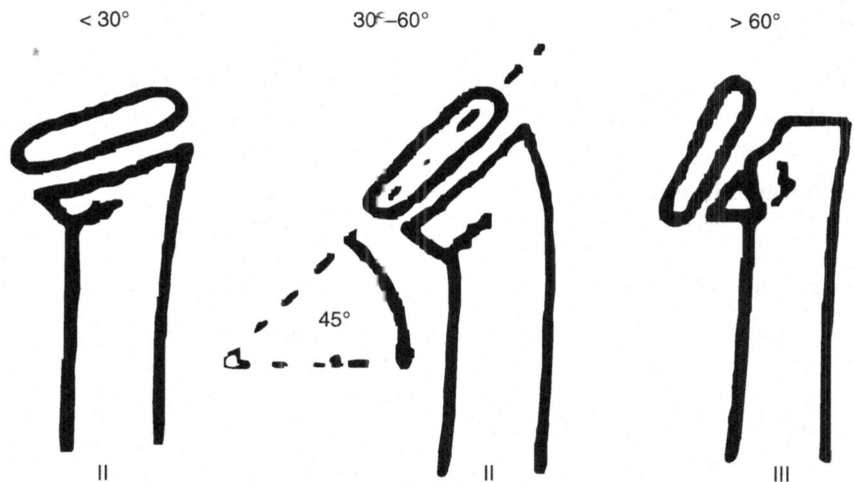

Fig. 3 The angle measured is the displacement of the superior articular surface of the radial head relative to a perpendicular radial shaft. Type 1 fractures are angled less than 30°. Type 2 fractures are angled between 30 and 60°. Type 3 fractures are angled more than 60° (Redrawn from O' Brien PI. Injuries involving the proximal radial epiphysis. Clin Orthop Relat Res. 1965;41:52)

Evaluation

- AP and lateral radiographs are usually sufficient. However, radiographs may underestimate the fragment size and extent of displacement as majority of the fragment is cartilaginous.
- Arthrogram may be done at surgery.
- Mostly posterolateral displacement with a transverse fracture line.

Classification (See Fig. 3)

- Type 1: Displacement <30°
- Type 2: Displacement 30–60°
- Type 3: Displacement >60°

Management

- Angulations <30° do not require reduction, only long arm cast immobilisation.
- Closed reduction is indicated for angulations >30°.
- Percutaneous wire or retrograde intramedullary fixation can be used for highly displaced fractures as reduction aids, when angulation >60°.
- Open reduction should be reserved for irreducible fractures as a last resort as it is associated with an increased rate of complications including non-union and avascular necrosis.

4.5.6 Monteggia Fractures

Monteggia lesion is the combined fracture of ulna and dislocation of radial head. It is important to recognise the combination because radial head dislocation is commonly missed.

Mechanism of Injury

- Fall on outstretched hand

Radiographs and Evaluation

- Line drawn from radial shaft and head should bisect the capitellum in any view.
- Always check the elbow and wrist x-rays in case of any "isolated" fracture of radius or ulna.
- Bado classification of Monteggia lesion:
  - Type 1: Anterior dislocation of radial head, most common
  - Type 2: Posterior dislocation of radial head
  - Type 3: Lateral dislocation of radial head
  - Type 4: Anterior, but associated with a radial neck or shaft fracture

Management

- Treatment principles: Correct ulnar deformity, restore ulna length and achieve congruent reduction of radiocapitellar joint.
- Closed reduction and cast immobilisation recommended for most.
- Surgical treatment of complete ulnar fractures recommended for unstable injuries, in setting of soft-tissue swelling and neurovascular concerns and in older patients.
  - IM nailing for transverse and short oblique fractures.
  - ORIF for long oblique and comminuted ulnar fractures.
- Cast immobilisation × 4–6 weeks, typically with forearm in supination.
  - Type 1 Bado is treated by closed reduction in flexion and elbow is immobilised in 110–120° flexion, neutral or slight supination.
    - Failure to obtain satisfactory alignment of ulnar fracture or reduction of radial head by closed means is an indication for surgery.
    - Boyd approach is preferred as it addresses both—radius and ulna.
  - Type 2 Bado is treated by closed reduction in extension and elbow is immobilised in extension.
  - Type 3 is treated by closed reduction in extension and elbow is immobilised in 110–120° of flexion if it is anterolateral. If posterolateral component, elbow is immobilised in 70–80° of flexion.

  - Type 4 principle of closed reduction is to convert type 4 to type 1 and then treat type 1. If unstable, the radial fracture may need intramedullary K-wire fixation.
  - Late manipulations up to 3 weeks after injury can be successful. Patients who present later may require open reduction of radial head with or without reconstruction of annular ligament. Osteotomy and realignment of proximal ulna may be done simultaneously.

4.5.7 Fractures of Both-Bone Forearm in Children

- 30–50 % of all paediatric fractures.
- Distal > middle >proximal.
- Most common: Open fractures and refractures.
- The remodelling potential of paediatric forearm fractures is considered to be most predictable in children less than 8–10 years of age.

Pathogenesis

- Single-bone forearm shaft fractures should raise suspicion regarding presence of a Galeazzi- or Monteggia-type injury.
- Injury that involves little rotational forces results in forearm fractures at nearly same level.

Classification, Evaluation and Management

- Plastic deformation.
  - Minimal deformity, limited forearm rotation.
  - Bowing with narrow interosseous space on x-rays.
- Greenstick fracture.
  - One cortex is fractured, opposite cortex is intact or with plastic deformation.
  - Rotational mechanism.
  - If alignment is unacceptable, closed reduction must be done.
- Complete fracture.

Treatment

Nonoperative

- Greenstick fracture patterns retain a degree of inherent stability; intentional completion of these fractures is not recommended. 10 % loss of reduction rate has been reported with greenstick fractures.
- Greenstick fractures often involve variable amounts of rotational deformity such that when the forearm is appropriately derotated, reduction of angulation occurs simultaneously.

- Apex volar greenstick fractures are considered to represent supination injuries that require a degree of pronation to affect reduction.
- Apex dorsal greenstick fractures are considered to be pronation injuries that require a degree of supination to aid reduction.
- Classic fingertrap and traction reduction techniques are probably best reserved for complete both-bone forearm fractures. When dealing with both-bone forearm fractures, respect should be paid to the level of fractures when choosing a relatively neutral, pronated or supinated forearm position.
- Estimated rotational malalignment should not exceed 45°.
- Undisplaced both-bone forearm fractures can be treated with cast. Above-elbow immobilisation is the rule.
- In displaced both-bone fractures with unacceptable deformity, closed reduction must be attempted.

Surgical Management

- Surgical indications: Irreducible or unstable fractures, open fractures, associated with vascular injury, multiple-injury patient, floating elbow, refracture.
- When complete fractures occur in children younger than 8–10 years of age with angulation of at least 20° in distal third, 15° in central third or 10° in the proximal third, risk–benefit discussions are appropriate regarding further efforts at fracture reduction and possible internal fixation.
- Complete forearm fractures in children older than 8–10 years should be evaluated very critically with the intention to accept no more than 10° of angulation at any level.

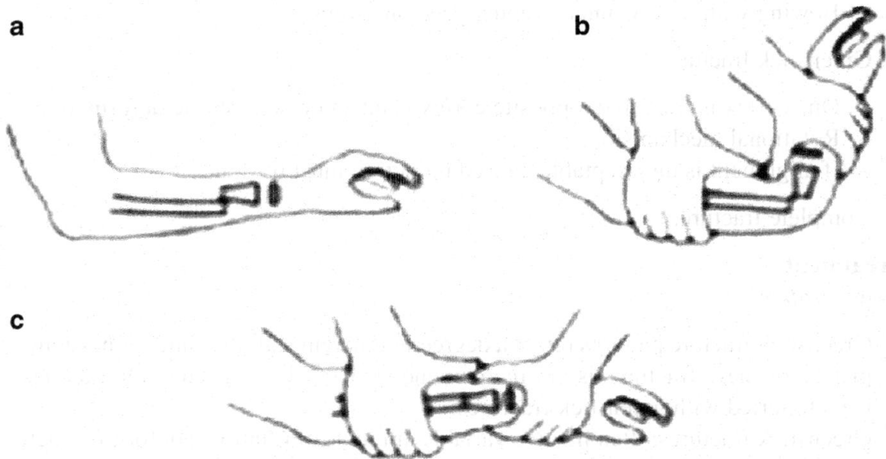

Fig. 4 Closed reduction manoeuvre for both-bone forearm fractures. The steps involve recreating the deformity and traction followed by reversal of deformity. (**a**) Deformity due to fracture. (**b**) Recreating the deformity. (**c**) Reversal of deforming forces

- Remodelling potential depends on the growth remaining, proximity to physis and deformity in plane of joint motion.
- Closed reduction requires adequate analgesia. Reduction manoeuvre (see Fig. 4) includes recreating the deformity, longitudinal traction and reversal of deformity. Cast should be well moulded.
- Fixation can be done with intramedullary nails or with plates in patients near skeletal maturity. In complete both-bone forearm fractures, the radius is routinely approached first as it is considered the more difficult bone to reduce. Physeal sparing entry points are used.

4.5.8 Distal Radius Epiphyseal and Metaphyseal Fractures

- 39 % of all physeal injuries.
- Peak age is between 10 and 14 years.

Mechanism of Injury

- Fall on outstretched hand.
- The injury pattern is often asymmetrical in that each bone fails in a different manner.

Fracture Patterns and Management

- Buckle or Torus Injuries
  - Minimally displaced and stable. Cast immobilisation for 3 weeks is usually adequate.
- Greenstick Injuries
  - Requires reduction if angulation is more than 20°
- Epiphyseal Injuries
  - Usually Salter–Harris types I and II. Significant degrees of displacement can be accepted as remodelling is rapid. Closed reduction can be achieved using traction–distraction method using finger trap.
  - Forceful late manipulations can result in physeal damage and growth plate arrest.
- Displaced Metaphyseal Fractures
  - Can be managed by closed reduction and cast immobilisation.
  - Careful follow-up is necessary for redisplacement.
  - Percutaneous pin fixation may be needed with concomitant ipsilateral fractures, in obese patients or with severe swelling.
  - Few injuries are irreducible as a result of soft-tissue interposition and open reduction and K-wire fixation may be necessary.

4.5.9 Hand Fractures

Introduction

Bimodal distribution.

- Infants and toddlers: Fingertip injuries.
- Adolescents: Sports-related fractures.

One-third of them are physeal (Salter–Harris II of border digits most common).

High-risk fractures for malunion; poor outcomes are associated with:

- Displaced articular fractures
- Physeal fractures of the distal phalanx
- Phalangeal neck fractures
- Open fracture

Specific Injuries

Seymour's Fracture

- Displaced physeal fracture of distal phalanx with nail bed laceration
- Failure of recognition: Infection, physeal arrest, nail plate deformity
- Treatment: Nail removal, incision and drainage, fracture reduction and stabilisation, nail bed repair

Phalangeal Neck Fractures

- True lateral radiograph is critical for diagnosis.
- Poor remodelling potential.
- Non-displaced fracture: Cast immobilisation, serial radiographs.
- Displaced fractures: Closed reduction and pinning.
- Consider osteoclasis in late-presenting cases.
- Established malunions: Subcondylar fossa reconstruction.

Phalangeal Shaft Fractures and Physeal Fractures

- Check for malrotation.
- Closed reduction recommended for malrotation or angulation >10°.
- Closed reduction, percutaneous pinning for unstable or malaligned fractures.

Unicondylar Fractures

- Non-displaced fractures—cast immobilisation, serial radiographs
- Displaced fractures—closed vs. open reduction and stabilisation with 2 points of fixation

Metacarpal Neck Fractures

- Large deformities well tolerated; high remodelling potential
- Non-displaced fractures: Cast immobilisation

- Unacceptable alignment: Closed reduction, cast immobilisation vs. pin fixation

Metacarpal Shaft Fractures

- Isolated diaphyseal fractures of central rays inherently stable
- Surgical indications: Open fractures, multiple fractures, unstable fractures with unacceptable alignment
- Treatment options: Percutaneous pinning, transmetacarpal pinning, screw fixation, plate fixation, IM fixation, external fixation

Salter–Harris III Fractures of the Thumb Proximal Phalanx

- Paediatric "gamekeeper's thumb"
- ORIF for displaced fractures

Bibliography

1. Flynn JC, Richards JF, Saltzman RI. Prevention and treatment of non-union of slightly displaced fractures of the lateral humeral condyle in children. J Bone Joint Surg Am. 1975;57:1087–92.
2. Gartland JJ. Management of supracondylar fractures of humerus in children. Surg Gynecol Obstet. 1959;109:145–54.
3. Jakob R, Fowles JV. Observations concerning fractures of the lateral humeral condyles in children. J Bone Joint Surg. 1975;40:430–6.
4. Lee BS, Esterhai JI, Das M. Fracture of distal radial epiphysis. Clin Orthop. 1983;1985:90–6.
5. Lincoln TL, Mubarak SJ. "Isolated" traumatic radial head dislocation. J Pediatr Orthop. 1994;14:454–7.
6. Patterson RF. Treatment of displaced transverse fractures of neck of radius in children. J Bone Joint Surg. 1934;16:695–8.
7. Price CT, et al. Malunited forearm fractures in children. J Pediatr Orthop. 1990;10:705–12.
8. Rang M. Children's fractures. Philadelphia: J.B Lippincott; 1983.
9. Reckling FW. Unstable fracture-dislocation of the forearm (Monteggia and Galeazzi). J Bone Joint Surg. 1982;64A:857–63.
10. Rockwood CA, Wilkins KE, King RE. Fractures in children. Philadelphia: J.B Lippincott; 1984.
11. Wedge JH, Robertson DE. Displaced fractures of neck of radius. J Bone Joint Surg. 1982;64 B:256.
12. Wiliamson DM, Coates CJ, Miller RK, Cole WG. Normal characteristics of the Baumann's angle: an aid in assessment of supracondylar fractures. J Pediatr Orthop. 1992;12:636–9.

5 Pelvic and Lower Limb Paediatric Trauma

Ashok Johari, Ratna Maheshwari, and Shalin Maheshwari

Take-Home Message

- Children younger than 36 months with a diaphyseal femur fracture should be evaluated for child abuse.
- In children between 6 months and 5 years with a diaphyseal femur fracture with less than 2 cm of shortening, early spica casting or traction with delayed spica casting is recommended.
- Rigid trochanteric entry nails, submuscular plating and flexible IMN are treatment options for children 11 years to skeletal maturity with diaphyseal femur fracture, but piriformis entry nails are not treatment option.
- The majority of paediatric and adolescent pelvis fractures are treated nonoperatively.
- Rapid application of an external fixator is occasionally indicated to close down the volume of the pelvis in open book injuries especially for haemodynamically unstable patients.
- The most important factor affecting outcome in neck femur fractures is likely the severity of vascular compromise sustained at the time of trauma.
- Urgent reduction of neck femur fractures appears to be responsible for improved outcomes.
- Surgical fixation of hip fractures (particularly Delbet II and III fractures) significantly decreases the risks of coxa vara and non-union.
- It is possible with any type of tibial fracture to develop compartment syndrome of the leg.
- Increasing need for pain medication has been shown to be one sign of developing compartment syndrome in children.
- Incidence of premature physeal arrest is high (52 %) in distal femoral physeal injuries; hence, parents must be warned.
- Because of the fact that ligaments in children are generally stronger than bone, tibial spine fractures, rather than ACL injuries, often occur in children.
- Tillaux fractures and triplane fractures both occur in the anterolateral distal tibial physis because of the order of distal tibial physeal closure (the central portion closes first, then the medial and finally the lateral).

5.1 Pelvic Fractures

Introduction

- Anatomic differences between skeletally immature and mature patients.
  - Triradiate cartilage is a physeal growth centre. Hence, there is potential for growth disturbance and its consequences.
  - Apophyseal growth centre prone for avulsion injuries.
  - Less brittle skeleton, hence greater energy absorption.
- Associated injuries.
  - Visceral: Bladder and urethra, bowel perforation, vascular injury, pulmonary contusion, cardiac contusion.
  - Skeletal: Long-bone fracture, skull and spine.

Evaluation Approximately half of all pelvic fractures identified on CT scan are not identified on plain AP pelvis radiographs. Inlet and outlet views have to be done. Abdominal and pelvic CT scan can be obtained while in scanner.

Classification The most common classification systems used for pelvic fractures are the Tile classification system and the Torode and Zieg classification system:

- Tile classification:
  - Type A (stable):

    A1: Does not involve the pelvic ring
    A2: Minimally displaced fractures of the pelvic ring

  - Type B (rotationally unstable but vertically stable):

    B1: Open book
    B2: Lateral compression, ipsilateral
    B3: Lateral compression, contralateral

  - Type C (rotationally and vertically unstable):
    C1: Unilateral
    C2: Bilateral
    C3: Associated with acetabular fracture
- Torode and Zieg classification:
  - Type I: Avulsions
  - Type II: Iliac wing fractures
  - Type III: Simple ring fractures without segmental instability
  - Type IV: Ring disruptions with segmental instability
- Regardless of the classification system used, it is essential to determine whether the pelvic fracture is stable.

Treatment

- Nonsurgical
  - The majority of paediatric and adolescent pelvis fractures are treated nonoperatively.
  - A1, A2, B1, B2 and B3 injuries are treated nonoperatively, except when associated with major haemorrhage or wide displacement greater than 3 cm.
  - Very young patients not able to ambulate with crutches or those who will not comply with activity restrictions or in significant discomfort can be immobilised in spica cast especially B1, B2 and B3 injuries.
- Surgical Indications
  - Rapid application of an external fixator is occasionally indicated to close down the volume of the pelvis in open book injuries especially for haemodynamically unstable patients. It can also be used in selective B2 and B3 injuries where nonoperative treatment does not seem adequate but where full ORIF is not indicated.
  - Surgery is most commonly indicated in adolescents with vertically unstable injuries or significantly displaced acetabular fractures.

Complications Malunion and non-union are extremely rare, though limb-length discrepancy may occur in vertically unstable fractures.

5.2 *Acetabular Fractures*

- Acetabular fractures in the skeletally immature will virtually always involve injury to triradiate cartilage.
- Premature physeal arrest of triradiate cartilage in a young patient will cause progressive dysplasia of the acetabulum.
- Imaging involves AP pelvis and Judet views:
  - Obturator oblique view: Useful to assess anterior column, obturator foramen and posterior wall
  - Iliac oblique view: Posterior column, iliac wing and anterior wall
  - CT scan: Helpful for preoperative planning
- Classification: Letournel and Judet classification is typically used as no paediatric specific fracture classification has received wide acceptance.
- Treatment:
  - Open reduction and internal fixation:
    - Fractures involving the major weight-bearing joint surface with greater than 2 mm displacement
    - Posterior wall fractures with associated hip instability

- Nonoperative treatment: All others.
- In case of displaced triradiate cartilage injuries, there are no concrete recommendations but open reduction and fixation can be considered for the markedly displaced triradiate injury.

5.3 *Fractured Neck of Femur*

Introduction

- Fractures of the femoral neck in children account for less than 1 % of all paediatric fractures.

Classification

- Delbet Classification (See Fig. 5)
  - Type I: Transphyseal, intracapsular, 50–100 % AVN rate
  - Type II: Transcervical, intracapsular, 40–60 % AVN, 10–20 % non-union
  - Type III: Cervicotrochanteric, extracapsular, 20–40 % AVN, 5–15 % non-union, coxa vara 20 %
  - Type IV: Intertrochanteric, extracapsular, <20 % AVN rates, coxa vara 10–30 %

Management

- The management guidelines for these fractures are dependent on a number of factors including age, degree of initial displacement, type of fracture, time to surgery and method of fixation.
- The most important factor is likely the severity of vascular compromise sustained at the time of trauma.

5.3.1 Management Guidelines

- *Diagnosis*:
  - Since most fractures of neck of femur in children are sustained as high-energy injuries, it is essential that the child be managed for ABCs and other visceral injuries.
  - The incidence of missed fractures of the neck femur in a polytrauma child is around 20–25 % in most series.
  - Important parameters which the treating surgeon should look for in a radiograph are amount of neck varus, direction of fracture line and degree of displacement. It is important to note that proximal metaphyseal fractures and stress fractures are not classifiable using the Delbet system.

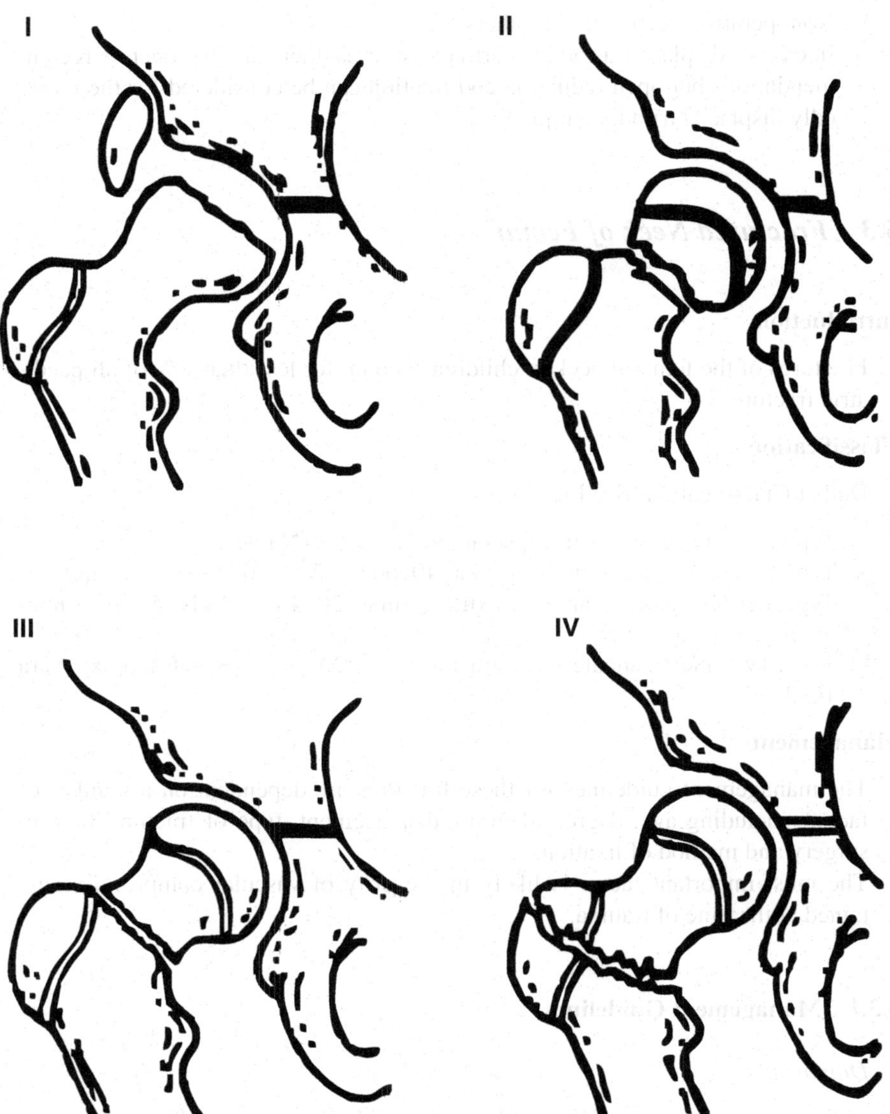

Fig. 5 Classification of femoral neck fractures. (1) Transphyseal with or without dislocation from the acetabulum. (2) Transcervical. (3) Cervicotrochanteric. (4) Trochanteric

– MRI is the single most important evaluation tool for an undisplaced fracture neck of femur in a child.
– Bone scan does not figure in the primary evaluation tool for paediatric femoral neck fractures but forms an important component in the diagnosis of stress fractures of the neck of femur in children.

- *Timing of treatment*:
  - Ideal treatment for displaced fractures is closed reduction and internal (rigid) fixation as soon as possible after injury. Delay in fixation is statistically shown to increase the risk of complications.
  - *Treatment*: The goal of treatment is anatomical reduction and fracture stabilisation. Definitive conservative management in a hip spica is now used in a very small group of children. Its indications are
    - Children less than 2 years of age with a fractured neck of femur
    - Children with undisplaced cervicotrochanteric and intertrochanteric fractures
    - Children with stress fractures of the neck of femur
      - *Method of reduction*:
      - Closed reduction is best carried out on a fracture table with the child under a general anaesthesia. The fracture is reduced in 20–30° of abduction, neutral extension and 10–12° of internal rotation.
      - *Rigid fixation*: Stabilisation can be achieved using 4 mm cancellous (cannulated) screws with extraphyseal placement of the screws. It is important to remember that the screws should be distal to the growth plate but no compromise should be made in achieving fracture stability. A lateral approach is used for inserting the screws. Alternatively smooth K wires can be used in the young child.
      - *Decompression*: Role of decompression is now considered to be controversial.
      - *Open reduction*:
      - If no angulation and less than 2 mm of displacement cannot be achieved by closed means, then open reduction by Watson-Jones approach can be done.
      - Factors in various series which appear to be responsible for improved results:
        - Emergent/urgent reduction: Absolutely within 24 h, within 12 h whenever possible
        - Anatomic reduction: Less than 2 mm of displacement
        - No angulation

Complications

- Coxa vara, delayed union and non-union, especially in patients treated without internal fixation.
- Other complications, including osteonecrosis, premature physeal closure and limb-length discrepancy, also occur and are more common with operative treatments.

5.4 Femoral Shaft Fractures

A. Epidemiology

- Child abuse is the cause of the vast majority of femur fractures before walking age.
- Although abuse must be considered in children up to 5 years of age, it is a less common cause of femur fractures after walking age.

B. Treatment
Goals of Treatment

- Timely union
- No rotational deformity
- Acceptable angulation: 20–30° sagittal and 10–20° frontal
- In between ages 2–10 years: 1–2 cm of overlap to counteract overgrowth
  - Nonsurgical:
    - Treatment with a Pavlik Harness or a spica cast is an option for infants 6 months and younger with diaphyseal femur fracture.
    - Spica casting is routinely performed in children age 6 months to 5 years with a diaphyseal femur fracture with less than 2 cm of shortening. This may be either immediate spica casting or traction followed by delayed spica casting.
    - When skeletal traction is used, it should be inserted into the distal femur rather than into the proximal tibia. (Proximal tibial traction pins risk damage to the tibial tubercle apophysis with resultant genu recurvatum.)
    - Shortening exceeding 2.5–3.0 cm is a relative contraindication and multiple trauma is an absolute contraindication to immediate spica casting.
  - Surgical treatment:
    - Indications: Most children older than 6 years are treated surgically, as are many younger multiple trauma patients.
    - Procedures:
      - Flexible intramedullary (IM) rodding is the treatment of choice for the vast majority of paediatric femoral shaft fractures. Comminuted or very distal or proximal fractures are harder to control with IM rods. Complication rates are higher in children >10 years of age.
      - External fixation has become less popular over the past 10 years. External fixation may be used for comminuted or segmental fractures. It has higher rates of delayed union and refracture than other forms of fixation.

- Open plating of femoral shaft fractures is rarely used in most centres because of the increased dissection required, the increased blood loss, the desire to avoid load-bearing implants and the presence of multiple stress risers following hardware removal.
- Submuscular bridge plating is becoming increasingly popular, especially for comminuted femoral shaft fractures. Insufficient data are currently available to assess outcomes accurately. Drawbacks for these devices are that they are load-bearing, there are many stress risers in the femoral shaft following hardware removal and there is a significant learning curve.
- Antegrade, rigid femoral nails are indicated in children with closed proximal femoral physes. In children with open physes, the risk of ON is up to 1–2 %.
- Trochanteric entry nails are gaining popularity for larger children (most commonly those older than 10 years and those with extensive comminution). These nails appear to cause abnormalities of proximal femoral growth (resulting in a narrow femoral neck), and the risk of ON is unknown.

C. Complications

- Limb-length discrepancy:
  - Typically 7–10 mm of ipsilateral overgrowth occurs in children who sustain a femur fracture between the ages of 2 and 10 years.
  - Limb-length discrepancy may occur as a result of either excessive overgrowth or excessive shortening at the time of fracture healing following cast treatment.
- Malunion:
  - Angular malunion is typically due to varus and/or procurvatum deformity, is unusual following surgical treatment and can be minimised following spica treatment by careful technique.
  - Torsional malunion is common but rarely of clinical consequence.
- Refracture is most common following external fixation and typically occurs following fixator removal. Refracture is most common following transverse or short oblique fractures.
- Delayed union and non-union are typically seen only after surgical treatment and are much more common when load-bearing devices (external fixators or plates) are used.
- ON of the femoral head has been reported following rigid antegrade nailing of femoral fractures in skeletally immature individuals with both piriformis fossa and trochanteric nail entry points.

5.5 Distal Femur Fracture

Introduction

Physeal injuries about the knee are 1–6 % of all physeal injuries in children.

Mechanism of Injury

- Usually hyperextension
- Occasionally a fall on hyperflexed knee

Presentation

- Tenderness over physis.
- Knee effusion.
- Inability to bear weight.
- Deformity.
- Always look for neurovascular injury.

Evaluation

- Non-displaced SH type I fractures may present with negative x-ray

Treatment *Goals*

- Restoration of growth plate in children with >2 years growth remaining
- Restoration of the articular surface

Management

- Salter–Harris types I and II: Closed reduction and casting or percutaneous fixation
- Salter–Harris types III and IV: Open reduction and percutaneous or internal fixation

Complications

- Incidence of premature growth arrest is high (52 %).
- Start range of motion early to avoid knee stiffness.

5.6 Tibial Fractures

- Because of the fact that ligaments in children are generally stronger than bone, tibial spine fractures, rather than ACL injuries, often occur in children.
- Proximal tibial metaphyseal fractures in children younger than 10 years typically grow into valgus in the first 6–12 months after injury. Observation is indicated in these cases because the genu valgum usually resolves spontaneously.

5.6.1 Tibial Shaft Fractures

Nonsurgical Treatment

- Most tibial fractures in children can be treated with reduction and casting. Acceptable alignment is not well defined. General guidelines are that shortening of less than 2 cm and angulation less than 10–15° are acceptable.
- Restore length, rotation and alignment.
- Tibial shaft without an associated fibular fracture tends to heal in slight varus and almost always can be treated nonoperatively.
- Toddler fractures are common accidental injuries in young children, typically sustained with a torsional mechanism. Non-displaced spiral tibial fractures may be managed with either a below- or above-knee cast with knee in slight flexion and weight bearing as tolerated, for 3 weeks.
- Healing takes 3–4 weeks for toddler fractures and 6–8 weeks for other tibial fractures.

Surgical Treatment

- Indications include open fractures, marked soft-tissue injury, unstable fractures, multiple trauma, >1 cm of shortening and unacceptable closed reduction (>10° of angulation), floating knee injuries.
- Fixation options include external fixation, intramedullary rod fixation and percutaneous pins or plates.

Complications

- When closed reduction is lost, it is typically due to a drift into varus for isolated tibial fractures and into valgus for combined tibial and fibular fractures.
- Delayed union and non-union are almost never seen in closed fractures but are more common following external fixation.
- Compartment syndrome, although relatively uncommon, can occur with open or closed fractures.

5.7 Tibial Tubercle Fractures

- This injury is typically found in teenage athletes involved in jumping sports and may follow Osgood–Schlatters syndrome.
- Watson-Jones described three types:

  Type 1, a small fragment of tibial tubercle is avulsed and displaced upward
  Type 2, the whole anterior portion of tibial tubercle is displaced upward
  Type 3, the fracture extends up to joint surface

- Nonsurgical treatment is rarely indicated, but it may be used in children with minimally displaced fractures (<2 mm) and no extensor lag.

- Surgical Treatment
  - Indications: Most children with these fractures require surgery. The only exceptions are those with minimally displaced fractures and no extensor lag. The knee extension mechanism must be restored.
  - Procedures: Surgery is via ORIF with screws. Screw fixation is done with avoidance of physis if possible. For type 3 fractures, the joint must be visualised to accurately reduce the joint surface and to assess for meniscal injury.

Complications: Compartment syndrome and genu recurvatum are both rare.

5.8 Anterior Tibial Spine (Tibial Eminence Fractures)

- If displaced can be associated with meniscal tears and MRI should be considered to evaluate.
- Displaced fractures should be treated with reduction and fixation that avoids the proximal tibial physis.
- The goal of surgical treatment is to prevent a block to motion (extension) and to minimise residual ACL laxity.

5.9 Distal Tibial Fractures

- An anatomic classification system is most typically used for ankle fractures. The Salter–Harris classification is commonly used for physeal fractures.
- A mechanistic classification system (typically, the Dias–Tachdjian classification) may be used. The Dias–Tachdjian classification is patterned after the Lauge–Hansen categorization of adult fractures and describes four main mechanisms: supination–inversion, supination–plantar flexion, supination–external rotation and pronation/eversion–external rotation.
- Medial malleolar Salter–Harris IV fractures have the highest rate of growth arrest of any ankle fracture and often result in varus ankle deformity and limb-length discrepancy.

5.9.1 Salter–Harris Type I

- Non-displaced SH type I fracture is treated with cast immobilisation. A below-knee cast worn for 3–4 weeks may suffice, with the first 2–3 weeks limited to non-weight bearing:
- Most displaced fractures can be treated with closed reduction and cast immobilisation. An above-knee non-weight-bearing cast is preferable initially, as this should reduce the risk of displacement after reduction.

5.9.2 Salter–Harris Type II Fractures

- Non-displaced fractures can be treated with cast immobilisation with an above-knee cast for 3–4 weeks.
- In case of displaced fractures, opinions differ as to what degree of residual displacement or angulation is unacceptable and requires open reduction. Incomplete reduction is usually caused by interposition of soft tissue between fracture fragments.
- If there is concern about redisplacement or stability, pins can be placed at that time.

5.9.3 Salter–Harris Types III and IV

- CT scans may be necessary to fully appreciate the degree of displacement.
- Non-displaced fractures can be treated with above-knee cast immobilisation.
- Displaced intra-articular fractures require anatomical reduction if possible. Failure to obtain this may result in articular incongruity and posttraumatic arthritis.
- If anatomical reduction cannot be obtained by closed methods, open reduction and internal fixation or mini-open arthroscopic reduction should be carried out.

5.9.4 Salter–Harris Type V Fractures

- Salter–Harris V fractures appear to be Salter–Harris I fractures on initial presentation and are noted to be type V fractures only retrospectively, when the child presents with a growth arrest and limb-length discrepancy.
- Because of the uncertain nature of this injury, no specific treatment recommendations have been formulated. Treatment is usually directed primarily towards the sequelae of growth arrest.

5.9.5 Juvenile Tillaux Fractures

- Tillaux fractures (as well as triplane fractures) occur in this location because the distal tibial physis closes centrally, then medially and then laterally.
- With external rotation of the foot, the anterior–inferior tibiofibular ligament avulses a fragment of bone of anterolateral tibia corresponding to the portion of distal tibial physis that is still open.
- Both below- and above-knee casts have been used.
- Fractures with more than 2 mm of displacement, especially those associated with articular incongruity, require closed or open reduction.

- Closed reduction is attempted by internally rotating the foot and applying direct pressure.
- If closed reduction is not successful, open reduction or percutaneous reduction can be done.
- Pins can be used for stabilisation of reduction.

5.9.6 Triplane Fracture

- This type of injury does not occur in children younger than 10 or older than 16.7 years.
- Radiographic views should include anteroposterior, lateral and mortise views. CT scans are very helpful.
- Non-displaced triplane fractures, those with less than 2 mm of displacement, as well as extra-articular fractures can be treated with long leg cast immobilisation with the foot in internal rotation for lateral fractures and in eversion for medial fractures.
- Fractures with more than 2 mm of displacement require reduction.
- Closed reduction of lateral triplane fractures is attempted by internally rotating the foot. Based on the mechanism of injury, the most logical manoeuvre for reduction of medial triplane fractures is abduction.
- If closed reduction is unsuccessful, open reduction is required. This can be accomplished through an anterolateral approach for lateral triplane fractures or through an anteromedial approach for medial triplane fractures.

5.9.7 Pilon Fractures

- Although these fractures are relatively rare in young patients, these injuries can be associated with severe soft-tissue swelling and oedema.
- Similar to the treatment in adults with these injuries, management of the soft tissues is critical, to prevent complications of skin loss, infection, wound healing problems, etc.
- Initial approaches may consist of application of external fixation or dressings to address swelling and oedema, with delay of surgical intervention for 5–15 days.
- Complications
  - Physeal arrest and growth disturbances
  - Usually occurs after SH type III and type IV fractures

Bibliography

1. Flynn JM, Skaggs DL, Sponseller PD, Ganley TJ, Kay RM, Leitch KK. The surgical management of pediatric fractures of the lower extremity. Instr Course Lect. 2003;52:647–59.

2. Gray DW. Trauma to the hip and femur in children. In: Sponseller PD, editor. OKU Pediatrics 2. Rosemont: American Academy of Orthopaedic Surgeons; 2002. p. 81–91.
3. Kay RM, Matthys GA. Pediatric ankle fractures: evaluation and treatment. J Am Acad Orthop Surg. 2001;9:268–78.

Part VI
Shoulder and Elbow

William Levine and Jonathan Danoff

Shoulder

Jonathan Danoff, Danielle Rome, Stephanie Gancarczyk, and William Levine

1 AC Joint Arthritis

Take-Home Message

- Radiographic evidence of AC joint arthritis must be correlated with clinical evidence of pain at the AC joint.
- Lidocaine injection test is highly specific for AC joint pathology and predicts success if surgery is indicated.
- Nonoperative management including activity modification is effective.
- Fastest return to full activity with arthroscopic techniques, but comparable long-term outcomes versus open surgery.

Definition

- Degeneration of the acromioclavicular joint (ACJ) that causes pain and disability in the shoulder

Etiology

- Primary osteoarthritis: degeneration secondary to large forces across the small joint surface area
  - Radiographic evidence of degeneration in the ACJ does not necessarily mean it is symptomatic. Sixty percent of elderly individuals have ACJ arthritis, but this is often asymptomatic.

J. Danoff, MD • D. Rome • S. Gancarczyk, MD • W. Levine, MD (✉)
Department of Orthopedic Surgery, Center for Shoulder, Elbow and Sports Medicine, New York Presbyterian/Columbia University Medical Center, New York, NY, USA
e-mail: wnl1@cumc.columbia.edu; wnl1@columbia.edu

C. Mauffrey, D.J. Hak (eds.), *Passport for the Orthopedic Boards and FRCS Examination*, DOI 10.1007/978-2-8178-0475-0_31

- Post-traumatic arthritis: superficial joint susceptible to trauma, associated with AC separations
- Distal clavicle osteolysis: secondary to repetitive stress (weight lifting; "weight lifter's shoulder")

Pathophysiology

- ACJ is a diarthrodial joint susceptible to degeneration and begins in the second decade.
- Arthritis characterized by sclerosis, osteophyte formation, subchondral cysts, and joint space narrowing.
- Distal clavicle osteolysis bone shows microscopic fractures, osteopenia, subchondral cysts, and distal clavicle erosions.

Radiographs

- Standard shoulder radiographs inadequate.
- Zanca view highlights the distal clavicle and AC joint.
- Normal ACJ space in young patient is 1–3 mm, but >60 years 0.5 mm.
- Distal clavicle osteolysis radiographs show relative osteopenia, loss of subchondral bone, increased size of the distal clavicle, and widening of joint space.
- Stress views not routinely used. Bone scan helpful in middle-age active patient with pain but no radiographic changes.
- MRI has low specificity but high sensitivity and must correlate to physical exam. Reactive bone edema in the distal clavicle/acromion (best seen on T2 images) best predictor of symptomatic AC joint.

Classification

- No true classification.
- Understanding etiology is key to determining treatment (primary OA, post-traumatic arthritis, distal clavicle osteolysis).

Treatment

- Treatment success directly related to ability of physician to distinguish AC joint pain from other sources of pain (subacromial, biceps, glenohumeral)
  - Selective AC joint anesthetic injection helpful to improve diagnostic accuracy

Nonoperative

- Activity modification (avoid inciting activity); if symptomatic during bench press exercise, encourage patient to decrease maximal weight to relieve symptoms.
- Heat therapy, NSAIDs.
- Intra-articular corticosteroid injections.
- Physical therapy (limited success unless coexistent impingement or restricted shoulder motion), rotator cuff strengthening.
- Recommended minimum 6 months of nonoperative treatment prior to surgery.

Operative

- Success of distal clavicle resection predicted by pain relief with intra-articular anesthetic injection.
- Regardless of technique used, resect 1 cm bone and ensure smooth distal clavicle from anterior to posterior ensuring no residual abutment (especially posterosuperior corner if performed arthroscopically).
- Outcomes are excellent for open or arthroscopic techniques and differ mainly in postoperative limitations (arthroscopic techniques enable faster return to activity).
- Distal clavicle resection contraindicated if history of AC separation higher than grade II.
- Preferential ligament preservation important – maintenance of superior AC joint capsule improves joint stability.
- High failure rate in workmen's compensation patients or those undergoing litigation.
- Open distal clavicle resection
  - Open distal clavicle resection allows for direct joint inspection to ensure no further impingement, preferred if open cuff repair is being performed.
  - Potential for weakness in the deltoid and trapezius which also delays return to sport.
  - Minimal shoulder motion allowed × 3 weeks, resistance exercises initiated at 6 weeks, and return to overhead activity at 3 months.
- Arthroscopic resection with subacromial approach or superior approach
  - Arthroscopic technique is technically more demanding and takes longer than open procedure.
  - Subacromial approach can be performed in conjunction with subacromial decompression for impingement.
  - Direct superior approach potentially avoids injury to the ACJ capsule and is preferred for distal clavicle osteolysis but is more difficult than subacromial approach if small joint space.
  - Both techniques allow immediate return to work, with sling for comfort for 2–3 days followed by permitted use of arm for ADLs, and for beginning of overhead activity after 3 weeks with return to full activity after 1–2 months.

Complications

- Inadequate resection is the most common cause of surgical failure, usually due to posterior distal clavicle abutment on the acromion, often seen as technical cause of failure in arthroscopic techniques secondary to uneven resection.
- Weakness or failure of deltoid/trapezius repair after open distal clavicle resection.
- If the ACJ is unstable, then poorer prognosis, conoid excision during surgery, or history of injury allows for increased mediolateral motion increasing chance for ACJ abutment and symptoms.
- If pain is not due to ACJ arthritis, then any surgical approach will fail to relieve pain, avoided by the use of lidocaine injection test.

Bibliography

1. Hossain S, Jacobs LG, Hashmi R. The long-term effectiveness of steroid injections in primary acromioclavicular joint arthritis: a five-year prospective study. J Shoulder Elbow Surg. 2008;17(4):535–8. Epub 2008/03/25.
2. Mall NA, Foley E, Chalmers PN, Cole BJ, Romeo AA, Bach BR, Jr. Degenerative joint disease of the acromioclavicular joint: a review. Am J Sports Med. 2013;41(11):2684–92. Epub 2013/05/08.
3. Rabalais RD, McCarty E. Surgical treatment of symptomatic acromioclavicular joint problems: a systematic review. Clin Orthop Relat Res. 2007;455:30–7. Epub 2006/12/13.
4. Shubin Stein BE, Ahmad CS, Pfaff CH, Bigliani LU, Levine WN. A comparison of magnetic resonance imaging findings of the acromioclavicular joint in symptomatic versus asymptomatic patients. J Shoulder Elbow Surg. 2006;15(1):56–9. Epub 2006/01/18.

2 Subacromial Impingement

Take-Home Message

- Etiology of this disease is debated (extrinsic versus intrinsic causes) and is likely multifactorial.
- Nonoperative treatment (steroid injections and physical therapy) often successful as first-line treatment.
- Operative intervention is controversial with regard to open versus arthroscopic, bursectomy alone or in conjunction with acromioplasty, and amount of acromioplasty; all operative treatments appear to show clinical improvement in literature.

Definition

- Compression of the contents of the subacromial space (rotator cuff tendons, bursa) by the anterior acromion, coracoacromial ligament, and acromioclavicular joint

Etiology

- Debate between primary causes of subacromial impingement, extrinsic versus intrinsic causes.
- Extrinsic causes: repetitive impingement of the humeral head and rotator cuff against the coracoacromial ligament causes bursitis and tendinopathy of the rotator cuff which further incites acromial spur formation on the anterolateral band.
- Intrinsic causes: partial versus full-thickness cuff tears (or weakness) increase in incidence with age due to natural degeneration versus traumatic tears leading to superior migration of the humeral head and glenohumeral joint narrowing the subacromial space and directly causing impingement of the greater tuberosity on the acromion and coracoacromial ligament which causes spur formation and tuberosity erosion.

Pathophysiology

- Bursitis, tendinopathy
- Acromial spur formation on the anterolateral band of the coracoacromial ligament
- Bursal-sided partial-thickness tears versus full-thickness tears of the supraspinatus
- Superior migration of the humeral head in the joint
- Secondary impingement: caused by underlying glenohumeral instability (decompression surgery will fail if not recognized)

Radiographs

- AP shoulder, true AP (Grashey view), scapular Y view (outlet), and axillary radiographs.
- Typical changes include AC joint osteophyte formation inferiorly, acromial enthesophytes, subchondral cysts or sclerosis in the humeral head around the greater tuberosity.
- Decreased acromiohumeral index (normal 7–8 mm).
- Outlet visualizes acromial morphology described by Bigliani et al.
- Axillary view shows the os acromiale (unfused acromial ossification center).
- MRI shows rotator cuff tears and degeneration and subacromial bursitis (thickness >3 mm, increased bursal fluid).

Classification

- Bigliani et al. described acromion morphology as seen on supraspinatus outlet view.
  - Type I: flat
  - Type II: curved
  - Type III: hooked, associated with impingement, highest incidence of rotator cuff tears
- Neer stages of impingement based on rotator cuff tendinopathy
  - Stage I: edema and hemorrhage of the bursa and cuff, patient <25 years old, reversible
  - Stage II: fibrosis and tendinitis of the cuff, patient 25–40 years old, activity-related pain
  - Stage III: AC spur and partial or complete cuff tear, patient >40 years old
- Two stages of impingement by Neer
  - Outlet impingement: coracoacromial arch impinges on the supraspinatus outlet.
  - Non-outlet impingement: due to thickening or hypertrophy of the rotator cuff tendons or bursa.

Treatment

- Operative and nonoperative management strategies equally efficacious

Nonoperative

- Activity modification
- Physical therapy shown to help improve pain and shoulder function, but no improvements in range of motion or strength noted; maximal improvement out to 1 year
- Subacromial injection with corticosteroid (NSAIDs inferior), notable improvement after 6 weeks

Operative

- Indicated after 6-month failed trial of nonoperative therapies
- Open anterior acromioplasty (Neer) versus arthroscopic subacromial decompression
  - Arthroscopic technique shown to have fast return to work and fewer days in the hospital although equally efficacious.
  - Open technique allows for direct cuff repair if necessary.
- Bursectomy alone versus anterior acromioplasty with bursectomy highly debated with both techniques showing decreased pain and improvements in functional scores
- Avoid coracoacromial ligament resection if massive tear

Complications

- Persistent pain, often secondary to incorrect initial diagnosis.
- If irreparable rotator cuff tear, excessive debridement of the coracoacromial ligament will lead to superior migration of the humeral head.
- Inadequate bone resection can lead to recurrent symptoms, whereas excessive bone resection can predispose to acromial fractures.
- Typical risks of arthroscopic portal creation includes injury to the suprascapular and axillary nerves.

Bibliography

1. Bigliani LU, Levine WN. Subacromial impingement syndrome. J Bone Joint Surg Am. 1997;79(12):1854–68. Epub 1997/12/31.
2. Bigliani LU, Morrison DS, April EW. The morphology of the acromion and its relationship to rotator cuff tears. Orthop Trans. 1986;10:228.
3. Davis AD, Kakar S, Moros C, Kaye EK, Schepsis AA, Voloshin I. Arthroscopic versus open acromioplasty: a meta-analysis. Am J Sports Med. 2010;38(3):613–8. Epub 2009/02/04.
4. Neer CS, 2nd. Anterior acromioplasty for the chronic impingement syndrome in the shoulder: a preliminary report. J Bone Joint Surg Am. 1972;54(1):41–50. Epub 1972/01/01.
5. Neer CS, 2nd. Impingement lesions. Clin Orthop Relat Res. 1983(173):70–7. Epub 1983/03/01.
6. Neer CS. Shoulder reconstruction. Philadelphia: Saunders; 1990. xi, 551 p.

3 Calcific Tendinopathy

Take-Home Message

- Calcium deposition in the rotator cuff tendon with unknown etiology, the supraspinatus is the most common location.
- Prevailing theory of reactive formation of calcium stages: pre-calcific, calcific (formative, resting, resorptive), and post-calcific.
- Acute pain in resorptive phase often resolves spontaneously with supportive care.
- Chronic pain in formative phase requires surgical intervention or extracorporeal shock-wave therapy.

Definition

- Self-limiting cell-mediated calcification within and around the living tendon followed by spontaneous phagocytic resorption and reconstitution of the normal viable tendon

Etiology

- Controversial mechanism with causative agent thought to be tissue hypoxia and local tissue pressure, no proven direct cause.
- Incidence 1.5× female versus male and increased if HLA-A1 antigen positive or coexistent insulin-dependent diabetes (30 %) (diabetics most likely to be asymptomatic), typically 30- to 50-year olds.
- Eighty percent occurrence in the supraspinatus, 25 % have rotator cuff tear.

Pathophysiology

- Calcium deposition within the tendon substrate causes cell-mediated inflammatory response which causes acute pain and secondarily leads to bursitis and thickening of the rotator cuff with secondary subacromial impingement.
- Degenerative calcification: tendon fiber degeneration mainly in the hypovascular zone manifests as tendonitis, and age-related wear leads to tenocyte necrosis with intracellular accumulation of calcium which leads to tendon calcification.
  - This theory has mainly been rejected as there is no noted increased incidence of this disease as patients age despite increasing number with rotator cuff pathology.
- Reactive calcification: prevailing theory, 3 stages, no definitive time course for each phase
  - Pre-calcific stage: fibrocartilaginous metaplasia of tenocytes turning into chondrocytes, painless

- Calcific stage: 3 phases
  - Formative: calcium crystal deposits form foci within tendon separated by fibrocartilage, chalk-like, ± pain
  - Resting: no further calcium deposition and no evidence of inflammation, ± pain
  - Resorptive: inflammatory cell-mediated reaction with increased vascularity around deposits with infiltration of macrophages and multinucleated giant cells, notable calcium deposit phagocytosis, form creamy calcium-containing pasty material that increases the intra-tendinous pressure, *++PAINFUL*
- Post-calcific stage: granulation tissue and remodeling with type III collagen replacing type I collagen, notable tendon healing, ± pain

Radiographs

- Plain film AP (evaluate supraspinatus, most common), internal (infraspinatus/teres minor) and external rotation (subscapularis), scapular Y (impingement) to localize calcium deposits
- CT helpful to confirm location of deposits as these can be difficult to see in plain films
- MRI useful for diagnosis of coexistent rotator cuff tear and subacromial bursitis or tendon edema

Classification

- DePalma and Kruper
  - Type I: resorptive phase, acute pain, fluffy-appearing deposits with poorly defined periphery with overlying streaks at the site where calcium deposits ruptured from the tendon into the subacromial bursa
  - Type II: formative phase, subacute or chronic pain, discrete homogeneous calcium deposits with uniform density and well-defined periphery
- Gärtner: evaluates appearance of calcium deposits on radiographs
  - Type I: homogeneous, defined borders
  - Type II: heterogeneous with sharp outline OR homogeneous without defined border
  - Type III: cloudy and translucent

Treatment

Nonoperative

- Physical therapy to maintain shoulder motion
- NSAIDs have unclear, unproven benefit.
- Subacromial corticosteroid injections.
- Needle lavage to release intra-tendinous pressure.
- Extracorporeal shock-wave therapy (ESWT).

Operative

- Open versus arthroscopic tendon debridement ± rotator cuff repair (if indicated)

  Resorptive Phase (Gärtner III)

- Spontaneous healing although length of time to heal varies; acute symptoms typically improve after 3–5 weeks, but time for complete resolution of radiographic appearance of calcium deposits ranges 3–10 years in 33 % of patients.
- Nonoperative therapy predominates with steroid injections for pain control and to decrease inflammation, needle lavage to decrease intra-tendinous pressure, and physical therapy to maintain motion.
- No indication for ESWT or surgery.

  Formative Phase (Gärtner I/II)

- Uncommon for symptoms to resolve with nonoperative management
- ESWT proven efficacious at high energy to target calcium deposits, best outcomes when combined with needle lavage
- Open or arthroscopic calcium deposit excision indicated if symptomatic, arthroscopic methods preferable
  - Recovery is longer if surgery is needed to allow for tendon healing, but this allows for rotator cuff repair if present.
  - Debate as to the level of aggressiveness with calcium debridement, if subacromial decompression is indicated and if it is necessary to explore the glenohumeral joint.

Complications

- Hematomas noted after ESWT
- Risk of creating a rotator cuff tear during arthroscopic or open calcium excision
- Secondary shoulder stiffness
- Typical risks of open shoulder surgery or arthroscopy

Bibliography

1. Cacchio A, Paoloni M, Barile A, Don R, De Paulis F, Calvisi V, et al. Effectiveness of radial shock-wave therapy for calcific tendinitis of the shoulder: single-blind, randomized clinical study. Phys Ther. 2006;86(5):672–82.
2. Galasso O, Amelio E, Riccelli DA, Gasparini G. Short-term outcomes of extracorporeal shock wave therapy for the treatment of chronic non-calcific tendinopathy of the supraspinatus: a double-blind, randomized, placebo-controlled trial. BMC Musculoskelet Disord. 2012;13:86
3. Le Goff B, Berthelot JM, Guillot P, Glémarec J, Maugars Y. Assessment of calcific tendonitis of rotator cuff by ultrasonography: comparison between symptomatic and asymptomatic shoulders. Joint Bone Spine. 2010;77(3):258–63.
4. Rizzello G, Franceschi F, Longo UG, Ruzzini L, Meloni MC, Spiezia F, et al. Arthroscopic management of calcific tendinopathy of the shoulder: do we need to remove all the deposit? Bull NYU Hosp Jt Dis. 2009;67(4):330–3.
5. Seil R, Litzenburger H, Kohn D, Rupp S. Arthroscopic treatment of chronically painful calcifying tendinitis of the supraspinatus tendon. Arthroscopy. 2006; 22(5):521–7.

4 Rotator Cuff Tear

Take-Home Message

- Result of extrinsic and intrinsic factors, impingement, and age-related degeneration.
- Partial
  - Bursal sided
  - Articular sided
- Full-thickness tear classification (Cofield, North America)
  - Small <1 cm
  - Medium 1–<3 cm
  - Large 3–<5 cm
  - Massive ≥5 cm
- Ellman classification is most commonly used to describe size and location of tear.
- Low-grade partial-thickness tears (<50 % thickness) can be debrided, while high-grade tears (>50 % thickness) or acute tears in young patients should be repaired.
- Full-thickness tears treated with primary repair may be amenable to direct tendon-to-bone healing or may require interval slide, marginal convergence techniques.
- Massive tear repair can be performed – negative prognostic factors include muscle atrophy (Goutallier 3 and 4 bad), level of retraction, and proximal humeral migration.

Definition

- Partial or complete detachment of one or more of the four muscle-tendon units (supraspinatus, infraspinatus, teres minor, subscapularis) that mobilize and dynamically stabilize the humeral head within the glenohumeral joint

Etiology

- Multifactorial with extrinsic and intrinsic causes that exacerbate one another
  - Extrinsic: acromioclavicular impingement or shoulder instability or trauma can cause tears that cause tendon degeneration that exacerbates disease and can also cause bursitis and tendon inflammation which worsens impingement and disease progression.
  - Intrinsic: normal aging, tendon overuse, and eccentric muscle loading leads to degeneration which can further cause glenohumeral instability and impingement leading to further tearing.

- Extrinsic causes (impingement) typically first show bursal-sided partial-thickness tears or intra-tendinous tears, while intrinsic causes lead to articular-sided tears.
- Known hypovascular zone near insertion of the supraspinatus predominantly in articular side may predispose to articular side tears.
- Common disease (not all symptomatic) with increasing incidence in elderly; unilateral rotator cuff tear and >65 years old associated with 50 % incidence of bilateral rotator cuff tear.
- Unclear in literature as to the natural history of partial-thickness tear progression, thought that partial-thickness tears increase strain on middle and bursal segments, which may lead tear progression.
- Spinoglenoid notch cysts may cause impingement of suprascapular nerve and impaired function of the infraspinatus which may masquerade as cuff tear.

Pathophysiology

- Partial or full thickness; small, medium, large, or massive tears.
- Inflammation and tendon swelling
- Loss of dynamic stability of the glenohumeral joint with poor coordination of the rotator cuff muscles and deltoid.
- Irreversible fatty atrophy and interfibrous fat infiltration of the rotator cuff muscle occur around 4 months after tear occurs.
- Cysts can form at cuff insertion if complete tear occurs.
- Articular-sided tears 2–3× are more common than bursal-sided tears.
- Overhead-throwing athletes usually present with partial-thickness tears on articular side of the supraspinatus and infraspinatus tendon.

Radiographs

- AP, scapular Y, and axillary views to evaluate joint for degenerative changes, subacromial spurs, cystic changes in the humeral head (suggests cuff tear), instability with superior migration of head, decreased acromiohumeral distance.
- Ultrasound helpful to dynamically test cuff and evaluate for tears.
- MRI/MRA is the most sensitive and specific; is the best method of visualizing size and shape of the tear, partial versus full thickness, and amount of retraction; and can also evaluate muscle atrophy; T2 images are the most useful; must confirm tear on coronal and sagittal views.
  - Shoulder in abduction and external rotation improves accuracy.

Classification

- Tear size description: small, <1 cm; medium, 1–3 cm; large, 3–5 cm; massive, ≥5 cm or involving 2 or more tendons
- Ellman classification system of partial-thickness rotator cuff tears describes size of tear and location
  - Size: I=< 3 mm (<25 % thickness), II=3–6 mm (25–50 % thickness), III=>6 mm (>50 % thickness)
  - Location: A=articular surface, B=bursal surface, C=interstitial

- Geometric classification (Davidson and Burkhart) guides treatment based on MRI findings
  - Type 1: crescent shaped, short and wide tear, mobile in medial/lateral direction, amenable to direct tendon-to-bone repair
  - Type 2: U shaped or L shaped, long and narrow, mobile in anterior/posterior direction, treat with marginal convergence
  - Type 3: massive contracted tear, long and wide, treated with interval slide technique and/or partial repair
  - Type 4: rotator cuff arthropathy, glenohumeral arthrosis and loss of acromiohumeral space, requires joint arthroplasty (see subsection on "Rotator Cuff Arthropathy")
- Goutallier classification: grading scheme to classify cuff muscle atrophy and assess potential ability to repair cuff, best assessed on sagittal T1 images
  - Grade 0 = normal
  - Grade 1 = some fatty streaks
  - Grade 2 = more muscle than fat
  - Grade 3 = equal muscle and fat
  - Grade 4 = more fat than muscle

Treatment

Nonoperative

- Useful in patients with minimal risk of progression to irreversible muscle/tendon changes (intact cuff with tendinitis especially associated with subacromial bursitis or impingement, small partial-thickness tears)
- Activity modification, avoid repeated forward flexion >90°
- Physical therapy, exercises to increase mobility and strengthen rotator cuff and periscapular musculature and improve shoulder stability
- Oral NSAIDs
- Subacromial or glenohumeral glucocorticoid or NSAID injections

Operative

- Any surgical repair where rotator cuff is re-approximated to the footprint takes 2–3 months to achieve biologic healing.
- Arthroscopic versus mini-open repair techniques used, historically open approaches were used.
- Partial-thickness rotator cuff tear
  - Debridement alone for low-demand patient with articular side tear <50 % tendon thickness with viable surrounding tissue.
  - Debridement with acromioplasty and subacromial decompression if bursal-sided tear and signs of mechanical impingement.
  - Tendon repair for manual laborer/athlete if bursal sided and >30 % thickness, acute repair better than delayed in this case.

  - PASTA (partial articular-sided supraspinatus tendon avulsion) tears should be repaired if >7 mm footprint is involved (violates >50 % footprint); however, this should be performed with great caution in overhead athletes as the tear is likely adaptive.

- Full-thickness rotator cuff tear
  - All-arthroscopic tendon repair comparable to open/mini-open repair.
  - Double-row suture anchor fixation superior to single row.
  - Chronic retracted tears may require interval slide and marginal convergence techniques to facilitate repair.

- Massive rotator cuff tear
  - Tendon debridement ± biceps tenotomy results in pain relief, can consider tuberoplasty, useful mainly in elderly, low-demand patient.
  - Subacromial decompression does not appear to be helpful when used with debridement without repair.
  - Tendon repair (w/ or w/o augmentation), outcomes are fair but high failure rate as tissue quality is poor, used in young patient and manual laborer.
  - Irreparable massive rotator cuff tear treated with tendon transfer of the latissimus dorsi to the greater tuberosity for posterosuperior tears of the supraspinatus/infraspinatus, or subcoracoid pectoralis major transfer for anterosuperior tears; these tendon transfer techniques are used in younger patient.
  - Ultimately results in rotator cuff arthropathy requiring reverse total shoulder arthroplasty.

Complications

- Tendon re-tear (rate of recurrence 11–94 %)
- Disruption of deltoid origin (gradual or acute)
- Stiffness/impaired range of motion (5–10 % of RCR patients)
- General complications of arthroscopy (postoperative infection/stiffness, foreign-body reaction)

Bibliography

1. Burks RT, Crim J, Brown N, Fink B, Greis PE. A prospective randomized clinical trial comparing arthroscopic single- and double-row rotator cuff repair: magnetic resonance imaging and early clinical evaluation. Am J Sports Med. 2009;37(4):674–82. Epub 2009/02/11.
2. Castricini R, Longo UG, De Benedetto M, Panfoli N, Pirani P, Zini R, et al. Platelet-rich plasma augmentation for arthroscopic rotator cuff repair: a randomized controlled trial. Am J Sports Med. 2011;39(2):258–65. Epub 2010/12/17.
3. Conway JE. Arthroscopic repair of partial-thickness rotator cuff tears and SLAP lesions in professional baseball players. Orthop Clin North Am. 2001;32(3):443–56. Epub 2002/03/13.

4. Davidson J, Burkhart SS. The geometric classification of rotator cuff tears: a system linking tear pattern to treatment and prognosis. Arthroscopy. 2010;26(3):417–24. Epub 2010/03/09.
5. Ellman H. Diagnosis and treatment of incomplete rotator cuff tears. Clin Orthop Relat Res. 1990;(254):64–74. Epub 1990/05/01.
6. Grasso A, Milano G, Salvatore M, Falcone G, Deriu L, Fabbriciani C. Single-row versus double-row arthroscopic rotator cuff repair: a prospective randomized clinical study. Arthroscopy. 2009;25(1):4–12. Epub 2008/12/30.
7. Lo IK, Burkhart SS. Double-row arthroscopic rotator cuff repair: re-establishing the footprint of the rotator cuff. Arthroscopy. 2003;19(9):1035–42. Epub 2003/11/11.
8. Lo IK, Burkhart SS. Current concepts in arthroscopic rotator cuff repair. Am J Sports Med. 2003;31(2):308–24. Epub 2003/03/19.
9. Oh JH, Kim SH, Ji HM, Jo KH, Bin SW, Gong HS. Prognostic factors affecting anatomic outcome of rotator cuff repair and correlation with functional outcome. Arthroscopy. 2009;25(1):30–9. Epub 2008/12/30.

5 Rotator Cuff Tear Arthropathy

Take-Home Message

- Rotator cuff insufficiency, degeneration of the glenohumeral joint, and superior migration of the humeral head associated w/ rotator cuff tear.
- Hamada classification grade 4 and 5 define CTA.
- Reverse shoulder arthroplasty is treatment of choice for patient >70 years old with pseudoparalytic shoulder with irreparable rotator cuff tear and pain.
- Hemiarthroplasty is procedure of choice if <70 years old with retained forward elevation >90°.

Definition

- Structural glenohumeral joint destruction associated with chronic rotator cuff tearing and superior migration of the humeral head

Etiology

- No single proven theory.
- Small full-thickness rotator cuff tears progress to massive rotator cuff tears and/or dysfunction leading to loss of fulcrum for abduction in the glenohumeral joint causing superior migration of the humeral head and abnormal articulation with

the acromion and eccentric compression against the glenoid and resultant cartilage degradation and joint destruction.
- Loss of range of motion and force transmission result in poor cartilage nutrition and disuse osteopenia which cause further degeneration.
- Also some consider that leakage of synovial fluid into periarticular space and loss of normal joint pressure lead to cartilage degradation due to hemorrhagic effusions and decrease of glycosaminoglycans, instability, and subluxation and considered that calcium phosphate crystals phagocytose by synovial cells and trigger release of MMPs which leads to cartilage degradation.
- Female > male, dominant side.

Pathophysiology

- Massive rotator cuff tear
- Thinning of the acromioclavicular joint ± subacromial spur with acetabularization of the glenoid and acromion
- Rounding of the greater tuberosity with femoralization of the humeral head
- Osteopenic humeral head
- Loss of humeral head cartilage with subchondral collapse of the humeral head
- Coracoid erosion
- Clavicle erosion
- Attritional rupture of the long head biceps tendon

Radiographs

- AP, scapular Y, and axillary views (notable findings include superior migration of humeral head with decreased AHI, osteophyte formation, glenohumeral distance decreases secondary to joint space narrowing, acetabularization, femoralization, superior glenoid wear, osteopenia of the acromion/proximal humerus/glenoid)
- CT: not required but useful to evaluate glenoid bone stock and quality
- MRI: not required but useful to visualize rotator cuff muscle atrophy/fatty infiltration and/or tear

Classification

- Hamada classification: describes progressive glenohumeral joint destruction secondary to rotator cuff tears; grade 4 and 5 represent cuff tear arthropathy.
  - Grade 1: acromiohumeral interval (AHI) >6 mm
  - Grade 2: AHI < 6
  - Grade 3: acetabularization of the acromion
  - Grade 4: narrowing of the glenohumeral joint w/ arthrosis
  - Grade 5: collapse of the humeral head

- Vistosky classification: describes humeral head position relative to the glenoid and stability (I = centered, II = decentered)
  - IA = centered, stable, minimal superior migration, dynamic stabilization maintained, stabilization by the coracoacromial arch w/ acetabularization of the CA arch and femoralization of the humeral head
  - IB = centered, medialized, minimal superior migration, compromised dynamic stabilization, stabilization by the CA arch w/ IA conditions and medial erosion of the glenoid
  - IIA = decentered, limited stable, superior translation, insufficient dynamic stabilization, minimum stabilization by the CA arch w/ acetabularization, femoralization, and superior medial erosion
  - IIB = decentered, unstable, anterior superior escape, no dynamic stabilization, no stabilization by the CA arch (deficient anterior structures)

Treatment

Nonoperative

If minimal joint line destruction (Vistosky type IA/IB), rest, physical therapy, oral analgesics

Operative

- Reverse total shoulder arthroplasty: indicated for patient >70 with a painful shoulder with irreparable rotator cuff tear associated with <90° forward elevation or pseudoparalysis of anterior elevation and/or abduction (Hamada grade 4 or 5), contraindicated if axillary nerve palsy (deltoid dysfunction), inadequate glenoid bone stock and/or poor glenoid bone quality, or history of shoulder infection
  - Improve external rotation/arm control w/ latissimus dorsi tendon transfer to the anterosuperior humeral head.
  - Goal is to medialize and distalize the center of rotation to the surface of the glenoid, which decreases shear forces on the glenoid while increasing deltoid tension to recruit more deltoid fibers for arm elevation. No effect on external rotation.

- Hemiarthroplasty: patient age <70 and active elevation >90°, head contained in the CA arch during overhead elevation; functional recovery inferior to reverse shoulder prosthesis
- Arthroscopic lavage and debridement: temporary pain relief (patient health too poor for more invasive surgical treatment)
- Glenohumeral arthrodesis: used if history of infection, severe deltoid deficiency, axillary nerve palsy (rare)
- Resection arthroplasty: used if chronic infection and loss of bone stock

Complications

- RTSA: dislocation, glenoid fracture, acromial spine fracture, hardware loosening, infection, periprosthetic humerus fracture, nerve injury, hematoma, notching is a significant occurrence, but long-term effect is unknown (grade 1, confined to pillar; grade 2, perforation to inferior screw; grade 3, over the lower screw; grade 4, extends under baseplate)
  - Highest complication rates when attempted for salvage procedure of prior revision arthroplasty or in setting of severe proximal humerus fracture
- Hemiarthroplasty: instability, cuff tear, ectopic ossification, glenoid and humeral component loosening, intraoperative fracture, infection, nerve injury
- Arthrodesis: nonunion, prominent hardware, malposition, infection, fracture of the humeral shaft

Bibliography

1. Boileau P, Watkinson DJ, Hatzidakis AM, Balg F. Grammont reverse prosthesis: design, rationale, and biomechanics. J Shoulder Elbow Surg. 2005;14(1 Suppl S):147S–61S. Epub 2005/02/24.
2. Favard L, Levigne C, Nerot C, Gerber C, De Wilde L, Mole D. Reverse prostheses in arthropathies with cuff tear: are survivorship and function maintained over time? Clinl Orthop Relat Res. 2011;469(9):2469–75. Epub 2011/03/09.
3. Feeley BT, Gallo RA, Craig EV. Cuff tear arthropathy: current trends in diagnosis and surgical management. J Shoulder Elbow Surg. 2009;18(3):484–94. Epub 2009/02/12.
4. Neer CS, 2nd, Craig EV, Fukuda H. Cuff-tear arthropathy. J Bone Joint Surg Am. 1983;65(9):1232–44. Epub 1983/12/01.
5. Nolan BM, Ankerson E, Wiater JM. Reverse total shoulder arthroplasty improves function in cuff tear arthropathy. Clin Orthop Relat Res. 2011;469(9):2476–82. Epub 2010/12/01.
6. Sirveaux F, Favard L, Oudet D, Huquet D, Walch G, Mole D. Grammont inverted total shoulder arthroplasty in the treatment of glenohumeral osteoarthritis with massive rupture of the cuff. Results of a multicentre study of 80 shoulders. J Bone Joint Surg Br. 2004;86(3):388–95. Epub 2004/05/06.
7. Stechel A, Fuhrmann U, Irlenbusch L, Rott O, Irlenbusch U. Reversed shoulder arthroplasty in cuff tear arthritis, fracture sequelae, and revision arthroplasty. Acta Orthop. 2010;81(3):367–72. Epub 2010/05/11.
8. Zumstein MA, Pinedo M, Old J, Boileau P. Problems, complications, reoperations, and revisions in reverse total shoulder arthroplasty: a systematic review. J Shoulder Elbow Surg. 2011;20(1):146–57. Epub 2010/12/08.

6 Glenohumeral Arthritis

Take-Home Message

- Articular cartilage damage of GH joint; secondary to osteoarthritis, rheumatoid or post-traumatic arthritis, avascular necrosis
- Walch classification of glenoid deformity: Type A1 = centered humeral head with flattened glenoid, A2 = centered humeral head with concentric glenoid wear, B1 = posteriorly subluxated and minor erosion, B2 = posteriorly subluxated w/ posterior erosion/biconcave appearance, C = retroversion > 25° with posteriorly subluxation and dysplasia
- Hemiarthroplasty for patients <50 years w/ normal/minimal glenoid involvement, inadequate glenoid bone, strenuous activity
- Total shoulder arthroplasty for patients >50 years w/ adequate glenoid bone, sedentary/moderate activity

Definition

- Loss of articular cartilage covering the humeral head and glenoid with variable degree of soft tissue contracture and bone erosion associated with limited shoulder motion

Etiology

- Primary osteoarthritis: cause unknown, likely remote/asymptomatic mechanical trauma triggering release of degradative enzymes/inflammatory mediators to the articular cartilage, final common pathway of all cases of osteoarthritis is articular cartilage compromise
- Secondary OA: single traumatic event versus repetitive microtrauma, instability, iatrogenic injury during prior joint surgery, and less commonly infection, osteonecrosis, gout, Paget's disease, rheumatoid disease, ochronosis, sickle cell disease, epiphyseal dysplasia
- Rheumatoid arthritis: influx of inflammatory cells (lymphocytes) into the joint and hypertrophic synovial tissue (forms pannus) that triggers release of cytokines, enzymes, and inflammatory mediators, resulting in joint destruction
- Avascular necrosis: subchondral collapse secondary to compromised blood supply leading to advanced cartilage destruction

Pathophysiology

- Progressive pain, stiffness, and loss of function
- Osteoarthritis: loss of external rotation, posterior subluxation, posterior glenoid bone loss, peripheral osteophytes especially at inferior humeral neck; rotator cuff and biceps intact in the majority of cases (95 %) and usually no evidence of subacromial impingement
  - Osteophytes and decreased joint stability increase friction at the joint resulting in additional cartilage damage, while increased stress on the bone leads to subchondral sclerosis (medial humeral head and posterior glenoid), cyst formation, and cartilage loss on superior or central head or involving entire head.

- Rheumatoid arthritis: regional osteopenia, central glenoid bone erosion, rotator cuff dysfunction/tearing seen in 30 % and long head of the biceps ruptured in 15 %, see joint space narrowing late in disease
- Trauma: humeral head or glenoid fractures or prominent hardware, tuberosity malunion/nonunion

Radiographs

- AP (plus with internal and external rotation views), true AP, and axillary views
  - Used to evaluate rotator cuff integrity (look for superior migration of head which may indicate cuff insufficiency) and glenoid bone stock on axillary view.
  - Primary OA: see subchondral sclerosis and cysts, osteophyte formation (inferior humerus), asymmetrical posterior joint space narrowing.
  - Post-traumatic arthritis: look for retained hardware or fractures (articular step-off, malunion, nonunion).
- CT: not required but useful to accurately classify glenoid bone erosion and quality.
- MRI: not typically necessary but can assess rotator cuff integrity (especially in rheumatoid arthritis case).
- Electromyography: assess post-traumatic/post-surgical nerve injuries.

Classification

- Walch classification: assessment of glenoid deformity
  - Type A, humeral head centered (A1 minor erosion, A2 major central erosion); B, posteriorly subluxated head (B1 minor posterior wear, B2 severe posterior wear with biconcave appearance); C, posteriorly subluxated w/ glenoid retroversion >25°, dysplastic glenoid

Treatment

Nonoperative

- Activity modification/avoidance
- Therapeutic/stretching exercises for flexibility
- NSAIDs
- Consideration for intra-articular corticosteroid injections early in disease process
- Close cooperation with rheumatologist critical to manage rheumatoid arthritis etiology with DMARDS, steroids, and methotrexate
- Little proven efficacy of chondroitin sulfate and nutritional supplements

Operative

- Resurfacing hemiarthroplasty: can be considered <50 years old, manual laborer with little glenoid wear; ultimately requires conversion to total shoulder arthroplasty secondary to glenoid arthrosis; advantage is this is bone preserving (theoretically)
- Stemmed hemiarthroplasty: patients <50 years with normal/minimal glenoid involvement, inadequate glenoid bone, and strenuous activity levels

- Biologic resurfacing of glenoid: can be done in young/active patients; use meniscal, fascia lata, dermal, or Achilles tendon allografts and capsular/fascia lata autografts; xenograft materials to cover the glenoid (no long-term data support efficacy of this procedure)
- Total shoulder arthroplasty (TSA): patients >50 years w/ adequate glenoid bone and moderate activity levels
  - Polyethylene glenoid component (most predictable pain relief, risk of progressive wear/loosening), allows for correction of glenoid incongruence or dysplasia.
  - Glenoid head height should be set to approximately 75 % radius of head.
  - For osteoarthritis, TSA compared to hemiarthroplasty, provides superior outcomes (pain, function, satisfaction, lower revision rate).
- Reverse total shoulder arthroplasty: see section on "Cuff Tear Arthropathy"
- Glenohumeral arthrodesis: rare, used if painful paralytic shoulder, septic arthritis, severe OA in young/highly active patients unfit for arthroplasty
- Open/arthroscopic debridement: rarely used, no benefit to removal of periarticular osteophytes, can be considered in young/active patients with congruent, centered joint and little evidence of osteophytes/sclerosis/cysts and for removal of intra-articular loose body or for synovectomy to treat synovial chondromatosis or pigmented villonodular synovitis

Complications

- Resurfacing and stemmed hemiarthroplasty: glenoid is not resurfaced so ultimately it can lead to arthritic change and require revision for pain, especially in young/active patient.
  - If inadequate bone stock risk bone collapse around implant and malposition leading to failure
- TSA: instability, rotator cuff tear or failed repair (leads to early glenoid component wear), glenoid/humeral component loosening, intraoperative fracture, axillary nerve injury, overstuffing joint leads to pain and stiffness and potential for a failed repair of subscapularis tendon, polyethylene wear.
- Arthrodesis: nonunion, prominent hardware, malposition, humeral shaft fracture.

Bibliography

1. Carroll RM, Izquierdo R, Vazquez M, Blaine TA, Levine WN, Bigliani LU. Conversion of painful hemiarthroplasty to total shoulder arthroplasty: long-term results. J Shoulder Elbow Surg. 2004;13(6):599–603. Epub 2004/12/01.
2. Chin PYK, Sperling JW, Cofield RH, Schleck C. Complications of total shoulder arthroplasty: are they fewer or different? J Shoulder Elbow Surg. 2006;15(1): 19–22.

3. Clinton J, Franta AK, Lenters TR, Mounce D, Matsen Iii FA. Nonprosthetic glenoid arthroplasty with humeral hemiarthroplasty and total shoulder arthroplasty yield similar self-assessed outcomes in the management of comparable patients with glenohumeral arthritis. J Shoulder Elbow Surg. 2007;16(5):534–8.
4. Coe MP, Greiwe RM, Joshi R, Snyder BM, Simpson L, Tosteson AN, et al. The cost-effectiveness of reverse total shoulder arthroplasty compared with hemiarthroplasty for rotator cuff tear arthropathy. J Shoulder Elbow Surg. 2012;21(10):1278–88. Epub 2012/01/24.
5. Elhassan B, Ozbaydar M, Diller D, Higgins LD, Warner JJ. Soft-tissue resurfacing of the glenoid in the treatment of glenohumeral arthritis in active patients less than fifty years old. J Bone Joint Surg Am. 2009;91(2):419–24. Epub 2009/02/03.
6. McNickle AG, L'Heureux DR, Provencher MT, Romeo AA, Cole BJ. Postsurgical glenohumeral arthritis in young adults. Am J Sports Med. 2009;37(9):1784–91. Epub 2009/06/11.
7. Radnay CS, Setter KJ, Chambers L, Levine WN, Bigliani LU, Ahmad CS. Total shoulder replacement compared with humeral head replacement for the treatment of primary glenohumeral osteoarthritis: a systematic review. J Shoulder Elbow Surg. 2007;16(4):396–402. Epub 2007/06/22.
8. Walch G, Badet R, Boulahia A, Khoury A. Morphologic study of the glenoid in primary glenohumeral osteoarthritis. J Arthroplasty. 1999;14(6):756–60. Epub 1999/10/08.
9. Wirth MA, Tapscott RS, Southworth C, Rockwood Jr CA. Treatment of glenohumeral arthritis with a hemiarthroplasty: a minimum five-year follow-up outcome study. J Bone Joint Surg A. 2006;88(5):964–73.

7 Avascular Necrosis

Take-Home Message

- Main blood supply to the humeral head is the anterolateral ascending branch of the anterior circumflex artery (branch off axillary artery), found 1 cm distal to inferior border of the pectoralis major, terminates as the arcuate artery (the posterior circumflex artery supplies the greater tuberosity and small portion of the posteroinferior humeral head).
- Cruess classification guides treatment (evaluation of humeral head and joint surface changes).
- Nonoperative management and core decompression useful for stage I and II with resurfacing for stage III and IV and total shoulder arthroplasty for stage V.

Definition

- Humeral head bone death and articular collapse secondary to compromise of the blood supply

Etiology

- Known predisposing factors: alcohol abuse, AIDS, sickle cell disease, corticosteroids, SLE, Gaucher's disease, pancreatitis, inflammatory bowel disease, trauma, infection, Caisson's ("the Bends"), chemotherapy, coagulation deficiencies, myeloproliferative disorder, thalassemia, radiation, pregnancy, organ transplants, idiopathic.
- Smoking increases incidence 3–5×, male-female (2:1).
- Main blood supply to the humeral head is the anterolateral ascending branch of the anterior circumflex artery (branch off axillary artery), found 1 cm distal to inferior border of the pectoralis major, terminates as arcuate artery (posterior circumflex artery supplies greater tuberosity and small portion of posteroinferior humeral head).

Pathophysiology

- Disease most commonly occurs in superomedial portion of the humeral head.
- Subchondral fracture and collapse with thick cartilage flaps with initial glenoid sparing.
- Articular surface collapse with abnormal articulation leading to glenoid degeneration and arthritis.
- Rotator cuff intact and long head biceps intact.
- No evidence of subacromial impingement.

Radiographs

- Complete shoulder series (AP, internal and external rotation views, scapular Y, axillary).
- MRI is the best method of assessing early stages of disease prior to bony collapse.
- Bone scan can be helpful but has low sensitivity.

Classification

- Cruess classification
  - I, normal x-ray with changes seen only on MRI; II, no collapse, subchondral sclerosis, osteopenia; III, crescent sign (subchondral fracture) without cartilage collapse; IV, articular collapse with flattening and early secondary osteoarthritis; V, degenerative changes include glenoid

Treatment

Nonoperative

- NSAIDs
- Activity modification (no overhead activity as disease is usually in the superomedial humeral head)

- Physical therapy with gentle motion and pendulums, but avoid resisted abduction
- Identify underlying cause (if possible) to avoid occurrence in other joints

Operative

- Core decompression: used in stages I and II, controversial for stage III, thought to reduce pressure in bone marrow while causing hyperemia and neovascularization to allow necrotic area to form new bone; variable results reported in the literature (better than that reported for femoral head core decompression), keep entry point lateral to the bicipital groove (risk of injury to the ascending branch of the anterior humeral circumflex artery)
- Arthroscopy: can be helpful for concurrent intra-articular visualization while using fluoroscopy for core decompression
- Hemiarthroplasty: stages III and IV, benefit shown as long as there are no glenoid arthritic changes
- Humeral head resurfacing: stages III and IV, can do total head resurfacing or subtotal resurfacing (replace only focal chondral defect while preserving normal cartilage)
- Total shoulder arthroplasty: used in stage III, IV, and V; most useful for stage V where the glenoid is involved

Complications

Core decompression: injury to the ascending branch of the anterior humeral circumflex artery can compromise blood supply to entire head accelerating disease.

- Typical complications for hemiarthroplasty, resurfacing, and total shoulder arthroplasty as reported in subsection "Glenohumeral Arthritis."

Bibliography

1. Chapman C, Mattern C, Levine WN. Arthroscopically assisted core decompression of the proximal humerus for avascular necrosis. Arthroscopy. 2004;20(9):1003–6. Epub 2004/11/05.
2. Cruess RL. Steroid-induced avascular necrosis of the head of the humerus. Natural history and management. J Bone Joint Surg Br. 1976;58(3):313–7. Epub 1976/08/01.
3. Cruess RL. Experience with steroid-induced avascular necrosis of the shoulder and etiologic considerations regarding osteonecrosis of the hip. Clin Orthop Relat Res. 1978;(130):86–93. Epub 1978/01/01.
4. Dines JS, Strauss EJ, Fealy S, Craig EV. Arthroscopic-assisted core decompression of the humeral head. Arthroscopy. 2007;23(1):103.e1–4. Epub 2007/01/11.
5. Lau MW, Blinder MA, Williams K, Galatz LM. Shoulder arthroplasty in sickle cell patients with humeral head avascular necrosis. J Shoulder Elbow Surg. 2007;16(2):129–34. Epub 2007/02/06.
6. Parsch D, Lehner B, Loew M. Shoulder arthroplasty in nontraumatic osteonecrosis of the humeral head. J Shoulder Elbow Surg. 2003;12(3):226–30. Epub 2003/07/10.

8 Adhesive Capsulitis

Take-Home Message

- Must rule out other shoulder pathologies.
- Nonoperative treatment predominates as majority regain motion and have decreased pain despite some residual deficits.
- Stage 1 and 2: physical therapy with gentle range of motion, home exercise program, and patient education.
- Stage 3 and 4: aggressive stretching exercises, no indication for steroid injections; if fail non-op, then proceed to arthroscopic capsular release and synovectomy with manipulation under anesthesia followed by persistent physical therapy.

Definition

- Painful shoulder with restricted passive and active range of motion at the glenohumeral joint secondary to progressive fibrosis and glenohumeral joint capsule fibrosis

Etiology

- Unknown cause.
- Associated with diabetes (increased with longer duration disease), thyroid dysfunction, Dupuytren's contractures, autoimmune disease, autonomic neuropathy, myocardial infarction.
- Females > males, 40–60 year old, non-dominant hand > dominant hand.
- Secondary adhesive capsulitis can mimic primary adhesive capsulitis but represents a stiff shoulder secondary to other coexistent shoulder pathology, and treatment should be tailored toward the primary pathology.

Pathophysiology

- Global capsular inflammation and fibrosis
- Synovitis
- Loss of axillary folds

Radiographs

- Complete shoulder series to rule out alternative pathology (locked posterior dislocation, rotator cuff tear, calcific tendonitis, osteoarthritis)
- Some use MRI to rule out other injuries but not required

Classification

- Neviaser and Neviaser described 4 stages
  - Stage 1: Inflammatory Stage
    - Gradual pain onset at deltoid insertion and capsular pain on deep palpation, complaints of night pain, loss of external rotation but most range of motion maintained.

  - Intra-articular anesthetic injection or regional block restores full motion.
  - Must exclude other disease processes (locked posterior dislocation, osteoarthritis, rotator cuff tear, calcific tendonitis).
  - Arthroscopic appearance: fibrinous synovial inflammatory reaction without adhesions or capsular contracture.
  - Biopsy: shows few inflammatory cells, hypervascularity, hypertrophic synovitis, but normal joint capsule.

- Stage 2: Freezing Stage

  - Primary complaint of night pain, motion restricted to forward flexion/abduction/internal and external rotation.
  - Intra-articular anesthetic injection or regional block does NOT restore full motion.
  - Arthroscopic appearance: christmas tree synovitis, axillary pouch begins to disappear.
  - Biopsy: hypertrophic and hypervascular synovitis with subsynovial scar formation.

- Stage 3: Frozen Stage (maturation)

  - Significant stiffness with pain at the limit of range of motion secondary to a mechanical block.
  - Intra-articular anesthetic injection or regional block does NOT restore any motion.
  - Arthroscopic appearance: complete loss of axillary recess with minimal synovitis.
  - Biopsy: dense, hypercellular collagenous tissue and fibrosis with a thin synovial layer.

- Stage 4: Thawing Stage (chronic)

  - Minimal pain with gradual, slow improvement in some shoulder motion
  - Arthroscopic appearance: mature adhesions mask intra-articular structures

Treatment

- Nonoperative treatment predominates especially early in the inflammatory and freezing stages. Majority of patient will regain near normal shoulder motion and have resolution of pain.
- Stage 1 and 2: physical therapy with gentle range of motion, home exercise program, patient education.
- Stage 3 and 4: persistent stretching exercises, steroid injections may or may not be helpful; if fail non-op, then proceed to arthroscopic capsular release and synovectomy with manipulation under anesthesia followed by persistent physical therapy.
- Levine et al. showed that failure to show improvement or range-of-motion regression after 4 months of supervised treatment are in more likely to fail nonoperative management, and surgical treatment may be necessary.

- Oral NSAIDs have no proven benefit for increasing shoulder motion although does decrease pain.
- Oral corticosteroid risks>benefits (no change in motion in long-term although short-term benefits).
- Intra-articular steroid injections provide short-term pain relief, good adjunct in early stages in conjunction with physical therapy, effectiveness of injection inversely proportional to symptom duration.
- Physical therapy can help prevent capsular contracture but does significantly improve motion acutely once lost.
- Suprascapular nerve blocks can help provide pain relief but no clear statistically significant improvement in shoulder motion (positive trend in literature).
- Hydrodilation shows improved pain relief but no effect on shoulder range of motion.
- Manipulation under anesthesia improves motion in short and long term.
- Arthroscopic capsular release and synovectomy successful for decreasing pain and improving shoulder motion and also can diagnose alternative intra-articular pathology.
  - Debate on how much of the capsule to release; we do not recommend releasing the intra-articular subscapularis tendon.
  - Rotator interval release increases external rotation, while posterior capsule release increases internal rotation.
- Open capsule release also successful but more historical.

Complications

- Manipulation under anesthesia: humerus fracture, labral tear, biceps tendon rupture, subscapularis rupture, dislocation.
- Open surgery can be complicated by stiffness secondary to approach.

Bibliography

1. Huang YP, Fann CY, Chiu YH, Yen MF, Chen LS, Chen HH, et al. Association of diabetes mellitus with the risk of developing adhesive capsulitis of the shoulder: a longitudinal population-based followup study. Arthritis Care Res. 2013;65(7):1197–202.
2. Jacobs LG, Smith MG, Khan SA, Smith K, Joshi M. Manipulation or intra-articular steroids in the management of adhesive capsulitis of the shoulder? A prospective randomized trial. J Shoulder Elbow Surg. 2009;18(3):348–53.
3. Jerosch J, Nasef NM, Peters O, Mansour AMR. Mid-term results following arthroscopic capsular release in patients with primary and secondary adhesive shoulder capsulitis. Knee Surg Sports Traumatol Arthrosc. 2013;21(5):1195–202.
4. Levine WN, Kashyap CP, Bak SF, Ahmad CS, Blaine TA, Bigliani LU. Nonoperative management of idiopathic adhesive capsulitis. J Shoulder Elbow Surg. 2007;16(5):569–73. Epub 2007/05/29.

5. Quraishi NA, Johnston P, Bayer J, Crowe M, Chakrabarti AJ. Thawing the frozen shoulder: a randomised trial comparing manipulation under anaesthesia with hydrodilatation. J Bone Joint Surg B. 2007;89(9):1197–200.
6. Shah N, Lewis M. Shoulder adhesive capsulitis: systematic review of randomised trials using multiple corticosteroid injections. Br J General Pract. 2007;57(541):662–7.
7. Vermeulen HM, Rozing PM, Obermann WR, Le Cessie S, Vlieland TPMV. Comparison of high-grade and low-grade mobilization techniques in the management of adhesive capsulitis of the shoulder: Randomized controlled trial. Phys Ther. 2006;86(3):355–68.
8. Yoon SH, Lee HY, Lee HJ, Kwack KS. Optimal dose of intra-articular corticosteroids for adhesive capsulitis: a randomized, triple-blind, placebo-controlled trial. Am J Sports Med. 2013;41(5):1133–9.

9 Glenohumeral Instability

Take-Home Message

- Careful history and physical exam to differentiate arm position at time of injury, and when instability occurs, this dictates requisite treatment.
- High re-dislocation rates for young athletes *after first time dislocation events.*
- Must distinguish multidirectional instability (mainly nonoperative treatment) from traumatic etiology (operative treatment).

Definition

Recurrent subluxation or dislocation of the glenohumeral joint secondary to a spectrum of pathologic conditions resulting in injury to the shoulder stabilizers

Etiology

- Traumatic: predictable pattern based on arm motion
  - Anterior dislocation with arm in abduction and external rotation
  - Posterior dislocation with arm in flexion, adduction, and internal rotation
- Atraumatic
  - Multidirectional instability (MDI)
- Acquired
  - Repetitive microtrauma
  - Athletes (overhead throwers, contact athletes)

Pathophysiology

- Disruption of static stabilizers (bony/articular anatomy, glenoid labrum, capsuloligamentous complex, negative intra-articular pressure) or dynamic stabilizers (rotator cuff, periscapular stabilizers, proprioception).
  - Inferior glenohumeral ligament (IGHL) deformation leads to subluxation and often fails at glenoid insertion (40 %).
  - Scapular muscle atrophy or rotator cuff tears.
- Associated with anteroinferior labral tear (Bankart) or glenoid rim fracture involving >25 % glenoid rim (bony Bankart), posteroinferior labral tear (reverse Bankart), anterior labroligamentous periosteal sleeve avulsion (ALPSA), glenolabral articular disruption (GLAD), humeral avulsion of the inferior glenohumeral ligament (HAGL).
- Impression fracture of the posterior superior humeral articular surface (Hill-Sachs lesion) or anterior superior surface (reverse Hill-Sachs).
- Mechanism of injury or position reproducing pain/apprehension symptoms is key to understanding injury
  - Anterior instability: arm in abduction and external rotation
  - Posterior instability: arm in flexion, adduction, and internal rotation
- Age of dislocation event predicts risk of recurrence: 95 % if <20 years old, 60 % if 20–25 years old, decreased risk of recurrence as age of initial dislocation increases.

Radiographs

- Anteroposterior (AP), lateral (scapular Y), and axillary views
  - Hill-Sachs lesion best seen on AP with internal rotation or Stryker notch view
  - Anterior glenoid fractures best seen on axillary view, look for bony Bankart
- CT scan helpful to further evaluate glenoid bony anatomy
- MRI arthrogram sensitive for labral lesions

Classification

- Voluntary versus involuntary subluxation or dislocation
- Traumatic versus atraumatic
- Type of instability commonly described by direction and degree of instability
  - Anteroposterior instability (graded 0–3 for humeral head translation)
    - 0 = normal motion, 1 = translation to rim, 2 = translation over rim with spontaneous reduction, 3 = locked dislocation over rim
  - Sulcus sign: estimate acromiohumeral interval with inferior stress to humerus
    - 1 = <1 cm interval, 2 = 1–2 cm interval, 3 = >2 cm interval

- Traumatic: TUBS (traumatic unilateral dislocations with a Bankart lesion)
  - >90 % recurrence rate, surgery indicated
- Atraumatic: AMBRI (atraumatic multidirectional bilateral shoulder dislocation/subluxation)
  - Rehabilitation often successful, if failed then inferior capsular shift or plication indicated

Treatment

Nonoperative

- Sling versus external rotation bracing for 3–6 weeks followed by rehabilitation stressing strengthening of periscapular muscle, rotator cuff, and deltoid
- MDI: treat with physiotherapy, lengthy rehabilitation focusing on closed kinetic chain exercises and scapular stabilization

Operative

- Labral lesion (Bankart repair)
- Glenoid deficiency (Bristow/Latarjet, bone block osteotomy, arthroplasty)
- Capsuloligamentous laxity (staple capsulorrhaphy, Putti-Platt, Magnuson-Stack, Boyd-Sisk)
  - Largely abandoned due to non-anatomic repair leading to excessive over-tightening anterior capsule can cause posterior instability and arthritis
- Capsular shift: for patients with MDI if failed extensive physical therapy
- Arthroscopic techniques largely equivalent to open procedures
  - Arthroscopic capsular plication highly effective for anterior shoulder instability.
  - Arthroscopic posterior capsulolabral reconstruction yields excellent outcomes in athletes with posterior instability.
- Open repair: advantageous if significant glenoid bone loss (large Hill-Sachs or significant glenoid bone loss >30 %, HAGL)

Complications

- Re-dislocation rates >90 % if young patient and nonoperative treatment.
- Over-tightening anterior capsule leads to posterior subluxation and glenohumeral arthritis.
- Loss of external rotation.
- Hardware failure or nonunion.
- Thermal capsular shrinkage no longer performed due to possible association with chondrolysis and longer-term results showing chondral damage and poor capsular tissue quality.

Bibliography

1. Ahmed I, Ashton F, Robinson CM. Arthroscopic Bankart repair and capsular shift for recurrent anterior shoulder instability: functional outcomes and identification of risk factors for recurrence. J Bone Joint Surg Am. 2012;94(14):1308–15. Epub 2012/07/20.
2. Bradley JP, Baker Iii CL, Kline AJ, Armfield DR, Chhabra A. Arthroscopic capsulolabral reconstruction for posterior instability of the shoulder: a prospective study of 100 shoulders. Am J Sports Med. 2006;34(7):1061–71.
3. Bradley JP, McClincy MP, Arner JW, Tejwani SG. Arthroscopic capsulolabral reconstruction for posterior instability of the shoulder: a prospective study of 200 shoulders. Am J Sports Med. 2013;41(9):2005–14. Epub 2013/06/28.
4. Jones KJ, Kahlenberg CA, Dodson CC, Nam D, Williams RJ, Altchek DW. Arthroscopic capsular plication for microtraumatic anterior shoulder instability in overhead athletes. Am J Sports Med. 2012;40(9):2009–14. Epub 2012/08/08.
5. Lafosse L, Lejeune E, Bouchard A, Kakuda C, Gobezie R, Kochhar T. The arthroscopic latarjet procedure for the treatment of anterior shoulder instability. Arthroscopy. 2007;23(11):1242.e1–5.
6. Larrain MV, Montenegro HJ, Mauas DM, Collazo CC, Pavón F. Arthroscopic management of traumatic anterior shoulder instability in collision athletes: analysis of 204 cases with a 4- to 9-year follow-up and results with the suture anchor technique. Arthroscopy. 2006;22(12):1283–9.
7. Lenters TR, Franta AK, Wolf FM, Leopold SS, Matsen Iii FA. Arthroscopic compared with open repairs for recurrent anterior shoulder instability: a systematic review and meta-analysis of the literature. J Bone Joint Surg A. 2007;89(2):244–54.
8. Mologne TS, Provencher MT, Menzel KA, Vachon TA, Dewing CB. Arthroscopic stabilization in patients with an inverted pear glenoid: results in patients with bone loss of the anterior glenoid. Am J Sports Med. 2007;35(8):1276–83.
9. Robinson CM, Howes J, Murdoch H, Will E, Graham C. Functional outcome and risk of recurrent instability after primary traumatic anterior shoulder dislocation in young patients. J Bone Joint Surg A. 2006;88(11):2326–36.
10. Warner JJP, Gill TJ, O'Hollerhan JD, Pathare N, Millett PJ. Anatomical glenoid reconstruction for recurrent anterior glenohumeral instability with glenoid deficiency using an autogenous tricortical iliac crest bone graft. Am J Sports Med. 2006;34(2):205–12.
11. Yiannakopoulos CK, Mataragas E, Antonogiannakis E. A comparison of the spectrum of intra-articular lesions in acute and chronic anterior shoulder instability. Arthroscopy. 2007;23(9):985–90.

10 SLAP and Biceps Tendon

Take-Home Message

- Abducted shoulder w/ maximum external rotation → increased force at base of biceps and labral strain → SLAP lesion
- Type I debridement of labral fraying; type III, debridement of bucket-handle tear; type II, IV, V reattachment of labrum (arthroscopy); distinguish between normal labral variation/aging and anatomic variants before repair (meniscoid superior labrum, sub-labral foramen, Buford complex)

Definition

- Detachment of the superior labrum extending from anterior to posterior about the biceps tendon, with or without involvement of the biceps tendon anchor

Etiology

- Compression loading of the flexed and abducted shoulder with forced external rotation
- Acute traumatic injury during a biceps traction load (arm acceleration during late-cocking phase of throwing or arm deceleration during follow-through phase of throwing), shearing forces on the superior biceps labral complex during a fall or in a restrained passenger in a motor vehicle crash
- Chronic repetitive injury (overhead motion)
  - Increased external rotation in late-cocking phase of overhead throw increases torsion forces at biceps root.
  - Posterior capsular contracture increases stress on the labrum.
  - Internal impingement.

Pathophysiology

- "Peel-back" mechanism (Burkhart and Morgan)
  - Abducted position: increased external and decreased internal rotation
  - Greater torsional loads across the superior labrum, the biceps tendon more posterior → medial displacement over glenoid
- SLAP lesion increases strain on the anterosuperior band of the inferior glenohumeral ligament w/ abduction and external rotation.
- Atrophy of the supraspinatus and infraspinatus muscle indicates ganglion cyst formation and suprascapular nerve compression, often associated with SLAP lesion.

Radiographs

- AP, true AP, scapular Y, axillary views to identify other pain sources
- MRI/MRA
  - Addition of gadolinium to MRI, and the shoulder in abduction and external rotation to improve accuracy.
  - Best seen in coronal oblique plane, irregular contrast extravasation into the superior labrum/biceps anchor, also axial cuts help evaluate displacement.
  - Sub-labral separation from glenoid up to 2 mm or more is normal.
- Arthroscopy = definitive diagnosis, must view from anterior and posterior portals
  - Type III and IV: bucket-handle tears, type II slap triad (sub-labral chondromalacia of the superior glenoid, frayed underside of the labrum, gap between the labrum and articular cartilage >5 mm)

Classification

- Snyder classification (types I–IV)
- Type I: fraying w/ localized degeneration on inner rim of the superior labrum
  - Superior labral/biceps anchor attachments intact
  - Associated with aging, most common asymptomatic pathology
- Type II: avulsion of the superior labrum from the superior glenoid tubercle at the biceps anchor (most common symptomatic pathology)
  - Anterior = labral avulsion from anterosuperior quadrant of the glenoid, most common in general population
  - Posterior = labral avulsion in posterosuperior quadrant, most common in throwers
  - Combined anterior and posterior = avulsion of both anterosuperior and posterosuperior quadrants
- Type III: bucket-handle tear of the superior labrum, normal biceps tendon attachment
- Type IV: bucket-handle tear of the superior labrum extending into the biceps tendon

Maffet, Gartsman, and Moseley classification (types V–VII), described SLAP lesions associated with instability

- Type V: Bankart lesion extending superiorly to biceps attachment
- Type VI: anterior or posterior labral flap +, type II biceps anchor avulsion
- Type VII: biceps attachment separation extending beneath the middle glenohumeral ligament

Powell, Nord, and Ryu further defined additional types (types VIII–X), described SLAP lesions with posterior extension

- Type VIII: type II w/ posterior labral extension
- Type IX: type II w/ circumferential labral tearing
- Type X: type II w/ posterior inferior labral separation

Treatment

Nonoperative

- Ice, NSAIDS
- Physical therapy: improve posterior capsular flexibility and strengthen rotator cuff and scapular stabilizers
- Growing enthusiasm for nonoperative management concurrent with decreased enthusiasm for operative management.

Operative

- If nonoperative methods fail for ≥6 months OR suprascapular nerve compression secondary to spinoglenoid notch cysts
- Arthroscopy
  - Type I: debridement of frayed edge
  - Type II: reattachment of the superior labrum
  - Type III: debridement of bucket-handle tear, careful to identify attachment site of MGHL to avoid inadvertent resection which would destabilize shoulder anteriorly
  - Type IV – <30 % of biceps tendon involved: debridement of labral tear and extension into the biceps; >30 %, biceps tenodesis and labral repair (young patient) and labral debridement and biceps tenotomy/tenodesis (patient >40 years old)
  - Types V, VI, and VII: reattachment of the superior labrum to correct glenohumeral shoulder instability
  - Type VI: debridement of flap
  - Types VIII, IX, X: reattachment of the labrum and debridement of flaps

Complications

Stiffness/loss of motion, can occur if the operated extremity inappropriately immobilized postoperatively for significant time period.

- Incorrect diagnosis: failure of repair if degeneration of the superior labrum is due to aging not a SLAP lesion (patients >40, w/ glenohumeral arthritis or rotator cuff tears).
- Failure to recognize normal anatomic variants of the anterior labrum (cordlike MGHL, large sub-labral foramen, Buford complex) can lead to loss of shoulder motion.
- Complications of arthroscopic repair: pain/postoperative impairment, failure of bioabsorbable tacks, synovitis and foreign-body granuloma formation, loose/broken hardware

Bibliography

1. Antonio GE, Griffith JF, Yu AB, Yung PS, Chan KM, Ahuja AT. First-time shoulder dislocation: High prevalence of labral injury and age-related differences revealed by MR arthrography. J Magn Reson Imaging. 2007;26(4):983–91. Epub 2007/09/27.
2. Boileau P, Parratte S, Chuinard C, Roussanne Y, Shia D, Bicknell R. Arthroscopic treatment of isolated type II SLAP lesions: biceps tenodesis as an alternative to reinsertion. Am J Sports Med. 2009;37(5):929–36. Epub 2009/02/21.
3. Brockmeier SF, Voos JE, Williams RJ, 3rd, Altchek DW, Cordasco FA, Allen AA, et al. Outcomes after arthroscopic repair of type-II SLAP lesions. J Bone Joint Surg Am. 2009;91(7):1595–603. Epub 2009/07/03.
4. Edwards SL, Lee JA, Bell JE, Packer JD, Bigliani LU, Ahmad CS, Levine WN, Blaine T. Non-operative treatment of superior anterior posterior labral tears: improvements in pain, function, and quality of life. Am J Sports Med. 2010;38:1456–61.
5. Franceschi F, Longo UG, Ruzzini L, Rizzello G, Maffulli N, Denaro V. No advantages in repairing a type II superior labrum anterior and posterior (SLAP) lesion when associated with rotator cuff repair in patients over age 50: a randomized controlled trial. Am J Sports Med. 2008;36(2):247–53. Epub 2007/10/18.
6. Friel NA, Karas V, Slabaugh MA, Cole BJ. Outcomes of type II superior labrum, anterior to posterior (SLAP) repair: prospective evaluation at a minimum two-year follow-up. J Shoulder Elbow Surg. 2010;19(6):859–67. Epub 2010/06/18.
7. Katz LM, Hsu S, Miller SL, Richmond JC, Khetia E, Kohli N, et al. Poor outcomes after SLAP repair: descriptive analysis and prognosis. Arthroscopy. 2009;25(8):849–55. Epub 2009/08/12.

11 Scapular Disorders: Serratus Palsy and Trapezius Palsy

Take-Home Message

- Serratus anterior palsy: paralysis of the serratus anterior muscle (disruption of the long thoracic nerve), treat with split pectoralis major transfer to inferior angle of the scapula
- Trapezius palsy: paralysis of the trapezius muscle (disruption of the cranial nerve XI, spinal accessory nerve), treat with Eden-Lange procedure (lateral transfer of the levator scapulae, rhomboid major, and rhomboid minor along the scapula)
- Scapular winging: medial winging in serratus palsy, lateral winging in trapezius palsy

Definition

- Serratus palsy: injury to long thoracic nerve resulting in paresis or paralysis of the serratus anterior and associated with medial scapular winging
- Trapezius palsy: injury to spinal accessory nerve resulting in paresis or paralysis of the trapezius muscle and associated with lateral scapular winging

Etiology

- Serratus palsy: injury to the long thoracic nerve (C5–7)
  - Neurapraxias due to blunt trauma causing traction over the second rib and traction and compression at inferior angle of the scapula (during general anesthesia/prolonged abduction)
  - Iatrogenic during radical mastectomy, first rib resection, trans-axillary sympathectomy, surgical positioning, and less commonly viral illness, Parsonage-Turner syndrome, isolated long thoracic neuritis, immunization, C7 nerve root lesions,
  - idiopathic
- Trapezius palsy: injury to the spinal accessory nerve (CN XI)
  - Cervical lymph node biopsy, injuries from trauma/traction or surgical procedures and rarely viral illness, acromioclavicular/sternoclavicular dissociation, post-carotid endarterectomy, post-catheterization of internal jugular vein

Pathophysiology

- Serratus palsy: medial and superior translation of the scapula with weakness and decreased forward elevation and abduction; secondarily results in subacromial impingement due to relative anterior rotation of the acromion; adhesive capsulitis can result from disuse.
- Trapezius palsy: downward and lateral translation of the scapula with progressive shoulder girdle pain, weakness of arm anterior elevation and abduction, eventual atrophy of the trapezius.

Radiographs

- AP, true AP, scapular Y, and axillary radiographs reveal structural alternative abnormalities (osteochondromas, cervical spondylosis, scoliosis)
- Electromyography confirms the muscles involved and the degree of denervation, also to assess function of the muscles to be transferred

Classification

- Scapular winging: (Kuhn, Plancher, and Hawkins)
  - Primary: neurologic (long thoracic nerve palsy with serratus anterior weakness, spinal accessory nerve palsy with trapezius weakness, dorsal scapular nerve palsy with rhomboid weakness), osseous (osteochondromas, fracture malunions), soft tissue (soft tissue contractures, muscular dystrophy, muscle avulsion or congenital agenesis, scapulothoracic bursitis)

  - Secondary: glenohumeral disorders (multidirectional instability and posterior instability)
  - Voluntary: seen in psychiatric patients or those looking for secondary gain

Treatment

- Serratus palsy

  - Nonoperative: all patients without penetrating trauma expect most cases resolve spontaneously w/in 1–2 years; ROM exercises to avoid glenohumeral stiffness, braces/orthotics to stabilize scapula to chest wall (controversial)
  - Operative: if no evidence of improvement over long term, then consider split pectoralis major transfer (dynamic transfer of sternal head of the pectoralis major to inferior angle of the scapula)
  - Scapulothoracic fusion is reserved in select cases as a salvage procedure in patients with previous failed pectoralis major transfers or in muscular dystrophies affecting multiple muscles (especially facioscapulohumeral "FSH" dystrophy)

- Trapezius palsy

  - Nonoperative: attempted for 1 year when nerve injury is initially missed and diagnosis delayed more than 6 months; physical therapy to strengthen remaining scapulothoracic muscles; shoulder orthotics but this will only help reduce the pain but does not result in return of function
  - Operative: with early detection nerve repair can be attempted, although majority are detected late; Eden-Lange procedure (lateral transfer of levator scapulae, rhomboid major, and rhomboid minor along scapula) with goal of scapula support/stabilization to shoulder girdle

Complications

- Pectoralis major transfer: seroma/infection, neurovascular injury, stiffness, scapular fracture through bone tunnel, graft loosening/loss of tension; breast asymmetry in female patients should be discussed preoperatively as possible complication
- Eden-Lange procedure: dysfunction due to failed integration of transferred muscles, pullout of transferred muscles (if immobilization is violated w/in 6 weeks period following surgery), injury to suprascapular nerve during dissection

Bibliography

1. Bigliani LU, Compito CA, Duralde XA, Wolfe IN. Transfer of the levator scapulae, rhomboid major, and rhomboid minor for paralysis of the trapezius. J Bone Joint Surg Am. 1996;78(10):1534–40. Epub 1996/10/01.
2. Borges CS, Ruschel PH, Ferreira MT. Pectoralis major to scapula transfer for patients with serratus anterior palsy. Tech Hand Up Extrem Surg. 2011;15(3):135–7. Epub 2011/08/27.

3. Elhassan B, Bishop A, Shin A. Trapezius transfer to restore external rotation in a patient with a brachial plexus injury. A case report. J Bone Joint Surg Am. 2009;91(4):939–44. Epub 2009/04/03.
4. Galano G, Bigliani LU, Ahmad CS, Levine WN. Surgical treatment of winged scapula. Clin Orthop. 2008;466(3):652–60.
5. Levy O, Relwani JG, Mullett H, Haddo O, Even T. The active elevation lag sign and the triangle sign: new clinical signs of trapezius palsy. J Shoulder Elbow Surg. 2009;18(4):573–6. Epub 2009/05/09.

Elbow

Jonathan Danoff, Danielle Rome, Stephanie Gancarczyk, and William Levine

1 Elbow Osteoarthritis

> **Take-Home Message**
> - Elbow osteoarthritis is characterized by osteophytes, capsular contracture, and preserved joint space/articular cartilage (early in disease).
> - Rettig classification for elbow osteoarthritis classifies arthritis development at ulnohumeral and radiocapitellar joints.
> - Surgical management: arthroscopic/open ulnohumeral arthroplasty, debridement, osteophyte removal, and capsular release.
> - Total elbow arthroplasty considered in patients >65 with low physical activity, avoided in young patients.

Definition

- Degenerative disease of the elbow joint characterized by osteophyte formation, capsular contracture, and loss of articular cartilage/joint space

Etiology

- Overuse: associated with manual laborers, weight lifters, throwing athletes; male > female, dominant elbow
- Rheumatoid arthritis: autoimmune, polyarticular systemic disease, causes synovitis and synovial tissue hyperplasia, soft tissue, and bone destruction, prevalence female > male, 35–50 years old on average

J. Danoff, MD • D. Rome • S. Gancarczyk, MD • W. Levine, MD (✉)
Department of Orthopedic Surgery, Center for Shoulder, Elbow and Sports Medicine, New York Presbyterian/Columbia University Medical Center, New York, NY, USA
e-mail: wnl1@columbia.edu; wnl1@cumc.columbia.edu

C. Mauffrey, D.J. Hak (eds.), *Passport for the Orthopedic Boards and FRCS Examination*, DOI 10.1007/978-2-8178-0475-0_32

- Post-traumatic arthritis: joint pain and dysfunction after an intra-articular fracture or dislocation about the elbow associated with malunion or nonunion; must rule out infectious etiology
- Osteochondritis dissecans (young patients)
- Synovial chondromatosis
- Valgus extension overload syndrome (overhead throwers)
- Trauma: untreated coronoid fractures, radial head injuries in children

Pathophysiology

- Articular degeneration with fragmentation of cartilaginous surfaces, loose body formation, capsular contracture, maintained joint space
  - Radiohumeral joint: high axial, shearing, and rotational stresses cause erosion of capitellum and hypertrophic callus formation on radial neck.
  - Ulnohumeral joint (advanced cases): central sparing of joint with noted fibrosis of anterior capsule and olecranon hypertrophy.
- Osteophytes on olecranon, coronoid process, and coronoid fossa
  - Posterior osteophytic impingement results in loss of elbow extension, flexion, and forearm rotation.
- Increased thickness of olecranon fossa bone and anterior/posterior fibrous tissue
- Rheumatoid arthritis: synovitis, elbow contracture, loss of end range of motion, laxity, ulnar or radial nerve compression, ligamentous laxity with instability with anterior displacement of radial head (at late stages)
- Post-traumatic arthritis: severe articular anatomy distortion with malunion/nonunion, possible infection, distortion of surrounding anatomy (if prior ulnar nerve transposition was performed at osteosynthesis), stiffness either at extremes or in mid-arc range of motion, associated ligamentous instability

Radiographs

- Radiographs including AP and lateral views to visualize osteophytes on olecranon fossa, coronoid and olecranon processes, loose bodies, radiocapitellar narrowing
  - Can consider a cubital tunnel view to assess for osteophytes/loose bodies causing ulnar nerve irritation
- CT can be considered for more accurate visualization of the location/size of osteophytes and loose bodies.
- MRI not typically obtained.
- EMG studies performed if concerned for neurologic symptoms, often ulnar neuritis from osteophyte impingement and elbow contractures.

Classification

- Rettig classification of osteoarthritis
  - Class I marginal osteophyte formation at ulnohumeral joint, normal radiocapitellar joint; class II, degenerative changes to ulnohumeral and

radiocapitellar joints with normal radiocapitellar joint alignment; class III: characteristics of class II disease with subluxation of radiocapitellar joint

- Mayo clinic classification of rheumatoid arthritis
  - Grade I, no joint space narrowing, periarticular osteopenia, mild-to-moderate synovitis; grade II, mild-to-moderate joint space narrowing with maintained articular architecture, synovitis unable to be controlled only with NSAIDs; grade III, variable amount of joint space narrowing, +/– cyst formation, loss of normal articular architecture, variable synovitis; grade IV, extensive joint space narrowing and articular architecture degeneration, subchondral bone loss and joint subluxation/ankylosis, minimal synovitis

Treatment

Nonoperative

- Mild pain, motion loss <15° can consider activity avoidance/modification.
- NSAIDS, corticosteroid injections, viscosupplementation.
- Occupational therapy helpful for pain relief, use gentle range-of-motion exercises.
- Moderate disease associated with end range-of-motion loss and contractures, requires static progressive splinting (if osteophytes limiting motion, then avoided because can worsen inflammation and pain).
- Rheumatoid arthritis typically treated with methotrexate, DMARDs, oral corticosteroids; these are highly successful and have helped avoid advanced stages of disease in many patients.

Operative

- Debridement, osteophyte excision, and anterior capsular release (+/– fenestration of olecranon fossa)
- Arthroscopic osteocapsular arthroplasty useful for patients <60 years with moderate/severe disease, maintained middle range of motion
- Open ulnohumeral arthroplasty use in advanced disease (Outerbridge-Kashiwagi, lateral column, or medial over-the-top approaches), may require ulnar nerve transposition if symptomatic and loss of range of motion <110°
- Rheumatoid arthritis: open/arthroscopic synovectomy (Mayo grade I/II/III with >90° arc of motion)
  - Radial head excision performed historically but often avoided as it serves as a main elbow stabilizer, can consider only if stable elbow and pro-supination maneuver elicits main symptoms
- Post-traumatic arthritis: usually young/active patient with moderate disease too severe for debridement, use interposition arthroplasty or hemiarthroplasty
  - Avoid total elbow arthroplasty given restrictions on activity and implant longevity.
- Total elbow arthroplasty: patients >65 years old with advanced disease and low physical demands with osteoarthritis or post-traumatic arthritis; in rheumatoid arthritis Mayo grade IV or arc of motion <90°

Complications

- Postoperative stiffness/infection
- Arthroscopic debridement: neurovascular injury especially if prior nerve transposition performed
- Total elbow arthroplasty: aseptic loosening, instability, triceps insufficiency, infection, instability (for more information see section "Elbow Arthroplasty")

Bibliography

1. Hattori Y, Doi K, Sakamoto S, Hoshino S, Dodakundi C. Capsulectomy and debridement for primary osteoarthritis of the elbow through a medial trans-flexor approach. J Hand Surg. 2011;36(10):1652–8. Epub 2011/08/30.
2. McLaughlin Ii RE, Savoie III FH, Field LD, Ramsey JR. Arthroscopic treatment of the arthritic elbow due to primary radiocapitellar arthritis. Arthroscopy. 2006;22(1):63–9.
3. Naqui SZ, Rajpura A, Nuttall D, Prasad P, Trail IA. Early results of the acclaim total elbow replacement in patients with primary osteoarthritis. J Bone Joint Surg. 2010;92(5):668–71. Epub 2010/05/04.
4. Rettig LA, Hastings Ii H, Feinberg JR. Primary osteoarthritis of the elbow: lack of radiographic evidence for morphologic predisposition, results of operative debridement at intermediate follow-up, and basis for a new radiographic classification system. J Shoulder Elbow Surg. 2008;17(1):97–105.
5. Wysocki RW, Cohen MS. Primary osteoarthritis and posttraumatic arthritis of the elbow. Hand Clin. 2011;27(2):131–7, v. Epub 2011/04/20.

2 Osteochondritis Dissecans of the Capitellum

Take-Home Message

- A localized osteochondral lesion with associated subchondral collapse, primarily affecting the dominant elbow of male throwing athletes and female gymnasts.
- Likely due to a combination of factors including repetitive trauma and subchondral ischemia.
- Should be distinguished from Panner's disease, which affects boys <10 years.
- Grading can be based on radiographs, MRI or arthroscopic findings. The most important factor to distinguish is whether the lesion is stable or unstable, as this can help to guide management.

Definition

- A localized osteochondral lesion that is characterized by an associated disruption of subchondral bone

Etiology

- The definitive etiology is unknown, though it has been thought to be due to repetitive trauma and ischemia.

Pathophysiology

- Dominant upper extremity of male throwing athletes and female gymnasts. Other associated sports include cheerleading, weight lifting, and tennis.
- Overuse or repetitive loading in these athletes can cause laxity in the medial elbow complex and predispose to compression at the radiocapitellar joint. In addition, the radiocapitellar joint experiences most of the axial compression forces at the elbow joint.
- In addition, it has been shown that the lateral capitellum has soft cartilage segments, which may be in part why this is the most reported location for OCD lesions in the elbow.
- In support of the vascular theory, repetitive compression to the capitellum may lead to subchondral ischemia and collapse, which in turn predisposes to cartilage fragmentation.
- The vascular supply to the capitellum is primarily by posterior end arteries.
- This should be distinguished from Panner's disease, an osteochondrosis of the entire capitellum seen in boys younger than 10 years old.

Radiographs

- AP and lateral views of the elbow with the opposite side obtained for comparison.
- Include an AP at 45° of flexion and oblique views of the elbow.
- Typical findings include an anterolateral lesion with cortical irregularity and a rim of sclerosis surrounding the lesion with or without loose bodies.
- CT and CT arthrography may be used to better delineate the bony anatomy of the lesion.
- MRI is used to assess the articular cartilage and to assess early OCD lesions.
- Contrast-enhanced MRI may be used to better assess the stability of a lesion, as an intervening fluid signal may be present. It is important to remember this will not always be present in unstable lesions.

Classification

- Based on AP radiographs, Minami et al.: grade 1, a visible translucent shadow; grade II, a split line or clear zone between the lesion and nearby subchondral bone; grade III, association with loose bodies.
- Based on MRI, Nelson et al.: grade 0, normal; grade 1, intact cartilage with signal changes; grade II, high signal breach of cartilage; grade III, thin rim of signal surrounding the fragment; grade IV, mixed or low signal loose body present.
- Based on arthroscopy, International Cartilage Repair Society: grade 1, stable lesions with a softened area covered by intact cartilage; grade II, partial discontinuity, but stable on probing; grade III, complete discontinuity, but remain located; grade IV, an empty defect with a dislocated fragment.

- The most important factor to distinguish is whether the lesion is stable or unstable, as this can help to guide management.

Treatment

Nonoperative

- Typically selected for patients with early, stable lesions.
- Primarily involves activity modification and duration is dictated by presence of symptoms.
- A follow-up MRI is usually obtained at 3–6 months.
- Rest is usually 3–6 weeks with gradual return to sports by 3–6 months.
- NSAIDs and braces have been proposed as beneficial, though there is no good clinical evidence to support these modalities of treatment.

Operative

- Indications include presence of loose bodies, mechanical symptoms, unstable lesions, and stable lesions that have failed 6 months of nonoperative management.
- Options include arthroscopic versus formal arthrotomy for removal of loose bodies, debridement, fragment excision, abrasion arthroplasty, microfracture, drilling, fragment fixation, bone grafting, and osteochondral autograft transplantation.
- Procedure selection is based on lesion characteristics.
- For acute lesions fixation can be considered, but the chance of a successful outcome is less predictable.
- For smaller lesions that no do not engage the radial head, microfracture or drilling can be considered.
- For large lesions that engage the radial head, osteochondral allograft or autograft should be considered. In particular, if a defect involves greater than 6–7 mm of the lateral column, grafting is the treatment of choice, as rebuilding the lateral column will prevent the radial head from engaging into the defect.
- Of note, if >30 % of the radial head is also involved, microfracture or drilling is the treatment of choice.
- Outcomes have been promising for both marrow stimulation and grafting groups, when patients are selected appropriately.
- Prognosis is best for patients with open growth plates, intact elbow range of motion, and localized disease. In addition, early-stage or stable and acute lesions have a better prognosis.
- Despite these treatments, approximately half of patients will develop radiocapitellar arthritis later in life.

Complications

- Persistent symptoms and poor functional outcome especially if chronic and lesion grade is underestimated and treated nonoperatively
- Loss of elbow range of motion
- Degenerative joint disease

Bibliography

1. Ahmad CS, ElAttrache NS. Treatment of elbow capitellar osteochondritis dissecans. Tech Shoulder Elbow Shoulder. 2006;7:169–74.
2. Ahmad CS, Vitale MA, ElAttrache NS. Elbow arthroscopy: capitellar osteochondritis dissecans and radiocapitellar plica. Instr Course Lect. 2011;60:181–90. Epub 2011/05/11.
3. Ruchelsman DE, Hall MP, Youm T. Osteochondritis dissecans of the capitellum: current concepts. J Am Acad Orthop Surg. 2010;18(9):557–67. Epub 2010/09/03.
4. Takahara M, Mura N, Sasaki J, Harada M, Ogino T. Classification, treatment, and outcome of osteochondritis dissecans of the humeral capitellum. J Bone Joint Surg Am. 2007;89(6):1205–14. Epub 2007/06/05.
5. Yadao MA, Field LD, Savoie 3rd FH. Osteochondritis dissecans of the elbow. Instr Course Lect. 2004;53:599–606. Epub 2004/05/01

3 Elbow Instability

Take-Home Message

- Elbow instability can be described as acute, recurrent, or chronic.
- Posterolateral rotatory instability is the most common type. Must recognize additional coronoid and/or radial head fractures.
- After closed reduction, nonoperative management should not be considered for patients with residual joint incongruity that can be seen after attempts have been made to hold reduction in a splint/cast.
- Operative correction follows a specific algorithm that includes assessing the lateral ligament complex and medial ligament complex.
- A hinged external fixator should be used for patients that still have instability after osseous fixation and ligamentous reconstruction.

Definition

- Failure of the static and dynamic constraints of the elbow that leads to joint incongruity and laxity.

Etiology

- Acute: posterolateral rotatory, valgus, varus-posteromedial rotatory
  - Posterolateral rotatory is the most common and can present as dislocation, fracture-dislocation, or fracture-subluxation.
  - Typically simple dislocations occur from falls onto an outstretched hand.
  - Fracture-dislocations tend to occur from a higher energy fall such as from a handlebar or bicycle or from a motor vehicle accident.

  - The mechanism of posterolateral dislocation is a fall onto an extended arm (in order to place the hand on the ground). On contact, the elbow flexes, resulting in an eccentric force on the medial head of the triceps primarily that causes an external rotation moment at the ulnohumeral joint.
  - The mechanism results in progressive soft tissue disruption. It starts laterally and progresses around anteriorly and posteriorly to end medially ("Horii circle").
  - If the coronoid and the radial head fail to rotate sufficiently away from the trochlea and the capitellum, they may fracture. This results in the "terrible triad."
  - Varus-posteromedial rotatory instability may present as an isolated coronoid fracture without a radial head fracture. This is because the mechanism is usually varus stress onto an axially loaded, flexed elbow, which causes LCL disruption and an anteromedial coronoid fracture.

- Recurrent:
  - May occur from inadequate treatment of an acute injury, connective tissue disorders, or iatrogenic injury during treatment for a different condition (such as debridement or release for lateral epicondylitis).
  - The most common type is recurrent posterolateral subluxation.

- Chronic

Pathophysiology

- The primary constraints of the elbow include the ulnohumeral articulation, the medial collateral ligament, and the lateral collateral ligament (especially the ulnar lateral collateral ligament).
- The secondary stabilizers include the radial head, common flexor and extensor origins, and the capsule.
- Muscles that cross the elbow and provide a compression force act as dynamic stabilizers.
- When these constraints fail under an excessive stress or load, elbow instability results.

Radiographs

- AP and lateral elbow radiographs should be obtained after reduction. If joint incongruity is noted, patients should be splinted or casted in a reduced position. Typically reduction can be achieved with flexion and pronation.
- CT scan can be obtained to better illustrate bony anatomy, assess size of fracture fragments, and define complexity of fracture patterns.

Classification

- Acute, recurrent, and chronic

Treatment

- In simple dislocations, an acute closed reduction is performed, typically with supination, traction, and then flexion. The patient is then splinted for approximately 1 week with the goal being early range of motion.
  - Frequent plain film imaging is obtained to assess for subluxation and joint congruity, as the presence of these abnormalities would warrant a change in treatment plan.
- When nonoperative management fails and there is persistent instability operative treatment is required. For posterolateral instability, the typical algorithm for operative treatment includes fracture fixation and lateral ligament complex reconstruction. If instability remains, the medial ligament complex should be evaluated and reconstructed. If the elbow remains unstable, a hinged external fixator should be placed.
  - Coronoid fractures require fixation, because the coronoid is an important anterior force-bearing surface of the elbow and important in stability. For small fragments, suture fixation is typically appropriate. For larger fragments, rigid fixation is needed.
  - Fractures of the radial head should try to be managed with open reduction and internal fixation. If the fragment has 3 or more parts, radial head replacement should be performed.

Complications

- Premature osteoarthritis due to joint incongruity
- Stiffness
- Persistent instability

Bibliography

1. Doornberg JN, Parisien R, Van Duijn PJ, Ring D. Radial head arthroplasty with a modular metal spacer to treat acute traumatic elbow instability. J Bone Joint Surg A. 2007;89(5):1075–80.
2. Giannicola G, Polimanti D, Sacchetti FM, Scacchi M, Bullitta G, Manauzzi E, et al. Soft tissue constraint injuries in complex elbow instability: surgical techniques and clinical outcomes. Orthopedics. 2012;35(12):e1746–53.
3. Lin KY, Shen PH, Lee CH, Pan RY, Lin LC, Shen HC. Functional outcomes of surgical reconstruction for posterolateral rotatory instability of the elbow. Injury. 2012;43(10):1657–61.
4. O'Driscoll SW. Stress radiographs are important in diagnosing valgus instability of the elbow. J Bone Joint Surg Am. 2002;84-A(4):686; author reply –7. Epub 2002/04/10.
5. Yu JR, Throckmorton TW, Bauer RM, Watson JT, Weikert DR. Management of acute complex instability of the elbow with hinged external fixation. J Shoulder Elbow Surg. 2007;16(1):60–7.

4 Lateral and Medial Epicondylitis

Take-Home Message

- Tendon degeneration following microtrauma at ECRB origin (lateral epicondyle)/flexor-pronator origin (medial epicondyle).
- Nonoperative management highly successful in majority of cases.
- Operative treatment includes open/arthroscopic excision of degenerative tendon with or without reattachment to epicondyle.

Definition

- Tendinosis at the musculotendinous origins of the lateral or medial epicondyle secondary to overuse injury

Etiology

- Lateral epicondylitis: forceful/repetitive forearm pronation-supination especially with elbow extension causes microtears in and weakens the extensor carpi radialis brevis (ECRB) tendon origin; exacerbated by resisted wrist extension and forearm supination
  - Associated with racket sports due to poor stroke mechanics (leading with flexed elbow, off-center striking of ball), increased loads in lateral muscle-tendon unit (improper racket weight, stringing, or grip size), increased force to extensor mass (increased ball momentum on hard courts)
- Medial epicondylitis: repetitive stress on flexor-pronator musculature (flexor carpi radialis and pronator teres) origin due to repetitive valgus forces at elbow (late-cocking/acceleration phase in throwing, follow-through phase in golf, top-spin in tennis); exacerbated by forced pronation and wrist flexion

Pathophysiology

- Stress/microtears at ECRB/flexor-pronator origin lead to tendon degeneration and inferior tissue ingrowth ("angiofibroblastic tendinosis").
  - Eventually the fraying/fibrillation cause macrotears and eventual rupture/avulsion.

Radiographs (Limited Use)

- AP view (full extension)/lateral view (90° flexion), can see calcification of epicondyle and rule out alternative pathologies.
- MRI shows tendon thickening/increased signal, high T2 signal in cystic areas in lateral epicondylitis (ECRB avulsions/mucoid degeneration).
- EMG can be useful to rule out posterior interosseous nerve compression.

Classification

- Epicondylar tendinosis (Nirschl)
  - Stage 1 = general inflammation, 2 = pathologic tissue alteration or angiofibroblastic degeneration, 3 = structural failure, 4 = stage 2 or 3 w/ fibrosis/calcification
- Arthroscopic classification of lateral epicondylitis (Baker et al.)
  - I = fraying of undersurface of ECRB w/o tearing, II = linear tearing (undersurface of ECRB/lateral capsule), III = partial/complete avulsions of ECRB origin

Treatment

Nonoperative

- Nonoperative management is successful in 95 % cases.
- Ice, NSAIDS, corticosteroid injections (danger of tendon rupture).
- Physical therapy with active and passive ROM exercises, wrist extensor, and rotator cuff strengthening (eccentric strengthening).
- Activity modification including correction of poor technique, improper equipment, use of counterforce bracing

Operative

- Attempt operative treatment after failure at least 3–6 months of nonoperative treatment
- Lateral epicondylitis: open, percutaneous, or arthroscopic release of ECRB
- Medial epicondylitis: open debridement of pathologic portions of flexor-pronator origin, reattachment at epicondyle

Complications

- Persistent pain/strength deficit
- Joint instability (risk of injury to lateral ulnar collateral ligament with arthroscopic debridement of ECRB)
- Hematoma, infection, nerve palsy or direct injury

Bibliography

1. Baker Jr CL, Murphy KP, Gottlob CA, Curd DT. Arthroscopic classification and treatment of lateral epicondylitis: two-year clinical results. J Shoulder Elbow Surg. 2000;9(6):475–82. Epub 2001/01/13.
2. Connell D, Datir A, Alyas F, Curtis M. Treatment of lateral epicondylitis using skin-derived tenocyte-like cells. Br J Sports Med. 2009;43(4):293–8. Epub 2009/02/20.
3. De Zordo T, Lill SR, Fink C, Feuchtner GM, Jaschke W, Bellmann-Weiler R, et al. Real-time sonoelastography of lateral epicondylitis: comparison of findings between patients and healthy volunteers. AJR Am J Roentgenol. 2009;193(1):180–5. Epub 2009/06/23.

4. Dunn JH, Kim JJ, Davis L, Nirschl RP. Ten- to 14-year follow-up of the Nirschl surgical technique for lateral epicondylitis. Am J Sports Med. 2008;36(2):261–6. Epub 2007/12/07.
5. Nirschl RP, Pettrone FA. Tennis elbow. The surgical treatment of lateral epicondylitis. J Bone Joint Surg Am. 1979;61(6A):832–9. Epub 1979/09/01.
6. Peerbooms JC, Sluimer J, Bruijn DJ, Gosens T. Positive effect of an autologous platelet concentrate in lateral epicondylitis in a double-blind randomized controlled trial: platelet-rich plasma versus corticosteroid injection with a 1-year follow-up. Am J Sports Med. 2010;38(2):255–62. Epub 2010/05/08.
7. Solheim E, Hegna J, Oyen J. Arthroscopic versus open tennis elbow release: 3- to 6-year results of a case–control series of 305 elbows. Arthroscopy. 2013;29(5):854–9. Epub 2013/02/08.
8. Thanasas C, Papadimitriou G, Charalambidis C, Paraskevopoulos I, Papanikolaou A. Platelet-rich plasma versus autologous whole blood for the treatment of chronic lateral elbow epicondylitis: a randomized controlled clinical trial. Am J Sports Med. 2011;39(10):2130–4. Epub 2011/08/05.

5 Distal Biceps Rupture

Take-Home Message

- Occurs when the biceps eccentrically contracts.
- Predisposed if tendon degeneration, poor vascularity, tendon impingement.
- Early surgical repair is key to regaining forearm supination and elbow flexion.
- Risk of neurapraxia, permanent nerve injury, and heterotopic ossification.

Definition

- Complete tear of the distal biceps tendon resulting in weakness of supination and elbow flexion

Etiology

- Eccentric contraction of biceps often when attempting to catch a falling load.
- Predominant in males, fourth to sixth decades, dominant extremity.
- 7.5× increased risk if smoker.
- Hypovascular zone in biceps tendon proximal to insertion point.
- During pronation can have tendon impingement on hypertrophic bone from the anterior margin of the radial tuberosity can contribute to failure.
- Prior injury or tendon degeneration can predispose to rupture.

Pathophysiology

- Disrupted distal biceps tendon lacks continuity and is retracted although lacertus fibrosis can be intact.

- Retraction of radial tuberosity can also have musculotendinous junction rupture or within tendon substance.
- If lacertus fibrosis intact, then tendon will not retract.
- Can have thickened, bulbous distal end of the tendon at rupture site with evidence of degeneration microscopically.

Radiographs

- XR elbow to evaluate for radial tuberosity bone avulsion or additional elbow fracture
- MRI not necessary but can be helpful to diagnose partial biceps tendon tears (differentiate from tendinosis and cubital bursitis), tears at the myotendinous junction, and measure retraction in chronic tears
- Ultrasound useful to visualize and confirm diagnosis

Classification

- Partial tear: incomplete tear of biceps tendon, can be due to preexisting pathologic degeneration within tendon
- Complete tear: tendon detachment from radial tuberosity
  - Acute (<4 weeks) versus chronic (>4 weeks)

Treatment

- Nonoperative management considered for low-demand patient or elderly with significant risks to surgery will have painless function but weakness notable to supination.
- Early surgical repair indicated for the majority of patients.
- Two-incision muscle-splitting technique (split ECU muscle and avoiding supinator dissection helps minimize synostosis formation) versus single anterior incision (interval between brachioradialis and pronator teres).
- Tendon fixation method: bone tunnel, suture anchor, intraosseous screw fixation, suspensory cortical button.
- Partial rupture: nonoperative treatment (NSAIDs, physical therapy); if unsuccessful and >50 % tendon torn, then prophylactic tendon release and repair as described for acute ruptures.
- Chronic rupture: requires extensile approach; if significant tendon retraction, then will require interposition grafting with autogenous tissue graft (semitendinosus tendon) or allograft (Achilles tendon).

Complications

- Single-incision technique has risk of radial nerve palsy (posterior interosseous "PIN") secondary to aggressive retraction, lateral antebrachial cutaneous nerve paresthesia common.
- Two-incision technique has risk of proximal radioulnar synostosis with loss of supination, also risk injury to PIN.
- Radial neck fracture if bone tunnel placed too proximal.
- Infection.
- Tendon re-rupture (highest risk in immediate postoperative period).

Bibliography

1. Idler CS, Montgomery 3rd WH, Lindsey DP, Badua PA, Wynne GF, Yerby SA. Distal biceps tendon repair: a biomechanical comparison of intact tendon and 2 repair techniques. Am J Sports Med. 2006;34(6):968–74. Epub 2006/02/16.
2. Jobin CM, Kippe MA, Gardner TR, Levine WN, Ahmad CS. Distal biceps tendon repair: a cadaveric analysis of suture anchor and interference screw restoration of the anatomic footprint. Am J Sports Med. 2009;37(11):2214–21. Epub 2009/07/23.
3. John CK, Field LD, Weiss KS, Savoie 3rd FH. Single-incision repair of acute distal biceps ruptures by use of suture anchors. J Shoulder Elbow Surg. 2007;16(1):78–83. Epub 2006/09/12.
4. Khan AD, Penna S, Yin Q, Sinopidis C, Brownson P, Frostick SP. Repair of distal biceps tendon ruptures using suture anchors through a single anterior incision. Arthroscopy. 2008;24(1):39–45. Epub 2008/01/10.
5. Sethi PM, Tibone JE. Distal biceps repair using cortical button fixation. Sports Med Arthroscopy Rev. 2008;16(3):130–5. Epub 2008/08/16.
6. Spang JT, Weinhold PS, Karas SG. A biomechanical comparison of EndoButton versus suture anchor repair of distal biceps tendon injuries. J Shoulder Elbow Surg. 2006;15(4):509–14. Epub 2006/07/13.
7. Wysocki RW, Cohen MS. Radioulnar heterotopic ossification after distal biceps tendon repair: results following surgical resection. J Hand Surg. 2007;32(8):1230–6. Epub 2007/10/10.

6 Elbow Arthroscopy

Take-Home Message

- A detailed knowledge of the surrounding anatomy is necessary to prevent iatrogenic injury to surrounding neurovascular structures.
- Remember to note the presence of a subluxing or previously transposed ulnar nerve.
- Useful for loose body removal, osteochondritis dissecans of the capitellum, extensor carpi radialis brevis debridement/release for lateral epicondylitis, radiocapitellar plica, debridement of osteoarthritis/synovitis, capsular release.

Introduction

- Due to technological advancements numerous conditions that once required open procedures may now be treated with a minimally invasive technique using elbow arthroscopy. However, given the many neurovascular structures in near proximity and the complex anatomy of the elbow, special attention should be paid to technique.

Anatomic Divisions

- Based on bony anatomy: anterior, posterior, and posterolateral
  - Anterior: coronoid, anterior trochlea, radial head, capitellum, medial and lateral condyles
  - Posterior: olecranon tip, olecranon fossa, posterior trochlea, medial and lateral gutters
  - Posterolateral: radial head, olecranon, capitellum, lateral gutter

Patient Positioning and Setup

Three options exist for patient positioning – supine, prone, or lateral decubitus.

- Supine – The designated arm is flexed to 90° and hung with traction equipment. This position allows easy access to the airway, orients anatomy in a standard manner, and allows easy conversion to an open procedure, if needed. However, it may be difficult to gain entry into the posterior compartment.
- Prone – The elbow is flexed 90° and held in a stationary arm support. While this allows easy access to the posterior compartment, it reverses the anatomic orientation and makes airway management more difficult.
- Lateral decubitus – The patient lies on the unaffected side and the designated arm is placed in a stationary arm holder. The operative arm is positioned with the shoulder forward flexed to 90° and internally rotated to 90°. This position allows easy access to all compartments and compromises airway management less than the prone position. It is important to limit the anterior support structures to avoid interference with arthroscopic tools. In addition, an axillary roll must be placed to protect neurovascular structures.

Portals

- IMPORTANT – The presence of a subluxing or previously transposed ulnar nerve should be noted, as it may require a small open medial exposure. Typically, a submuscular transposition is an absolute contraindication for the medial portal.
- Proximal anteromedial portal – 2 cm above the medial epicondyle and 1 cm anterior to intermuscular septum. At-risk structures include the medial antebrachial cutaneous nerve and the ulnar nerve.
- Proximal anterolateral portal – 2 cm proximal to the lateral epicondyle and directly anterior to the surface of the humerus. At-risk structures include the posterior antebrachial cutaneous nerve and the radial nerve proper, which can be moved further out of the field with elbow flexion.
- Anterolateral portal – 3 cm distal and 2 cm anterior to the lateral epicondyle. Risk to neurovascular structures is significant but decreases with a more proximally placed portal.
- Posterolateral portal – Anywhere from the tip of the olecranon to 3 cm proximal in the posterolateral gutter.
- Direct posterior portal – Splits the triceps 3 cm proximal to the olecranon tip. Neurovascular structures at risks include the medial and posterior antebrachial cutaneous nerves and ulnar nerve.

- Soft spot portal – Located at the center of the triangle made by the radial head, lateral epicondyle and olecranon tip. The neurovascular structure most at risk is the posterior antebrachial cutaneous nerve. This portal is most useful for access to the radiocapitellar joint.

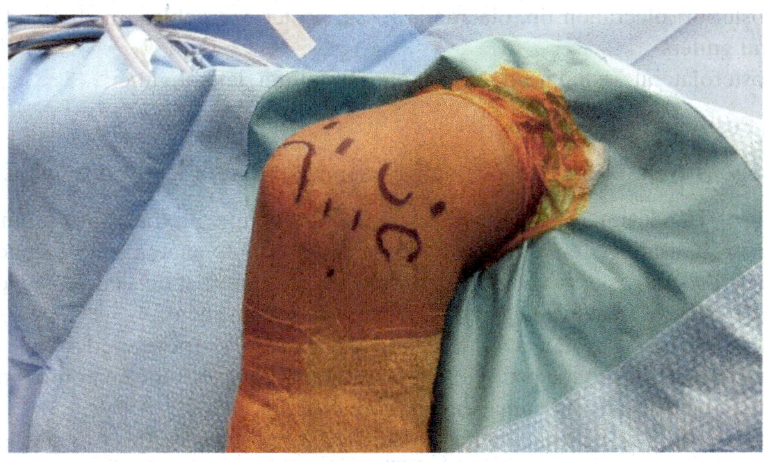

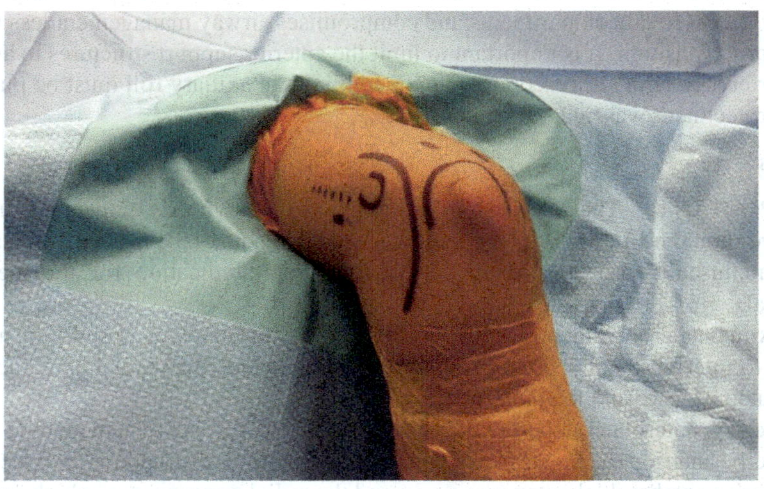

Technique Pearls

- Important landmarks should all be drawn out prior to the start of the procedure to aid with positioning and keep the performing surgeon aware of the ulnar nerve. The landmarks include the following: medial and lateral epicondyles, radial head, and olecranon.

- Typically the standard 4.0 mm 30° arthroscope is used, but a smaller 2.7 mm arthroscope may be necessary when working on young or smaller patients or in the radiocapitellar joint.
- Side-vented inflow cannulas may cause fluid extravasation and should be avoided. An elastic bandage is wrapped around the forearm to further reduce the effect of fluid extravasation.
- The joint is distended with approximately 15–25 cc of sterile saline to increase the bone/articular surface to neurovascular structure distance. Of note, this does not significantly change the capsule to neurovascular structure distance.

Applied Technique

- Loose body removal
- Osteochondritis dissecans – capitellum
- ECRB debridement/release for lateral epicondylitis
- Radiocapitellar plica
- Arthritis/synovitis
- Capsular release

Complications

- Iatrogenic nerve injury or chondral injury
- Collateral ligament injury

Bibliography

1. Ahmad CS, Vitale MA. Elbow arthroscopy: setup, portal placement, and simple procedures. Instr Course Lect. 2011;60:171–80. Epub 2011/05/11.
2. Dodson CC, Nho SJ, Williams 3rd RJ, Altchek DW. Elbow arthroscopy. J Am Acad Orthop Surg. 2008;16(10):574–85. Epub 2008/10/04.

7 Elbow Arthroplasty

Take-Home Message
- Indications: advanced arthritis/articular incongruity secondary to intra-articular distal humerus fractures with contracture, elderly/inactive patients
- Contraindications: prior or current infection, paralysis of upper extremity, inadequate soft tissue sleeve, noncompliance w/ postoperative restrictions
- Bryan-Morrey approach and linked, semi-constrained implants preferred

Definition

- Surgical reconstruction of the elbow joint replacing the ulnohumeral articulation of the elbow joint with a prosthesis

Indications

- Arthritic pain/instability
  - Osteoarthritis: patients >65 years w/ painful arc of motion and low physical demands
  - Rheumatoid arthritis: advanced cases (grade III/IV): severe articular cartilage destruction
  - Post-traumatic arthritis: patients >65 years with low physical demands and significant articular incongruity/instability after an attempted osteosynthesis of an intra-articular fracture/dislocation
- Acute trauma
  - Highly comminuted (or unable to obtain stable fixation) distal humerus fracture in an elderly (>65 years old)/low-demand patient, large, post-traumatic bone defects
- Reconstruction after tumor resection

Contraindications

- Absolute: active infection, upper extremity paralysis, lack of soft tissue sleeve for coverage, poor patient compliance with postoperative activity limitations
- Relative: remote history of elbow infection, neurologic injury involving elbow flexors

Radiographs

- AP and lateral elbow radiographs obtained to assess the degree of joint destruction
- Preoperative planning to measure humeral bow and medullary canal diameter, and ulnar medullary canal diameter/angulation; if prior total shoulder arthroplasty, must assess for canal length and consider using short-stem humeral component
- Cervical spine radiographs (+/− MRI) obtained preoperatively in a patient with rheumatoid arthritis to rule out coexistent cervical spine pathology
- CT scan obtained if acute/post trauma to assess degree of articular or metaphyseal comminution and bone defects

Surgical Considerations

- Total elbow arthroplasty: prosthetic replacement of the distal humerus and proximal ulna articulations; can use linked (semi-constrained) versus unlinked (resurfacing)
- Hemiarthroplasty: distal humerus replaced while preserving ulna/radial head articulations; can be considered in acute trauma setting with intact/repairable collateral ligaments
- Interposition arthroplasty: ulnohumeral joint recontouring, release elbow contractures, collateral ligament reconstruction, hinged external fixator applied at end of procedure; considered in post-traumatic arthritis and when the patient is too young or highly active and poor candidate for restrictions required in total elbow arthroplasty

Postoperative Care/Restrictions

- Elbow splinted for 24–36 h in full extension followed by open-chain active-assisted range-of-motion exercises
- Hemovac used to evacuate hematoma
- Restrictions: no pushing or overhead activities ×3 months; no repetitive lifting >5 lb (or single event >10 lbs) weight restriction for lifetime

Complications

- Infection, aseptic loosening, short/long term mechanical failure, triceps weakness/avulsion, ulnar nerve injury, periprosthetic fracture, deep venous thrombosis, stiffness/impingement, instability (problematic in unlinked prosthesis)

Bibliography

1. Celli A, Morrey BF. Total elbow arthroplasty in patients forty years of age or less. J Bone Joint Surg Am. 2009;91(6):1414–8. Epub 2009/06/03.
2. Day JS, Lau E, Ong KL, Williams GR, Ramsey ML, Kurtz SM. Prevalence and projections of total shoulder and elbow arthroplasty in the United States to 2015. J Shoulder Elbow Surg. 2010;19(8):1115–20. Epub 2010/06/18.
3. Jenkins PJ, Watts AC, Norwood T, Duckworth AD, Rymaszewski LA, McEachan JE. Total elbow replacement: outcome of 1,146 arthroplasties from the Scottish Arthroplasty Project. Acta Orthop. 2013;84(2):119–23. Epub 2013/03/15.
4. Kodde IF, Van Riet RP, Eygendaal D. Semiconstrained total elbow arthroplasty for posttraumatic arthritis or deformities of the elbow: a prospective study. J Hand Surg. 2013;38(7):1377–82.
5. McKee MD, Veillette CJH, Hall JA, Schemitsch EH, Wild LM, McCormack R, et al. A multicenter, prospective, randomized, controlled trial of open reduction-internal fixation versus total elbow arthroplasty for displaced intra-articular distal humeral fractures in elderly patients. J Shoulder Elbow Surg. 2009;18(1):3–12.
6. Prasad N, Dent C. Outcome of total elbow replacement for distal humeral fractures in the elderly: a comparison of primary surgery and surgery after failed internal fixation or conservative treatment. J Bone Joint Surg B. 2008;90(3):343–8.
7. Sperling JW, Cofield RH, Schleck CD, Harmsen WS. Total shoulder arthroplasty versus hemiarthroplasty for rheumatoid arthritis of the shoulder: results of 303 consecutive cases. J Shoulder Elbow Surg. 2007;16(6):683–90.

8 Athletic Injuries of the Elbow: MCL Tears

Take-Home Message

- Athletic injuries to the elbow can be classified as medial tension injuries, lateral compression injuries, extension overload injuries, and/or tendinopathies
- The MCL is composed of three bundles – the anterior, posterior, and oblique bundles. The anterior bundle is the primary stabilizer to valgus stress.
- MCL reconstruction with a tendon graft is the primary mode of surgical correction.

Definition

- The elbow withstands high forces, especially in athletes that participate in activities that cause repetitive microtrauma, such as baseball players, tennis players, gymnasts, etc. Typically, the injuries fall within medial tension injuries, lateral compression injuries, extension overload injuries, and/or tedonopathies.

Etiology

- The causes are widespread and diverse. The etiologies can be divided based on localization of pain.
  - Medial – medial collateral ligament (MCL) injury, medial epicondylitis
  - Lateral – osteochondritis dissecans, lateral epicondylitis, radial nerve entrapment, ulnar neuropathy
  - Anterior – pronator teres syndrome, distal biceps rupture
  - Posterior – posteromedial impingement, olecranon stress fracture
- The MCL is composed of an anterior, posterior, and oblique bundle. It originates at the anteroinferior aspect of the medial humeral epicondyle and inserts onto the sublime tubercle of the ulna.
- The anterior bundle is the most important static stabilizer for valgus stability at 20–120° of flexion. Outside this range of motion, the primary stabilizer is the osseous constraint of the olecranon and the trochlea.
- Most common is a chronic injury due to repetitive medial tension stress that causes microtrauma to the MCL ligament and eventual incompetence.
- Acute rupture or acute-on-chronic injury is also possible. Common injury in throwing athletes who present with decreased throwing velocity.
  - There are six phases to the overhead throw, which are as follows: windup, early cocking, late cocking, acceleration, deceleration and follow-through. Maximum valgus torque occurs during late cocking.

Pathophysiology

- Medial elbow instability to valgus load.
- Usually presents with episodic medial elbow pain, and patients may develop ulnar neuritis over time.

Radiographs

- Elbow radiographs (AP, oblique, and lateral) with or without stress views are standard. An oblique axial view with the elbow in 110° of flexion is used to better visualize posterior medial olecranon osteophytes. Findings may include calcifications within the substance of the MCL and spurs at the location of origin or insertion, posterior osteophytes, and/or loose bodies.
- MRI is the study of choice and useful in evaluating the extent of ligament injury and also for evaluating chondral injury.

Classification

- Acute, acute on chronic, and chronic

Treatment Complications

Nonoperative

- NSAIDs
- Activity modification
- Rehabilitation – The focus should be on strengthening of the flexor-pronator mass and shoulder musculature. A formal throwing program usually is not initiated until at least 3 months after injury.

Operative

- MCL repair should be considered only for those with acute traumatic avulsion.
- MCL reconstruction with a tendon graft is the primary mode of surgical correction. It is useful for those who have failed nonoperative management and may be used in partial or complete tears.
- Various techniques have been described including figure-of-8 reconstruction (such as the Jobe technique), triangular graft reconstruction (such as the Docking technique), interference screw fixation, and suture anchor fixation.
- Access to the ulnar insertion site at the sublime tubercle can be via a flexor-pronator mass takedown or a flexor carpi ulnaris splitting technique. The latter is preferred because it decreases injury to the flexor muscles, which act as secondary stabilizers of the elbow.
- Ulnar nerve transposition should be considered with a subluxing nerve or for those that present with symptoms of ulnar neuropathy.
- Patients are usually placed in a postoperative splint, then transitioned to a hinged elbow brace in 1 week. Full range of motion is usually restored over the course of 5–6 weeks.

Complications

- Ulnar neuropathy
- Medial antebrachial cutaneous nerve injury

Bibliography

1. Cain Jr EL, Andrews JR, Dugas JR, Wilk KE, McMichael CS, Walter 2nd JC, et al. Outcome of ulnar collateral ligament reconstruction of the elbow in 1281 athletes: results in 743 athletes with minimum 2-year follow-up. Am J Sports Med. 2010;38(12):2426–34. Epub 2010/10/12.
2. Jones KJ, Osbahr DC, Schrumpf MA, Dines JS, Altchek DW. Ulnar collateral ligament reconstruction in throwing athletes: a review of current concepts. AAOS exhibit selection. J Bone Joint Surg Am. 2012;94(8):e49. Epub 2012/04/21.
3. Savoie FH, Morgan C, Yaste J, Hurt J, Field L. Medial ulnar collateral ligament reconstruction using hamstring allograft in overhead throwing athletes. J Bone Joint Surg Am. 2013;95(12):1062–6. Epub 2013/06/21.

9 Elbow Neuropathies

Take-Home Message

- At risk for injury at the level of the elbow include the radial nerve, PIN, median nerve, anterior interosseous nerve, and ulnar nerve
- Most common compressive neuropathy of the upper extremity is cubital tunnel syndrome (compression of the ulnar nerve)
- Nonoperative management is successful in majority of the cases and usually requires 3–6 months for resolution of symptoms
- Space-occupying lesions require operative excision

Definition

- Cubital tunnel syndrome: compressive neuropathy of the ulnar nerve at the cubital tunnel
- PIN compression syndrome: compressive neuropathy of the posterior interosseous nerve (PIN) at the radial tunnel presenting with an isolated motor palsy
- Radial tunnel syndrome: compressive neuropathy of the PIN within the radial tunnel presenting with pain only and no weakness
- Pronator syndrome: compressive neuropathy of the median nerve associated with pain and paresthesias
- Anterior interosseous nerve syndrome: compressive neuropathy of the anterior interosseous nerve (AIN) associated with motor weakness or paralysis

Etiology

- Nerve ischemia secondary to altered blood circulation from tissue pressure increases.
- Can be secondary to external compression on the nerve from direct trauma, soft tissue swelling/inflammation, elbow flexion, osteofibrous tunnels, muscular hypertrophy, tumors (ganglia, lipomas), osteophytes, aneurysms, rheumatoid pannus.
- Repetitive stress on the nerve via compression, contusion, or traction.
- Anconeus epitrochlearis in cubital tunnel syndrome is a rare anatomic anomaly in athletes.

Pathophysiology

- Demyelination, axonal loss, and intraneural fibrosis can be seen in chronic compression injury.
- Cubital tunnel syndrome: sites of compression include (1) arcade of Struthers, (2) medial intermuscular septum, (3) medial epicondyle, (4) cubital tunnel covered by Osborne's ligament, and (5) flexor-pronator aponeurosis.
- Radial tunnel syndrome/PIN compression syndrome: sites of compression include (1) fibrous bands connecting the brachioradialis and brachialis at the level of the radiocapitellar joint, (2) leash of Henry, (3) proximal edge of ECRB, (4) arcade of Fröhse, and (5) distal edge supinator.

  - PIN compression syndrome: weakness of wrist and finger extensors.
  - Radial tunnel syndrome: pain only disturbance 3–4 cm distal to lateral epicondyle in area of mobile wad and radial tunnel; must differentiate from lateral epicondylitis.

- Pronator syndrome: sites of compression include (1) lacertus fibrosus, (2) between two heads of the pronator teres, (3) proximal fibrous arch of the flexor digitorum superficialis, and (4) ligament of Struthers (if present in 1–2 % population).

  - Aching pain and paresthesias result

- Anterior interosseous nerve (AIN) syndrome: sites of compression include (1) deep head of pronator teres, (2) flexor digitorum superficialis, and (3) presence of Gantzer's muscle.

  - Weakness of paralysis of flexor pollicis longus, flexor digitorum profundus to the index and middle fingers, and pronator quadrates; no sensory loss but can have pain along nerve course.

Radiographs

- Elbow radiographs (AP and lateral) can be used to rule out alternative pathology.
- MRI may be helpful to look for soft tissue masses that can cause compression.
- Electrodiagnostic testing most commonly used to confirm diagnosis.

Classification

- Seddon: describes clinical and pathologic findings

  - Type 1 = neurapraxia (impaired function without anatomic discontinuity), type 2 = axonotmesis (axonal injury with distal degeneration with maintained nerve alignment and supporting tissue structures including epineurium and perineurium), type 3 = neurotmesis (complete disruption in nerve structure)

- Sunderland

  - First degree = impaired function without anatomic discontinuity, second degree = axonal injury with distal degeneration with maintained nerve alignment and supporting tissue structures including epineurium and perineurium, third degree = nerve fiber disruption in endoneurium but with maintained epineurium and perineurium, fourth degree = nerve fiber disruption with only epineurium intact, fifth degree = complete nerve transection

Treatment

Nonoperative

- Nonoperative management successful in the majority of cases for these neuropathies
- Rest, activity modification, avoid elbow extension (radial tunnel syndrome) or flexion (cubital tunnel syndrome) for long periods of time

- Splinting at night or full time
- Oral NSAIDs
- Corticosteroid injections

Operative

- If there is a space-occupying lesion, then operative excision is usually indicated; otherwise, often attempt nonoperative management for >6 months prior to proceeding to operative intervention.
- Cubital tunnel syndrome:
  - In situ decompression can be done open versus endoscopic.
  - Medial epicondylectomy.
  - Anterior transposition (subcutaneous, intramuscular, submuscular).
- PIN compression syndrome and radial tunnel syndrome: surgical decompression of the radial tunnel at all five sites of possible compression.
- Pronator syndrome/AIN syndrome: surgical exploration of the median nerve/AIN and decompression.

Complications

- Nerve injury
- Hematoma at dissection and decompression locations
- Inadequate release
- Nerve subluxation
- Scar formation with formation of new site of compression

Bibliography

1. Ahčan U, Zorman P. Endoscopic decompression of the ulnar nerve at the elbow. J Hand Surg. 2007;32(8):1171–6.
2. Andreisek G, Crook DW, Burg D, Marincek B, Weishaupt D. Peripheral neuropathies of the median, radial, and ulnar nerves: MR imaging features. Radiographics. 2006;26(5):1267–87.
3. Bartels RH, Verhagen WI, van der Wilt GJ, Meulstee J, van Rossum LG, Grotenhuis JA. Prospective randomized controlled study comparing simple decompression versus anterior subcutaneous transposition for idiopathic neuropathy of the ulnar nerve at the elbow: part 1. Neurosurgery. 2005;56(3):522–30; discussion –30. Epub 2005/02/26.
4. Bencardino JT, Rosenberg ZS. Entrapment neuropathies of the shoulder and elbow in the athlete. Clin Sports Med. 2006;25(3):465–87.
5. Clavert P, Lutz JC, Adam P, Wolfram-Gabel R, Liverneaux P, Kahn JL. Frohse's arcade is not the exclusive compression site of the radial nerve in its tunnel. Orthop Traumatol Surg Res. 2009;95(2):114–8.
6. Hariri S, McAdams TR. Nerve injuries about the elbow. Clin Sports Med. 2010;29(4):655–75.
7. Huisstede BMA, Miedema HS, Van Opstal T, De Ronde MTM, Kuiper JI, Verhaar JAN, et al. Interventions for treating the posterior interosseus nerve syndrome: a systematic review of observational studies. J Peripher Nerv Syst. 2006;11(2):101–10.

8. Macadam SA, Gandhi R, Bezuhly M, Lefaivre KA. Simple decompression versus anterior subcutaneous and submuscular transposition of the ulnar nerve for cubital tunnel syndrome: a meta-analysis. J Hand Surg. 2008;33(8):1314.e1–2.
9. Ulrich D, Piatkowski A, Pallua N. Anterior interosseous nerve syndrome: retrospective analysis of 14 patients. Arch Orthop Trauma Surg. 2011;131:1561–5.
10. Zlowodzki M, Chan S, Bhandari M, Kalliainen L, Schubert W. Anterior transposition compared with simple decompression for treatment of cubital tunnel syndrome: a meta-analysis of randomized, controlled trials. J Bone Joint Surg A. 2007;89A(12):2591–8.

10 Stiff Elbow

Take-Home Message

- The functional range-of-motion arcs are 30–130° of flexion/extension and 50° of supination to 50° of pronation. Patients will notice disability when these arcs are lost.
- The key is prevention.
- It is unclear if continuous passive motion (CPM) is important to maintain results and limit joint effusion postoperatively.

Definition

- The functional range-of-motion arch of the elbow is 30–130° of extension/flexion and 50° of supination to 50° of pronation with notable loss of motion and disability when these 100° range-of-motion arcs are lost.

Etiology

- Arthritis: osteoarthritis, inflammatory arthritis, post-traumatic arthritis
- Trauma: distal humerus fracture, elbow fracture-dislocation, etc.
- Acquired soft tissue contracture: burn injury, postoperative scar
- Congenital syndrome: arthrogryposis, cerebral palsy
- Infectious

Pathophysiology

- Highly variable given the various causes of elbow stiffness.
- Despite the high variability in cause, stiffness can be summed up in four stages. It is important to note these four stages can arise after initial injury and after correction.
  - Bleeding: joint capsule distension will cause pain and resistance to range of motion.
  - Edema.
  - Granulation tissue.
  - Fibrosis: occurs when granulation tissue matures and forms rigid scar tissue.

- A detailed neurovascular exam should be conducted and ulnar nerve function should be recorded, as postoperative ulnar neuropathy can occur as a complication of elbow stiffness treatment.

Radiographs

- AP, lateral, and oblique radiographs should be part of the standard workup.
- CT may be obtained to better illustrate the bony topography.
- With these studies focus should be on identifying loose bodies, heterotopic ossification, joint incongruity, fracture nonunion, etc.
- Typically, MRI is of little diagnostic help, unless tumor is a suspected diagnosis.

Classification

- Kay: based on the structure impeding elbow range of motion
  - Soft tissue contracture
  - Soft tissue contracture with ossification
  - Non-displaced articular fracture with soft tissue contracture
  - Displaced intra-articular fracture with soft tissue contracture
  - Post-traumatic bony bars
- Morrey: classifies elbow stiffness as extrinsic, intrinsic or mixed
  - Extra-articular or extrinsic: skin, muscle, capsule, collateral ligament, heterotopic ossification
  - Intra-articular or intrinsic: articular malalignment, intra-articular adhesions, cartilage degeneration, loose bodies, osteophyte formation
  - Mixed: extrinsic contractures developing as a result of intrinsic pathology

Treatment

- Goals of treatment include improving range of motion (and thereby functioning in activities of daily living) and decreasing pain.

Nonoperative

- Outcomes improve when treatment is initiated early.
- The keyword is prevention. If a patient presents with elbow trauma, a congenital syndrome, or soft tissues injury, healthcare providers should start thinking about elbow stiffness prevention from day one.
- Once stiffness is present, the goal of nonoperative management is plastic deformation of soft tissue through stress relaxation.
- Use of an adjustable static splint is ideal as it can be placed in many different positions.
- Therapy should involve active and passive exercise with avoidance of further soft tissue trauma, inflammation, and significant pain, because these could lead to further stiffness. Continuous passive motion (CPM) is a useful tool.

- For the reasons just described, manipulation under anesthesia is a controversial treatment option.
- More recently, the beneficial role of botulism toxin A in preventing elbow stiffness has been explored.

Operative

- Considered after a failure of nonoperative management.
- It is important to document an accurate range-of-motion arc preoperatively. If maximum flexion is less than 90° ulnar nerve transposition is recommended if significant motion is re-gained due to concern for postoperative ulnar nerve neuropathy.
- The surgical options are often based on the origin of the elbow stiffness. However, there are a few more general treatments.
- An arthroscopic release can be performed. The three options include capsular release, capsulotomy, and capsulectomy. Capsulectomy is most successful, but also the most technically demanding and dangerous to nearby neurovascular structures.
- Open capsular release is an option. Medial and/or lateral approaches are the most common methods of entry. The lateral approach is termed "the column procedure."
- After release, CPM is often used to maintain range of motion. It is encouraged to start within the first few days, because it mobilizes fluid out of the affected joint.
- Other options include loose body removal, osteophyte resection, and distraction interposition arthroplasty and total elbow arthroplasty.

Complications

- Ulnar neuropathy
- Other iatrogenic nerve injuries
- Recurrent stiffness

Bibliography

1. Araghi A, Celli A, Adams R, Morrey B. The outcome of examination (manipulation) under anesthesia on the stiff elbow after surgical contracture release. J Shoulder Elbow Surg. 2010;19(2):202–8.
2. Ćefo I, Eygendaal D. Arthroscopic arthrolysis for posttraumatic elbow stiffness. J Shoulder Elbow Surg. 2011;20(3):434–9.
3. Gundlach U, Eygendaal D. Surgical treatment of posttraumatic stiffness of the elbow: 2-year outcome in 21 patients after a column procedure. Acta Orthop. 2008;79(1):74–7.
4. Singh H, Nam KY, Moon YL. Arthroscopic management of stiff elbow. Orthopedics. 2011;34(6):167

Part VII
Wrist and Hand

Steven Maschke and Abhishek Julka

Wrist

Abhishek Julka and Steven Maschke

1 Wrist

Abhishek Julka and Steven Maschke

Take-Home Message

- Potential spaces in the hand communicate and may transmit infection across the hand.
- Wrist arthrosis is treated with motion-preserving procedures such as PRC or limited to complete wrist fusion. Limited fusions necessitate articulating surfaces on non-fused bones to be intact, i.e., no radiolunate arthrosis with capitolunate fusion.
- The TFCC stabilizes the DRUJ and is vascularized in its peripheral 1/3. Tears destabilizing the DRUJ and in the vascularized portion warrant repair.
- SL ligament tears and scaphoid nonunions result in predictable patterns of arthrosis managed similarly with motion-preserving procedures vs. fusions.

A. Julka, MD (✉)
Professor, Department of Orthopedic Surgery, University of Wisconsin, Madison, Wisconsin, USA
e-mail: julka.4@gmail.com

S. Maschke, MD
Cleveland Clinic, Department of Orthopedic Surgery, Abu Dhabi, UAE
e-mail: maschks@ccf.org

C. Mauffrey, D.J. Hak (eds.), *Passport for the Orthopedic Boards and FRCS Examination*, DOI 10.1007/978-2-8178-0475-0_33

Definition

- Dorsal compartments: 6 extensor compartments
  - APL, EPB
  - ECRL, ECRB
  - EPL
  - EDC, EIP
  - EDM
  - ECU
- Bursas of the hand
  - Radial bursa: thumb MCP joint to the proximal edge of the TCL (transverse carpal ligament)
    - Deep to FDP at the wrist
  - Ulnar bursa: small finger MCP joint to proximal edge of TCL
    - Deep to FDP at the wrist
- Spaces of the hand
  - Deep:
    - Parona's space: potential space between PQ fascia and FDP tendons where radial and ulnar bursa communicate
      - Infections may track from ulnar to radial bursa via this space
    - Thenar: bound by thenar musculature radially and a vertical septum originating from the third MC ulnarly
    - Midpalmar: bound radially by the third MC septum described above and ulnarly by hypothenar septum
    - Hypothenar: located between hypothenar septum and hypothenar musculature
    - Thenar, midpalmar, and hypothenar spaces bound distally by web
  - Superficial:
    - Interdigital space: loose connective tissue between fingers (web)
    - Subaponeurotic space: between extensor tendons and metacarpal periosteum dorsally
    - Subcutaneous: soft connective tissue on hand dorsum
- Dorsal compartment tendinopathy:
  - De Quervain's: first dorsal compartment tendinopathy
  - Intersection syndrome: second dorsal compartment tendinopathy

- Patterns of arthrosis:
  - SNAC: scaphoid nonunion advanced collapse
    - Arthrosis due to progression of altered kinematics and wrist loading from scaphoid nonunion
  - SLAC: scapholunate advanced collapse
    - Arthrosis due to progression of altered kinematics and wrist loading due to scapholunate dissociation
- Kienbock disease:
  - Lunate necrosis and fragmentation
- DRUJ: distal radioulnar joint
- TFCC: triangular fibrocartilage complex
  - Stability implied by articular congruity and TFCC
  - Composed of volar and dorsal radioulnar ligaments, articular disc, ulnocarpal ligaments, and ECU subsheath
  - Stabilizes DRUJ and function in ulnocarpal load transmission
  - Deep attachment on fovea at ulnar styloid base

Etiology

- Infection: penetrating injury, extension of infection from flexor tendon synovitis
- De Quervain's: new lactating mothers. Repeated thumb abduction and ulnar deviation. Anatomic anomaly of separate EPB compartment.
- Intersection syndrome: common in rowers and weight lifters
- Kienbock's: likely multifactorial
- DRUJ:
  - Fall on extended pronated hand often associated with distal radius fractures
  - Fractures within 7.5 cm of distal radius articular surface at high risk of DRUJ injury

Pathophysiology

- Collar button abscess: forms volar and dorsal in the interdigital space
  - Abducted finger posture differentiates this from a dorsal or volar subcutaneous abscess.
  - May begin with a break in web skin.
  - Tight volar skin causes dorsal tracking and prominence of infection.
- Parona's space: typically a continuation of radial or ulnar bursa infection
- Thenar space:
  - Posture of thumb abduction
  - Difficulty with thumb range of motion
  - Most common deep space infection

- Midpalmar space:
  - Midpalmar fullness and loss of concavity
  - Flexed posture of digits
- De Quervain's:
  - Inflammation within the first dorsal compartment due to overuse or anatomic anomaly of separate APL and EPB compartments
  - Presents and swelling and tenderness adjacent to the radial styloid
  - Pain with thumb flexion and ulnar deviation (Finkelstein's test)
- Intersection syndrome:
  - Inflammation within second dorsal compartment
  - Edema and tenderness is 4–5 cm proximal to the radial styloid in contrast to De Quervain's
- Instability:
  - DISI: scapholunate dissociation leads to lunate extension which characterizes the deformity.
  - VISI: lunotriquetral dissociation leads to lunate flexion.
  - Static change in posture of the lunate requires LT or SL ligament disruption as well as loss of secondary stabilizers.
- Scaphoid
  - Scaphoid has retrograde blood supply increasingly disrupted with more proximal fractures.
  - Unstable fractures (proximal pole, displaced, angulated, comminuted) require fixation.
  - Nonunion leads to progressive arthrosis (SNAC wrist).
- Kienbock disease:
  - Presumed avascular necrosis due to multiple factors.
  - Ulnar variance is not definitively a factor in disease development.
- TFCC:
  - Vascular supply present in periphery and absent centrally.
  - Functional TFCC tear may result due to ulnar styloid base fracture.
  - Ulnar styloid tip fracture leaves TFCC intact and does not require fixation.
- SLAC:
  - Scapholunate ligament injury → progressive diastasis, flexion of the scaphoid and extension of the lunate → progressive arthrosis

Imaging

- Infection:
  - Hand and wrist radiographs to rule out osteomyelitis or foreign body
  - MRI and US to determine extent and depth of involvement
- Instability:
  - DISI:
    - SL angle > 60° on lateral X-ray
    - Scaphoid ring sign on AP
  - VISI:
    - SL angle < 30°
    - Lunate flexion
- Kienbock disease:
  - X-ray: lunate sclerosis, fracture lines, disintegration, and collapse in later stages
  - MRI: decreased signal on T1 imaging
  - CT: demonstrates fracture lines and bony architecture
- TFCC:
  - MR arthrogram: dye extravasation to the DRUJ
- DRUJ:
  - True lateral X-ray: demonstrates subluxation
  - Pronation, supination, and neutral CT: can be done with both wrists to demonstrate DRUJ incongruity

Classification

- Instability
  - General classification
    - Carpal instability dissociative: loss of normal alignment and interconnection within bones in same carpal row, i.e., scapholunate dissociation
    - Carpal instability non-dissociative: instability among carpal rows or within the radiocarpal joint
    - Carpal instability complex: combination of the above
    - Carpal instability adaptive: instability stemming from extrinsic malalignment (distal radius malunion)
  - Based on lunate posture
    - DISI: lunate extension
    - VISI: lunate flexion

- Kienbock disease: Lichtman
  - Stage 1: no radiographic abnormality. Changes noted on MRI.
  - Stage 2: increased sclerosis on X-ray without collapse
  - Stage 3A: lunate collapse with maintained carpal height
  - Stage 3B: lunate collapse with carpal collapse and loss of carpal height
  - Stage 4: arthrosis (midcarpal or radiocarpal)
- Arthrosis:
  - SLAC/SNAC- Watson
    - Radial styloid-scaphoid arthrosis
    - Entire scaphoid facet arthrosis
    - Scaphocapitate, lunocapitate
    - Addition of radiolunate
- TFCC Tear: Palmer classification
  - Type 1 – traumatic
    - 1A: central perforation
    - 1B: ulnar avulsion
    - 1C: distal avulsion
    - 1D: radial avulsion
  - Type 2 – degenerative

Treatment

- Abscess:
  - Irrigation, debridement, and culture directed antibiotics
  - Incisions left partially open
  - Soaks and dressing changes initiated following debridement
  - Collar button abscess: volar and dorsal incisions for decompression
  - Parona's space: decompression with or without decompression of adjacent infected bursas
  - Midpalmar space: volar curvilinear incision
  - Thenar space: combined volar and dorsal incisions typically
  - Hypothenar space: longitudinal incision along the radial border of the hypothenar musculature
  - Dorsal subcutaneous or subaponeurotic space: one or two longitudinal incisions
- Tendinopathy:
  - De Quervain's:
    - Splinting with or without cortisone injection
    - Operative release of first dorsal compartment and all subcompartments
    - Lactating mothers: nonoperative treatment. Typically resolve when lactation concludes

- Intersection syndrome:
  - Splinting in wrist extension, modifying activities
  - Cortisone injection in second compartment
  - Operative release of the second compartment (rarely needed)
- Instability:
  - SL disruption:
    - Partial ligament tear: arthroscopic debridement or pinning
    - Complete tear:
      - Acute: open ligament repair, pinning
      - Chronic: SL ligament reconstruction with or without capsulodesis if malalignment reducible
        - All capsulodesis procedures result in loss of wrist ROM.
        - Post reconstruction, previous radiographic deformity/malalignment recurs over time.
      - Chronic non-reducible: arthrodesis
- Scaphoid nonunion:
  - Open treatment with bone grafting and screw fixation
- Arthrosis:
  - Preserved lunate facet and capitate cartilage: proximal row carpectomy
  - Preserved lunate facet and arthritic capitate: scaphoid excision, radial styloidectomy, four-corner fusion
  - Loss of lunate facet cartilage: limited radiolunate fusions vs. total wrist fusion
  - Wrist fusion position: 15° of extension, slight ulnar deviation
- Kienbock disease:
  - Various procedures without agreement on natural history or gold standard for treatment
  - Stage 1, 2: nonoperative, immobilization
  - Stage 3A: revascularization procedures, joint leveling
    - Shortening preferred to lengthening to decrease risk of nonunion.
    - Level wrists may benefit from capitate. shortening.
  - Stage 3B: restoration of scaphoid posture via limited carpal fusion
  - Stage 4: salvage with wrist fusion, arthroplasty, or PRC
- DRUJ:
  - Acute instability: if reduces with forearm rotation. Immobilize in supination/pronation for 6 weeks. Inability to maintain reduction warrants pinning proximal to DRUJ for 4–6 weeks.

- TFCC:
  - 1A:
    - Nonoperative. Arthroscopic debridement if nonoperative fails
  - 1B:
    - Stable DRUJ: nonoperative with immobilization
    - Unstable DRUJ: peripheral repair of TFCC or ulnar styloid
  - 1C:
    - Nonoperative with immobilization
    - Arthroscopic or open repair if the above fails
  - 1D:
    - Repair if symptomatic

Complications

- Infection: recurrence, stiffness, contracture
- De Quervain's release: volar subluxation of first dorsal compartment tendons
- Scaphoid nonunion: increasing arthrosis following a SNAC progression
- Scapholunate dissociation: increasing arthrosis following a SLAC progression
- Wrist fusions: nonunion, incomplete relief of pain

Bibliography

1. Beredjiklian PK. Kienböck's disease. YJHSU. 2009;34:167–175. doi:10.1016/j.jhsa.2008.10.012.
2. Ilyas AM, Ilyas A, Ast M, Schaffer AA, Thoder J. De quervain tenosynovitis of the wrist. J Am Acad Orthop Surg. 2007;15:757–64.
3. Kuo CE, Wolfe SW. Scapholunate instability: current concepts in diagnosis and management. J Hand Surg Am. 2008;33:998–1013. doi:10.1016/j.jhsa.2008.04.027.
4. Sachar K. Ulnar-sided wrist pain: evaluation and treatment of triangular fibrocartilage complex tears, ulnocarpal impaction syndrome, and lunotriquetral ligament tears. J Hand Surg Am. 2008;33:1669–79. doi:10.1016/j.jhsa.2008.08.026.
5. Weiss KE, Rodner CM. Osteoarthritis of the wrist. YJHSU. 2007;32:725–46. doi:10.1016/j.jhsa.2007.02.003.

2 Wrist Instability

Abhishek Julka and Steven Maschke

Take-Home Message

- Extrinsic wrist ligaments connect radius to carpus where as intrinsic ligaments connect adjacent carpal bones.
- SL disruption with attenuation results in flexion of the scaphoid, lunate extension, and progressive arthrosis.
- Perilunate dislocation is a high-energy injury that requires anatomic reduction and pinning often with volar and dorsal approaches.
- Midcarpal instability is uncommon and characterized by a "clunk" with radial deviation/extension due to pathologic transition of the proximal row from flexion to extension.

Definition

- Extrinsic ligaments: connect radius/ulna to the carpus
  - Volar: listed radial to ulnar
    - Radioscaphocapitate: originating at lateral radial margin traversing the waist of the scaphoid inserting on the capitate body
    - Long radiolunate: originating at volar radius traveling obliquely to insert upon the lunate
    - Short radiolunate: originates at the medial radius margin and travels vertically to insert on the lunate
    - Ulnar-capitate ligament: originates at the base of ulnar styloid and travels obliquely to capitate insertion
    - Ulnolunate ligament: originates at volar TFCC and travels vertically to the lunate
    - Ulnotriquetral ligament: originates at volar TFCC and travels vertically to the triquetrum
  - Dorsal:
    - Dorsal radiocarpal ligament: connects dorsal radius and triquetrum
- Intrinsic ligaments: connect adjacent carpal bones
  - Scapholunate interosseous ligament:
    - Three segments: volar, proximal (membranous), dorsal (strongest)
    - Dorsal segment most crucial to stability

- Lunotriquetral interosseous ligament:
  - Three segments: volar (strongest), proximal (membranous), dorsal
  - Volar segment most crucial to stability
    - Wrist instability:
      - DISI: dorsal intercalated segmental instability
      - VISI: volar intercalated segmental instability

Etiology

- DISI: secondary to scapholunate ligament tear with loss of secondary stabilizers
- VISI: secondary to lunotriquetral ligament tear with loss of secondary stabilizers
- Midcarpal: etiology unclear

Pathophysiology

- Instability:
  - DISI: scapholunate dissociation leads to lunate extension which characterizes the deformity.
  - VISI: lunotriquetral dissociation leads to lunate flexion.
  - Static change in posture of the lunate requires lunotriquetral or scapholunate ligament disruption as well as loss of secondary stabilizers.
- Carpal instability dissociative:
  - LT ligament tear:
    - Isolated LT disruption rare
    - Typically associated with perilunate dislocation
  - SL ligament tear:
    - Acute injury usually high energy
    - Pathologic changes to scaphoid and lunate posture require disruption of secondary stabilizers along with SL ligament.
    - Loss of balancing flexion force on the lunate results in extension and eventual DISI posture.
- Carpal instability non-dissociative:
  - Radiocarpal: three types
    - Ulnar translocation: radiocarpal ligament rupture or attenuation leading to ulnar translocation of entire carpus
    - Radial translocation: ulnocarpal ligament rupture or loss of radial height postfracture
    - Radiocarpal dislocation: due to rupture of extrinsic radiocarpal ligaments or radial styloid fracture with associated volar dislocation
- Carpal instability complex:
  - Perilunate dislocation is a progressive injury beginning with SL disruption and ending with perilunate dislocation.

- Lesser arc: ligamentous injury resulting in dislocation of the carpus with lunate remaining in lunate fossa.
- Greater arc: ligament injury with fracture typically through scaphoid or triquetrum resulting in dislocation described above.
- Axial instability: longitudinal disruption of the carpus due to high-energy crushing mechanism

- Midcarpal instability
  - Between proximal row and either radius or distal row.
  - "Clunk" occurs during going from ulnar deviation and flexion to radial deviation extension due to loss of smooth transition of flexion/extension among carpal rows.
  - Often associated with generalized laxity.

Imaging

- Instability:
  - DISI:
    - SL angle > 60° on lateral X-ray
    - Scaphoid ring sign on AP
  - VISI:
    - SL angle < 30°
    - Lunate flexion

Classification

- Instability:
  - General classification
    - Carpal instability dissociative: loss of normal alignment and interconnection within bones in same carpal row, i.e., scapholunate dissociation
    - Carpal instability non-dissociative: instability among carpal rows or within the radiocarpal joint
    - Carpal instability complex: combination of the above
    - Carpal instability adaptive: instability stemming from extrinsic malalignment (distal radius malunion)
  - Based on lunate posture
    - DISI: lunate extension
    - VISI: lunate flexion
  - Mayfield classification of perilunate dislocation:
    - SL ligament disruption
    - Disruption of lunocapitate articulation
    - Lunotriquetral ligament disruption
    - Lunate dislocation

Treatment

- Instability
  - Carpal instability dissociative:
    - SL disruption:
      - Partial ligament tear: arthroscopic debridement or pinning
      - Complete tear:
        - Acute: open ligament repair, pinning
        - Chronic: SL ligament reconstruction with or without capsulodesis if malalignment reducible
          - All capsulodesis procedures result in loss of wrist ROM.
          - Post reconstruction, previous radiographic deformity/malalignment recurs over time.
        - Chronic non-reducible: arthrodesis
    - LT disruption:
      - Acute injury: pinning and immobilization
      - Chronic: arthrodesis, arthroscopy with debridement
  - Carpal instability non-dissociative:
    - Radiocarpal: three types
      - Ulnar translocation: no large series. Ligament repair largely unsuccessful. Arthrodesis is an option.
      - Radial translocation: rare diagnosis without established gold standard treatment.
      - Radiocarpal dislocation: ORIF radial styloid.
  - Carpal instability complex:
    - Closed reduction percutaneous pinning if ideal alignment attained closed
    - Open reduction, pinning, acute interosseous ligament repair if closed reduction is nonanatomic
    - Volar and dorsal approach often required
  - Midcarpal instability:
    - Nonoperative with immobilization
    - Operative treatment: capsular reinforcement, ligamentous reconstructions, limited arthrodesis
    - No agreement on gold standard treatment

Complications

- Scapholunate dissociation: increasing arthrosis following a SLAC progression
- LT Injury: LT synovitis, arthrosis
- LT arthrodesis: high nonunion rate

Bibliography

1. Cooney WP, Garcia-Elias M, Dobyns JH, Linscheid RL. Anatomy and mechanics of carpal instability. Surg Rounds Orthop. 1989;3:15–24.
2. Garcia-Elias M, Lluch AL, Stanley JK. Three-ligament tenodesis for the treatment of scapholunate dissociation: indications and surgical technique. YJHSU. 2006;31:125–134.
3. Gelberman RH, Cooney WP, Szabo RM. Carpal instability. Instr Course Lect. 2001;50:123–36.
4. Lichtman DM, Wroten ES Understanding midcarpal instability. YJHSU. 2006;31:491–98. doi:10.1016/j.jhsa.2005.12.014.
5. Mayfield JK, Johnson RP, Kilcoyne RK. Carpal dislocations: pathomechanics and progressive perilunar instability. YJHSU. 1980;5:226–41.

Hand

Abhishek Julka and Steven Maschke

1 Trigger Finger

Abhishek Julka and Steven Maschke

Take-Home Message

- Corticosteroid injection and splinting first-line therapy for trigger digit.
- Injection less effective in diabetics.
- Preserve A2 and A4 pulleys in fingers and thumb oblique pulley in release.
- Persistent triggering following release should warrant evaluation of Camper's chiasm and triggering at A3.
- Small but reported risks of nerve injury, recurrence, and bowstringing.

Definition

- Mechanical entrapment of flexor tendons due to a mismatch between tendon size and pulley apparatus.

Etiology

- Primary trigger digit: Trigger finger without underlying systemic condition
- Secondary trigger digit: Trigger finger with presence of diabetes or other systemic comorbidity

A. Julka, MD (✉)
Professor, Department of Orthopedic Surgery, University of Wisconsin, Madison, Wisconsin, USA
e-mail: julka.4@gmail.com

S. Maschke, MD
Cleveland Clinic, Department of Orthopedic Surgery, Abu Dhabi, UAE
e-mail: maschks@ccf.org

C. Mauffrey, D.J. Hak (eds.), *Passport for the Orthopedic Boards and FRCS Examination*, DOI 10.1007/978-2-8178-0475-0_34

- Triggering at A3: Due to FDP enlargement at camper's chiasm
  - Common in RA

Pathophysiology

- Pulley hypertrophy, fibrocartilaginous metaplasia of pulley and apposing flexor tendon surface, tenosynovitis (RA)

Radiographs

- Helpful in nonclassic presentations

Classification

- Grade I (pre-triggering): Pain, occasional catching, tenderness at A1 pulley
- Grade II (active): Triggering which can be resolved actively
- Grade III (passive): Triggering requiring passive manipulation for resolution
- Grade IV (contracture): Fixed flexion contracture of PIP. Un-correctable

Treatment

- Nonoperative:
  - Splinting in extension or slight MP flexion
  - Corticosteroid injections:
    - Less efficacious in diabetics
    - More effective than splinting alone
    - Worse prognosis with young patients, diabetics, and multiple digit pathology
- Surgical:
  - Typically A1 pulley release alone.
  - RA patients may require A3 pulley release or resection of one FDS slip.
  - Preserve A2 and A4 in fingers and oblique pulley in thumb to avoid bowstringing.
  - Release may be done percutaneously or open.

Complications

- Digital nerve injury, bowstringing, and recurrence

Bibliography

1. Baumgarten KM. Corticosteroid injection in diabetic patients with trigger finger. A prospective, randomized, controlled double-blinded study. J Bone Joint Surg Am. 2007;89:2604. doi:10.2106/JBJS.G.00230.
2. Gilberts ECAM, Beekman WH, Stevens HJPD, Wereldsma JCJ. Prospective randomized trial of open versus percutaneous surgery for trigger digits. J Hand Surg Am. 2001;26:497–500. doi:10.1053/jhsu.2001.24967.
3. Rozental TD. Trigger finger: prognostic indicators of recurrence following corticosteroid injection. J Bone Joint Surg Am. 2008;90:1665. doi:10.2106/JBJS.G.00693.
4. Ryzewicz M, Wolf JM. Trigger digits: principles, management, and complications. YJHSU. 2006;31:135–46. doi:10.1016/j.jhsa.2005.10.013.

2 Thumb Carpometacarpal Joint

Abhishek Julka and Steven Maschke

Take-Home Message

- Volar oblique (beak) ligament provides the primary restraint to the thumb CMC joint.
- Articular degeneration begins volar and progresses radial and dorsal.
- Stabilization procedures have high failure rates in late stage arthrosis.
- CMC arthrodesis indicated in young patients projecting strenuous hand use.

Definition

- Trapezium: Biconcave articular surface.
- Arthrosis of the first carpometacarpal joint commonly known as CMC arthrosis or basilar joint arthrosis. The second most common arthrosis of the hand following the DIP; it is most common in females 40–50.

Etiology

- Most common in women
- CMC laxity due to congenital (Ehler-Danlos), traumatic, or anatomic etiologies
- Loss of articular congruity (Bennett's fracture)

Pathophysiology

- Deep anterior oblique ligament (AOL, beak ligament): Connects volar ulnar trapezium to the volar ulnar aspect of the metacarpal
  - Restraint dorsal translation of the thumb metacarpal during pinch.
  - Attenuation or incompetence is linked to basilar joint instability and subsequent arthrosis.
- Bennett's fractures occur through bone attached to AOL making the ligament functionally incompetent.
- Decreased bony congruency may predispose to development of instability → arthrosis.
- Progression of cartilage degeneration: Volar radial trapezium/volar metacarpal → dorsal trapezium/radial metacarpal.

Radiographs

- AP of the wrist to visualize other areas of arthrosis.
- Robert's view: True AP of the basilar joint obtained in full forearm pronation with thumb resting on the X-ray cassette.
- Lateral radiographs of the CMC articulation.
- Findings are detailed in Eaton's staging system.

Classification

- Eaton classification:
  - Stage I: Radiographic signs of synovitis such as widening. No signs of arthrosis
  - Stage II: Joint space narrowing. Osteophytes <2 mm
  - Stage III: Substantial joint space narrowing with sclerosis, osteophytes >2 mm and cyst formation
  - Stage IV: Marked basilar joint degeneration with scaphotrapezial arthrosis

Treatment

- Surgical:
  - Stage 1–2:
    - Volar ligament reconstruction: Reconstruction successful in early stages failing largely with presence of cartilage degeneration (stage 3 or 4).
    - Metacarpal extension osteotomy: Redirects load to preserved dorsal articular surface.
    - Contraindications: Dorsal articular degeneration, extension deformity >10°, substantial laxity or un-reducible subluxation.
  - Stage 3–4:
    - Trapeziometacarpal arthrodesis:
      - Young patients placing strenuous and repetitive loads
      - Position of fusion: 30° of palmar abduction, 20° of radial deviation and pronation
    - Trapeziectomy: Excision of the trapezium. Small percentage of procedures complicated by proximal migration and weakness.
    - Trapeziectomy with ligament reconstruction and tendon interposition (LRTI): Multiple tendon grafts, i.e., FCR and APL; palmaris used to reconstruct the AOL through a metacarpal bone tendon. Remaining tendon is placed into the space between scaphoid and first metacarpal.
      - MCP joint laxity:
        - Addressed to prevent zigzag deformity and collapse with pinch.
        - Options: Stabilizing procedures, i.e., volar capsule reefing and arthrodesis.
        - MCP arthrodesis: Position at 20° flexion, 5° abduction, and 5° pronation.
      - Concomitant STT arthrosis is treated with trapezoid hemi-resection or arthrodesis.

    - Arthroplasty: Hemi-arthroplasty and total joint arthroplasty options available. Complications of loosening particularly in younger patients.
  - Prospective trials have found no difference between trapeziectomy with or without ligament reconstruction.
- Nonoperative:
  - Splinting in abduction
  - Activity modification
  - Corticosteroid injection: Long-term benefit debated

Complications

- Dorsal surgical approach: Radial sensory nerve injury (neuropraxia, neuroma)
- Trapeziectomy with or without ligament reconstruction: Weakness, proximal migration of first metacarpal, graft extrusion
- CMC arthrodesis: 10 % rate of nonunion
- Arthroplasty: Loosening primarily in younger patients
- Patient dissatisfaction
- Silicone interposition: Synovitis, fragmentation of foreign material

Bibliography

1. Belcher HJ, Nicholl JE. A comparison of trapeziectomy with and without ligament reconstruction and tendon interposition. J Hand Surg Br. 2000;25:350–6. doi:10.1054/jhsb.2000.0431.
2. Forthman CL. Management of advanced trapeziometacarpal. YJHSU. 2009;34:331–4. doi:10.1016/j.jhsa.2008.11.028.
3. Froimson AI. Tendon arthroplasty of the trapeziometacarpal joint. Clin Orthop Relat Res. 1970;70:191–9.
4. Wajon A, Carr E, Edmunds I, Ada L. Surgery for thumb (trapeziometacarpal joint) osteoarthritis. Cochrane Database Syst Rev. 2009;(4):CD004631. doi:10.1002/14651858.CD004631.pub3.

3 Ring Avulsion Injury

Abhishek Julka and Steven Maschke

Take-Home Message

- Ring avulsion occurs due to force generated by a ring onto the digit.
- Zone of injury is larger than it appears visually due to avulsion mechanism.
- Class 2 injuries may require vein grafts due to often long segments of damage to arteries.
- Class 3 injuries are treated with the considerations given to all replants.

Definition

- Ring avulsion: Soft tissue and bony digital injury due to pull on a ring.

Etiology

- Commonly occurs with the ring finger by a variety of mechanisms.
- Force required to disrupt soft tissue and bone is far less than that required to disrupt the ring.

Pathophysiology

- Injury can entail soft tissue alone to complete amputations of the finger.
- Zone of injury is larger than visually appreciated.
- Major risk factor is wearing a ring.

Radiographs

- Standard X-rays of the finger and amputated part for pre-op planning.

Classification

- Urbaniak
  - Class 1: Circulation adequate
  - Class 2: Circulation inadequate
  - Class 3: Complete degloving or complete amputation
- Kay
  - Class 1: Circulation adequate with or without bony injury
  - Class 2: Circulation inadequate without bony injury
    - Arterial only injury
    - Venous only injury
  - Class 3: Circulation inadequate with bony injury
  - Class 4: Complete amputation

Treatment

- Through debridement of all devitalized tissue.
- Avulsion mechanism denotes worse prognosis than sharp laceration/amputation.
- Better outcomes with 2-vein repair than 1.
- Better outcomes with 2-artery repair vs. 1.
- Digits requiring nerve repair show poor recovery of sensibility most achieving protective sensation.
- Urbaniak classification:
  - Class 1: Require soft tissue closure or reconstruction alone
    - May require full-thickness skin graft to avoid contracture
  - Class 2: Arterial and venous repair
    - Often requires vein grafting due to avulsion type injury to the arteries
  - Class 3: Consideration of amputation versus replantation
    - Follow treatment algorithm and indications discussed in replantation chapter.

Complications

- Cold intolerance, contractures, decreased sensibility, failure of replant or revascularization, revision procedures

Bibliography

1. Kay S, Werntz J, Wolff TW. Ring avulsion injuries: classification and prognosis. YJHSU. 1989;14:204–13.
2. Nissenbaum M. Class IIA ring avulsion injuries: an absolute indication for microvascular repair. YJHSU. 1984;9:810–5.
3. Sanmartin M, Fernandes F, LaJoie AS, Gupta A. Analysis of prognostic factors in ring avulsion injuries. J Hand Surg Am. 2004;29:1028–37. doi:10.1016/j.jhsa.2004.07.015.
4. Urbaniak JR, Evans JP, Bright DS. Microvascular management of ring avulsion injuries. YJHSU. 1981;6:25–30.

4 Replantation

Abhishek Julka and Steven Maschke

Take-Home Message
- Mechanism of injury is largely indicative of prognosis.
- Red line and ribbon sign represent avulsion and therefore convey a large zone of injury.
- Amputated part should not be submerged not placed on ice directly as this increases injury.
- Order for replantation is the following: osseous fixation, tendon repair, venous then arterial repair or vice versa, followed by nerve repair

Definition

- Replantation: Reattachment of a part that is completely severed from the body.

Etiology

- Wide array of mechanisms from industrial to recreational use of table saws.

Pathophysiology

- Indications and Contraindications
  - Indications:
    - Any amputation in children
    - Thumb amputation
    - Multiple digit amputations
      - Thumb takes precedence.
      - Thumb and 1–2 digits for opposition are ideal.
    - Single digit distal to FDS insertion
    - Hand amputation through palm
  - Contraindications:
    - Relative:
      - Avulsion injury
        - Markers of avulsion injury
          - Ribbon sign: Vessel curls much like a ribbon representing intimal injury. Requires vein grafting to bypass zone of injury.
          - Red line sign: Multiple skin hematomas along the path of the vessel represent disruption of cutaneous branches of avulsed vessel.

        - Zone 2 single digit amputations
        - Segmental amputation
        - Prolonged ischemia time

    - Absolute

        - Patient factors: Noncompliance, mental disability, comorbidities precluding surgery
        - Life-threatening injury precluding anesthesia/operation

- Ischemia time:

    - Digits: 12 h warm and 24 h cold
    - 6 h warm and 12 h cold ischemia time for proximal amputation with increasing muscular component

Radiographs

- Amputated and residual limb X-rays to identify bone defects or loss

Classification

- Mechanism:

    - Guillotine: Better prognosis
    - Crush or avulsion: Worse prognosis

Treatment

- Amputated part:

    - Wrap in saline-soaked gauze and immerse in cold water.
    - Do not submerge in water.
    - Placing over ice results in frostbite injury.

- Pre-op care:

    - Patient hydration and warming
    - Tetanus and open fracture antibiotics

- Operative treatment:

    - Amputated part may be prepared on the back table.
    - Expose residual digit with ulnar and radial midaxial incisions.
    - Locate and tag arterial, venous, and neural structures for later repair.
    - Order of repair: Skeletal fixation, extensor tendon repair, flexor tendon repair, and artery and nerve repair, followed by dorsal vein repair.

        - Some prefer to repair the dorsal veins following extensor tendon repair as it is the most difficult aspect of the case.
        - Two veins and at least one artery repair is ideal.
        - Bathing vessels in lidocaine or papaverine reduces vasospasm.

    - Bone shortening and vein grafting used when vessels end do not appose tension free.

- Artery-only repair feasible for distal digit replants
  - Nail bed bleeding protocols to prevent congestion
  - Require 5–7 days hospitalization and 1–4 units blood transfusion
- Post-op care:
  - Anticoagulation, warming, restriction of nicotine, and monitoring
  - Leech application for venous congestion
    - *Aeromonas hydrophila* infection: Ciprofloxacin or Bactrim prophylaxis
  - ROM started per 7–10 days once viability is consistent

Complications

- Infection, cold intolerance, stiffness, pain, nonunion, prolonged anesthetic with complex reconstruction, blood transfusion

Bibliography

1. Boulas HJ. Amputations of the fingers and hand: indications for replantation. J Am Acad Orthop Surg. 1998;6:100–5.
2. Erken HY, Takka S, Akmaz I. Artery-only fingertip replantations using a controlled nailbed bleeding protocol. YJHSU. 2013;38:2173–9. doi:10.1016/j.jhsa.2013.08.110.
3. Urbaniak JR, Roth JH, Nunley JA, Goldner RD, Koman LA. The results of replantation after amputation of a single finger. J Bone Joint Surg Am. 1985;67:611–9.

5 Flexor Tendon Injuries

Abhishek Julka and Steven Maschke

Take-Home Message

- Dual blood supply through arterial contribution and diffusion.
- Zone 2 contains FDS and FDP and has the most guarded outcomes.
- Number of core sutures crossing repair site is directly related to repair strength.
- Quadrigia and lumbrical plus result from over advancement or proximal migration of FDP tendon, respectively.
- Early motion promotes increased tensile strength and decreased adhesions and improves tendon nutrition.

Definition

- Complete or partial laceration to finger and thumb flexor tendons.

Etiology

- Most commonly traumatic
- Attritional ruptures due to prominent hardware, bone, or inflammatory disease
- Mannerfelt lesion: FPL rupture due to bony prominence within the carpal tunnel

Pathophysiology

- Tendon nutrition:
  - Arterial: longitudinal vessels in the palm
  - Interosseous: vessels at tendon insertion and digital arteries via vincula to FDS and FDP
  - Synovial fluid: diffusion within tendon sheath
- Tendon healing: Three phases
  - Inflammatory – 48–72 h
  - Proliferative – Fibroblast proliferation, collagen production. Up to 4 weeks
  - Remodeling – 112 days

Radiographs

- AP, lateral, and oblique radiographs to identify fractures, foreign bodies, or FDP avulsions.

Classification

- Verdan:
  - Zone 1 – Distal to FDS insertion

  - Zone 2 – FDS insertion to distal palmar crease
  - Zone 3 – Distal palmar crease to distal transverse carpal ligament (TCL)
  - Zone 4 – Overlies the carpal tunnel
  - Zone 5 – Proximal TCL to the musculotendinous junction

- FDP avulsion: Leddy and Packer

  - Type 1: Retraction into palm (repair within 7 days)
  - Type 2: Retraction to PIP (repair possible up to 6 weeks)
  - Type 3: Large bone fragment avulsion with retraction to distal A4 pulley (early ORIF)

Treatment

- Contraindications: Severe injury with soft tissue loss or crush injury.
- Primary repair:

  - Zone 1:

    - <1 cm of distal tendon: → Advancement and repair to bone with suture anchor or interosseous suture and dorsal button
    - >1 cm of distal tendon: → Tendon repair

  - Zone 2:

    - Ideally 4 strand or greater core suture repair with or without epitendinous suture
    - FDS slip excision reduces work of flexion substantially

  - Zone 3–5:

    - Core and epitendinous suture in a similar fashion to zone II with improved outcomes

  - Surgical Technique Pearls:

    - Approached tendon via window between A2–A4 pulleys.
    - Complete release of A2, A4, or both results in bowstringing and decreased tendon excursion and flexor lag.
    - 50 % of A2 and A4 pulleys can be released without compromised tendon excursion.
    - Thumb: Preservation of the oblique pulley is paramount.
    - Ideal repair: Atraumatic technique with strength for early digital motion
    - Core suture: Strength of repair is directly proportional to strands of suture crossing the repair site

      - At least a 4 strand repair is for early range of motion protocols. Ideally placed 1 cm from the tendon edge

    - Epitendinous suture: Augments repair strength by 30 %
    - Flexor sheath repair: No benefit

- Partial tendon laceration:
    - >60 % laceration: → Repaired
    - <60 % laceration: → Debrided to prevent triggering
- Late tendon reconstruction:
    - Two stage
        - Stage 1: Silicone rod insertion
        - Stage 2: Silicone rod removal with tendon graft insertion within implant-generated sheath
- Rehabilitation:
    - Tendon excursion: Decreases adhesions, improves repair tensile strength, and improves tendon nutrition.
    - Children unable to participate in therapy: Immobilize for 4–6 weeks followed by active motion protocol with therapy
    - Repair weakest at 10–12 days
    - Active motion protocol:
        - Requires compliant patient
        - Typically begin with passive flexion and active holding of a fist
            - Dorsal blocking splint limits wrist extension.
            - Progressing to active motion and discontinuation of the splint at 6 weeks.
    - Passive motion protocol:
        - Less compliant or more tenuous repairs
        - Provide excursion of flexor tendon without activation of flexor musculature
        - That is, Duran, Kleinert

Complications

- Repair rupture, stiffness, and bowstringing
- Quadrigia: Limited excursion of adjacent digits due to over advancement of FDP zone 1 laceration >1 cm
    - May occur with over tensioned graft reconstruction
- Lumrical plus: Paradoxical IP extension with attempted flexion due to increased lumbrical tone caused by proximally retracted FDP tendon
    - May occur with graft reconstruction that is too loose

Bibliography

1. Freilich AM, Chhabra AB. Secondary flexor tendon reconstruction, a review. YJHSU. 2007;32:1436–42. doi:10.1016/j.jhsa.2007.08.018.

2. Lilly SI, Messer TM. Complications after treatment of flexor tendon injuries. J Am Acad Orthop Surg. 2006;14:387–96.
3. Strickland J. Flexor tendon injuries: I. Foundations of treatment. J Am Acad Orthop Surg. 1995;3:44–54.
4. Strickland J. Flexor tendon injuries: II. Operative technique. J Am Acad Orthop Surg. 1995;3:55–62.

6 Dupuytren Disease

Abhishek Julka and Steven Maschke

Take-Home Message
- Typically effects males in their 50s of northern European descent.
- Primary collagen type in pathologic tissue is type III.
- The myofibroblast is the predominant cell type in pathologic tissue.
- Spiral and retrovascular cords displace the neurovascular structures volar and central.
- Surgical treatment is initiated at MCP flexion contracture >30°.

Definition
Fibromatosis of palmar and digital fascia.

Etiology
- Autosomal dominant with variable penetrance
- Presents in 50s–60s age group
- Northern European descent
- 7:1 Male to female ratio
- Possible factors are androgens and ischemia due to microvascular disease

Pathophysiology
- Dupuytren fascia: Contains type III collagen vs. type I in non-pathologic palmar fascia.
- Myofibroblast is the predominant cell type present.
- Abnormal concentration of PDGF, TGF-B, EGF (epidermal growth factor) found in pathologic tissue
- Pretendinous cord: Fibrosis of pretendinous band. Causes MCP contracture.
- Central, lateral digital, and spiral cords cause PIP contracture.
- Spiral cord: May volarly and centrally displace neurovascular bundle.
- Natatory cord: Derived from natatory ligament. Causes 2nd, 3rd, and 4th web space contracture.

- Retrovascular cord: Causes DIP contracture, displaces neurovascular structure centrally and volarly.
- Cleiland ligament dorsal to neurovascular structures and not affected.
- Grayson's ligament volar to neurovascular structures and affected.
- Fibromatosis generally proceeds clinically with skin dimpling, formation of nodules of myofibroblast nodules (Dupuytren's nodules), formation of pathologic chords with subsequent contracture formation.
- Long-standing flexed posture may lead joint contracture that does not correct with cord resection.

Radiographs

- None required for classic presentation

Classification

- Tubiana classification: Degree of passive extension deficit
  - Stage 1: 0–45°
  - Stage 2: 45–90°
  - Stage 3: 90–135°
  - Stage 4: >135°
- Iselin classification:
  - Stage 1: Nodules, no contracture
  - Stage 2: MCP contracture alone
  - Stage 3: MCP and PIP contracture
  - Stage 4: Stage 3 + DIP hyperextension

Treatment

- Not required till 30° flexion contracture noted or + table top test
- Nonoperative:
  - Needle fasciotomy: Percutaneous division of cords under local anesthesia
  - Best for MCP contracture. High rate of recurrence
  - Enzymatic fasciotomy: *Clostridium histiolyticum* collagenase injection into cord followed by passive manipulation
    - Complications: Tendon ruptures, skin tears, and postinjection edema
- Operative:
  - Segmental or radical fasciectomy with or without skin resection.
  - If skin is excised, the defect may be closed, left open (McCash Technique), or covered with skin graft.
  - PIP contractures addressed with manipulation or release.
    - Less than full ROM expected
  - High rate of recurrence.

Complications

- Operative treatment:
  - Neuropraxia with contracture correction
  - Wound complications
  - Dupuytren contracture recurrence. Rate approximately 30 %.
  - Vascular compromise
  - Postoperative digital contracture
- Nonoperative:
  - Joint contractures
  - Enzymatic fasciotomy: Tendon ruptures, skin tears, and postinjection edema

Bibliography

1. Hughes TB Jr, Mechrefe A, Littler JW, Akelman E. Dupuytren's disease. J Am Soc Surg Hand. 2003;3:27–40. doi:10.1053/jssh.2003.50005.
2. Hurst LC, Badalamente MA, Hentz VR, Hotchkiss RN, Kaplan FTD, Meals RA, Smith TM, Rodzvilla J. Injectable collagenase clostridium histolyticum for Dupuytren's contracture. N Eng J Med. 2009;361:968–79.
3. McCash CR, The open palm technique in Dupuytren's contracture, Br J Plast Surg. 1964 Jul;17:271–80.
4. Strickland JW, Leibovic SJ. Anatomy and pathogenesis of the digital cords and nodules. Hand Clin. 1991;7:645–57; discussion 659–60.
5. Tubiana R, Thomine JM, Brown S. Complications in surgery of Dupuytren's contracture. Plast Reconstr Surg. 1967;39:603–12.

Miscellaneous Conditions Affecting the Wrist and/or the Hand

Abhishek Julka and Steven Maschke

1 Compression Neuropathies

Abhishek Julka and Steven Maschke

Take-Home Message

- Median nerve compression is supported by a latency >4.5 s and reduction of amplitude and velocity across the wrist.
- Loss or presence of sensation in the dorsal ulnar cutaneous nerve distinguishes between proximal or distal compression.
- Parsonage turner presents with severe pain, variable sensory/motor abnormalities, followed by resolution of pain within weeks. It typically self resolves over 1–2 years.
- The addition of tenosynovectomy, neurolysis, and transverse carpal ligament lengthening has shown no benefit in carpal tunnel release.

Definitions

- Compressive neuropathy: Mechanical compression of a peripheral nerve resulting in pathologic alteration to its function.
- Nerve conduction studies:
  - Latency: Measure of speed of conduction for motor or sensory nerves along the fastest fibers.

A. Julka, MD (✉)
Professor, University of Wisconsin Department of Orthopedic Surgery,
e-mail: julka.4@gmail.com

S. Maschke, MD
Cleveland Clinic, Department of Orthopedic Surgery,
e-mail: maschks@ccf.org

C. Mauffrey, D.J. Hak (eds.), *Passport for the Orthopedic Boards and FRCS Examination*, DOI 10.1007/978-2-8178-0475-0_35

  - Conduction Velocity: Measure of rate of conduction across a determined segment of the nerve.
  - Amplitude: Measure of height of action potential. Relates to number of conducting axons.

- EMG:
  - Insertional activity: Muscle electrical activity upon needle insertion. Positive sharp waves in acute denervation, electrical silence in chronic denervation without reinnervation.
  - Fibrillation potentials: Earliest sign of denervation. Most sensitive indicator of nerve compression.
  - Motor unit potentials: Generated by voluntary muscle contraction
    - Decreased motor unit recruitment or activation denotes denervation.
- EMG/NCS limitations
  - Does not test small or unmyelinated nerve fibers, i.e., pain and temperature.
  - Latency examines fastest conducting fibers only. Normal latency can be present with many but not all of the nerve fibers affected.
  - May be normal up to 6 weeks following complete nerve injury.

Etiology

- *Median nerve*:
  - Proximal to distal: Ligament of Struthers. between two heads of pronator teres, FDS, compression from accessory muscle (Gantzer's) described but rare.
  - Carpal Tunnel:
    - Edematous state, i.e., pregnancy, renal disease, decreased tunnel volume with flexor tenosynovitis, posttraumatic hematoma. Work-related etiologies debated.
    - Rare: Hereditary neuropathies, i.e., CMT and HNPP.
    - Pronator syndrome:
      - Compression of median nerve in the forearm presenting as isolated sensory symptoms.
      - Compression due to pronator teres, under ligament of Struthers, FDS origin.
      - Resisted forearm pronation, long finger flexion, or elbow flexion can reproduce symptoms.
    - AIN Syndrome:
      - Compressive or unprompted loss of AIN function presenting as loss of FPL and index finger FDP function.
    - Parsonage-Turner syndrome: Brachial plexus neuritis typically progresses from several weeks of severe pain to loss of motor function. Isolated AIN palsy is common.

- *Ulnar nerve*:
  - Differential for intrinsic atrophy: Cervical root compression, motor neuron disease, i.e., amyotrophic lateral sclerosis and Guillain-Barre
    - Compression at elbow:
      - Flexion decreases space in the cubital tunnel and increases interneural pressure
      - Motor conduction velocity <50 m/s across the elbow diagnostic
      - Multiple sites of compression: Medial head of tricep, medial intermuscular septum, arcade of Struthers, cubital tunnel, between heads of FCU
    - Guyon's canal:
      - Zone 1: Commonly ganglion cyst
      - Zone 2: Ganglion cyst or hook of hamate fracture
      - Zone 3: Ulnar artery thrombosis
- *Radial Nerve*:
  - Wartenburg's syndrome: Superficial radial nerve compression as its transitions volar to dorsal between ECRL and BR muscles.
    - Etiology: Compressive accessories (wrist watch), repeated supination/pronation activities, localized inflammation (DeQuervein's).
    - Examination: Decreased sensation dorsal thumb, index finger, first dorsal web space. Positive Tinel's, reproduction of symptoms with ulnar deviation.
  - Radial Tunnel: Formed laterally by BR and ECRL, medially by bicep and brachialis, and posteriorly by the capsule of the radiocapitellar joint.
    - Clinical diagnosis, pain with palpation over tunnel, concomitant lateral epicondylitis common. Typically no electrodiagnostic findings.
  - Posterior interosseous nerve: Compression due to elbow synovitis (RA), mass, iatrogenic injury with bicep tendon repair.
    - Clinically presents as loss of extensor function with ECRL and BR maintained. That is, attempted wrist extension results in radial deviation.

Pathophysiology

- *Nerve compression*:
  - Acute changes due to compression related to transient ischemia.
  - Superficial nerve fibers affected first followed by deeper fibers.
  - Nerve topography dictates progression of symptoms (sensory vs. motor).
  - Progression in chronic compression:
    - Compression → restricted circulation, → neural edema, → perineural fibrosis, → demyelination, → axonal degeneration.

Radiographs

- AP and lateral X-rays of the wrist may demonstrate bony abnormality.
- AP and lateral X-rays of the elbow may demonstrate a supracondylar process, medial humeral condyle osteophytes, signs of RA.

Classification

- Seddon classification:
  - Neuropraxia: Disruption of myelin.
  - Axonotmesis: Axonal disruption with variable retention of connective tissue elements.
  - Neurotmesis: Disruption of entire nerve.
- Sutherland classification:
  - Further classification of axonotmesis into three distinct types based on increasing damage to connective tissue elements. Questionable clinical relevance.
- Guyon's canal zones:
  - Zone 1: Proximal aspect of canal. Mixed sensory and motor nerve compressions.
  - Zone 2: Distal radial aspect of canal. Deep motor branch compression.
  - Zone 3: Distal ulnar aspect of canal. Sensory branch compression.

Treatment

- NCS/EMG limitations
  - Does not test small or unmyelinated nerve fibers, i.e., pain and temperature.
  - Latency examines fastest conducting fibers only. Normal latency can be present with many, but not all of the nerve fibers affected.
  - May be normal up to 6 weeks following complete nerve injury.
- Nonoperative:
  - Carpal tunnel: Night time neutral wrist splints, corticosteroid injections proven short-term benefit and prediction of response to surgery
  - Cubital tunnel: Activity modification, elbow pad and splints preventing full flexion and decreasing further nerve trauma or compression, nerve glides, and FCU stretching
  - Wartenberg's: Limitation of supination/pronation activities, avoidance of compression, corticosteroid injections
  - Guyon's canal compression: Avoidance of compression
  - Parsonage-Turner syndrome: Supportive treatment. Self-resolving

- Operative:
  - Carpal tunnel: Carpal tunnel release. No difference with addition of tenosynovectomy, neurolysis, or lengthening of transverse carpal ligament.
  - Cubital tunnel: Cubital tunnel release in situ is gold standard.
  - Transposition only for nerve subluxation (instability) or failed in situ release. May resect a portion of medial head of triceps if needed.
  - Wartenburg's: Radial sensory nerve decompression between ECRL and BR tendons.
  - Guyon's canal: Decompression with removal of offending agent. That is, aneurysm excision, pisiform excision, ganglion excision, and hook of hamate excision.
  - PIN: Decompression, rare and debated.

Complications

- Iatrogenic nerve injury and incomplete recovery with all nerves

Bibliography

1. Andersen JH, Thomsen JF, Overgaard E, Lassen CF, Brandt LPA, Vilstrup I, Kryger AI, Mikkelsen S. Computer use and carpal tunnel syndrome: a 1-year follow-up study. JAMA. 2003;289:2963–9. doi:10.1001/jama.289.22.2963.
2. Cranford CS, Ho JY, Kalainov DM, Hartigan BJ. Carpal tunnel syndrome. J Am Acad Orthop Surg. 2007;15:537–48.
3. Elhassan B, Steinmann SP. Entrapment neuropathy of the ulnar nerve. J Am Acad Orthop Surg. 2007;15:672–81.
4. Lubahn JD, Cermak MB. Uncommon nerve compression syndromes of the upper extremity. J Am Acad Orthop Surg. 1998;6:378–86.
5. Shum C, Parisien M, Strauch RJ, Rosenwasser MP. The role of flexor tenosynovectomy in the operative treatment of carpal tunnel syndrome. J Bone Joint Surg Am. 2002;84-A:221–5.

2 Tumors

Abhishek Julka and Steven Maschke

Take-Home Message

- A detailed history and physical examination including regional lymph node examination are necessary for any mass concerning for malignancy.
- <2 cm soft, mobile superficial masses may undergo excisional biopsy.
- Fractures through enchondromas are treated with standard fracture management then treatment of the enchondroma following fracture healing.
- Glomus tumor is hallmarked by cold sensitivity, tenderness, and subungual discoloration.

Definition

- Ganglion: Soft tissue, mucoid-filled mass.
- Mucoid cyst: Cyst overlying the DIP joint in the digits.
- Epidermal inclusion cyst: Keratin production due to subcutaneous deposition of epidermal cells.
- Enchondroma: Benign cartilage tumor.
- Giant cell tumor of the tendon sheath: A localized form of PVNS.
- Glomus tumor: A benign tumor of perivascular smooth muscle cells located in glomus bodies.
- Glomus body: Prominent in subungual area. Responsible for temperature and blood flow regulation.
- Osteochondroma: Benign tumor of bone and cartilage adjacent to the epiphysis.
- Schwannoma: Benign tumor of Schwann cell.
- Synovial chondromatosis: Cartilage metaplasia of tenosynovial or synovial tissue.
- Osteoid osteoma: Benign often self-resolving tumor of bone.

Etiology

- Ganglion:
  - Due to mucoid degeneration and often arise from joint below.
  - Dorsal: Scapholunate articulation.
  - Volar: Radioscaphoid or scaphotrapezial articulation.
- Mucoid cyst: Typically originates from a degenerative DIP articulation.
- Epidermal inclusion cyst: Penetrating trauma.
- Enchondroma: Idiopathic or associated with syndromes.
- Giant cell tumor of the tendon sheath: Idiopathic.
- Glomus tumor: Idiopathic.
- Osteochondroma: Solitary lesion rare in the hand. Typically associated with a syndrome.
- Schwannoma or neurofibroma: Idiopathic or associated with neurofibromatosis when multiple.
- Synovial chondromatosis: Idiopathic.
- Osteoid osteoma: Idiopathic.

Pathophysiology

- Ganglion
  - Most common soft tissue mass in the hand.
  - May cause pain due to compression of overlying structures.
- Mucoid cyst:
  - Skin thinning common as is underlying osteophyte.

- Epidermal inclusion cyst:
  - Deeply deposited epidermal tissue produces a slow growing mass of keratin.
  - Solid mass on tactile surfaces of the hands.
  - Can cause bony erosion as it expands.
- Enchondroma:
  - Benign cartilaginous tumor often presents in the hand.
  - Most common primary bone tumor of the hand.
  - Proximal phalanx and metacarpals are most common.
  - Symptoms are due to mass effect and occasional fracture.
  - Hypercellularity and cellular atypia common in pathologic specimen unlike enchondromas elsewhere which are hypocellular and lack atypia.
  - Syndromes with multiple enchondromas:
    - Ollier's
    - Maffuci's: Above with the addition of hemangiomas
    - High rate of malignant transformation to chondrosarcoma
    - New pain, new or rapid growth, and aggressive radiographic findings warrant biopsy
- Chondrosarcoma:
  - Giant cell tumor of the tendon sheath:
  - Second most common soft tissue mass of the hand.
  - Slow growing, firm mass often presents overlying the DIP joint of the radial three digits.
  - Histologic similarity to PVNS.
  - May involve bone in chronic cases.
- Glomus tumor: Growth of perivascular smooth muscle cells of the glomus body
  - Clinically presents as subungual lesion, cold hypersensitivity, and exquisite tenderness to palpation
- Osteochondromas:
  - Typically occur in the hand with syndromes of multiple osteochondromas
  - Pathology similar to lesions elsewhere
  - Medullary canal continuous with lesion
  - Cartilage cap present
- Schwannoma:
  - Histologically composed of two areas:
    - Antoni A: A hypercellular area
    - Antoni B: A hypocellular area

- Typically eccentrically located and well circumscribed.
- Pathology is due to nerve compression.
- Distinctly separable from the nerve fibers.
- Examination will demonstrate a mobile, soft mass, with a possible Tinel's sign.
- Stain S-100 positive.
- Malignant transformation in rare cases.

- Neurofibroma:
  - Distinguished form schwannoma histologically by the addition of fibroblasts and perineural cells.
  - Not easily separable from nerve fibers, intertwined within the nerve.
  - Multiple lesions associated with neurofibromatosis and higher rate of malignant transformation.
- Epithelioid sarcoma: Rare sarcoma.
  - One of the most common primary sarcomas in the hand.
  - Presents as a nodule or firm mass. Occasional ulceration and drainage.
  - Lymphatic involvement is common as is recurrence.
- Synovial chondromatosis:
  - Pain, stiffness, and swelling due to mass effect of metaplastic tissue
  - May be intra-articular or extend to the tenosynovium
- Osteoid osteoma:
  - Similar to lesion in other locations
  - Small nidus that produces prostaglandins
  - History of pain particularly at night and relief with NSAIDs

Radiographs

- Standard radiographs obtained
  - Calcifications within mass may be present.
  - Vascular lesion: Phleboliths
  - Chondral lesions
  - Periosteal reaction
  - Cortical destruction/invasion
    - Tumor or infection
  - Giant cell tumor of tendon sheath: Bony erosions
  - Enchondroma: Central, expansive, lytic lesion with punctate calcification
  - Osteoid osteoma: Central nidus
  - Giant cell tumor: Expansive, lytic, poorly marginated, locally aggressive epiphyseal lesion

- CT Scan with contrast
  - Demonstrate bony extent of lesion
  - Helpful with pre-op planning for complex lesions
  - Osteoid osteoma: Nidus visualized surrounded by sclerotic bone
- MR with contrast
  - Demonstrate soft tissue extent of lesion
  - Visualize synovial chondromatosis that is not yet ossified
- MR angioram:
  - Extent of vascular lesion
- Bone scan
  - Nonspecific marker of osteoblastic activity.
  - Sensitive but nonspecific.
  - Whole body scan can evaluate for metastatic disease.

Classification

- Benign
  - Latent: Without change overtime
  - Active: Continued growth retrained by anatomic boundaries
  - Locally aggressive: Continued growth beyond anatomic boundaries
- Sarcoma: Enneking classification
  - Grade: Histologic appearance
    - G0 (benign), G1 (low), G2 (high)
  - Location:
    - T1 (intra-compartmental), T2 (extra-compartmental)
  - Metastases:
    - M0 (none), M1 (present)

Treatment

- Evaluation for etiology
  - Detailed history and examination.
  - Pulsation, thrill, or engorgement with dependency may support vascular lesion.
  - Growth, pain, skin changes, and regional lymphatic enlargement may support malignancy.
  - Family history or multiple lesions may support hereditary condition.

- Surgical treatment:
  - Small (<2 cm), mobile, superficial, soft tissue masses may undergo excisional biopsy.
  - Masses not qualifying under "a":
    - Incisional biopsy.
    - Longitudinal incisions.
      - Can be incorporated into later resection.
    - Meticulous hemostasis.
    - Single compartment approach.
    - Frozen section + cultures prior to definitive resection.
      - If frozen section indeterminate, close wound and plan re-operation when permanent section is analyzed.
  - Epidermal inclusion cyst: Surgical resection.
  - Ganglion cyst: Surgical resection with capsular excision.
  - Mucoid cyst: Surgical resection with debridement of underlying osteophyte. Overlying skin excised when attenuated severely.
  - Giant cell tumor of tendon sheath: Marginal excision of mass. Recurrence rate is high.
  - Glomus tumor: Nail is removed, tumor excised, and nail bed repaired.
  - Synovial chondromatosis: Excision. Recurrent rate is low.
  - Enchondromas:
    - Excison if symptomatic.
    - Fracture: Allow healing of fracture then address lesion.
    - Surgical treatment is curettage with bone grafting.
    - Do not use autograft from the lesion itself.
  - Chondrosarcoma:
    - Surgical resection
  - Osteochondroma:
    - Excision if symptomatic
  - Osteoid osteoma:
    - Excision if no resolution with time
  - Giant cell tumor:
    - Curretage and bone grafting.
      - Adjuvant treatment decreases recurrence
    - Resection and reconstruction if extensive involvement.
    - Amputation considering in fingers with extensive involvement.
    - Recurrence rate is high.

- Epithelioid sarcoma:
  - Wide resection versus more proximal amputation

Complications

- Recurrence
- Positive margin resection
- Misdiagnosis
- Malignant transformation

Bibliography

1. Angelides AC, Wallace PF. The dorsal ganglion of the wrist: its pathogenesis, gross and microscopic anatomy, and surgical treatment. YJHSU. 1976;1:228–35.
2. Plate A-M, Lee SJ, Steiner G, Posner MA. Tumorlike lesions and benign tumors of the hand and wrist. J Am Acad Orthop Surg. 2003;11:129–41.
3. Plate A-M, Steiner G, Posner MA. Malignant tumors of the hand and wrist. J Am Acad Orthop Surg. 2006;14:680–92.
4. Simon MA, Finn HA. Diagnostic strategy for bone and soft-tissue tumors. Instr Course Lect. 1994;43:527–36.
5. Thornburg LE. Ganglions of the hand and wrist. J Am Acad Orthop Surg. 1999;7:231–8.

3 Rheumatoid Arthritis

Abhishek Julka and Steven Maschke

Take-Home Message

- Medical management of the disease is the first-line treatment for synovitis in tendons or joints.
- Surgical management must take into account future progression of disease and address underlying mechanical etiologic factors resulting in the pathology.
- Periarticular erosions and osteopenia and joint subluxation are radiographic hallmarks.

Definition

- An inflammatory polyarticular arthritis causing erosive deterioration of various tissues in the body among which are the joints and soft tissues of the hand.

Etiology

- Autoimmune.
- Genetic factors have been identified.
- Precise cause unknown.

Pathophysiology

- Extensor apparatus: Testable components affected in RA
  - Lateral bands: Formed by trifurcation of the extensor tendon over proximal phalanx.
  - Oblique retinacular ligament (ORL): Connects flexor sheath overlying the proximal phalanx to terminal extensor tendon. Links PIP and DIP flexion/extension.
  - Triangular ligament (TL): Connects conjoined lateral bands over middle phalanx. Prevents volar subluxation of lateral bands.
  - Transverse retinacular ligament (TRL): Connects flexor sheath and lateral aspect of conjoined lateral bands. Prevents dorsal subluxation of lateral bands.

- Finger deformities
  - Swan neck deformity:
    - Etiology: DIP, PIP, or MCP initiated
      - PIP synovitis → *PIP hyperextension*, → stretch of TRL, → lateral band dorsal subluxation, → decreased extension force → *DIP flexion*
      - Terminal extensor tendon attritional rupture, → *DIP flexion*, → extensor force transmits to PIP, → *PIP hyperextension*
      - MCP volar/ulnar subluxation, → intrinsic tightness, → *PIP hyperextension,* → progress to PIP initiated *DIP flexion*
  - Boutonniere deformity: PIP flexion and DIP extension
    - Etiology: PIP initiated
      - PIP synovitis, → central slip and triangular ligament attenuation, → volar subluxation of lateral bands, → *PIP flexion,* → *DIP Extension*, → compensatory MCP extension
    - MCP deformity
      - Volar subluxation, MCP ulnar deviation
      - Factors:
        - Synovitis → attenuation of volar plate, radial sagittal band, attenuation of collateral ligaments →
        - Increasing flexion force: Intrinsic contractures, extensor tendon ruptures
        - Concurrent wrist deformity: Radial deviation

- Vaughn-Jackson syndrome:
  - Etiology: Ulnar head prominence (caput ulnae) due to volar radiocarpal subluxation and carpal supination. Results in attritional extensor tendon ruptures.
    - Differential for loss of extension in RA: Tendon rupture, MCP dislocation, sagittal band rupture PIN palsy
- Arthrosis
  - Etiology: Cytokine and pannus initiated cartilage erosion and ligamentous attenuation
    - Hand: MCP and IP joints are classically involved.
    - Wrist: Radiocarpal, midcarpal, radioulnar, or any combination.
    - Characteristic wrist deformity: Loss of carpal height, ulnar translation of carpus, carpal supination with resultant ulnar head prominence.
- Tenosynovitis
  - Dorsal or volar wrist commonly
    - Dorsal: More clinically apparent than volar
  - Often first sign of RA
  - Tendon ruptures through infiltration and compression ischemia
  - May cause carpal tunnel syndrome
- Flexor tendon ruptures:
  - Less common
  - FPL most common
  - Progress radial to ulnar typically starting
  - Mannergelt syndrome: FPL rupture due to erosion of distal scaphoid through volar capsule

Radiographs

- Standard AP, lateral radiographs to identify degree of arthrosis and erosion.
- Findings include peri-articular erosion, peri-articular osteopenia, joint subluxation or dislocation.

Classification

- Swan neck deformity: Nalebuff classification
  - Type 1 – PIP joint flexible.
  - Type 2 – Limited PIP flexion when MCP held extended. Intrinsic tightness.
  - Type 3 – Reduced PIP flexion despite MCP position.
  - Type 4 – PIP joint arthrosis.

- Boutonniere deformity – Nalebuff classification
  - Type 1 (mild): Deformity passively correctable.
  - Type 2 (moderate): Fixed deformity without arthrosis.
  - Type 3 (severe): Fixed deformity with arthrosis.

Treatment

- Swan neck deformity:
  - Nonoperative: Figure of 8 splint.
  - Operative:
    - Type 1: DIP Fusion, PIP static, or dynamic restraint procedures (sublimis sling, lateral band tenodesis).
    - Type 2: PIP or DIP initiated treated with ulnar intrinsic tendon release. MCP initiated deformity treated with arthroplasty with or without intrinsic release.
    - Type 3: Address ligaments maintaining lateral bands in dorsal position and joint contracture, i.e., lateral bands, triangular ligament, dorsal capsule, collateral ligaments, and extensor tendon.
    - Type 4: PIP arthrodesis or arthroplasty.
- Boutonnier deformity:
  - Nonoperative: Splinting
  - Operative:
    - Type 1: DIP extension is most limiting. Treat DIP extension with terminal tendon tenotomy. Resulting mallet deformity is well tolerated.
    - Type 2: Attain full PROM nonoperatively or via surgery with contracture release and central slip reconstruction.
    - Type 3: Arthrodesis or arthroplasty.
- Vaughn-Jackson syndrome:
  - Goal: Restore extensor tendon function and address cause (ulnar head).
  - Tendon transfers with or without end-to-side transfer of ruptured tendon to adjacent intact extensor.
  - Ulnar head resection (Darrach).
  - Sauve-Kapandji viable option:
    - DRUJ Fusion with creation of a ulna pseudoarthrosis proximal to the fusion allowing rotation.
  - Ular head arthroplasty:
    - Mixed results with instability being problematic.

- Wrist arthrosis:
  - Arthrodesis
    - Limited vs. total
    - Depends on quality of articular surfaces particularly midcarpal articulation
    - Limited arthrodesis contraindicated with pancarpal arthrosis
  - Arthroplasty
    - Option for pancarpal arthrosis in low demand patients
- MCP deformity:
  - MCP arthorplasty: Non-reconstructable painful MCP deformity/arthrosis
- Tenosynovectomy
  - Indications: Failure of medical management >4 months
  - Dorsal: More common
  - Volar: In setting of carpal tunnel syndrome
- Tendon ruptures:
  - Mannergelt syndrome: FPL rupture due to erosion of distal scaphoid through volar capsule
    - Ring FDS tendon transfer
    - Autograft reconstruction of tendon

Complications

- Partial wrist arthrodesis: Progressive ulnar translocation deformity
- Caput ulnae: Progressive tendon ruptures
- Darrach: Worsening ulnar translocation of carpus, proximal stump instability, and symptomatic convergence

Bibliography

1. Abboud JA, Beredjiklian PK, Bozentka DJ. Metacarpophalangeal joint arthroplasty in rheumatoid arthritis. J Am Acad Orthop Surg. 2003;11:184–91.
2. Boyer MI, Gelberman RH. Operative correction of swan-neck and boutonniere deformities in the rheumatoid hand. J Am Acad Orthop Surg. 1999;7:92–100.
3. Papp SR, Athwal GS, Pichora DR. The rheumatoid wrist. J Am Acad Orthop Surg. 2006;14:65–77.
4. Rozental TD. Reconstruction of the rheumatoid thumb. J Am Acad Orthop Surg. 2007;15:118–25.

Part VIII
Lower Limb Reconstruction

Thomas P. Sculco and Michael B. Cross

Hip Reconstruction

Michael B. Cross, Thomas P. Sculco, Brandon J. Erickson, Alexander Christ, Wayne G. Paprosky, Benjamin F. Ricciardi, Bryan D. Haughom, Jared M. Newman, Aleksey Dvorzhinskiy, Michael Hellman, Matthew P. Abdel, and Benjamin McArthur

1 Principles of Total Hip Arthroplasty

Brandon J. Erickson, Michael Cross

Take-Home Message

- Preoperative planning is essential to obtain consistent, reproducible outcomes and to restore leg lengths and offset.
- Generally, the goal of acetabular component position should be *35–45° of abduction and 10–25° anteversion.*
- The goal of femoral component position should be *10–15° of anteversion.*
- Cementless hips (particular acetabular components) have decreased rates of aseptic loosening compared to cemented components in younger patients.
- Cemented or hybrid fixation carries the risk of fat embolism syndrome, intraoperative hypoxia, and hypotension.

M.B. Cross, MD (✉) • T.P. Sculco MD • A. Christ, MD • B.F. Ricciardi, MD
J.M. Newman, MD • A. Dvorzhinskiy, BS
Department of Orthopaedic Surgery, Hospital for Special Surgery, 535 E 70th Street, 10021, New York, USA
e-mail: crossM@HSS.EDU

B.J. Erickson, MD • W.G. Paprosky, MD • B.D. Haughom, MD • M. Hellman, MD
Department of Orthopaedic Surgery, Rush University Hospital, 1611 W Harrison Street, Chicago, IL 60612, USA

M.P. Abdel, MD
Department of Orthopaedic Surgery, Mayo Clinic, 4111 W Circle Drive, Rochester, MN 55901, USA

B. McArthur, MD
Department of Orthopaedic Surgery, Washington Orthopaedics and Sports Medicine, 5215 Loughboro Rd, Washington DC, 20016, USA

C. Mauffrey, D.J. Hak (eds.), *Passport for the Orthopedic Boards and FRCS Examination*, DOI 10.1007/978-2-8178-0475-0_36

Definitions

Primary arc range – arc of motion prior to impingement and subsequent dislocation.
Excursion – distance a head must displace to dislocate.
Press-fit (*underream*) – prepare the cup or canal 1–2 mm smaller than the implant diameter to allow the bone to expand.
Line to line – bone is prepared to actual size of implant.

Radiography

- Preoperative: AP Pelvis, AP/lateral hip (cross-table or frog lateral).
  - AP views should be taken with hip/foot in 10°–15° of internal rotation to get true AP view of femoral neck offset (assuming normal anteversion of 10°–15°).

Templating

- Order is the same as surgery – acetabular side first, then femoral component second
  - Acetabular side:
    - Draw horizontal reference line through base of both teardrops.
    - Mark the ilioischial line, teardrop, and superolateral margin of acetabulum.
    - Place cup template at 40°+/–10° of abduction with the medial border at the ilioischial line, ensuring there is adequate lateral bone coverage.
    - If templating for a cemented cup, allow for 2–3 mm cement mantle.
    - Mark center of rotation of cup and compare to contralateral side.
    - Special consideration is necessary for protrusio acetabuli or a lateralized or dysplastic acetabulum.
  - Femoral side:
    - Goal – restore femoral offset and optimize limb length.
    - Determine limb length discrepancy by measuring distance from lesser trochanter (or tip of greater trochanter) to horizontal reference line – compare this to discrepancy seen on physical exam (measure from ASIS to medial malleolus to determine limb length or use block testing which measures *functional* leg length discrepancy).
      - During templating, if the center of rotation of the femur is superior to that of the acetabulum, you will increase limb length; conversely if it is inferior, you will shorten the limb.
    - When templating width of stem, for cementless proximally fitted stem, you want optimal contact between the lateral and medial endosteal cortices of the proximal femur.
      - For fully porous-coated stems, it's necessary to obtain optimal endosteal contact in the diaphysis.
      - In cemented stems, allow for a 2 mm circumferential cement mantle.

  - Restoring offset – goal is to restore offset of normal hip.
    - If templated center of rotation of the prosthetic head is medial to the cup, this will produce an increased offset. Conversely, if it's lateral to the cup, there will be decreased offset.

Hip Stability

- Component design and alignment
  - Assess stability intraoperatively by taking hip through extreme ROM.
  - Design:
    - Primary arc range – arc of motion prior to impingement and dislocation; determined by head-neck ratio (*larger ratio = greater arc ROM before impingement*) – *narrow neck tapers* (*e.g., 12/14*) *have a more favorable head-neck ratio* and therefore are more stable than a neck with a collar/skirt.
    - Excursion – distance a head must displace to dislocate (smaller the excursion, the easier a hip will dislocate); this distance is *one half the femoral head diameter* (28 mm head has an excursion of 14 mm).
  - Alignment – THA femoral head is smaller than native, causing decreased stability and ROM.
    - You want the THA primary arc ROM within the center of the patient's functional ROM. This way there will be some stability if the primary arc ROM is exceeded.
    - If the THA is malaligned, the primary arc is not centered, leading to excessive hip excursion on one side of the arc of ROM.

Types of Fixation

- Cup position should be: abduction of 35°–45° and anteversion of 10°–25°.
- Femoral stem should have 10°–15° anteversion.
- Stem can often be placed in the patient's anatomic version, unless the patient has excessive anteversion or femoral retroversion.
- Cemented – essentially a static fixation without potential to remodel.
  - Mechanical stability of cemented implants increases with worsening osteoporosis as the cement is better able to interdigitate with more porous bone.
  - Historically a cement mantle of 2 mm circumferentially around implant was recommended; more recently the two thirds rule is often applied.
    - Two thirds of the canal is filled with the implant, and one third is filled with cement.
    - Cement mantle defects (bone touches prosthesis) create an area of concentrated stress, leading to earlier loosening.
  - Stiff implants are preferred to avoid bending/torsional forces on cement mantle.

- Cementless (biologic) – dynamic biologic fixation with ability to remodel.
  - Arguably, should not be used in bone that was previously irradiated as this bone will have decreased bone ingrowth/ongrowth, leading to aseptic failure.
  - Initially ingrowth requires the implant to be in contact with cortical (not cancellous) bone, surface coating/ongrowth surface +/– with hydroxyapatite (osteoconductive; rapidly closes gaps), and rigid fixation (micromotion less than *150 um*) to allow bone in/ongrowth.
    - Rigid fixation is achieved by one of two techniques:
      - Press-fit (underream) – prepare the cup 1–2 mm smaller than the implant diameter to allow the bone to expand (generates hoop stresses around implant to prevent motion) when the implant is inserted – common for acetabular preparation depending on the system used.
      - Line to line – bone is prepared to actual size of implant.
  - Porous coating
    - Metallic surface has pores (sized between *50–350 um*) into which bone can grow.
      - If pore size is too big/small, bone ingrowth will be suboptimal.
      - Deeper pores allow increased bone ingrowth.
      - *40–50%* of surface should be porous to allow bone to fill a significant amount of the stem.
        - Less porosity inhibits bone ingrowth, and excessive porosity increases risk of the porous-coated surface shearing off.
  - Grit blasted
    - Abrasive spray roughens up metal surface, producing hills and valleys on surface into which bone can grow and produce a stable construct
    - Bone *ongrowth* increases with increasing surface roughness (distance between peak and valley on surface).
    - Unlike the porous-coated implant where bone grows into the prosthesis, bone only grows onto the prosthesis with grit blasted (or plasma spray) implants.
      - This necessitates a larger area of coating to obtain stability.

Complications

- Loosening
  - Aseptic femoral/acetabular loosening is a primary reason for revision THA.
    - In cemented THA, the acetabular component often fails.
    - In cementless THA, the femoral component more often fails.

  - Evaluate with radiographs – presence of following predicts loosening.
    - *Presence of radiolucent lines around the components*
    - *Prosthesis fracture*
    - *Presence of a pedestal*
    - *Subsidence or change in the position of the components over time when looking at successive radiographs*
    - *Lack of spot welds*
    - *Lack of medial calcar blunting*
- Dislocation – cited at 1–2 % (some cite up to 9 %) after primary and up to 25 % after revision
- Leg-length discrepancy
  - *True discrepancy* – transverse ischial line on AP pelvis radiograph shows a discrepancy.
  - *Apparent discrepancy* – leg length is restored and is equal as measured by a the transverse ischial line; however, because of abductor contracture or scoliosis, the operative leg feels different.
    - This will resolve unless it is secondary to severe scoliosis.
    - Do not use a shoe lift for at least *3–6 months after surgery*.
  - *Most common reason for litigation after total hip replacement.*
- Stress shielding – bone density loss in proximal femur over time in a patient with a well-fixed implant.
  - Caused by stiff implants (stiffness increases with the stem radius (r^4) and with round, solid stems) bearing majority of stress/weight.
    - Hollow/tapered and fluted stems are less stiff.
  - Usually with cementless femoral components.
  - Most common with fully porous-coated stems.
- Fat embolism syndrome – *rapid onset of hypotension and hypoxia* shortly after cemented implant is inserted.
  - Most commonly seen when inserting the cemented stem (i.e., during femoral preparation) as opposed to the cup.
  - Fat is forced out of bone and into the venous system by the increase in intramedullary pressure.
    - Fat droplets reach lungs and act as small emboli, preventing oxygenation of blood returning to the lungs.
    - Vasodilatation, leading to hypotension, also occurs.
    - Seen more commonly in elderly patients (usually because they have cardiopulmonary disease and have osteoporotic, porous bone which allows fat to escape more easily).

Bibliography

1. Barrack RL. Dislocation after total hip arthroplasty: implant design and orientation. J Am Acad Orthop Surg. 2003;11(2):89–99. Epub 2003/04/03.
2. Corten K, Bourne RB, Charron KD, Au K, Rorabeck CH. Comparison of total hip arthroplasty performed with and without cement: a randomized trial. A concise follow-up, at twenty years, of previous reports. J Bone Joint Surg Am. 2011;93(14):1335–8. Epub 2011/07/28.
3. Della Valle AG, Padgett DE, Salvati EA. Preoperative planning for primary total hip arthroplasty. J Am Acad Orthop Surg. 2005;13(7):455–62. Epub 2005/11/08.
4. Emerson Jr RH. Increased anteversion of press-fit femoral stems compared with anatomic femur. Clin Orthop Relat Res. 2012;470(2):477–81. Epub 2011/07/26.
5. Kiernan S, Hermann KL, Wagner P, Ryd L, Flivik G. The importance of adequate stem anteversion for rotational stability in cemented total hip replacement: a radiostereometric study with ten-year follow-up. Bone Joint J. 2013;95-B(1):23–30. Epub 2013/01/12.
6. Ritter MA, Harty LD. Fat embolism in revision total hip arthroplasty. J Arthroplasty. 2002;17(8):1063–5. Epub 2002/12/13.
7. Takenaga RK, Callaghan JJ, Bedard NA, Liu SS, Klaassen AL, Pedersen DR. Cementless total hip arthroplasty in patients fifty years of age or younger: a minimum ten-year follow-up. J Bone Joint Surg Am. 2012;94(23):2153–9. Epub 2012/12/12.

2 Tribology

Alexander Christ

Take-Home Message

- Tribology is the study of friction, wear, and lubrication.
- The most common type of wear in total joint arthroplasty is *adhesive wear*.
- Three-body wear is a type of *abrasive wear*.
- Although 200 times smoother, prosthetic joints do not have as low a friction coefficient as native joints due to the complex interactions between articular cartilage and synovial fluid, which contains *hyaluronate* molecules that allow it to act as a non-Newtonian fluid.

Definitions

Tribology: the study of friction, wear, lubrication, and their interrelationships. Derived from Greek term “*tribos*,” meaning rubbing

Bio-tribology: the study of tribology of biologic systems, in this case synovial joints, with the goal of understanding these systems and developing medical interventions to address pathology

History

Early 1500s, da Vinci first relates friction as ratio of transverse force to axial load.
1699 Amontons describes friction as independent of contact area.
1781 Coulomb describes friction independent of velocity of surfaces.
1962 Charnley performs total hip arthroplasty with stainless steel femoral head and ultra-high-molecular-weight polyethylene cup.
1966 Jost publishes landmark report first coining term "tribology."
1973 Dowson opens field of bio-tribology with the study of lubricants in nature.

Basic Principles *Friction* – defined as the resistance when two bodies slide across each other. The coefficient of friction, μ, relates the transverse resistive load to axial loading. All surfaces exhibit some roughness (small variations in surface height), and the projections of a surface are referred to as asperities. Friction is formed as asperities slide past each other and deform.

Wear – the fundamental microscopic process by which material is removed from a surface. This can be mechanical or chemical. Wear mechanisms are often classified as follows:

Abrasive: hard particles/protuberances are forced to move against and along each other. *Three-body wear* is the most common form of abrasive wear in arthroplasty, where loose bodies between the two surfaces cause accelerated polyethylene wear.
Adhesive: generated by the sliding of one surface along another, where asperities fuse and are subsequently ruptured. This is the most common form of wear in arthroplasty.
Fatigue: occurs when the surface of a material is deformed by cyclic loading. This type of wear is asymmetric.
Fretting: caused by small amplitude oscillatory movement between contact surfaces.
Erosive: caused by particles that impinge on a surface or edge and remove material.
Corrosive: due to chemical reaction on a wearing surface. Most common form is oxidation, where metal oxides have much different shear strengths and tend to flake away.

Lubrication – a material included between surfaces that reduces friction. Three basic modes:

Fluid Film: two surfaces separated by a thin fluid layer so that asperities do not contact.
Boundary layer: monolayer of lubricant molecules absorb to each surface. This occurs at low velocities and high loading.
Mixed: between the extremes of fluid film and boundary.

Running-in – occurs when newly machined surfaces experience a decrease in friction coefficient as they go from mixed to fluid film lubrication. This has been demonstrated in metal-on-metal prostheses.

Characteristics of Joints

Native Joint

Articular cartilage – 65–80 % water, 10–20 % collagen (type II), and 4–7 % aggrecan

Surface roughness of 1–6.0 μm, coefficient of friction 0.005–0.02 for knees, and 0.01–0.04 for hips

Lubricated by synovial fluid, which is non-Newtonian (nonconstant viscosity) due to long-chain hyaluronate molecules, making it a much more effective lubricant.

Rheumatoid synovial fluid loses hyaluronate molecules (less effective lubricant).

Osteoarthritic synovial fluids maintain hyaluronate component (still an effective lubricant).

Continual loading causes fatigue damage and interfacial wear.

Prosthetic Joint

Much smoother than native joint (~0.0025 μm) but similar coefficient of friction 0.015–0.03.

Lubrication provided by third-space fluid and lymphatic sources.

Also experience fatigue damage and interfacial wear.

Metal-on-metal joints undergo a running-in period, while ceramic on ceramic does not.

Bearing Surfaces

Materials

Polymers – the most commonly used is cross-linked ultra-high-molecular-weight polyethylene.

Ceramics – aluminum oxide and zirconia-toughened aluminum.

Metals – cobalt-chrome-molybdenum alloys.

Combinations

Hard on soft: metal or ceramic head with poly cup

Hard on hard: ceramic on ceramic or meta on metal

Simulation

Wear Screening Device

Provides information exclusively on intrinsic features of materials.

Do not represent geometry of biomaterials.

Inadequate at predicting in vivo wear rates.

Much faster and cheaper.

Wear Joint Device

Real prostheses tested in an environment simulating physiological conditions.
Multiple parameters: degrees of freedom (DOF), stations, loading, ball-cup position, lubrication fluid, and temperature.
Two-axis simulator reproduces flexion/extension and abduction/adduction.
Three-axis simulator adds internal/external rotation but is more expensive and computationally more complicated.

Bibliography

1. Affatato S, Spinelli M, Zavalloni M, Mazzega-Fabbro C, Viceconti M. Tribology and total hip joint replacement: current concepts in mechanical simulation. Med Eng Phys. 2008;30(10):1305–17.
2. Bhushan B. Definition and history of tribology. In: Principles and applications of tribology. New York: Wiley; 1999.
3. Davin JP. Biotribology. Hoboken: Wiley; 2010.
4. Dowson D. Bio-tribology. Faraday Discuss. 2012;156:9–30; discussion 87–103.
5. Mazzucco D, Spector M. The role of joint fluid in the tribology of total joint arthroplasty. Clin Orthop Relat Res. 2004;429:17–32.
6. Norris JA, Stabile KJ, Jinnah RH. An introduction to tribology. J Surg Orthop Adv. 2008;17(1):2–5.

3 Osteolysis and Wear

Michael B. Cross, Wayne G. Paprosky

Take-Home Message

- Osteolysis occurs from a cellular response to wear debris and particles.
- Osteolysis is best diagnosed using serial x-rays after total hip arthroplasty.
- C-reactive protein (CRP) and erythrocyte sedimentation rate (ESR) should be performed to rule out a septic joint prior to any revision for osteolysis.
- The 4 main indications to revise a patient for polyethylene wear are: severe pain, instability, full-thickness polyethylene wear, and rapid and progressive osteolysis seen on serial x-rays.

Definitions Osteolysis – bone loss secondary to a cellular response to wear debris and particles

Etiology Cellular response to wear debris and particles, most commonly from *polyethylene* (*macrophages*) but can also occur from *metal particles* (*lymphocytes*)

Pathophysiology

Progressive wear of the polyethylene liner generating ~1 μm particles.
Macrophages engulf the particles and activate osteoclasts.
Osteoclastic response to wear particles (most commonly polyethylene).
Bone resorption.

Radiology

Prior x-rays, including the initial postoperative x-ray are helpful.
AP pelvis, cross-table lateral (or frog lateral), and Judet views.
CT scan or MRI is also helpful to determine extent of osteolysis.

Classification

Type I: stable and well-positioned modular cup with an intact locking mechanism
Type II: any of the following, unstable (loose) cup, poorly positioned acetabular component, nonmodular cup, and poor track record of the cup

Indications With any revision THA, deep infection should be ruled out preoperatively by obtaining an erythrocyte sedimentation rate (ESR) and C-reactive protein (CRP).

If ESR or CRP is elevated, a hip aspiration should be performed to obtain a cell count with differential and aerobic/anaerobic cultures.

The indications to manage polyethylene wear and osteolysis:

- Severe pain, instability, full-thickness polyethylene wear with metal head articulating with the metal socket, and/or rapid and progressive osteolysis seen on serial x-rays

Treatment Yearly monitoring of radiographs until indications for surgery are met
Once surgery indications are met:

Type I: polyethylene liner exchange with larger head if possible
Type II: requires acetabular component revision

Prior to surgery, one must find out the implant manufacturer, size of the shell, femoral stem type, and femoral head size allowed with acetabular component size.

Complications Main complication is dislocation after head and liner exchange.

Bibliography

1. Maloney WJ, Herzwurm P, Paprosky W, Rubash HE, Engh CA. Treatment of pelvic osteolysis associated with a stable acetabular component inserted without cement as part of a total hip replacement. J Bone Joint Surg Am. 1997;79(11):1628–34.

2. Maloney WJ, Paprosky W, Engh CA, Rubash H. Surgical treatment of pelvic osteolysis. Clin Orthop Relat Res. 2001;393:78–84.
3. McArthur B, Cross M, Geatrakas C, Mayman D, Ghelman B. Measuring acetabular component version after THA: CT or plain radiographs? Clin Orthop Relat Res. 2012;470(10):2810–8.
4. Puri L, Lapinski B, Wixson RL, Lynch J, Hendrix R, Stulberg SD. Computed tomographic follow-up evaluation of operative intervention for periacetabular lysis. J Arthroplasty. 2006;21(6 Suppl 2):78–82.
5. Restrepo C, Ghanem E, Houssock C, Austin M, Parvizi J, Hozack WJ. Isolated polyethylene exchange versus acetabular revision for polyethylene wear. Clin Orthop Relat Res. 2009;467(1):194–8.
6. Schmalzried TP, Fowble VA, Amstutz HC. The fate of pelvic osteolysis after reoperation. No recurrence with lesional treatment. Clin Orthop Relat Res. 1998;350:128–37.
7. Southwell DG, Bechtold JE, Lew WD, Schmidt AH. Improving the detection of acetabular osteolysis using oblique radiographs. J Bone Joint Surg Br. 1999;81:289–95.
8. Stulberg SD, Wixson RL, Adams AD, Hendrix RW, Bernfield JB. Monitoring pelvic osteolysis following total hip replacement surgery. An algorithm for surveillance. J Bone Joint Surg Am. 2002;84-A(Suppl 2):116–22.
9. Talmo CT, Kwon YM, Freiberg AA, Rubash HE, Malchau H. Management of polyethylene wear associated with a well fixed modular cementless shell during revision total hip arthroplasty. J Arthroplasty. 2011;26(4):576–81.

4 Polyethylene Manufacturing

Benjamin F. Ricciardi

Take-Home Message

- Ultra-high-molecular-weight Polyethylene is a *long-chain polymer of ethylene.*
- Primary fabrication includes *direct compression molding or ram extrusion.*
- Sterilization methods include *radiation, ethylene oxide, and gas plasma.*
- *Radiation results in cross-linking through free radical production.* These free radicals can be quenched with *annealing* or *remelting.*
- *Highly cross-linked polyethylene* (*UHMWPE*) *has decreased wear* but worse mechanical properties (lower fracture toughness) than conventional polyethylene in vitro and in total hip arthroplasty at medium-term follow-up.

Definitions

- *Polyethylene*: a long-chain *polymer* of the monomer hydrocarbon ethylene
- Ultra-high-molecular-weight polyethylene (UHMWPE): long polyethylene polymer with molecular weight of between *1* and *6 million g/mol in molecular weight*

Fabrication Methods

- UHMWPE is primary polyethylene traditionally used with orthopedic devices.
- Three primary methods of UHMWPE fabrication:
  - *Direct molding* – resin is placed in mold that compresses to create component. Also called net shape molding.
  - *Ram extrusion* – resin is first extruded under heat and pressure into a cylindrical bar, which is then machined into final component.
  - *Compression molding* – resin first molded into large sheet, which is then machined to create final component.
- *Direct compression molding*: combines compression molding with direct molding to create polyethylene component directly from a mold under high heat and pressure.

Sterilization and Degradation

- Until 1995, UHMWPE was sterilized for clinical use with low-dose (25– 40 kGy) gamma radiation in air and packaged in air.
- *Gamma irradiation in air created free radicals that are prone to oxidize* in the polyethylene with treatment and shelf aging, causing *early and rapid degradation of physical, chemical, and mechanical properties, leading to catastrophic failure*. As a result, alternative sterilization methods were created.
- Alternative sterilization methods that reduce oxidation: *gamma radiation with inert or low oxygen package ethylene oxide gas plasma*

Cross-Linking

- *Radiation* can create *cross-linking within the polyethylene* through recombination of free radicals (not seen in ethylene oxide or gas plasma sterilization alone).
  - Advantage: *cross-linking reduces abrasive and adhesive wear* of polyethylene.
  - Disadvantage: may *decrease tensile strength and resistance to crack propagation.*
  - Type of radiation (gamma, electron beam), dose (50–100 kGy), atmosphere (air, argon, nitrogen), and postradiation treatment (annealing, remelting, sequential radiation) can all influence amount of cross-linking and effect on mechanical properties.

- Postradiation processing: helps to *reduce residual free radicals* left after radiation, preventing degradative effects.
  - *Remelting*: *heating above melting temperature* (>*140* °*C*). Eliminates all free radicals but decreases mechanical properties through reduced crystallinity.
  - *Annealing*: heating to *just below melting temperature*. Leaves more free radicals than remelting but has less effect on mechanical properties, and thus, it is thought a thinner polyethylene can be tolerated.
  - *Vitamin E*: antioxidant that may protect against oxidation and avoid need to melt polyethylene.
- First-generation highly cross-linked HMWPE: postirradiation remelting or annealing performed to quench free radicals.
- Second-generation highly cross-linked HMWPE: tried to improve remelting effect on mechanical properties or annealing with residual free radicals. All avoid melting. Includes sequential annealing and irradiation, vitamin E, and mechanical deformation with annealing.

Clinical Results: THA

In vitro: mechanical testing revealed *decreased wear of highly cross-linked polyethylene* versus conventional polyethylene. Additionally, highly cross-linked polyethylene linear wear rates appear independent of head size, unlike conventional polyethylene, where increased head size creates more volumetric wear.

In vivo: Lower femoral head penetration rates, significantly reduced volumetric wear, and reduced rates of radiographic osteolysis with highly cross-linked polyethylene for acetabular components up to 13 years follow-up.

Clinical Results: TKA

In vitro: mechanical testing revealed decreased wear of highly cross-linked polyethylene versus conventional polyethylene. *Smaller, more biologically active particles produced by wear of highly cross-linked polyethylene* in knee simulator relative to conventional polyethylene.

In vivo: Less clinical evidence for reduced wear or osteolysis with highly cross-linked polyethylene in TKA. *Post fracture may be a concern given reduced mechanical properties* in posterior-stabilized knee designs. Need more clinical evidence to determine the benefits.

Bibliography

1. Crowninshield RD, Muratoglu OK; Implant Wear Symposium 2007 Engineering Work Group. How have new sterilization techniques and new forms of polyethylene influenced wear in total joint replacement? J Am Acad Orthop Surg. 2008;16(Suppl 1):S80–5.

2. Digas G, Kärrholm J, Thanner J, Malchau H, Herberts P. The Otto Aufranc Award. Highly cross-linked polyethylene in total hip arthroplasty: randomized evaluation of penetration rate in cemented and uncemented sockets using radiostereometric analysis. Clin Orthop Relat Res. 2004;429:6–16.
3. D'Lima DD, Hermida JC, Chen PC, Colwell Jr CW. Polyethylene cross-linking by two different methods reduces acetabular liner wear in a hip joint wear simulator. J Orthop Res. 2003;21(5):761–6.
4. Engh Jr CA, Hopper Jr RH, Huynh C, Ho H, Sritulanondha S, Engh Sr CA. A prospective, randomized study of cross-linked and non-cross-linked polyethylene for total hip arthroplasty at 10-year follow-up. J Arthroplasty. 2012;27(8 Suppl):2–7.e1.
5. Engh CA, Sychterz CJ, Engh Jr CA. Conventional ultra-high molecular weight polyethylene: a gold standard of sorts. Instr Course Lect. 2005;54:183–7.
6. Hopper Jr RH, Young AM, Orishimo KF, Engh Jr CA. Effect of terminal sterilization with gas plasma or gamma radiation on wear of polyethylene liners. J Bone Joint Surg Am. 2003;85-A(3):464–8.
7. Kurtz SM, Muratoglu OK, Evans M, Edidin AA. Advances in the processing, sterilization, and crosslinking of ultra-high molecular weight polyethylene for total joint arthroplasty. Biomaterials. 1999;20(18):1659–88.
8. Lachiewicz PF, Geyer MR. The use of highly cross-linked polyethylene in total knee arthroplasty. J Am Acad Orthop Surg. 2011;19(3):143–51.
9. Li S, Burstein AH. Ultra-high molecular weight polyethylene. The material and its use in total joint implants. J Bone Joint Surg Am. 1994;76(7):1080–90.
10. McCalden RW, MacDonald SJ, Rorabeck CH, Bourne RB, Chess DG, Charron KD. Wear rate of highly cross-linked polyethylene in total hip arthroplasty. A randomized controlled trial. J Bone Joint Surg Am. 2009;91(4):773–82.
11. Micheli BR, Wannomae KK, Lozynsky AJ, Christensen SD, Muratoglu OK. Knee simulator wear of vitamin E stabilized irradiated ultrahigh molecular weight polyethylene. J Arthroplasty. 2012;27(1):95–104.
12. Muratoglu OK, Merrill EW, Bragdon CR, O'Connor D, Hoeffel D, Burroughs B, Jasty M, Harris WH. Effect of radiation, heat, and aging on in vitro wear resistance of polyethylene. Clin Orthop Relat Res. 2003;417:253–62.
13. Sychterz CJ, Orishimo KF, Engh CA. Sterilization and polyethylene wear: clinical studies to support laboratory data. J Bone Joint Surg Am. 2004;86-A(5):1017–22.

5 Surgical Management of the Young Adult with Hip Pain

Bryan D. Haughom, Jared M. Newman

Take-Home Message

- Hip pain encompasses a wide differential diagnosis including neurologic, gynecologic, urologic, gastrointestinal, and musculoskeletal etiologies.

- Surgical treatment of hip pain is largely centered upon management of bony deformity, and the pathology can be categorized as primarily acetabular (undercoverage vs. overcoverage) as well as femoral (abnormal version vs. abnormal head-neck offset).
- Radiographic evaluation is crucial in determining the fundamental underlying pathology.
- Goals of surgery are to create a stable painless hip and to prevent cartilage degeneration.

Background

- Hip pain in a young adult or an adult patient may encompass a wide spectrum of disorders, ranging from neurologic, gynecologic, urologic, gastrointestinal, and orthopedic.
- Abnormalities of the bony femoroacetabular joint, including both primary femoral-sided and acetabular-sided disease.
- *Acetabular dysplasia* – can be broken into three broad categories:
  - Overcoverage (i.e., pincer deformity)
  - Undercoverage (i.e., classic hip dysplasia)
  - Abnormal acetabular version
- *Femoral dysplasia* – abnormal proximal femoral geometry can include abnormalities of the following:
  - Femoral neck version
  - Femoral head-neck offset (i.e., CAM deformity).
- Persistent hip pain in a young adult (<50 years of age) is often due to an underlying bony abnormality (femoral or acetabular).
- Bony abnormalities of the hip joint may represent an untreated condition from birth/youth, or it may be the sequalae of previously diagnosed and/or treated hip dysplasia.
- Underlying bony pathology (i.e., hip dysplasia) is thought to account for a large share of the young adult hip arthritis seen by arthroplasty surgeons.
- An increasing effort to diagnose and treat these conditions prior to degenerative changes is encouraged, though definitive proof of a true causative relationship is lacking.
- Traditional open, minimally invasive open, and arthroscopic techniques are described to address the myriad of conditions that are associated with adult hip dysplasia.

Etiology

- The etiology of bony hip disease is diverse. Primary femoral and acetabular-sided disease has been described; however, often both exist concurrently.

- Many disorders have been described as etiologies of dysplasia including developmental hip dysplasia, acetabular retroversion, acetabular protrusio, proximal femoral valgus, Legg-Calvé-Perthes disease, and chronic slipped capital femoral epiphysis to name a few.
- More subtle abnormalities including mild acetabular dysplasia, focal acetabular overcoverage, and CAM deformities with time may also lead to early onset hip pain.

Pathophysiology

- The fundamental pathology at play in is a mismatch between the sphericity of the femoral head and the congruence of the acetabulum.
- Relative undercoverage (i.e., classic dysplasia) may result in a decreased contact area and increased loads over a smaller effective area.
- Relative overcoverage, in the case of the acetabulum, or an aspherical femoral head, in the case of a CAM lesion, may lead to impingement of the soft tissue labrum.
- In response to the underlying bony abnormalities, muscular, postural, capsular adaptation, and cartilage degeneration may ensue which may lead to pain.
- Patients often present with complains of the insidious onset of groin pain (particularly with flexion adduction and internal rotation (FADDIR), and flexion abduction and external rotation (FABER)).
- Physical examination may demonstrate decreased or asymmetric hip range of motion (particularly in internal rotation) as well as hip abductor weakness and possibly leg length discrepancy. Provocative tests (i.e., impingement tests such as the FADDIR and FABER tests) may reproduce the pain.

Radiography

- Standard radiographs include an anteroposterior (AP) view of pelvis as well as AP and lateral views of the hip. Alternative views such as the Dunn lateral and the false profile view have been advocated as well.
- Advanced imaging including CT and MRI scans may provide information about the three-dimensional bony architecture (CT scan) and the capsulolabral structures (MRI scan).
- Radiographic measurements include:
  - *Alpha angle*
    - Angle formed between the axis of the femoral neck, the center of the femoral head, and the point at which the femoral head becomes aspherical.
    - May be measured on all views.
    - CAM deformity is defined as alpha angle >55°.
  - *Center-edge angle (CEA)*
    - Angle formed between a perpendicular to the axis of the pelvis (i.e., a line connected between the ischial tuberosities) and the lateral margin of the acetabular dome.

    - Pincer deformity is defined as CEA > 39°.
    - Classic hip dysplasia is defined as CEA < 20°.
      - Mild hip dysplasia: 20–25°
  - *Acetabular index (Tonnis angle)*
    - Measured on AP pelvis radiograph.
    - Angle formed between a horizontal line at the apex of the acetabular tear drop and the lateral edge of the acetabulum.
    - Abnormal values include >10° and <0°.
- Additional radiographic findings
  - *Crossover Sign*
    - Measured on the AP pelvis radiograph
    - An indication of acetabular retroversion

Classification

- Femoroacetabular impingement is measured quantitatively by the aforementioned measurements. No true classification systems are employed.
- Classic hip dysplasia on the other hand has several classification systems that quantify the severity.
- *Crowe classification*
  - Class I: femoral head proximal displacement <10 % or femoral head subluxation <50 %
  - Class II: femoral head proximal displacement 10–15 % or femoral head subluxation 50–75 %
  - Class III: femoral head proximal displacement 15–20 % or femoral head subluxation <75–100 %
  - Class IV: femoral head proximal displacement >20 % or femoral head subluxation >100 %
- *Hartofilakidis classification*
  - Dysplasia (type A): femoral head is contained within the bony acetabulum with some degree of subluxation.
  - Low dislocation (type B): femoral head articulates with a false acetabulum that partially involves the true acetabulum to a varying degree.
  - High dislocation (type C): femoral head is completely dislocated from true acetabulum but rather articulates with separate (posterior/superior) false acetabulum.

Treatment

- Treatment options for the spectrum of adult hip pathology, from classic hip dysplasia to femoroacetabular impingement, are broad and varied. Primarily acetabular, primarily femoral, and combined approaches are described. Moreover, both open and arthroscopic treatment options have both been described with reasonable success.

- Whether in the case of classic dysplasia where abnormal loading patterns lead to increasing contact forces and wear or in the case of FAI where bony abnormalities are thought to create labral and cartilage wear, the goal of surgical treatment is to create a stable painless hip and delay or altogether halt the progression to osteoarthritis.
- *Classic hip dysplasia*
  - Fundamental pathologies at play are a relative acetabular undercoverage (anterior/lateral) and often abnormal acetabular version. Surgical treatment aims to correct the overall alignment of the acetabulum.
  - Patients should have no evidence of radiographic osteoarthritis and painless passive ROM (>90° flexion, >30° abduction).
  - The primary surgical treatment option in the skeletally mature patient is the periacetabular osteotomy (PAO). This open surgical procedure is often performed via a Smith-Peterson approach. It allows for medialization of the hip as well as large corrections in acetabular version and lateral undercoverage (i.e., tilt).
  - The goal of the operation is to restore normal acetabular parameters (i.e., acetabular index, lateral center edge angle, and version). Care is taken to prevent overcorrection and subsequent acetabular retroversion.
- *Femoroacetabular impingement (FAI)*
  - As previously mentioned, FAI represents a large spectrum of disease. Primary acetabular (i.e., pincer), femoral (i.e., CAM), and mixed pathologies are often encountered.
  - Arthroscopic and open procedures have both been described and have shown excellent short-term results, though long-term results are lacking.
  - Arthroscopic procedures utilize a traction table in conjunction with intraoperative fluoroscopy. Arthroscopic techniques allow for both femoral osteochondroplasty (CAM) and acetabular rim trimming (pincer lesion) as well as labral repair.
  - Open surgical approaches have been described with and without surgical hip dislocation. Similar to arthroscopic techniques, both femoral and acetabular bony abnormalities as well as soft tissue issues may be addressed. Both anterolateral (Watson-Jones) and anterior (Smith- Peterson) approaches have been described.
  - Surgical treatment aims to decompress the femoral as well as the acetabular regions of impingement. Moreover, attempts to address the resultant labral and cartilage damage are undertaken as well.
- *Resultant femoral deformity*
  - As previously described, a multitude of conditions (e.g., Legg-Calvé-Perthes and slipped capital femoral epiphysis) may leave patients dysplastic proximal femurs and impingement.

- Surgical treatments have been developed which address the underlying bony abnormalities. These have been used in conjunction with acetabular reorientation osteotomies.
- These procedures typically require surgical hip dislocation and have been performed with a combined lateral and Smith-Peterson approach as well as a isolated Watson-Jones approach.
- Proximal femoral osteotomies include both femoral neck and intertrochanteric, depending on pathology in question. These procedures produce flexion, internal rotation, and valgus to correct the underlying deformity. Additionally femoral osteochondroplasties are often performed to eliminate impingement.
- Unfortunately high rates of avascular necrosis (15–35 %) have been described in the setting of femoral neck osteotomies however.

Bibliography

1. Beck M, Kalhor M, Leunig M, Ganz R. Hip morphology influences the pattern of damage to the articular cartilage: femoroacetabular impingement as a cause of osteoarthritis of the hip. J Bone Joint Surg Br. 2013; 7(2):79–90.
2. Clohisy JC, Barrett SE, Gordon JE, et al. Periacetabular osteotomy for the treatment of severe acetabular dysplasia. J Bone Joint Surg Am. 2005;87: 254–9.
3. Clohisy JC, Beaulé PE, O'Malley A, Safran MR, Schoenecker P. AOA symposium: hip disease in the young adult. Current concepts of etiology and surgical treatment. J Bone Joint Surg Am. 2008;90(10):2267–81.
4. Clohisy JC, Zebala LP, Nepple JJ, Pashos G. Combined hip arthroscopy and limited open osteochondroplasty for anterior femoroacetabular impingement. J Bone Joint Surg Am. 2010;92(8):1697–706.
5. Cross MB, Maak TG, Fabricant P, Kelly BT. Impingement (Acetabular Side). Clin Sports Med. 2011;30(2):379–90.
6. Cross MB, Shindle MK, Kelly BT. Arthroscopic anterior and posterior labral repair: a case report and review of the literature. HSS J. 2010;6(2):223 [Epub ahead of print, March 3, 2010].
7. Crowe JF, Mani VJ, Ranawat CS. Total hip replacement in congenital dislocation and dysplasia of the hip. J Bone Joint Surg Am. 1979;61:15–23.
8. Ganz R, Horowitz K, Leunig M. Algorithm for femoral and periacetabular osteotomies in complex hip deformities. Clin Orthop Relat Res. 2010;468(12): 3168–80.
9. Hartofilakidis G, Stamos K, Karachalios T, Ioannidis TT, Zacharakis N. Congenital hip disease in adults: classification of acetabular deficiencies and operative treatment with acetabuloplasty combined with total hip arthroplasty. J Bone Joint Surg Am. 1996;78:683–92.
10. Jaberi FM, Parvizi J. Hip pain in young adults: femoroacetabular impingement. J Arthroplasty. 2007;22(7 Suppl 3):37–42.

11. Jamali AA, Mladenov K, Meyer DC, et al. Anteroposterior pelvic radiographs to assess acetabular retroversion: high validity of the "cross-over-sign". J Orthop Res. 2007;25:758–65.
12. Larson CM. Arthroscopic management of pincer-type impingement. Sports Med Arthros. 2010;18(2):100–7.
13. Laude F, Sariali E, Nogier A. Femoroacetabular impingement treatment using arthroscopy and anterior approach. Clin Orthop Relat Res. 2009;467: 747–57.
14. Matheney T, Kim YJ, Zurakowski D, et al. Intermediate to long-term results following the Bernese periacetabular osteotomy and predictors of clinical outcome. J Bone Joint Surg Am. 2009;91:2113–23.
15. Murphy SB, Kijewski PK, Millis MB, Harless A. Acetabular dysplasia in the adolescent and young adult. Clin Orthop Relat Res. 1990;261:214–23.
16. Nötzli HP, Wyss TF, Stoecklin CH, Schmid MR, Treiber K, Hodler J. The contour of the femoral head-neck junction as a predictor for the risk of anterior impingement. J Bone Joint Surg Br. 2002;84:556–60.
17. Nunley RM, Prather H, Hunt D, Schoenecker PL, Clohisy JC. Clinical presentation of symptomatic acetabular dysplasia in skeletally mature patients. J Bone Joint Surg Am. 2011;93 Suppl 2:17–21.
18. Philippon MJ, Schenker ML. A new method for acetabular rim trimming and labral repair. Clin Sports Med. 2006;25(2):293–7.
19. Rebello G, Spencer S, Millis MB, Kim YJ. Surgical dislocation in the management of pediatric and adolescent hip deformity. Clin Orthop Relat Res. 2009;467(3):724–31.
20. Reynolds D, Lucas J, Klaue K. Retroversion of the acetabulum. A cause of hip pain. J Bone Joint Surg Br. 1999;81:281–8.
21. Sankar WN, Neubuerger CO, Moseley CF. Femoral anteversion in developmental dysplasia of the hip. J Pediatr Orthop. 2009;29(8):885–8.
22. Schoenecker PL, Clohisy JC, Millis MB, Wenger DR. Surgical management of the problematic hip in adolescent and young adult patients. J Am Acad Orthop Surg. 2011;19(5):275–86.
23. Shore BJ, Novais EN, Millis MB, Kim YJ. Low early failure rates using a surgical dislocation approach in healed Legg-Calvé-Perthes disease. Clin Orthop Relat Res. 2012;470(9):2441–9.
24. Steppacher SD, Huemmer C, Schwab JM, Tannast M, Siebenrock KA. Surgical hip dislocation for treatment of femoroacetabular impingement: factors predicting 5-year survivorship. Clin Orthop Relat Res. 2014;472(1): 337–48.
25. Sugano N, Noble PC, Kamaric E, Salama JK, Ochi T, Tullos HS. The morphology of the femur in developmental dysplasia of the hip. J Bone Joint Surg Br. 1998;80(4):711–9.

6 Nonarthroplasty Options

Aleksey Dvorzhinskiy, Michael B. Cross

Take-Home Message

- Total hip arthroplasty (THA) is not an ideal solution for some young/active patients or those who have had multiple failed arthroplasties on the hip.
- *Femoral/pelvic osteotomies* correct known mechanical deformities in young patients, which lead to osteoarthritis. The results are dependent on correct indications, minimal osteoarthritis, and surgical technique.
- *Hip arthrodesis* fuses severely diseased joints to relieve pain in patients who are young and active and have healthy neighboring joints. Results are dependent on proper fusion positioning, surgical technique, and minimal disease in neighboring joints. Conversion to THA is usually performed later in life due to eventual pain in neighboring joints and produces adequate results.

6.1 Femoral/Pelvic Osteotomy

Introduction

- THA is the primary surgical procedure used in the treatment of osteoarthritic hip joints.
- High failure rates and insufficient longevity of THA make delay of this procedure advantageous.
- Numerous studies suggest that *OA is largely caused by preexisting anatomical deformities* (e.g., hip dysplasia, slipped capital femoral epiphysis, Legg-Calve-Perthes disease, etc.)
  - Excessive, unevenly distributed loads cause damage to cartilage and lead to OA.
- Correction of a known deformity can therefore prevent or delay the need for THA.
  - Preferable in younger, more active patients.
- Corrective femoral/pelvic osteotomy can *treat early or low-grade OA* or be used in its *prevention.*
  - The goal is to postpone or obviate the need for THA.
  - Success of the procedure is inversely correlated with progression of disease.

Evaluation of the Patient

- Selection: *radiographic evidence of a correctable mechanical problem in the hip joint in a patient at a young physiologic age with little/no signs of osteoarthritis present.*
- Presenting symptoms include pain, weakness of ipsilateral limb, and instability.
- Pain typically mild, related to weight bearing and relieved with rest.
- Good preoperative range of motion (ROM) correlates with better outcomes.
- Absolute contraindications
  - *Severely limited ROM (<60° of flexion)*
  - Neuropathic arthropathy
  - Severe osteoporosis
  - Inflammatory disease
  - Infection
- Relative contraindications
  - Mild-moderate stiffness
  - Advanced age
  - Moderate OA
  - Morbid obesity

Femoral Osteotomies

- Indicated for treatment of primarily *femoral disorders*
- Classified in reference to final geometry of the proximal femur in the frontal plane (varus vs. valgus)
  - Varus intertrochanteric osteotomy
    - Indications: coxa valga, sometimes coexisting with mild acetabular dysplasia or leg length discrepancy (longer ipsilateral leg)
    - Ideal patient: spherical femoral head, little/no acetabular dysplasia, eccentric sourcil, neck-shaft angle >135° valgus
    - *Ideal medial displacement of osteotomy*: *10–15 mm*
    - Disadvantages: *shortening of the leg*, *Trendelenburg gait, and prolonged abductor weakness*
  - Valgus intertrochanteric osteotomy
    - Indications:
      - Femoral neck nonunions: converts shear forces into compressive stresses that increase possibility of union.
      - Coxa vara (shaft angle <120°)
  - Flexion, internal rotation proximal femoral osteotomy
    - Indications:
      - Slipped capital femoral epi hysis causing hip impingement/osteoarthritis

Pelvic Osteotomies

- Indicated for the treatment of *primarily acetabular disorders*
- Can be combined with femoral osteotomies in patients with deformities encountered on both sides of the hip joint
  - *Reconstructive osteotomies* (*redirect acetabulum*)
    - Indicated for hip dysplasia in *young adults which is present with minimal or no symptoms* and before the development of OA
    - After osteotomy, femur continues to articulate with hyaline cartilage.
      - *Single innominate*: one osteotomy, limited reorientation.
      - *Double innominate*: adds second osteotomy to single innominate, reorientation still limited.
      - *Triple innominate*: several options, three osteotomies. Avoids lateralization of the hip and improves amount of correction.
      - *Spherical*: osteotomy around joint, large corrections can be made with less instability. Risks: *avascular necrosis of the acetabulum*, penetration of the joint.
      - *Periacetabular* (*Bernese*): Five osteotomies. Advantages: one surgical incision, *large, multidimensional corrections possible, low risk of avascular necrosis*, maintenance of posterior column integrity, diameter of true pelvis intact (unimpaired vaginal deliveries).
  - *Salvage osteotomies* (*do not redirect acetabulum*)
    - Provide additional support to the femoral head by forcing the femur to articulate with the hip capsule (*fibrocartilage rather than hyaline*).
    - Indicated in *adults* (*<50*) with moderate-severe symptoms, limited hip motion *but >60° flexion* and mild-moderate OA.
      - *Chiari*: medial displacement of ilium proximal to joint capsule.
      - *Shelf*: local bone graft onto the anterolateral aspect of ilium to augment deficient lateral margin of acetabulum.

6.2 Hip Arthrodesis (Fusion)

Introduction

- Uncommon procedure used to treat advanced hip degeneration in young patients.
  - Achieves rigid internal fixation through bone apposition at the fusion site.
- THA will likely fail in these patients due to its lack of durability over a long life expectancy.
  - Arthrodesis permits eventual conversion to THA albeit with some morbidity

- Indications:
  - *Advanced hip degeneration in a young patient (e.g., 30 years of age) with a desire to maintain a high activity level* (i.e., manual labor)
    - Etiology is commonly post-traumatic/postinfectious as *normal adjacent joints* (ipsilateral knee, contralateral hip, lumbar spine) *are required.*
  - Advanced hip degeneration in patient in whom a THA is contraindicated or would have a high complication rate
    - That is, history of sepsis, multiple revisions of failed THA, etc.
- Contraindications:
  - Degenerative/dysplastic disease in adjacent joints (ipsilateral knee, contralateral hip, lumbar spine)
  - Major limb-length discrepancy (>2.0 cm)
    - Requires adjustments in surgical procedure
  - *Active infection of the joint (absolute CI)*

Surgical Techniques

- *Arthrodesis position is CRITICAL* for minimizing deterioration of neighboring joints regardless of surgical procedure chosen.
  - *25–30° flexion*
  - *0–5° adduction*
  - *5–10° lower extremity external rotation*
    - Cobra plating through lateral approach with trochanteric osteotomy
      - *Reliable fusion.*
      - Avoidance of postoperative cast immobilization.
      - Stripping of abductor muscles *negatively affects gait after THA conversion.*
      - Risk of *instability with deficient bone stock.*
    - Plating through an anterior approach to hip
      - *Spares hip abductors*
      - *Less bone stock needed for stability*
      - Less reliable fusion as reported by one study with a limited number of patients
    - Double-plating technique (*both frontal and lateral plates*)
      - Suited for unreduced dislocations, avascular bony surfaces, hips operated on multiple times, and poor patient compliance
      - Commonly performed in two stages

Results

- Depend on:
  - Proper surgical technique
  - Final hip positioning
  - Minimal limb length discrepancy
  - Patient selection (minimal disease in adjacent joints)
- Assessment:
  - Functional outcomes (gait, activities of daily living, sexual activity)
    - Majority report resolution of pain
    - Sizable minority of patients report difficulties with sexual activity and activities of daily living, e.g., dressing
  - Effect on adjacent joints
    - Contralateral hip: patient's arthritic/dysplastic mobile hips had inferior functional outcomes as compared to patients with normal hips.
    - Ipsilateral knee and lower back demonstrate greater instability and arthritic changes as a result of hip fusion.
    - *Most common reason for conversion to THA is pain in contralateral hip, lumbar spine, and ipsilateral knee caused by abnormal gait secondary to hip fusion.*
- Conclusion:
  - Arthrodesis achieves lasting relief of hip pain in most patients at the cost of long-term issues in adjacent joints.
  - Conversion to THA is performed most often to alleviate pain in adjacent joints. In patients >50 at time of conversion, survival of prosthesis is comparable to a primary replacement

Bibliography

1. Beaulé PE, Matta JM, Mast JW. Hip arthrodesis: current indications and techniques. J Am Acad Orthop Surg. 2002;10(4):249–58. Review.
2. Pogliacomi F, De Filippo M, Costantino C, Wallensten R, Soncini G. 2006: the value of pelvic and femoral osteotomies in hip surgery. Acta Biomed. 2007;78(1):60–70. Review.

7 The Difficult Primary Total Hip Arthroplasty

Michael Hellman, Jared M. Newman

> **Take-Home Message**
> - The difficult primary total hip arthroplasty requires extensive preoperative planning with the understanding that some complications are inevitable.
> - Lengthening of the leg *>4 cm* carries a higher risk of *sciatic nerve palsy*.

Definition When likelihood of intraoperative difficulties, perioperative complications or premature failure is higher than normal for a THA.

Selected Anatomical Abnormalities *Preoperative Leg Length Discrepancy*

Definition: Shortening of the femur/tibia or cephalad displacement of the femoral head relative to the true acetabulum.
Measurements: length of limb is measured clinically from ASIS to ipsilateral medial malleolus or umbilicus to medial malleoli.
Complications related to excessive lengthening:

Mechanical – vaulting limp, pelvic obliquity, and low back pain

Physiologic – postoperative nerve palsy (femoral and *sciatic*)

Lengthening Principles:

Typically should not lengthen more than 4 cm
Amount of lengthening that is tolerated is proportional to patient's height (i.e., taller patients generally tolerate more lengthening).
Amount of lengthening tolerated is dependent on when patient's length discrepancy occurred (i.e., chronic limb length inequality is harder to lengthen without a shortening osteotomy).
If acetabular component is placed in its anatomic position, a shortening femoral osteotomy may be required.
Lengthening or shortening greater than or equal to 2 cm, trochanteric osteotomy and repositioning must be considered (e.g., sliding trochanteric osteotomy).
If soft tissue contractures are present, one can perform: (1) a complete capsulotomy, (2) adductor tenotomy, and (3) z-lengthening of tensor fascia lata (TFL).
Inspect and palpate the sciatic nerve while lengthening in the operating room.
Indications for SSEP monitoring can include planning >2 cm lengthening, developmental hip dysplasia, significant prior surgery, infection, and trauma.

Excessive Femoral Anteversion

Definition: anteversion significantly greater than the normal (~15°)
Measurements: can estimate femoral anteversion with a true lateral of the hip, but gold standard is with a CT and measuring with reference to the posterior femoral condyles

Complications of Uncorrected Excessive Femoral Anteversion:

Impingement of prosthetic neck or greater trochanter
Anterior dislocation
Limited external rotation

Excessive Anteversion Correction Principles:

Templating a stem for the metaphysis of an anteverted neck does not allow for retroversion.

If anteversion cannot be corrected with a smaller broach size, straight cemented should be considered.

Use a burr to sculpt the posteromedial endosteal cortex if necessary.

Acetabular Dysplasia

Radiographic definition: center edge angle <25° suggests acetabular undercoverage; <20° suggests severe undercoverage.

Complications Related to Acetabular Hypoplasia:

Femoral nerve and profunda femoris artery are often in abnormal locations.
Higher risk of sciatic nerve palsy when reconstructing the acetabulum.

Principals of Correcting Acetabular Positioning in the Setting of Acetabular Dysplasia:

Cementless acetabular cups fixated with screws will usually suffice.

Smaller cup sizes (<50 mm OD) are usually necessary.

The apex of the acetabular recess must be more craniad than the lateral lip of the acetabulum (preserve the lateral acetabulum while reaming).

Structural support graft may be necessary.

Classification *Acetabular Bony Defects*
Classification (AAOS)

- Type I (segmental): loss of part of the acetabular rim or medial wall
- Type II (cavitary): substantial volumetric loss in bone of the acetabular cavity
- Type III (combined): combination of segmental and cavitary deficiencies
- Type IV (pelvic discontinuity): complete separation between the superior and inferior acetabulum
  - A: discontinuity with mild segmental or cavitary loss
  - B: discontinuity with moderate to severe segmental or cavitary loss
  - C: discontinuity with prior pelvic irradiation

Common Complications

- Early failure
- Graft resorption
- Acetabular cup loosening
- Acetabular malpositioning

Principles of Filling Acetabular Bony Defects

- Most small- to moderate-sized defects can use a cementless acetabulum with dome screws.
- Large superior defects may require allograft support with reconstruction plates, oblong-shaped acetabular cups, or proximal placement of acetabular components.
- Type II cavitary defects may require particulate allograft or autograft.
- Type III defects with intact pelvic columns may require oversized acetabular cups with particulate allograft or autograft.
- Pelvic discontinuity may require structural allograft, jumbo cup with distraction technique, metal protrusio rings, cages, or mesh.

Selected Conditions *Acetabular Protrusio (Medial Wall Deficiency)*

Radiographic definition – femoral head migrates medial to Kohler's line.

Etiology – ankylosing spondylitis, idiopathic, infection, metabolic bone disease, osteomalacia, osteoporosis, Paget's disease, rheumatoid arthritis, rickets, trauma, and tumor.

Pathoanatomy: femoral head migrates medially and superiorly.

Principles of reconstruction – center of rotation should be restored from its abnormal medial position to a more normal lateral position.

Techniques of reconstruction – see principals of filling acetabular bony defects.

Ankylosis/Hip Arthrodesis

Indications – debilitating low back or hip pain, functional deficit due to hip malposition, knee problems, and painful pseudarthrosis.

Pathoanatomy – dependent on original diagnosis. Soft-tissue contractures due to dense scar tissue, worry about loss of bone stock (TB, pyogenic infection, physeal arrest causing hypoplasia).

Principles of reconstruction – center of rotation of hip in an anatomic location placing the hip abductors at the greatest mechanical advantage.

Techniques of reconstruction – will likely require a greater trochanter osteotomy and an in situ femoral neck cut. See lengthening principals.

Post-Traumatic Hip Replacement

Pathoanatomy – significant abnormalities about the greater and lesser trochanters, metaphysis may be present. May be a cortex spike in canal blocking insertion of femoral component. May have significant acetabular bone loss.

Principles of reconstruction – allow adequate time for fracture healing before attempting to convert to THA.

Techniques of reconstruction: have proper tools for removal of retained hardware; screw holes represent stress risers; burrs to remove sclerotic bone are often necessary.

Developmental Hip Dysplasia

Indications for surgery – significant hip pain, substantial interference with ordinary functioning, and major leg-length discrepancy.

Pathoanatomy – excessive acetabular anteversion, hypoplastic acetabulum and femur; center of rotation is usually elevated and laterally displaced.

Crowe's classification

- Based on 3 anatomic landmarks: height of pelvis, medial head-neck junction in affected hip, and inferior margin of acetabulum
- Crowe I: subluxation <50 % or proximal dislocation <0.1 % of the pelvic height
- Crowe II: subluxation 50–75 % or proximal dislocation of 10–15 % of pelvic height
- Crowe III: subluxation 75–100 % or proximal dislocation of 15–20 % of pelvic height
- Crowe IV: subluxation >100 % or proximal dislocation of >20 % of pelvic height

Principles of reconstruction – best place for acetabular reconstruction is where the normal hip should have developed; consider femoral shortening.

In general, in Crowe I and IV, the cup should be placed in the anatomic position; in Crowe II and III, a modified higher hip center can be used.

Juvenile Rheumatoid Arthritis

Definition – inflammatory polyarticular arthritis at less than 16 years

Pathoanatomy – acetabular cavity and femoral head may be hypoplastic; protrusio, ankylosis, or subluxation may be present.

Principles of reconstruction – must use both AP and lateral radiographs for planning because diaphysis is significantly smaller on the lateral; usually bone is hypervascular, and the possibility of transfusion is high.

Bibliography

1. Argenson JN, Flecher X, Parratte S, Aubaniac JM. Anatomy of the dysplastic hip and consequences for total hip arthroplasty. Clin Orthop Relat Res. 2007;465:40–5.
2. Baghdadi YM, Larson AN, Sierra RJ. Restoration of the hip center during THA performed for protrusio acetabuli is associated with better implant survival. Clin Orthop Relat Res. 2013;471(10):3251–9.
3. Barrack RL, Newland CC. Uncemented total hip arthroplasty with superior acetabular deficiency. Femoral head autograft technique and early clinical results. J Arthroplasty. 1990;5(2):159–67.

4. Clohisy JC, Beaulé PE, O'Malley A, Safran MR, Schoenecker P. AOA symposium: hip disease in the young adult. Current concepts of etiology and surgical treatment. J Bone Joint Surg Am. 2008;90(10):2267–81.
5. Crowe JF, Mani VJ, Ranawat CS. Total hip replacement in congenital dislocation and dysplasia of the hip. J Bone Joint Surg Am. 1979;61:15–23.
6. D'Antonio JA, Capello WN, Borden LS, Bargar WL, Bierbaum BF, Boettcher WG, Steinberg ME, Stulberg SD, Wedge JH. Classification and management of acetabular abnormalities in total hip arthroplasty. Clin Orthop Relat Res. 1989;243:126–37.
7. Edwards BN, Tullos HS, Noble PC. Contributory factors and etiology of sciatic nerve palsy in total hip arthroplasty. Clin Orthop Relat Res. 1987;218:136–41.
8. Gates III HS, Poletti SC, Callaghan JJ, McCollum DE. Radiographic measurements in protrusio acetabuli. J Arthroplasty. 1989;4(4):347–51.
9. Haidukewych GJ, Berry DJ. Hip arthroplasty for salvage of failed treatment of intertrochanteric hip fractures. J Bone Joint Surg Am. 2003;85-A(5):899–904.
10. Hamadouche M, Kerboull L, Meunier A, Courpied JP, Kerboull M. Total hip arthroplasty for the treatment of ankylosed hips : a five to twenty-one-year follow-up study. J Bone Joint Surg Am. 2001;83-A(7):992–8.
11. Kilgus DJ, Amstutz HC, Wolgin MA, Dorey FJ. Joint replacement for ankylosed hips. J Bone Joint Surg Am. 1990;72(1):45–54.
12. Kitsoulis PB, Stafilas KS, Siamopoulou A, Soucacos PN, Xenakis TA. Total hip arthroplasty in children with juvenile chronic arthritis: long-term results. J Pediatr Orthop. 2006;26(1):8–12.
13. Kobayashi S, Saito N, Nawata M, Horiuchi H, Iorio R, Takaoka K. Total hip arthroplasty with bulk femoral head autograft for acetabular reconstruction in developmental dysplasia of the hip. J Bone Joint Surg Am. 2003; 85-A(4):615–21.
14. Krych AJ, Howard JL, Trousdale RT, Cabanela ME, Berry DJ. Total hip arthroplasty with shortening subtrochanteric osteotomy in Crowe type-IV developmental dysplasia. J Bone Joint Surg Am. 2009;91(9):2213–21.
15. Lai KA, Shen WJ, Huang LW, Chen MY. Cementless total hip arthroplasty and limb-length equalization in patients with unilateral Crowe type-IV hip dislocation. J Bone Joint Surg Am. 2005;87(2):339–45.
16. Li J, Wang Z, Li M, Wu Y, Xu W, Wang Z. Total hip arthroplasty using a combined anterior and posterior approach via a lateral incision in patients with ankylosed hips. Can J Surg. 2013;56(5):332–40.
17. Liu R, Li Y, Bai C, Song Q, Wang K. Effect of preoperative limb-length discrepancy on abductor strength after total hip arthroplasty in patients with developmental dysplasia of the hip. Arch Orthop Trauma Surg. 2014;134(1):113–9.
18. Malviya A, Walker LC, Avery P, Osborne S, Weir DJ, Foster HE, Deehan DJ. The long-term outcome of hip replacement in adults with juvenile idiopathic arthritis: the influence of steroids and methotrexate. J Bone Joint Surg Br. 2011;93(4):443–8.

19. Marega L. The management of version abnormalities and angular deformities in developmental dysplasia of the hip. Orthopedics. 2005;28(9 Suppl):s1097–9.
20. Matsushita A, Nakashima Y, Fujii M, Sato T, Iwamoto Y. Modular necks improve the range of hip motion in cases with excessively anteverted or retroverted femurs in THA. Clin Orthop Relat Res. 2010;468(12):3342–7.
21. Miki H, Sugano N. Modular neck for prevention of prosthetic impingement in cases with excessively anteverted femur. Clin Biomech (Bristol, Avon). 2011;26(9):944–9.
22. Murphy SB, Simon SR, Kijewski PK, Wilkinson RH, Griscom NT. Femoral anteversion. J Bone Joint Surg Am. 1987;69(8):1169–76.
23. Paxton Jr ES, Keeney JA, Maloney WJ, Clohisy JC. Large acetabular defects can be managed with cementless revision components. Clin Orthop Relat Res. 2011;469(2):483–93.
24. Reikerås O, Haaland JE, Lereim P. Femoral shortening in total hip arthroplasty for high developmental dysplasia of the hip. Clin Orthop Relat Res. 2010;468(7):1949–55.
25. Rosenstein AD, Diaz RJ. Challenges and solutions for total hip arthroplasty in treatment of patients with symptomatic sequelae of developmental dysplasia of the hip. Am J Orthop (Belle Mead NJ). 2011;40(2):87–91.
26. Swanson MA, Huo MH. Total hip arthroplasty in the ankylosed hip. J Am Acad Orthop Surg. 2011;19(12):737–45.
27. Yun AG, Figgie M, Dorr LD, Scott RD. Hip disease in juvenile rheumatoid arthritis. Orthopedics. 2006;29(3):233–9.
28. Zhang H, Huang Y, Zhou YX, Zhou YX, Lv M, Jiang ZH. Acetabular medial wall displacement osteotomy in total hip arthroplasty: a technique to optimize the acetabular reconstruction in acetabular dysplasia. J Arthroplasty. 2005;20(5):562–7.

8 Revision Total Hip Arthroplasty

Matthew P. Abdel

Take-Home Message

- The most common indications for revision total hip arthroplasty (THA) include osteolysis, polyethylene wear, aseptic loosening, instability, and infection.
- Infection must be ruled out before proceeding with revision THA.
  - ESR, CRP, and aspiration (*WBC count above 1,700–3,000 cells/μL and/or neutrophil count >65–80 %*).
- Dislocation is the most common complication of revision THA.

Indications for Revision

- Septic
- Aseptic
  - Osteolysis
  - Polyethylene wear
  - Loosening
  - Instability
  - Malpositioned components
  - Adverse local tissue response
    - Metal-on-metal (MoM) articulations
    - Modular necks

Assessment

- History
  - Previous infection, draining wound, or revision procedure?
  - Query most recent antibiotic use.
  - Symptoms
    - *Groin pain → acetabulum*
    - *Thigh pain → femoral component*
    - *Start-up pain → component loosening*
    - *Night pain or pain at rest → infection*
- Physical examination
  - Appearance of wound
  - Range of motion (ROM)
  - Strength (particularly hip flexors and hip abductors)
- Laboratory analysis
  - ESR
  - CRP
  - CBC with differential
  - Aspiration
    - Obtain if infectious laboratories are not normal.
    - Send aspiration for cell count with differential and cultures.
    - Increased suspicion if WBC count is above *1,700–3,000 cells/μL and/or neutrophil count >65–80 %.*

Imaging

- Radiographs
  - AP pelvis
  - Orthogonal views of the involved hip

  - Full-length femur radiographs vs. hip-to-ankle radiograph
  - *Judet views if concerned about columns and/or pelvic discontinuity*
  - Prior radiographs
    - Pre-index surgical intervention radiographs
    - Immediate radiograph after primary procedure
- Computerized tomography (CT)
  - Useful to determine extent of bone loss and osteolysis (usually underestimated by radiographs)
  - Allows for accurate assessment of component position (particularly version)
- Magnetic resonance imaging (MRI) with metal suppression technique
  - Essential in any suspected adverse local tissue reaction case (i.e., MoM, modular necks, etc.)
  - Helpful to assess abductor
  - May also provide information about component positioning

Classifications

- Acetabular deficiency
  - *AAOS classification* of acetabular bone loss
    - Type I (segmental): loss of part of the acetabular rim or medial wall
    - Type II (cavitary): substantial volumetric loss in bone of the acetabular cavity
    - Type III (combined): combination of segmental and cavitary deficiencies
    - Type IV (pelvic discontinuity): complete separation between the superior and inferior acetabulum
      - A: discontinuity with mild segmental or cavitary loss
      - B: discontinuity with moderate to severe segmental or cavitary loss
      - C: discontinuity with prior pelvic irradiation
    - Type V (arthrodesis): hip arthrodesis
  - *Paprosky classification* of acetabular bone loss
    - Type I: Mild deformity with an intact rim; no femoral head migration; no ischial osteolysis; intact Kohler's line
    - Type II: <3 cm of femoral head center migration
      - A: Superior dome bone lysis but with an intact superior rim; no ischial osteolysis; intact Kohler's line
      - B: Loss of superior rim but with superolateral migration; mild ischial osteolysis; intact Kohler's line
      - C: Loss of superior dome with destruction of the medial wall; mild ischial osteolysis; disrupted Kohler's line

- Type III: > 3 cm of femoral head center migration
  - A: significant superior bone loss with superolateral cup migration; moderate ischial osteolysis; intact Kohler's line
  - B: significant bone loss with superomedial cup migration; severe ischial osteolysis; disrupted Kohler's line

- Femoral deficiency
  - *AAOS classification* of femoral bone loss
    - Type I (segmental): loss of supportive femoral cortical shell
    - Type II (cavitary): loss of endosteal bone with intact cortical shell
    - Type III (combined): combination of segmental and cavitary bone deficiencies
    - Type IV (malalignment): loss of normal femoral geometry due to prior surgery, trauma, or disease
    - Type V (stenosis): narrowing of the canal due to trauma, hardware, or bony hypertrophy
    - Type VI (femoral deficiency): loss of femoral integrity from fracture or nonunion
  - *Paprosky classification* of femoral bone loss
    - Type I: minimal metaphyseal bone loss
    - Type II: extensive metaphyseal bone loss but with intact diaphysis
    - Type III
      - A: extensive metadiaphyseal bone loss, with at least 4 cm of intact diaphyseal cortical bone
      - B: extensive metadiaphyseal bone loss, with less than 4 cm of intact diaphyseal bone loss
    - Type IV: extensive metadiaphyseal bone loss with a nonsupportive diaphysis

Treatment

- General
  - Acetabular component only
    - Porous-coated hemispherical cup with screws
      - Standard sizing
      - Jumbo cup (at least 6 mm larger than primary component)
    - Porous-coated hemispherical cup with screws and augmentation
      - Tantalum metal augments
      - Bone graft (structural allograft vs. cancellous bone chips)
      - Reconstruction cage

- Femoral component only
  - Primary total hip arthroplasty (THA) stem
  - Uncemented extensively porous-coated stem
  - Uncemented modular fluted, tapered stem
  - Modular oncology components (i.e., proximal femoral replacement)
  - Alternatives
    - Cemented stems
    - Impaction bone grafting
    - Allograft prosthetic composite (APC)
- Both acetabular and femoral components (combination of above techniques)
- Femoral head and liner exchange
  - Indication: eccentric wear of the polyethylene with stable acetabular and femoral component.
    - Pain
    - Instability
    - Rapid, progressive osteolysis
  - Outcome: dislocation is most common complication.
- Two-stage explant and reimplantation
  - Most common treatment method for infections in the USA
  - Requires thorough irrigation and debridement (key portion of procedure), followed by antibiotic spacer placement and IV antibiotics (6 weeks)
  - Reimplant after drug holiday (additional 2–6 weeks) and return of inflammatory markers to normal levels

Complications

- Dislocation (most common)
- Infection
- Nerve palsies
  - Sciatic
  - Femoral (often related to retractor placement)
- Periprosthetic fracture
  - Intraoperative
  - Postoperative
- VTE
  - PE
  - DVT
- Limb length inequalities

Bibliography

1. Berry DJ. Antiprotrusio cages for acetabular revision. Clin Orthop Relat Res. 2004;(420):106–12.
2. Burstein G, Yoon P, et al. Component removal in revision total hip arthroplasty. Clin Orthop Relat Res. 2004;(420):48–54.
3. Della Valle CJ, Berger RA, et al. Cementless acetabular reconstruction in revision total hip arthroplasty. Clin Orthop Relat Res. 2004;(420):96–100.
4. Della Valle C, Parvizi J, et al. Diagnosis of periprosthetic joint infections of the hip and knee. J Am Acad Orthop Surg. 2010;18(12):760–70.
5. Sheth NP, Nelson CL, et al. Acetabular bone loss in revision total hip arthroplasty: evaluation and management. J Am Acad Orthop Surg. 2013;21(3):128–39.
6. Valle CJ, Paprosky WG. Classification and an algorithmic approach to the reconstruction of femoral deficiency in revision total hip arthroplasty. J Bone Joint Surg Am. 2003;85-A(Suppl 4):1–6.

9 Common Complications

Benjamin McArthur

Take-Home Message

- *Infection*:
  - Diagnosis may require multiple adjunct tests (including synovial fluid WBC and %PMNs, synovial fluid culture, and serum CRP and ESR).
  - Gold standard treatment of chronic; deep infection is 2-stage revision.
- *Instability*:
  - In the early postoperative setting, nonoperative management and closed reduction are recommended; must obtain an x-table lateral x-ray to determine direction of dislocation prior to reduction.
  - Patient-specific factors and surgical technique may both contribute.
  - Recurrent instability (>3 dislocations) often requires surgical management.
- *Periprosthetic Fractures*:
  - Vancouver classification is most widely utilized and is useful for descriptive purposes as well as treatment plan.
  - If the stem is loose, then revising the femoral component is always necessary.

- *Osteolysis*:
  - Osteoclast activation via inflammatory cytokines results in periprosthetic bone resorption.
  - Revision for polyethylene wear should be performed in the setting of severe pain secondary to synovitis from particle debris, rapidly progressive polyethylene wear on serial radiographs and symptoms or gross instability from excessive wear.
- *Venous Thromboembolism*
  - Clinical signs of DVT and PE are often subtle requiring a high index of suspicion and adjunct studies (e.g., lower extremity venous Doppler and CT angiography of the chest).
  - Guidelines for appropriate prophylaxis should be followed to reduce risk symptomatic DVT or PE. Recent changes to ACCP guidelines have brought AAOS and ACCP recommendations into better agreement.
- *Neurologic Injury*
  - High-risk populations include: DDH, revision surgery, history of prior surgery (such as acetabular ORIF), and females.
  - Conservative measures and observation are most often recommended unless an obvious, correctable cause of injury, such as an aberrantly placed screw or expanding hematoma can be identified.
- *Vascular Injury*
  - Aberrant screw placement, anterior or inferior capsular release, and aggressive anterior retraction are the most common causes.
  - Awareness of vascular anatomy is paramount to prevention of this dangerous complication.

Infection

- Classification:
  - Positive intraoperative cultures after revision surgery
  - Early acute: discovered within ~30 days of index surgery
  - Late hematogenous: seeding of a previously uninfected implant during bacteremia, resulting in late onset acute infection
  - Late indolent: long standing, discovered more than 1 month after index surgery

- Diagnosis:
  - Clinical history: Pain is most common symptom (may or may not be worse with movement), febrile illness, and wound drainage
  - Adjunct studies:
    - ESR/CRP: sensitivity of ~91 and 95 %, respectively
    - Radiographs: early or rapid osteolysis, as well as periosteal reaction should raise suspicion
    - Nuclear medicine: dual-tracer study with tagged WBC (indium) scan more specific than Tc-99 alone
    - Synovial fluid aspirate:
      - Cell count >1,700
      - Differential >64 % neutrophils
      - Culture (+)
  - Mayo criteria: any 1 of the following defines a PJI
    - Two or more (+) cultures of the same organism from preoperative aspirate or intraoperative tissue samples
    - Intraoperative histopathology with evidence of acute inflammation, >10 PMN per HPF
    - Gross purulence
    - Sinus tract in communication with prosthesis
- Treatment
  - Irrigation, debridement, modular component exchange (e.g., polyethylene), and retention of implanted components:
    - Typically indicated in early acute and within 2 weeks of acute hematogenous infection
    - May be a salvage for late indolent infection in which patient cannot medically tolerate complete revision
  - One-stage revision: removal of components and any cement, when present followed by thorough irrigation and debridement and reimplantation of components
    - May be useful in comorbid patients who are unlikely to withstand 2-stage reconstruction
  - Two-stage revision: removal of components and any cement when present, thorough irrigation and debridement, insertion of antibiotic cement spacer (4 g antibiotic recommended per bag of cement, though protocol differs by institution)
    - ~6 weeks of IV antibiotics
    - Second-stage revision can be performed after repeat aspiration (done 2 weeks after antibiotics are stopped) is negative; *gold standard for treatment of late, deep infection.*

  - Antibiotic suppression: lifelong oral antibiotic suppression
    - After multiple failed revisions
    - After limited debridement in comorbid patient

Instability

- Incidence: 2–3 % after primary THA, closer to 10 % after revision
  - Increased risk in alcoholic patients, neurologically impaired, patients with rheumatoid arthritis, female gender, and history of prior surgery.
  - Posterior approach without posterior repair predisposes to posterior instability.
  - Larger femoral heads in revision THR decrease postoperative dislocation.
- Mechanisms:
  - Abductor dysfunction: most important variable in THA stability, functions as "rotator cuff" of the hip; compressive force imparts stability.
    - Causes:
      - Denervation or injury from exposure
      - Inadequate restoration of lever arm via leg length and offset
      - Trochanteric fracture and/or nonunion
      - Necrosis from metal and/or polyethylene wear particles
    - Progressive weakness and atrophy from deconditioning
  - Capsular laxity or failure of capsular repair
    - Especially important with posterior approach, repair of short external rotators and capsular soft tissue as well as quadratus have been noted to enhance stability.
  - Impingement: ROM-induced contact between femoral and acetabular components and/or trochanteric bone impinging with the acetabular component to lever the head out of cup
    - Bony impingement: May be caused by residual osteophytes on the femur or acetabulum or decreased offset after reconstruction (i.e., trochanter impinges on the acetabular component)
    - Component impingement: contact between neck of femoral component and rim of cup
      - Primary arc: degrees of motion present before component neck impinges on rim of cup.
      - Head-neck ratio: Major determinant of primary arc; larger head-neck ratio allows for a greater arc of motion before impingement.

- Excursion distance: distance head will translate after impingement before levering out.
  - Determined primarily by the radius of the head and presence or absence of an elevated liner
- Component alignment: Goal is to maintain primary arc within patients functional ROM so that impingement does not occur with daily activities.
  - Traditional "safe zone" of 40° inclination +/– 10 and 15° anteversion +/– 10 associated with decreased incidence of instability

- Treatment:
  - Nonoperative: Successful in 2/3 of dislocations that occur within 3 months of surgery; less successful in late dislocations.
    - Obtain a x-table lateral x-ray to determine component position and determine direction of dislocation.
    - To reduce a posterior dislocation, flex, adduct, internally rotate, and pull traction.
    - To reduce an anterior dislocation, extend the hip, and externally rotate the hip while pulling longitudinal traction.
    - Debated options for management after closed reduction include:
      - Reinstitution of full posterior hip precautions
      - Abduction bracing
      - Casting
      - Knee immobilizer (for posterior dislocation)
  - Operative methods: indicated after failed nonoperative management (often after 3 dislocations but may proceed sooner if grossly malpositioned components); obtain x-table lateral or CT scan to determine component positioning prior to deciding operative treatment.
    - Correction of component malpositioning: most frequently encountered malposition is acetabular retroversion.
    - Larger head: increase primary arc.
    - Dual mobility component: head is constrained within a mobile bearing polyethylene, increases effective head-neck ratio.
    - Constrained component: head locks into fixed polyethylene, requires significant force to dislocate.
      - Increased force transmission to components associated with risk for earlier fixation failure
      - Recommended for cases of a well-fixed and well-positioned acetabular component.
      - Constrained component use prior to osseointegration can cause early failure and loosening.

Periprosthetic Fractures

- Classification: Vancouver classification is most widely utilized.
  - *Vancouver A*: trochanteric fractures
    - A_g: greater trochanter
    - A_l: lesser trochanter
  - *Vancouver B*: fractures at the level of the stem or tip of the stem
    - B_1: well-fixed component
    - B_2: loose component
    - B_3: severe proximal osteolysis, minimal proximal bone stock, and loose component
  - *Vancouver C*: fracture well distal to the tip of the stem with well-fixed stem
- Treatment
  - A_g: Nonoperative with abduction precautions (i.e., no active abduction); can consider open reduction, internal fixation (ORIF) with large displacement and abductor dysfunction
  - A_l: Nonoperative unless the calcar is compromised requiring a calcar replacing prosthesis
  - B1: Open reduction internal fixation with retention of components +/– cortical strut allograft
  - B2: Revision to longer stemmed femoral component with diaphyseal fixation distal to the fracture + ORIF
  - B3: Revision with structural strut allograft, tumor prosthesis such as proximal femoral replacement or alloprosthetic composite (APC), + ORIF
  - C: ORIF

Osteolysis

- Pathophysiology:
  - Particle induced:
    - Particulate debris from articulation (including metal ions, cement, and especially polyethylene) is phagocytosed by macrophages (or lymphocytes in the case of metal debris).
    - Proinflammatory cytokines TNF-α and IL-1β signaling cascade are initiated.
    - Osteoclast activation and recruitment occur, and periprosthetic bone is resorbed.
  - Fluid pressure induced: Fluid pressure and flow around a prosthesis have also been noted to induce bone resorption in animal models in the absence of particles. The signaling cascade involved in this pathway is less well defined.

- Classification:
  - Zones of osteolysis
    - *Gruen Zones*: zones of resorption around the femoral stem numbered 1–7 progressing counterclockwise around the stem from superolateral (greater trochanter) to superomedial (lesser trochanter)
    - *DeLee-Charnley zones*: zones of resorption around the acetabular component. Numbered 1–3 progressing from superolateral (ilium) to inferomedial (ischium)
  - Paprosky classification of bone loss
    - Femur:
      - *Type I*: minimal loss of metaphyseal cancellous bone, intact diaphysis.
      - *Type II*: extensive loss of metaphyseal bone, intact diaphysis.
      - *Type IIIA*: metaphysis nonsupportive, ≥4 cm of intact diaphysis proximal to isthmus for fixation.
      - *Type IIIB*: metaphysis nonsupportive, <4 cm of intact diaphysis proximal to isthmus.
      - *Type IV*: extensive metadiaphyseal damage with widened femoral canal, isthmus is nonsupportive.
    - Acetabulum: based on 4 variables
      - Migration of hip center of rotation relative to superior obturator line
      - Degree of teardrop destruction
      - Ischial osteolysis
      - Integrity of Kohler's line

Type	Center of rotation migration	Ischial osteolysis	Kohler's line	Teardrop
I	None	None	Intact	Intact
IIA	Mild (<3 cm)	None	Intact	Intact
IIB	Moderate (<3 cm)	Mild	Intact	Intact
IIC	Mild (<3 cm)	Mild	Disrupted	Moderate lysis
IIIA	Severe (>3 cm)	Moderate	Intact	Moderate lysis
IIIB	Severe (>3 cm)	Severe	Disrupted	Severe lysis

- Management:
  - Well-fixed prosthesis with evidence of osteolysis and no symptoms:
    - Close monitoring with more frequent follow-up and radiographs.

- Reasons for revising a component for polyethylene wear include: severe pain, symptoms or evidence of instability, rapidly progressive osteolysis in which the surgeon has determined delaying revision may compromise component fixation or result in fracture.
  - Treatment consists of liner exchange (if components are modular and exchangeable) +/– morselized bone grafting with either allograft or autograft to fill the osteolytic defects.

- Loose prosthesis:
  - Femoral component revision:
    - *Proximal porous-coated stem*: rarely advisable in revision for osteolysis except for Paprosky I or II defects only.
    - *Fully porous-coated stem*: Paprosky II or IIIA with minimum of 4 cm scratch fit in diaphyseal bone.
    - *Modular fluted tapered stem*: Paprosky II (S-ROM), IIIA or IIIB defects, able to gain stable fixation with smaller segment of diaphyseal press fit.
    - *Nonmodular, tapered, fluted stem*: Paprosky II, IIIA, IIIB; particularly useful for IIIB defects with intact lesser trochanter anatomy but <4 cm of isthmus; flutes allow for rotational stability and require only 2 cm of isthmus for stability.
    - *Impaction bone grafting*: Paprosky IIIA, IIIB, or IV if defect contained, technically demanding, allows reconstitution of bone stock.
    - *Alloprosthetic Composite* Paprosky IV defects, technically demanding, allows fixation of abductors to proximal femoral allograft, improved bone stock.
    - *Proximal femoral replacement*: Paprosky IV defects in elderly or low physical demand patients
  - Acetabular component:
    - *Noncemented hemispheric cup*: Paprosky I, II , or IIIA defects; column and some rim support required; supplement with screws; most commonly used treatment option for revision THA.
    - *Impaction grafting and cemented cup*: may restore bone stock for simple cavitary defects.
    - *Structural allograft*: bulk allograft (i.e., femoral head) may restore bone stock, but resorption and loss of fixation can be problematic; infection risk is also higher.
    - *Modular porous metal augments*: allow for biologic fixation, augments screwed to pelvis, unitized to porous-coated cup with cement.
    - *Ring and cage*: roof reinforcement ring or anti-protrusio cages can be used as scaffold with fixation into ilium and/or ischium in conjunction with bone grafting. Cup cemented into cage.

- *Cup cage*: porous-coated cup with or without porous metal augments and spanning ilioischial cage, can be used for Paprosky IIIA, IIIB, and pelvic discontinuity.
- *Oblong cup*: may be useful for superior rim defects.
- *Custom triflange*: CT-based 3D model of pelvis used to create custom porous-coated flanges which allow for rigid fixation of columns, as opposed to flexible cage. Rigid fixation may aid in healing of discontinuity.
- In setting of an *acute discontinuity*, treatment can be *plate fixation and hemispherical acetabular component*; in setting of *chronic discontinuity*, some recommend using a *distraction technique*, with augments and a *jumbo acetabular component*.

Venous Thromboembolism: Deep Venous Thrombosis (DVT) and/or Pulmonary Embolism (PE)

- Most frequent complication following major orthopedic surgery
  - Without prophylaxis, incidence: 50 % DVT, 20 % PE, 2 % fatal PE
- Diagnosis:
  - Clinical exam: limited sensitivity and specificity
    - DVT: classic signs of calf tenderness, swelling, and pain with forced dorsiflexion are present in <30 % of patients.
    - PE: dyspnea noted in ~80 %, chest pain in ~60 %, both in 45 %.
  - Additional studies
    - DVT: Doppler ultrasound or venography
    - PE:
      - EKG: sinus tachycardia most common, also can see new right bundle branch block, inverted T-waves in V1–V3, or "S1Q3T3" pattern, which is less common but considered characteristic
      - ABG: pulmonary alveolar-arterial oxygen gradient >20 mmHg
        CXR: primarily rules out other etiology for hypoxia. The classic focal hyperlucency "Westermark's Sign" is rarely seen.
      - CT chest with IV contrast: allows for rapid diagnosis. May be problematic for patients with contrast allergy or impaired renal function.
      - Ventilation/perfusion scan: nuclear medicine scan identifies mismatch between ventilation and perfusion and assesses probability of PE.
- Treatment
  - Therapeutic anticoagulation: typically at least 3 months for DVT and 6 for PE
    - Coumadin: inhibits vitamin K-dependent factors: II, VII, IX, and X. Also inhibits protein C and S resulting in transient hypercoagulable state at initiation of treatment. Oral administration requires monitoring with PT/INR to titrate dose.

  - Unfractionated heparin: binds antithrombin III and potentiates its effects on thrombin and factor Xa. Intravenous administration requires frequent monitoring with PTT to titrate rate.
  - Low-molecular-weight heparin similar to UF heparin, less effect on thrombin. Subcutaneous injection, does not require monitoring; however, wound complications and bleeding is more common.
  - Factor Xa inhibitors: fondaparinux is a synthetic heparin pentasaccharide administered subcutaneously. Rivaroxaban is a recently approved factor Xa inhibitor which is administered orally.
  - Direct thrombin inhibitors: primarily utilized in the setting of thrombosis related to heparin-induced thrombotic thrombocytopenia (HITT).

– Inferior vena cava filter: advocated by some for a subset of patients.

  - Significant hemorrhagic complications or contraindications to therapeutic anticoagulation
  - Recurrent thromboembolic events in spite of appropriate anticoagulation
  - Lacking physiologic reserve and high risk of mortality with further embolic insult
  - Prolonged immobilization (i.e., pelvic fractures/trauma), especially if undergoing multiple procedures requiring frequent interruptions in pharmacologic anticoagulation

- Prophylaxis guidelines: previously conflict existed between ACCP and AAOS guidelines; however, recent changes in 2012 have brought guidelines into better agreement. Grade of recommendation is based on quality of literature support.

Summary of ACCP 9th, 2012 Edition Recommendations

Grade	Recommendation
1B	Administer one of the following for a minimum of 10–14 days post-op: LMWH; fondaparinux; dabigatran[a], apixaban[a], and rivaroxaban; low-dose unfractionated heparin; adjusted-dose vitamin K antagonist; and aspirin
1B	In patients who decline injections: use apixaban[a] or dabigatran[a]
1B	Do not use Doppler (or duplex) ultrasonography screening before hospital discharge
1C	Use portable, battery-powered, intermittent pneumatic compression device* (IPCD) that records wear time. To be worn for 18 h daily
2B	Extend thromboprophylaxis up to 35 days
2C/2B	Use of LMWH in preference to the other agents
2C	Patients receiving pharmacologic prophylaxis: add IPCD during hospital stay
2C	Patients at increased bleeding risk: IPCD or no prophylaxis
2C	Do not use IVC filter placement for primary prevention in patients with contraindications to pharmacologic and mechanical thromboprophylaxis

[a]Not FDA approved for DVT prophylaxis for total joint replacement

Neurologic Complications: Overall Incidence 1–3 %

- Patients at higher risk:
  - DDH, especially if lengthening >2–3 cm
  - Female gender
  - Revision THR
  - Other prior hip surgery (e.g., acetabular ORIF for fracture)
- Mode of injury:
  - Usually unknown (47 %).
  - Compression: errant or overly aggressive retraction.
  - Ischemia: excessive perineural dissection may put blood supply at risk.
  - Traction: Intraoperative positioning or leg lengthening.
  - Direct trauma or laceration: least common mechanism.
- Nerves affected:
  - Sciatic: Most commonly affected
    - Peroneal division more susceptible to injury than tibial resulting in post-op foot drop.
    - Posterior retraction, posterior column hardware removal, screw penetration of sciatic notch, and leg lengthening are common culprits.
  - Femoral: Second most common
    - Excessive retraction levering off of anterior acetabular wall can induce injury.
    - Ensuring retractor placement deep to iliopsoas tendon is protective.
  - Obturator: relatively uncommon
    - May present late as groin or inguinal pain
  - Superior gluteal: associated with direct lateral or anterolateral approach
    - Intrasubstance division of the gluteus medius greater than 3–4 cm proximal to the tip of the trochanter can result in denervation.
  - Lateral femoral cutaneous: associated with direct anterior approach
    - May present as transient or permanent anterior thigh numbness.
    - Painful neuralgia, "meralgia paresthetica" is rare but can be a source of severe and persistent pain.
- Acute Management
  - Decrease any neural tension:
    - Sciatic nerve: typically knee is flexed with hip mostly extended or only minimally flexed.
    - Femoral nerve: flex hip and knee.

  - Imaging as indicated:
    - Critically assess radiographs for evidence of direct injury, such as errant screw placement.
    - MRI if concern exists for expanding hematoma: typically characterized by initially normal neuroexam which progressively declines, often with increasing pain.
  - Reoperation
    - May be indicated if correctable cause of injury is noted such as aberrant screw placement or expanding hematoma
  - Supportive
    - Pain control for neuralgia
    - Appropriate bracing as indicated
      - AFO for sciatic nerve foot drop
      - Drop lock knee brace for femoral nerve deficit and quad weakness
      - Abduction orthosis for superior gluteal nerve injury and abductor dysfunction
- Prognosis
  - 40 % of patients asymptomatic in 1–2 years
  - 45 % with mild deficit
  - 15 % with major motor or sensory deficit
  - Better prognosis with incomplete injury pattern and some early recovery
  - Worse prognosis with painful dysesthesia and complete motor and sensory block

Vascular Injury: Reported Incidence 0.1–0.2 %

- Increased risk in patients with vascular grafts or atherosclerosis
- External iliac vessels
  - Screw placement in the anterosuperior quadrant
  - Excessively medial placement of retractor over anterior acetabular rim.
    - More proximal placement is protective as greater iliopsoas muscle belly may be interposed between retractor and vessels.
- Common femoral vessels
  - Excessively medial placement of anterior acetabular retractor
  - Anteromedial capsular release from a posterior approach
- Obturator vessels
  - Division of inferior capsule during acetabular exposure
  - Inferior acetabular retractor placement
- Superior gluteal
  - Screw penetration of the sciatic notch

Bibliography

1. Barrack RL. Neurovascular injury: avoiding catastrophe. J Arthroplasty. 2004;19(4 Suppl 1):104–7. Review. PubMed PMID: 15190562.
2. Barrack RL. Current guidelines for total joint VTE prophylaxis: dawn of a new day. J Bone Joint Surg Br. 2012;94(11 Suppl A):3–7. doi:10.1302/0301-620X.94B11.30824. Review. PubMed PMID: 23118370.
3. Brown GA. Venous thromboembolism prophylaxis after major orthopaedic surgery: a pooled analysis of randomized controlled trials. J Arthroplasty. 2009;24(6 Suppl):77–83. doi:10.1016/j.arth.2009.06.002. Epub 2009 Jul 22. Review. PubMed PMID: 19628366.
4. DeHart MM, Riley Jr LH. Nerve injuries in total hip arthroplasty. J Am Acad Orthop Surg. 1999;7(2):101–11. Review. PubMed PMID: 10217818.
5. Della Valle CJ, Di Cesare PE. Complications of total hip arthroplasty: neurovascular injury, leg-length discrepancy, and instability. Bull Hosp Joint Dis. 2001–2002;60(3–4):134–42. Review. PubMed PMID: 12102400.
6. Della Valle CJ, Paprosky WG. The femur in revision total hip arthroplasty evaluation and classification. Clin Orthop Relat Res. 2004;420:55–62. PubMed PMID: 15057079.
7. Della Valle CJ, Steiger DJ, Di Cesare PE. Thromboembolism after hip and knee arthroplasty: diagnosis and treatment. J Am Acad Orthop Surg. 1998;6(6):327–36. Review. PubMed PMID: 9826416.
8. Duncan CP, Masri BA. Fractures of the femur after hip replacement. Instr Course Lect. 1995;44:293–304. Review. PubMed PMID: 7797866.
9. Fahlgren A, Bostrom MP, Yang X, Johansson L, Edlund U, Agholme F, Aspenberg P. Fluid pressure and flow as a cause of bone resorption. Acta Orthop. 2010;81(4):508–16. doi:10.3109/17453674.2010.504610. PubMed PMID: 20718695; PubMed Central PMCID: PMC2917576.
10. Gaski GE, Scully SP. In brief: classifications in brief: Vancouver classification of postoperative periprosthetic femur fractures. Clin Orthop Relat Res. 2011;469(5):1507–10. doi:10.1007/s11999-010-1532-0. Review. PubMed PMID: 20809166; PubMed Central PMCID: PMC3069264.
11. Haake DA, Berkman SA. Venous thromboembolic disease after hip surgery. Risk factors, prophylaxis, and diagnosis. Clin Orthop Relat Res. 1989;242:212–31. Review. PubMed PMID: 2468437.
12. Hanssen AD, Rand JA, Osmon DR. Treatment of the infected total knee arthroplasty with insertion of another prosthesis. The effect of antibiotic-impregnated bone cement. Clin Orthop Relat Res. 1994;309:44–55. PubMed PMID: 7994976.
13. Johnson AJ, Zywiel MG, Stroh A, Marker DR, Mont MA. Serological markers can lead to false negative diagnoses of periprosthetic infections following total knee arthroplasty. Int Orthop. 2011;35(11):1621–6. doi:10.1007/s00264-010-1175-5. Epub 2010 Dec 23. PubMed PMID: 21181540; PubMed Central PMCID: PMC3193961.

14. Leone JM, Hanssen AD. Management of infection at the site of a total knee arthroplasty. Instr Course Lect. 2006;55:449–61. Review. PubMed PMID: 16958480. Joint Replacement Arthroplasty. 4th ed. Philadelipia: Lipincott Williams & Wilkins, 2011. 653–735. Print.
15. Lewinnek GE, Lewis JL, Tarr R, Compere CL, Zimmerman JR. Dislocations after total hip-replacement arthroplasties. J Bone Joint Surg Am. 1978;60(2):217–20. PubMed PMID: 641088.
16. Manganelli D, Palla A, Donnamaria V, Giuntini C. Clinical features of pulmonary embolism. Doubts and certainties. Chest. 1995;107(1 Suppl):25S–32. Review. PubMed PMID: 7813325.
17. Masri BA, Meek RM, Duncan CP. Periprosthetic fractures evaluation and treatment. Clin Orthop Relat Res. 2004;420:80–95. Review. PubMed PMID:15057082.
18. Merkel KD, Erdmann JM, McHugh KP, Abu-Amer Y, Ross FP, Teitelbaum SL. Tumor necrosis factor-alpha mediates orthopedic implant osteolysis. Am J Pathol. 1999;154(1):203–10. PubMed PMID: 9916934; PubMed Central PMCID: PMC1853441.
19. Nachbur B, Meyer RP, Verkkala K, Zürcher R. The mechanisms of severe arterial injury in surgery of the hip joint. Clin Orthop Relat Res. 1979;141:122–33. PubMed PMID: 477093
20. Palestro CJ. Radionuclide imaging after skeletal interventional procedures. Semin Nucl Med. 1995;25(1):3–14. Review. PubMed PMID: 7716556.
21. Pellicci PM, Bostrom M, Poss R. Posterior approach to total hip replacement using enhanced posterior soft tissue repair. Clin Orthop Relat Res. 1998;355:224–8. PubMed PMID: 9917607.
22. Schmalzried TP, Amstutz HC, Dorey FJ. Nerve palsy associated with total hip replacement. Risk factors and prognosis. J Bone Joint Surg Am. 1991;73(7):1074–80. PubMed PMID: 1874771.
23. Schmalzried TP, Noordin S, Amstutz HC. Update on nerve palsy associated with total hip replacement. Clin Orthop Relat Res. 1997;344:188–206. Review. PubMed PMID: 9372771.
24. Segawa H, Tsukayama DT, Kyle RF, Becker DA, Gustilo RB. Infection after totalknee arthroplasty. A retrospective study of the treatment of eighty-one infections. J Bone Joint Surg Am. 1999;81(10):1434–45. PubMed PMID: 10535593.
25. Sheth NP, Nelson CL, Springer BD, Fehring TK, Paprosky WG. Acetabular bone loss in revision total hip arthroplasty: evaluation and management. J Am Acad Orthop Surg. 2013;21(3):128–39. doi:10.5435/JAAOS-21-03-128. PubMed PMID: 23457063.
26. Trampuz A, Hanssen AD, Osmon DR, Mandrekar J, Steckelberg JM, Patel R. Synovial fluid leukocyte count and differential for the diagnosis of prosthetic knee infection. Am J Med. 2004;117(8):556–62. PubMed PMID: 15465503.

Knee Reconstruction

Robert Burns, Natalie L. Zusman, Michael B. Cross, Alexander S. McLawhorn, Rachel M. Frank, Bryan D. Haughom, Peter K. Sculco, Matthew P. Abdel, Brandon J. Erickson, Michael Hellman, Nicolas M. Fort, and Natalie L. Zusman

R. Burns, BS (✉) • N.L. Zusman, BS
Hospital for Special Surgery New York, New York, USA

M.B. Cross, MD
Department of Adult Reconstruction, Hospital for Special Surgery, New York, NY, USA

A.S. McLawhorn, MD, MBA
Department of Orthopaedic Surgery, Hospital for Special Surgery, New York, NY, USA

R.M. Frank, MD
Department of Orthopaedic Surgery, Rush University Medical Center, Rush University Medical Center Chicago, IL, USA

B.D. Haughom, MD
Department Orthopaedic Surgery, Rush University, Chicago, IL, USA

P.K. Sculco, MD
Adult Reconstruction Joint Replacement, Hospital for Special Surgery, New York, NY, USA

M.P. Abdel, MD
Department Orthopaedic Surgery, Mayo Clinic, Rochester, MN, USA

B.J. Erickson, MD
Rush University Medical Center, Chicago, IL, USA

M. Hellman, MD
Rush University Medical Center, Chicago, IL, USA

N.M. Fort, BS
Weill Cornell Medical College, New York, NY, USA

N.L. Zusman, BS

C. Mauffrey, D.J. Hak (eds.), *Passport for the Orthopedic Boards and FRCS Examination*, DOI 10.1007/978-2-8178-0475-0_37

1 Principles of Total Knee Arthroplasty

Robert Burns, Natalie L. Zusman and Michael B. Cross

Take-Home Message

- The primary goal in total knee arthroplasty (TKA) procedures is to provide patients with pain relief and improve function through implantation of a stable prosthesis.
- Variations in implant designs include posterior stabilized (PS), cruciate retaining (CR), bicruciate substituting (BCS), and ACL/PCL retaining.
- Basic principles of TKA: balance of the soft tissues, equalization of flexion and extension gaps, and restoration of the mechanical axis, joint line, and patellofemoral alignment and mechanics.

Indications and Contraindications

- Primary indication: end-stage degenerative osteoarthritis (primary, posttraumatic, secondary to avascular necrosis, osteochondritis, or sepsis).
- Additional indications include inflammatory arthropathies, osteonecrosis, tumor, and fracture.
- Contraindications: preexisting sepsis or infections (including osteomyelitis) either at knee or distant site and severe vascular disease.

Radiography

- Plain radiographs of the knee should include weight-bearing anteroposterior (AP), lateral (at 30° of flexion), PA flexed (or alternatively a tunnel view), and merchant views of the involved knee, as well as a long-leg hip-to-ankle standing AP radiograph of both limbs to assess asymmetry and mechanical and anatomic limb axes.
- AP and lateral plain radiographs of the hips may be indicated in the context of symptoms of groin pain, stiffness, or limited range of motion or may be indicated for severe knee pain with normal knee radiographs.
- Magnetic resonance imaging (MRI) may be indicated to evaluate meniscal and ligament integrity.

Templating

- The purpose of preoperative templating is to assist the surgeon in selecting an appropriate implant design and size of the femoral and tibial component, as well as assess the patient's deformity and mechanical versus anatomic axis.
- Tibiofemoral angles: Assess the degree of malalignment and/or deformity using a standing AP radiograph:
    - Anatomic tibiofemoral angle: angle formed from the shaft axis of the femur to the tibia

  - Mechanical: angle formed from the femoral mechanical axis to the tibial shaft axis

- The goal is to template for placing the tibial component at 90° to the anatomic-mechanical axis to model the normal joint line during the gait cycle.

Implant Designs

- *Total knee replacement*: The two most common implant designs are the posterior stabilized (PS) and cruciate retaining (CR). Meta-analyses have shown no difference in implant type with regard to postoperative extension angle, patient satisfaction, complications (such as anterior knee pain), short- and long-term knee society outcomes (pain and function), as well as similar prosthesis survivorship. The most significance difference between the two implant designs is the *greater flexion angle and increased range of motion in the PS design as compared to the CR design.*
  - *Posterior-stabilized implant*

Advantages	Disadvantages
Less technically demanding	Patella clunk syndrome (esp early designs)
Increased range of motion	Tibial post fracture
Predictable knee kinetics	Impingement
Restricted axial rotation and condylar translation	

  - *Cruciate-retaining implant*: indicated for patients with a functional posterior cruciate ligament, younger age, and more active lifestyle

Advantages	Disadvantages
Bone preservation	Sagittal laxity/tightness
	Potential paradoxical rollback
Increased proprioception	Less flexion
	Tibial bearing damage (shear)

Implant Fixation

- *Cemented:* A static fixation without osseointegration potential that provides immediate mechanical stability in the acute postoperative period. Cemented implants are indicated for patients with poor bone quality.
- *Non-cemented:* Biologic interface between the native bone and the implant. A non-cemented implant may be indicated in patients with adequate bone quality. Two non-cemented implant options include hydroxyapatite coating or high-porosity trabecular metal, which function by encouraging bony ingrowth at the implant-bone interface. Traditionally, non-cemented components had a high failure rate, especially on the tibial side.
- *Hybrid fixation:* The femoral (or tibial) component is cementless, while the tibial (or femoral) and patellar components are cemented.

Surgical Approaches

- *Medial parapatellar approach*:
  - Overview: most common approach
  - Advantages:
    - Good exposure to all three compartments.
    - Facilitates difficult primary TKA and is recommended for revision TKA.
    - Rectus snip can be easily used in cases of a difficult exposure.
  - Disadvantages: potential disruption to extensor mechanism
- *Midvastus approach*:
  - Overview:
    - Vastus medialis fibers split parallel.
    - Patellar eversion.
  - Advantages:
    - Preservation of the patellar vasculature
    - Preservation of the vastus medialis insertion on quadriceps tendon
    - Potentially allows for accelerated rehabilitation
    - Reduced need for lateral retinacular release
  - Disadvantages:
    - Disruption of the vastus medialis.
    - Articular surface exposure can be inferior in obese patients compared to separating the vastus medialis and quadriceps.
  - Contraindications:
    - Less than 80° of preoperative knee motion
    - Hypertrophic arthritis
    - Previous high tibial osteotomy
    - Obesity
- *Subvastus ("southern") approach*:
  - Overview:
    - Incision is made inferior to the vastus medialis.
    - Elevation of the vastus medialis from the medial intermuscular septum.
    - Patellar eversion.
  - Advantages:
    - Preservation of the patellar vasculature
    - Preservation of the extensor mechanism

    - Reduced need for lateral retinacular release
    - Earlier clinical recovery
  - Disadvantages:
    - Exposure is less predictable.
    - Increased difficulty everting patella.
  - Contraindications:
    - Obesity
    - Muscular thighs
    - Patients with marked deformity in knee
    - Revision TKA
    - Previous knee arthrotomy

- *Lateral parapatellar approach*:
  - Overview:
    - Primary indication is severe valgus deformity (common deformity in rheumatoid arthritis).
    - Lateral arthrotomy starts lateral to the quadriceps tendon and extends 1–2 cm lateral to the patella and through the medial edge of Gerdy's tubercle, ending in the anterior compartment fascia.
    - Iliotibial band release/lengthening.
    - Medial patellar eversion.
  - Advantages:
    - Direct exposure to the pathological features of the valgus deformity
    - Improved patellar tracking via preservation of the *vastus medialis*
    - *No need for lateral release*
    - Minimal risk of patellar avascular necrosis because of preservation of medial blood supply
  - Disadvantages:
    - Difficult to address medial pathology.
    - The *common peroneal nerve* is at risk for damage during this approach.
    - The *lateral meniscus* may be incised accidentally if arthrotomy is performed too close to the joint line.
    - Increased difficulty medially everting the patella.
  - Contraindications:
    - Fixed varus deformity

Complications

- *Arterial injury*: The prevalence of arterial injury following TKA is 0.03–0.17 % and most commonly involves the popliteal artery. The major risk factor is preexisting peripheral arterial disease, and the risk is compounded by the use of a tourniquet during the procedure.*Arthrofibrosis:* Stiffness after TKA, also termed arthrofibrosis, prevalence ranges in the literature from 1 to 25 %. Proposed risk factors include poor preoperative range of motion, previous operations, diabetes, depression, and poor patient education; perioperative, surgeon technique and operative time; and postoperative, infection and poor pain control and patient compliance with physiotherapy.
- *Aseptic loosening*: Aseptic loosening is one of the most common reasons for revision TKA and is best diagnosed by radiographic presence of radiolucent lines around the components, periprosthetic fractures, and *changes in component positions in successive radiographs.*
- *Mortality*: Incidence of mortality has been reported as 0.2 % at 20 days and 1.6 % at 1 year postoperative. Independent predictors of mortality include increased patient age, diabetes, and simultaneous bilateral TKA.
- *Peroneal nerve injury*: The prevalence of common peroneal nerve palsy is 0.3–9.5 %, although these numbers are thought to be underestimates of the true prevalence given the wide spectrum of nerve injury presentations. Controversy surrounds proposed risk factors, but some are thought to be younger age, higher body mass index, preoperative valgus deformity, preoperative flexion contracture, and duration of perioperative tourniquet use.

Bibliography

1. American Association of Orthopedic Surgeons Board of Directors. Treatment of osteoarthritis of the knee: evidence based guideline 2nd ed. American Academy of Orthopaedic Surgeons; 2013. Website. http://www.aaos.org/research/guidelines/GuidelineOAKnee.asp. Accessed 15 Jul 2014.
2. Bercik MJ, Joshi A, Parvizi J. Posterior cruciate-retaining versus posterior-stabilized total knee arthroplasty: a meta-analysis. J Arthroplasty. 2013;28(3):439–44.
3. Brown TE, Harper BL, Bjorgul K. Comparison of cemented and uncemented fixation in total knee arthroplasty. Orthopedics. 2013;36(5):380–7.
4. Chmell MJ, Moran MC, Scott RD. Periarticular fractures after total knee arthroplasty: principles of management. J Am Acad Orthop Surg. 1996;4(2):109–16.
5. Feeley BT, Gallo RA, Sherman S, Williams RJ. Management of osteoarthritis of the knee in the active patient. J Am Acad Orthop Surg. 2010;18(7):406–16.
6. Hoppenfeld S, deBoer P, Buckley R, editors. Surgical exposures in orthopaedics: the anatomic approach. 4th rev. ed. Philadelphia: Lippincott Williams & Wilkins; 2009.

7. Hsu HP, Garg A, Walker PS, et al. Effect of knee component alignment on tibial load distribution with clinical correlation. Clin Orthop Relat Res. 1989;248: 135–44.
8. Li N, Tan Y, Deng Y, Chen L. Posterior cruciate-retaining versus posterior-stabilized total knee arthroplasty: a meta-analysis of randomized controlled trials. Knee Surg Sports Traumatol Arthrosc. 2014;22(3):556–64.
9. Lie SA, Engesaeter LB, Havelin LI, et al. Early postoperative mortality after 67,548 total hip replacements: Causes of death and thromboprophylaxis in 68 hospitals in Norway from 1987 to 1999. Acta Orthop Scand. 2002;73:392–9.
10. Lonner JH, Lotke PA. Aseptic complications after total knee arthroplasty. J Am Acad Orthop Surg. 1999;7:311–24.
11. Nelson CL, Kim J, Lotke PA. Stiffness after total knee arthroplasty. J Bone Joint Surg Am. 2005;87(S1):264–70.
12. Ranawat CS Padgett DF, Ohashi Y. Total knee arthroplasty for patients younger than 55 years. Clin Orthop Relat Res. 1989;249:27–33.
14. Schinsky MF, Macaulay W, Parks ML. Nerve injury after primary total knee arthroplasty. J Arthroplasty. 2001;16(8):1048–54.
15. Smith DF, McGraw RW, Taylor DC, et al. Arterial complications and total knee arthroplasty. J Am Acad Orthop Surg. 2001;9:253–7.
16. Williams DH, Garbur DS, Masri BA. Total knee arthroplasty: Techniques and results. BCMJ. 2010;52(9):447–54.

2 Prosthesis Mechanical Alignment, Q Angle

Alexander S. McLawhorn

Take-Home Message

- Restoration of neutral mechanical alignment requires perpendicular cuts to the mechanical axes of the femur and the tibia.
- Femoral component should be lateralized and placed parallel to the neutral rotational axis of the femur (i.e., epicondylar axis) or externally rotated 3° relative to the posterior condylar axis (if using a posterior referencing system); preoperative valgus deformity may require more external rotation of the femoral component if using a posterior referencing system.
- Q angle should be minimized by avoiding internal rotation of the tibial and femoral components, by lateralizing the femoral component, and by placing the patellar component superior and medial.

Alignment Goals

- *Restore near-neutral mechanical coronal alignment* to the lower extremity.
  - Accepted range of coronal alignment is ±*3° from neutral (0°).*
- Mechanical axis should pass through the *central 1/3* of the knee.
- Minimize Q angle.

Preoperative Radiographic Evaluation

- *Standing* AP, flexed PA (the Rosenberg view), hip-to-knee standing alignment, and merchant and lateral radiographs of bilateral knees.
- Identify medial or lateral joint space gapping (can be a sign of collateral ligament insufficiency), subluxation of femur on the tibia (on AP and/or lateral), and bone defects.
- Anticipate the need for ligament releases to balance the knee and/or ↑ prosthetic constraint for MCL/LCL incompetence.
- *Standing full-length radiographs* (AP and lateral) assist in *determining femoral valgus cut angle* if femoral or tibial deformity is present or in very tall (>190 cm) or short (<152 cm) patients.
- Excessive *preoperative deformity and femoral bowing* ↑ risk of postoperative *malalignment.*
- *Merchant* view evaluates *patellofemoral articulation* and articular congruence (patellar tilt).
- Preoperative patellar tilt predicts risk of postoperative tilt.

Long-Leg Alignment

- *Mechanical axis* of limb passes from *center of femoral head to center of ankle* (i.e., center of plafond).
- Normally passes through central 1/3 to slightly medial of knee joint; if passes medial 1/3 = varus alignment; if passes lateral 1/3 = valgus alignment.
- Quantified by *mechanical axis deviation (MAD)*, measured as perpendicular distance from center of knee to mechanical axis of the limb:
  - Normal MAD: *8 ± 7 mm medial to center of knee*
  - Varus MAD: >15 mm medial to center of knee
  - Valgus MAD: >10 mm lateral to center of knee
- *Anatomic tibiofemoral angle* formed by line bisecting femoral diaphysis and a second line bisecting tibial diaphysis; normal angle: *5–7° valgus.*
- *Mechanical tibiofemoral angle* formed by mechanical axes of femur and tibia (see below); normal angle: *1 ± 2° varus.*
- Postoperative neutral mechanical axis permits even load distribution across medial and lateral condyles of prosthesis.

Femoral Alignment

- *Anatomic axis of femur (AAF)* defined by a line bisecting femoral diaphysis.
  - Determines entry point of femoral intramedullary cutting guide, which parallels anatomic axis.
  - Normal distal femur is in *5–7° of anatomic valgus.*
- *Mechanical axis of femur (MAF)* defined by line from center of femoral head to intersection of anatomic axis and intercondylar notch.
- *Valgus cut angle (VCA)* defined as difference between AAF and MAF; normal angle: ~*6°*.
- Template VCA on standing full-length AP radiograph.
- VCA perpendicular to mechanical axis of femur and limb.
- Since proximal femoral offset does not vary significantly from patient to patient, *VCA tends to vary with patient height*; *tall* patients require *VCA <5°*; *short* patients require *VCA >7°*.
- Consider VCA of 3° in valgus knees to "overcorrect" alignment; however, this is surgeon preference rather than an accepted rule.

Tibial Alignment

- *Anatomic axis of tibia (AAT)* defined by line that bisects tibial diaphysis.
- Determines entry point for tibial intramedullary cutting guide.
- *Normal tibia in 2–3° of anatomic varus.*
- *Mechanical axis of tibia (MAT)* defined by line from center of tibia plateau to center of ankle; *usually coincident with AAT, unless tibial deformity.*
- Proximal tibia cut should be perpendicular to mechanical axis of tibia.

Limb Alignment and Implant Survival

- *>3° of tibial component varus* risks early implant failure, usually through medial plateau bone collapse.
- *>8° of femoral component valgus* contributes to early implant failure.
- Historically superior implant survivorship and patient satisfaction for neutral to slightly valgus limb alignment (between 2.5° and 7.4° of *anatomic valgus*).
- Recent literature questions whether modern implant survivorship is improved for TKA aligned ±*3° from neutral (0°)*.
- Excessive *preoperative* malalignment (>8° of varus or >11° of valgus) has ↑ risk of failure; can be incompletely mitigated by postoperative neutral alignment.
- *Soft tissue balance* is also key factor in load distribution across prosthesis and for implant survival.

Q Angle

Anatomy

- *Q angle* is defined as angle between line from anterior-superior iliac spine (ASIS) to center of patella (axis of quadriceps) and second line from center of patella to tibial tuberosity (axis of patellar tendon).
- Normal angle: *11 ± 7°*.
- Varies with patient height; *greater in short patients; less in tall patients.*
- *Larger Q angles ↑ lateral subluxation forces on the patella*; risk for pain, mechanical symptoms, accelerated wear, and dislocation.

Intraoperative Management

Femoral Component

- Can use a combination of anteroposterior (Whiteside's line), transepicondylar, or posterior condylar axes to assess axial femoral rotation.
- *Anteroposterior axis (Whiteside's line)* defined as a perpendicular line from center of trochlear groove to intercondylar notch and the neutral rotational axis (i.e., transepicondylar axis).
- *Transepicondylar axis (TEA)* defined as line connecting medial sulcus (insertion of MCL) and lateral epicondyle; some believe TEA may most consistently produce a balanced flexion gap but is difficult to determine intraoperatively.
- *Posterior condylar axis* defined as line tangent to posterior condyles; in normal knee, 3° internally rotated relative to transepicondylar axis; if lateral femoral condyle hypoplastic, referencing posterior condylar axis internally rotates femoral component.
- Internal rotation of femoral component ↑ Q angle.
- Medialization of femoral component ↑ Q angle.

Tibial Component

- Place tibial component in neutral rotation, centered over *medial 1/3 of tibial tubercle.*
- Internal rotation of tibial component ↑ Q angle, by causing relative external rotation of the tibial tubercle.
- Medialization of tibia component ↑ Q angle.

Patellar Component

- Implant superiorly on patella and/or medialize.
- Medialization ↓ Q angle, but smaller patellar component needed.
- Perform lateral release, if intraoperative lateral subluxation of patella observed during trialing:
  - Required less often with medialization of component.
  - Release the tourniquet prior to performing a lateral release, as tourniquets may cause false subluxation of the patella.

Postoperative Assessment

- *CT scan* is best for assessing malrotation of femoral and tibial components.
  - AP axis of *femoral component* should be perpendicular to *TEA*, and posterior condylar axis of prosthesis should be parallel to TEA:
    - Mild internal rotation (IR) ≤3°.
    - Moderate IR 4–6°.
    - Severe IR ≥6°.
    - ≥4° of IR may benefit from early revision.
  - *Tibial component* rotation defined as angle between a line bisecting the tibial tubercle and a line drawn perpendicular to the posterior aspect of the tibial insert:
    - *Up to 18° of IR* can be normal, based on this measurement technique.
    - ≥27° of IR is usually abnormal and symptomatic.

Bibliography

1. Arima J, Whiteside LA, McCarthy DS, White SE. Femoral rotational alignment, based on the anteroposterior axis, in total knee arthroplasty in a valgus knee. A technical note. J Bone Joint Surg Am. 1995;77(9):1331–4.
2. Bargren JH, Blaha JD, Freeman MA. Alignment in total knee arthroplasty. Correlated biomechanical and clinical observations. Clin Orthop Relat Res. 1983;173:178–83.
3. Berend ME, Ritter MA, Meding JB, Faris PM, Keating EM, Redelman R, Faris GW, Davis KE. Tibial component failure mechanisms in total knee arthroplasty. Clin Orthop Relat Res. 2004;428:26–34.
4. Berger RA, Rubash HE, Seel MJ, Thompson WH, Crossett LS. Determining the rotational alignment of the femoral component in total knee arthroplasty using the epicondylar axis. Clin Orthop Relat Res. 1993;(286):40–7.
5. Bindelglass DF, Cohen JL, Dorr LD. Patellar tilt and subluxation in total knee arthroplasty. Relationship to pain, fixation, and design. Clin Orthop Relat Res. 1993;(286):103–9.
6. Bonner TJ, Eardley WG, Patterson P, Gregg PJ. The effect of post-operative mechanical axis alignment on the survival of primary total knee replacements after a follow-up of 15 years. J Bone Joint Surg Br. 2011; 93(9):1217–22.
7. Cates HE, Ritter MA, Keating EM, Faris PM. Intramedullary versus extramedullary femoral alignment systems in total knee replacement. Clin Orthop Relat Res. 1993;(286):32–9.
8. Deakin AH, Basanagoudar PL, Nunag P, Johnston AT, Sarungi M. Natural distribution of the femoral mechanical-anatomical angle in an osteoarthritic population and its relevance to total knee arthroplasty. Knee. 2012; 19(2):120–3.
9. Fang DM, Ritter MA, Davis KE. Coronal alignment in total knee arthroplasty: just how important is it? J Arthroplasty. 2009;24 (6 Suppl):39–43.

10. Hofmann AA, Tkach TK, Evanich CJ, Camargo MP, Zhang Y. Patellar component medialization in total knee arthroplasty. J Arthroplasty. 1997;12(2):155–60.
11. Hsu RW, Himeno S, Coventry MB, Chao EY. Normal axial alignment of the lower extremity and load-bearing distribution at the knee. Clin Orthop Relat Res. 1990;(255):215–27.
12. Jeffery RS, Morris RW, Denham RA. Coronal alignment after total knee replacement. J Bone Joint Surg Br. 1991;73(5):709–14.
13. Lewonowski K, Dorr LD, McPherson EJ, Huber G, Wan Z. Medialization of the patella in total knee arthroplasty. J Arthroplasty. 1997;12(2):161–7.
14. Mahaluxmivala J, Bankes MJ, Nicolai P, Aldam CH, Allen PW. The effect of surgeon experience on component positioning in 673 press fit condylar posterior cruciate-sacrificing total knee arthroplasties. J Arthroplasty. 2001; 16(5):635–40.
15. Mantas JP, Bloebaum RD, Skedros JG, Hofmann AA. Implications of reference axes used for rotational alignment of the femoral component in primary and revision knee arthroplasty. J Arthroplasty. 1992;7(4):531–5.
16. Marx RG, Grimm P, Lillemoe KA, Robertson CM, Ayeni OR, Lyman S, Bogner EA, Pavlov H. Reliability of lower extremity alignment measurement using radiographs and PACS. Knee Surg Sports Traumatol Arthrosc. 2011; 19(10):1693–8.
17. McGrory JE, Trousdale RT, Pagnano MW, Nigbur M. Preoperative hip to ankle radiographs in total knee arthroplasty. Clin Orthop Relat Res. 2002;(404): 196–202.
18. McPherson EJ. Patellar tracking in primary total knee arthroplasty. Instr Course Lect. 2006;55:439–48.
19. Mullaji AB, Shetty GM, Lingaraju AP, Bhayde S. Which factors increase risk of malalignment of the hip-knee-ankle axis in TKA? Clin Orthop Relat Res. 2013;471(1):134–41.
20. Nagamine R, Whiteside LA, White SE, McCarthy DS. Patellar tracking after total knee arthroplasty. The effect of tibial tray malrotation and articular surface configuration. Clin Orthop Relat Res. 1994;(304):262–71.
21. Nam D, Maher PA, Robles A, McLawhorn AS, Mayman DJ. Variability in the relationship between the distal femoral mechanical and anatomical axes in patients undergoing primary total knee arthroplasty. J Arthroplasty. 2013;28(5): 798–801.
22. Nicoll D, Rowley DI. Internal rotational error of the tibial component is a major cause of pain after total knee replacement. J Bone Joint Surg Br. 2010;92 :1238–44.
23. Parratte S, Pagnano MW, Trousdale RT, Berry DJ. Effect of postoperative mechanical axis alignment on the fifteen-year survival of modern, cemented total knee replacements. J Bone Joint Surg Am. 2010;92(12):2143–9.
24. Petersen TL, Engh GA. Radiographic assessment of knee alignment after total knee arthroplasty. J Arthroplasty. 1988;3(1):67–72.

25. Pietsch M, Hofmann S. Early revision for isolated internal malrotation of the femoral component in total knee arthroplasty. Knee Surg Sports Traumatol Arthrosc. 2012; 20 (6):1057–63.
26. Rand JA, Coventry MB. Ten-year evaluation of geometric total knee arthroplasty. Clin Orthop Relat Res. 1988;232:168–73.
27. Rhoads DD, Noble PC, Reuben JD, Tullos HS. The effect of femoral component position on the kinematics of total knee arthroplasty. Clin Orthop Relat Res. 1993;(286):122–9.
28. Ritter MA, Faris PM, Keating EM, Meding JB. Postoperative alignment of total knee replacement. Its effect on survival. Clin Orthop Relat Res. 1994;(299):153–6.
29. Ritter MA, Davis KE, Meding JB, Pierson JL, Berend ME, Malinzak RA. The effect of alignment and BMI on failure of total knee replacement. J Bone Joint Surg Am. 2011;93(17):1588–96.
30. Ritter MA, Davis KE, Davis P, Farris A, Malinzak RA, Berend ME, Meding JB. Preoperative malalignment increases risk of failure after total knee arthroplasty. J Bone Joint Surg Am. 2013;95(2):126–31.
31. Srivastava A, Lee GY, Steklov N, Colwell Jr CW, Ezzet KA, D'Lima DD. Effect of tibial component varus on wear in total knee arthroplasty. Knee. 2012;19(5):560–3.
32. Whiteside LA, Arima J. The anteroposterior axis for femoral rotational alignment in valgus total knee arthroplasty. Clin Orthop Relat Res. 1995;(321):168–72.

3 Ligament Balancing: Coronal and Sagittal

Rachel M. Frank and Michael B. Cross

Take-Home Message

- Ligament balancing is critical for successful TKA outcomes.
- Sagittal imbalances in *either* the flexion or extension gap can be corrected with altering the *femur* and/or soft tissues, whereas imbalances in *both* the flexion and extension gap can be corrected by altering the *tibia* and/or polyethylene thickness.
- Coronal plane balancing can be achieved by *gradually*, stepwise releasing the contracted *medial* (for *varus* deformity) or *lateral* (for *valgus* deformity) soft tissues.
- An intraoperative flexion contracture can be managed by releasing the posterior capsule and posterior osteophytes and/or resecting more distal femur.
- In general, soft tissues are contracted on the concave side of the deformity and loose/attenuated on the convex side.

Definitions

- "Balanced knee":
  - Full ROM (however the passive *flexion* achievable *postoperative* is dependent on *preoperative motion*)
  - Symmetric medial/lateral balance at full extension, midflexion, and 90° flexion
  - Near-neutral varus/valgus mechanical alignment in extension and flexion
  - Balanced flexion/extension gap without medial/lateral tightness or laxity
  - Well-tracking patella
  - Correct rotation balance between components
- Coronal plane balancing → correcting varus/valgus deformity
- Sagittal plane balancing → correcting (equalizing) flexion/extension gap
- *Gap balancing technique* → Bony resection on the tibia and femur is determined by the intraoperative tension of the ligaments.
- *Measured resection technique* → Bony resection on the tibia and femur is made first, and the ligaments are balanced depending on the bony resection.

Etiology of a Poorly Balanced Knee

- Coronal plane imbalance: Medial or lateral ligamentous complexes become tight and/or stretched depending on deformity.
- Sagittal plane imbalance: Often caused by a progressive flexion contracture deformity from a tight posterior capsule, tight hamstrings, or large posterior osteophytes; improper intraoperative tibial and femoral bone resection can lead to intraoperative sagittal plane imbalance.

Radiography

- Standard AP, lateral, merchant views + the Rosenberg view (45° flexion PA view)
- Bilateral long-leg standing axis films to assess overall limb alignment

Treatment Operative

- Coronal Balancing
  - Varus deformity:
    - Lateral structures on convex side of deformity → attenuated.
    - Medial structures on concave side of deformity → contracted.
    - Goal → Release medial structures, and tighten lateral structures.
    - A near-neutral alignment after the bony resections should be achieved prior to performing soft tissue releases.
    - Algorithm for a gradual medial release:
      - Remove *osteophytes*, meniscus + *capsule* attachments on the medial side of the tibia.
      - Release *deep MCL*:

        - Do *not* release superficial MCL → will result in valgus instability requiring a constrained prosthesis or repair with augmentation.
    - Can release posteromedial corner (*semimembranosus and posteromedial capsule*).
    - Can consider partial superficial MCL release, but should be used with extreme caution:
        - Posterior oblique portion → Release if tight in extension.
        - Anterior portion → Release if tight in flexion.
- Valgus deformity:
    - Lateral structures on concave side of deformity → contracted
    - Medial structures on convex side of deformity → attenuated
    - Goal → Release lateral structures, and tighten medial structures.
    - A near-neutral alignment after the bony resections should be achieved prior to performing soft tissue releases.
    - Lateral release:
        - Remove *osteophytes*, lateral *capsule*.
        - Release *iliotibial band (ITB)* if tight in *extension*.
        - Release *popliteus*/posterolateral corner if tight in *flexion*.
        - Release *lateral collateral ligament (LCL)* if tight in *flexion and extension* → may require a constrained prosthesis.
    - If the *MCL* is *incompetent*, a *constrained* total knee arthroplasty will be required.
    - When releasing the posterolateral corner, be cautious of the *peroneal nerve*.
    - The *inside-out technique* can be used using lamina spreaders and/or tensors to determine which structures are tight on the lateral side of the knee and thus which need releasing.

- *Sagittal Balancing*
    - Traditional teaching in TKA has focused on obtaining equal flexion/extension gap → tibial insert stable through entire arc of motion.
    - Pearls:
        - Symmetric gap (*flexion and extension*) → Adjust *tibia (or polyethylene)*.
        - *Asymmetric* gap → Adjust *femur*.
        - Adjusting femoral component size alters anteroposterior (AP) diameter:
            - Will help with *flexion* gap
            - Does *not* affect prosthesis height → thus does *not* affect extension gap
    - Flexion contracture:
        - Posterior structures on concave side of deformity → contracted.
        - Goal → Carefully release posterior structures.

- Posterior release → can more safely be performed in flexion to allow popliteal artery to fall further out of field:
  - Remove *posterior osteophytes*.
  - Pierce/release *posterior capsule* (e.g., off the posterior femoral condyles).
  - Consider *medial/lateral gastrocnemius* release or *hamstring releases* in rare situations.

– *Strategies for achieving equal flexion and extension gaps:*

- Tight in flexion, tight in extension → Cut more tibia.
- Loose in flexion, loose in extension → Use thicker PE or thicker tibial insert.
- Tight in flexion, balanced in extension → Downsize femoral component.
  - Can also:
    - Release or resess the PCL (for cruciate-retaining designs).
    - Increase the posterior slope in tibia.
    - Resect more posterior femoral condyle (i.e., anteriorize the femoral component).
    - Release posterior capsule (use with caution as this may affect extension gap as well).
- Tight in flexion, loose in extension → Downsize femoral component and use thicker tibial insert.
- Balanced in flexion, tight in extension → Resect more distal femur or release posterior capsule (again, releasing the posterior capsule may also loosen the flexion space).
- Balanced in flexion, loose in extension → Augment distal femur, or distalize the joint line (will require a revision component if augments are used); may also downsize the femoral component (or anteriorize the femoral component) and increase the thickness of the polyethylene.
  - Remember → Altering femoral component size does *not* affect extension gap.
- Loose in flexion, tight in extension → Resect more distal femur, and upsize femoral component.
  - In revisions, can use thinner distal femoral augmentation.
- Loose in flexion, balanced in extension → Upsize femoral component, or increase the size of posterior augments (in revisions).
  - Can also posteriorize femoral component (may require an augment), provided that doing so will not notch the anterior femoral cortex.

Complications

- Correction of severe combined deformity of *valgus + flexion contracture* can lead to *peroneal nerve palsy* from over-lengthening a previously contracted nerve:
  - At baseline in these patients, nerve on concave side → tight
  - With correction of alignment, nerve put on even more stretch
  - Treat in the recovery with immediate knee flexion and removal of dressing:
    - Allow up to 3 months for return of function.
    - Although recovery of function can occur, *complete nerve recovery* occurs in less than *30 %* of patients.
- Posterior release can lead to *popliteal artery injury*.
- A *flexion contracture* present postoperatively, which was corrected intraoperatively, is often due to tight *hamstring* tendons.
- Not balancing flexion gap (if left too loose) in a posterior-stabilized (PS) knee can lead to cam-post dislocation, resulting in a *posterior knee dislocation*.

Arthroplasty Salvage Options for Knees That Have Instability Not Correctable by Soft Tissue Balancing

- *Coronal plane* instability (varus/valgus) – can be treated with a *constrained* prosthesis with a thicker post.
- *Anteroposterior instability with an incompetent extensor mechanism* – requires a *hinge*-type prosthesis with *extensor mechanism reconstruction*.
  - Knee arthrodesis can also be considered.
- *Global* knee instability requires a *hinge*-type prosthesis.

Bibliography

1. Ahn JH, Back YW. Comparative study of two techniques for ligament balancing in total knee arthroplasty for severe varus knee: medial soft tissue release vs. bony resection of proximal medial tibia. Knee Surg Relat Res. 2013; 25:13–8.
2. Babazadeh S, Stoney JD, Lim K, Choong PF. The relevance of ligament balancing in total knee arthroplasty: how important is it? A systematic review of the literature. Orthop Rev (Pavia). 2009;1:e26.
3. Brooks P. Seven cuts to the perfect total knee. Orthopedics. 2009;32(9).
4. Clarke HD, Scott WN. Knee: axial instability. Orthop Clin North Am. 2001;32:627–37, viii.
5. Dennis DA, Komistek RD, Kim RH, Sharma A. Gap balancing versus measured resection technique for total knee arthroplasty. Clin Orthop Relat Res. 2010;468:102–7.

6. Gonzalez MH, Mekhail AO. The failed total knee arthroplasty: evaluation and etiology. J Am Acad Orthop Surg. 2004;12:436–46.
7. Manson TT, Khanuja HS, Jacobs MA, Hungerford MW. Sagittal plane balancing in the total knee arthroplasty. J Surg Orthop Adv. 2009;18:83–92.
8. Mihalko WM, Saleh KJ, Krackow KA, Whiteside LA. Soft-tissue balancing during total knee arthroplasty in the varus knee. J Am Acad Orthop Surg. 2009;17:766–74.
9. Morgan H, Battista V, Leopold SS. Constraint in primary total knee arthroplasty. J Am Acad Orthop Surg. 2005;13:515–24.
10. Verdonk PC, Pernin J, Pinaroli A, Ait Si Selmi T, Neyret P. Soft tissue balancing in varus total knee arthroplasty: an algorithmic approach. Knee Surg Sports Traumatol Arthrosc. 2009;17:660–6.
11. Whiteside LA, Mihalko WM. Surgical procedure for flexion contracture and recurvatum in total knee arthroplasty. Clin Orthop Relat Res. 2002:189–95.
12. Yercan HS, Ait Si Selmi T, Sugun TS, Neyret P. Tibiofemoral instability in primary total knee replacement: a review, part 1: basic principles and classification. Knee. 2005;12:257–66.

4 Implant Designs in TKA

Bryan D. Haughom and Michael B. Cross

Take-Home Message

- TKA implant designs range from relatively *unconstrained* (*cruciate retaining and posterior stabilized*) to more *constrained designs* (*non-hinged and hinged*). Every effort is made to minimize the amount of constraint needed in both primary and revision settings.
- Regardless of design (i.e., degree of constraint), a successful arthroplasty requires stable fixation, near-neutral mechanical alignment, and adequate soft tissue balancing.
- Each design has its unique complications, e.g., *cruciate retaining* (*PCL rupture or late PCL insufficiency*) and *posterior stabilized* (*cam jump (dislocation), post impingement, patellar clunk, and post fracture*).
- With increasing constraint, there is an increasing risk of aseptic loosening due to the increased strain at the interface.

Background

- A number of design options are available in TKA including unconstrained (posterior cruciate ligament [PCL] retaining, i.e., cruciate retaining (CR) and p*osterior stabilized (PS)*) and more *constrained* (with both *hinged and non-hinged* varieties) designs.

- Debate continues with regard to the ideal primary arthroplasty implant, with the PCL remaining at the heart of the controversy. Surgeons are divided into those who routinely sacrifice the PCL, those who retain it, and those who decide based upon the pathology.
- Most surgeons attempt to utilize the least amount of constraint as necessary to provide a stable, well-balanced knee.
- Long-term studies show excellent outcomes (>90 % survival at 10 years) with the use of both cruciate-retaining and posterior-stabilized knees in the setting of primary TKA.
- Constrained TKA plays a more prominent role in the revision setting.
- Despite the continued debate, most surgeons would agree that the most important factors in long-term outcomes are implant stability, restoration of a near-neutral mechanical axis, and soft tissue balancing.

Concepts in Knee Arthroplasty Design

- *Posterior cruciate ligament*:
  - *Primarily functions in the sagittal* plane, preventing relative *posterior subluxation of the tibia*
  - *Secondary* stabilizer to *resist varus angulation and external tibial rotation at 90°*
  - Facilitates *femoral rollback* in knee flexion
- *Femoral rollback*:
  - Characterized by relative posterior translation of the tibiofemoral contact point with knee flexion
    - Occurs primarily on the *lateral* side of the knee
  - Facilitated by the *PCL* in *CR* implants
  - Effectively created by tibial *post-cam* contact in *PS* implants
- *Constraint*:
  - Defined as design elements that provide stability to the knee that offset instability secondary to soft tissue deficiency.
  - Constrained options exist for the *coronal* (i.e., *high tibial post and/or wider post* designs) and *sagittal* (i.e., *hinged* components) instability.
  - Typically reserved for complex primary and revision TKA.
  - Instability is the cause of ~10–25 % of failed TKA, highlighting the importance of appropriately balancing and when necessary utilizing adequate constraint.

Design Options

- In *in*creasing degree of constraint, design options include:
  - Cruciate-retaining (CR) TKA
  - Posterior-stabilized (PS) TKA

- Constrained (non-hinged) TKA
- Constrained (hinged) TKA

Cruciate-Retaining (CR) TKA

- Central to the CR design is the preservation of the PCL. Additional design modifications include a *PCL cut out on the tibial tray* and a *flatter tibial tray* to facilitate femoral rollback.
- Advantages:
  - Retention of a native "central stabilizer" (PCL).
  - Stress is transferred to native tissue, as opposed to the tibial post (in the PS design), potentially avoiding post wear.
  - *Conservation of bone*:
    - Radiographically, one should look for a *lack of a box* on *lateral* radiograph.
  - More consistent joint line (to facilitate PCL tensioning).
  - Preservation of proprioceptive fibers.
  - Some evidence suggests improved function with certain motions (i.e., stair climbing, kneeling, squatting).
- Disadvantages:
  - Some evidence suggests potential for *paradoxical motion* (anterior translation) though this is controversial.
  - Attention should be paid to avoiding over-tightening flexion gap (with PCL retention) which can lead to increased wear:
    - Tibial resection requires greater slope than PS designs.
  - Late instability can develop with rupture of the PCL:
    - Presents with difficulty with stairs, instability, hyperextension, and/or recurrent effusions
  - Relative contraindications:
    - Large deformity correction (flexion contracture or varus/valgus >15°).
    - Inflammatory arthritis.
    - Prior patellectomy (potential increased anteroposterior instability).
    - All of these are debated however in the literature.

Posterior-Stabilized (PS) TKA

- Central to the design of a PS knee is the sacrifice of the PCL. A tibial post articulates with a femoral cam during flexion to facilitate femoral rollback. Additionally, the tibial post serves to prevent posterior tibial subluxation (and resultant "cam jump" or dislocation). Tibial polyethylene is characteristically more congruent in PS designs.

- Advantages:
  - Proponent of PS knees argues balancing is performed with greater ease in comparison to CR knees.
  - Theoretically less "sliding" wear with cam-post flexion kinematics as opposed to CR designs.
  - Some contend deformity correction (large flexion contracture, varus/valgus >15°) easier with PS design.
  - No concern of ligamentous laxity in the setting of inflammatory arthritis or prior PCL injury.
  - Can be used in prior patellectomy patients.
  - Historically was believed that *higher flexion* can be achieved with PS designs:
    - Now most recognize that the biggest determinate of *postoperative flexion angle* is the amount of *preoperative motion.*
- Disadvantages:
  - *Greater bone resection*:
    - The flexion gap increases with PCL sacrifice, resulting in greater femoral resection to adequately balance.
    - Can lead to an elevated joint line and risk of patella baja
  - Risk for elevated joint line (as above)
  - Risk of *dislocation*:
    - Femoral cam jump typically occurs in high flexion (with or without a varus/valgus force). It is characterized by the tibial post translating out of the confines of the femoral cam and posterior subluxation of the tibia. Often caused by a loose flexion gap:

      (a) Treatment is initially *closed reduction.*
      (b) *Revision* required for *recurrent instability.*
  - *Tibial post fracture/wear:*
    - PS designs rely upon cam-post articulation; however, inherent stresses are placed. Polyethylene post is at risk of wear (particularly in hyperextension). Can result in increased osteolysis from post wear.
  - *Patellar clunk*: *pain and audible clunk* associated with the entrapment of hypertrophied nodule (scar) at the proximal pole of the patella in the box. Distinct complication of *earlier PS designs.* Typically occurred at *30–45° flexion.*

Cruciate Retaining Versus Posterior Stabilized

- Despite the fervent dogma surrounding the use of PS and CR knees, studies have shown excellent long-term outcomes with regard to implant survival and patient function in both designs.

Constrained (Non-hinged) TKA

- The primary design features of a constrained non-hinged TKA is a high central post, wider post, and a deep femoral cam box; this acts to provide varus/valgus constraint.
- All constrained (non-hinged) designs are by definition posterior-stabilized designs as well.
- Important implant in complex primary and revision TKA.
- Indications:
  - Severe coronal deformity (particularly valgus deformity)
  - Collateral ligament insufficiency/deficiency
  - Recurrent instability (either midflexion, extension, or flexion in the coronal plane) in the setting of a standard PS or CR implant
  - Persistent flexion/extension imbalance
- Disadvantages:
  - Larger intercondylar notch bone cut needed to facilitate larger tibial post. Results in more bone loss and potential difficulty with revision surgery
  - Increased constraint:
    - *Increased stress* placed at implant-bone/implant-cement *interface*, resulting in *higher risk of aseptic loosening*
    - More stress placed on longer post-cam articulation, with *increased risk of post fracture and polyethylene wear*
  - The use of *stemmed* components to decrease stress at the interface

Constrained (Hinged) TKA

- Hinged TKA components are the most constrained components available on the market. They are characterized by a *linked* articulation at the *tibiofemoral joint*, which controls *sagittal and coronal motion*. Many designs possess a *rotating platform* which allows for *axial rotation.*
- Indications:
  - Severe collateral ligament deficiency
  - Hyperextension instability (i.e., recurvatum)
  - Massive bone loss: periarticular tumor resection, infection, high-energy periarticular trauma, and neuropathic joint
  - Global instability with dislocation
  - Deficient extensor mechanism (including when performing an extensor mechanism allograft)
- Advantages:
  - Affords global stability *(coronal and sagittal)* in the face of soft tissue deficiency
  - Can be used in situations of massive bone loss

- Disadvantages:
  - Risk of *aseptic loosening* is greater with increasing degree of constraint. Higher forces transmitted to bone-cement/bone-implant interface.
  - *Large degree of bone resection* is necessary to implantation. Subsequent revision surgery is more difficult.

  Requires the use of stems.

5 Patellofemoral Joint

Rachel M. Frank

Take-Home Message
- Isolated PF arthritis is often caused by PF instability.
- PF arthritis most commonly occurs in conjunction with TF arthritis, rather than in isolation.
- Treatment options vary, but ultimately many patients require TKA.

Definitions

- Main function of patella → *improve mechanical advantage* of extensor mechanism by increasing lever arm of quadriceps
- Q angle → angle from ASIS to center of patella to tibial tuberosity
  - *Males → 11–17°*
  - *Females → 14–20°*
- Maximum patellofemoral contact → 90° of knee flexion

Etiology

- PF arthritis occurs most commonly with tibiofemoral arthritis rather than in isolation.
- *Risk factors for patella instability* leading to PF arthritis:
  - Patella alta.
  - Trochlear dysplasia.
  - Excessive lateral patellar tilt.
  - Increased Q angle causes lateral shift of patella → increases contact force at PF joint and can lead to patella instability.
  - *Miserable malalignment syndrome* → combination of femoral anteversion, genu valgum, and external tibial torsion:
    - Leads to increased Q angle

- History of inflammatory arthritis (i.e., rheumatoid arthritis).
- History of trauma (i.e., patella fracture).

Pathophysiology

- Changes in articular cartilage → increased water content, increased IL-1 content, increased matrix metalloproteinase (plasmin, stromelysin) levels, increased chondrocyte activity and proliferation, decreased proteoglycan quantity, and decreased collagen quantity and stiffness.
- Changes in subchondral bone → increased thickness, osteophyte development, osteochondral junction breakdown, cyst formation, and microfracture formation.
- Patella cartilage is thick but thought to be less stiff and more compressible than other joints.

Radiography

- Standard AP, lateral, and merchant views:
  - Blumensaat's line (lateral view) → corresponds to roof of intercondylar notch.
    - With knee flexed to 30, line should touch inferior pole of patella.
  - Insall-Salvati ratio (lateral view) → ratio of patellar length (superior to inferior poles) to patella tendon length (inferior pole of patella to tibial tubercle):
    - Normal: between *0.8 and 1.2* (<0.8 suggests patella alta; >0.8 suggests patella baja).
  - Sulcus angle (merchant view) → formed by medial/lateral condyles and deepest point of sulcus, measurement of trochlear depth; *>138° indicates PF dysplasia.*
- Bilateral long-leg standing axis films to assess alignment and Q angle.
- MRI can be helpful in documenting status of patellar/trochlear cartilage to determine appropriateness for cartilage restoration procedures in early disease states.

Treatment

- Nonoperative:
  - Weight loss
  - NSAIDs
  - Injections → corticosteroid ± hyaluronic acid
  - Patella bracing/strapping
  - Physical therapy → quadriceps strengthening (focus on vastus medialis oblique (VMO))
  - Activity modification → avoid provocative knee flexion (deep squatting, stairs)
- Operative:
  - Arthroscopic debridement → controversial
  - Patellofemoral arthroplasty (PFA):

  - Relative indications → *isolated PF compartment disease*, normal alignment, and PF tracking; often performed in younger patients
  - Contraindications: inflammatory arthritis, poor patient understanding of the procedure and risks of future degeneration of the tibiofemoral joint, and severe patellar malalignment or maltracking
  - Improvements in trochlear design from inlay to onlay style have decreased incidence of postoperative patellar instability:
    - Onlay trochlear implant is placed perpendicular to AP axis of femur, so component rotation is not affected by native trochlear inclination.
- TKA:
  - With patella resurfacing:
    - Maintain a post-cut patellar thickness of greater than 12 mm to decrease risk of postoperative fracture.
    - Avoid overstuffing the patella to decrease risk of anterior knee pain.
  - Strict attention to rotational alignment of tibial/femoral components.
  - Aggressive lateral release if necessary (however, often times not required once alignment is corrected).
  - Avoid performing maneuvers that increase the Q angle including:
    - Internal rotation of the tibial component
    - Internal rotation of the femoral component
    - Lateral placement of the patellar component
    - Inferior placement of the patellar component
    - Medial placement of the femoral component
- Patellectomy:
  - Rarely performed due to 25–50 % reduction in knee extension strength and increased tibiofemoral contact forces
- Tibial tubercle osteotomy ± lateral release (for early OA):
  - Anteriorization (Maquet osteotomy)
  - Anteromedialization (AMZ, Fulkerson osteotomy):
    - *Anteriorization* → elevates distal extensor mechanism and shifts *patellar contact forces proximally*
    - *Medialization → decreases lateral force vector*
    - *Contraindicated* in patients with significant medial facet OA (as well as medial femoral condyle OA)
- Cartilage restoration (for focal grade IV osteochondral defects in young patients):
  - Microfracturing
  - Autologous chondrocyte implantation (ACI):
    - Improved outcomes when performed concurrently with AMZ compared to when performed in isolation

    - Osteochondral allograft/autograft:
        - Regardless of lesion size, better than microfracture and ACI if there is subchondral bone marrow edema present on MRI
- Patellectomy:
    - Salvage, last resort only

Treatment Algorithm

- Young patient with isolated patellar or trochlear defect → realignment + cartilage restoration
- Young patient with mild PF disease → nonoperative management
- Young patient with severe, isolated PF disease → consider PFA versus TKA
- Patient with severe PF disease + mild-moderate TF disease → TKA

Complications

- PFA → implant failure and poor outcomes with early implant design.
    - Progressions of *tibiofemoral arthritis* and *patellar malalignment/instability* are *common causes of PFA failure*.
    - Patella fracture.
    - Adverse reactions to metal debris in joint (rare with nonmetal-backed patellas).

Bibliography

1. Beitzel K, Schottle PB, Cotic M, Dharmesh V, Imhoff AB. Prospective clinical and radiological two-year results after patellofemoral arthroplasty using an implant with an asymmetric trochlea design. Knee Surg Sports Traumatol Arthrosc. 2013;21:332–9.
2. Farr J, Covell DJ, Lattermann C. Cartilage lesions in patellofemoral dislocations: incidents/locations/when to treat. Sports Med Arthrosc. 2012;20: 181–6.
3. Gomoll AH, Minas T, Farr J, Cole BJ. Treatment of chondral defects in the patellofemoral joint. J Knee Surg. 2006;19:285–95.
4. Lonner JH, Bloomfield MR. The clinical outcome of patellofemoral arthroplasty. Orthop Clin North Am. 2013;44:271–80.
5. Mihalko WM, Boachie-Adjei Y, Spang JT, Fulkerson JP, Arendt EA, Saleh KJ. Controversies and techniques in the surgical management of patellofemoral arthritis. Instr Course Lect. 2008;57:365–80.
6. Morris MJ, Lombardi Jr AV, Berend KR, Hurst JM, Adams JB. Clinical results of patellofemoral arthroplasty. J Arthroplasty. 2013;28(9 Suppl):199–201.
7. Pascual-Garrido C, Slabaugh MA, L'Heureux DR, Friel NA, Cole BJ. Recommendations and treatment outcomes for patellofemoral articular cartilage defects with autologous chondrocyte implantation: prospective evaluation at average 4-year follow-up. Am J Sports Med. 2009;37 Suppl 1:33S–41S.

8. Preston CF, Fulkerson EW, Meislin R, Di Cesare PE. Osteotomy about the knee: applications, techniques, and results. J Knee Surg. 2005;18:258–72.
9. Walker T, Perkinson B, Mihalko WM. Patellofemoral arthroplasty: the other unicompartmental knee replacement. Instr Course Lect. 2013;62:363–71.

6 Wear in TKR: Thickness, Geometry, Kinematics, Polyethylene Sterilization, and Machining

Peter K. Sculco

Take-Home Message

- Polyethylene wear dependent on contact stress – combination of load, contact area, and PE thickness.
- PE minimum thickness is 8 mm.
- Conformity of PE to femoral component geometry: highly conforming → higher contact area → lower stress → less wear.
- PCL retaining TKR: PE flat to allow more sliding versus PCL substituting use post-cam mechanism to ensure femoral rollback versus mobile-bearing PE highly conforming but higher backside wear.
- Sterilization of PE with gamma irradiation: irradiation → free radicals → cross-linking of PE chains.
- Sterilization in air is bad → oxidation of PE → decreased toughness and rapid clinical failure.
- Direct compression molding of PE has smoother finish and lower wear rate than a machined PE component.

Types of PE Wear in TKR and PE Thickness

Four modes of wear in TKR:

Mode 1: articulation between intended bearing surfaces.

Mode 2: primary bearing surface against nonintended second surface (in TKR, if femoral component penetrates through a PE tibial bearing and rubs against tibial baseplate).

Mode 3: third body wear: contaminant particles directly abrade one or both of the primary surfaces (cement debris).

Mode 4: two secondary (nonprimary) surfaces rubbing together (backside wear between inferior surface of PE and tibial baseplate).

Wear damage (changes in appearance of PE)

Seven patterns of surface damage: embedded debris, scratching, pitting, burnishing, surface deformation, abrasion, and delamination. Delamination is seen in PE that has undergone oxidation.

Types of wear: steady-state linear (number of cycles) and time dependent (fatigue and delamination after accumulation of many cycles)

PE thickness: 8 mm is minimum PE thickness.

Contact stress increases with thinner PE design and results in greater wear. Catastrophic failure of PE if thickness less than 4 mm. No change in stress pattern once PE is 8 mm in thickness.

PE Articular Geometry

Conformity between tibial and femoral articulating surfaces has both sagittal and coronal geometries. As radius of femoral and tibial surfaces coincides, the articular conformity increases.

Most TKR design is a single radius for each condyle of femoral component and a single, slightly larger radius for each tibial plateau. Coronal (frontal) conformity limits internal/external rotation usually highly conforming (not much rotation in normal knee).

High conformity (deep dished PE): large contact areas → lower contact stresses → more constraint → less wear.

Downside: may not allow for physiologic movement (rotation).

Low conformity (flat PE) allows more physiologic motion.

Downside: smaller contact areas → higher contact stresses → greater sliding → higher wear rates.

Mobile bearing has high conformity → larger contact area → reduced wear compared to fix bearing but potential increase in 3rd body wear from metallic tray and inferior PE surface.

PE Kinematics

Motion pattern in a TKR: rolling, sliding, and rotation.

Design goal: Replicate femoral rollback → increase flexion.

Posterior cruciate-retaining (CR) TKR:

PCL tension → posterior femoral translation.
PE insert has flat surface that allows sliding.
Flat PE shape has large contact area, which lowers stress.

Posterior-stabilized (PS) cruciate-substituting TKR:

PE has a post-cam mechanism and more posterior femoral rollback with flexion than CR.
Downside: wear or fracture of post (rare).

Mobile bearing (MB): The design goal is to allow more normal joint kinematics with high conformity, larger contact areas, lower contact stresses, and presumably less wear.

PE Sterilization

PE sterilized with gamma irradiation between 3 and 3.5 Mrads.

Initially in the 1970s, gamma irradiated in air → oxygen led to oxidation of PE → breaks PE bonds → reduced toughness → fatigue cracking and delamination of PE → clinical failure.

Currently, gamma irradiation and packaging performed in argon, nitrogen, or a vacuum environment.

Gamma irradiation also produces free radicals which cross-links PE chains → improve wear resistance but decrease ductility (highly cross-linked has higher risk for post fracture).

PE Machining

Two types of PE fabrication

- Compression molding:

  Molding PE powder directly into PE shape
  Surface finish smooth, no machining marks
  0.05 mm wear/year in vitro

- Machined

  Made from stock PE material. Cylindrical ram-extruded bars or large sheets of PE
  Implant machined into final shape
  May generate subsurface cracking that predisposes to delamination
  0.11 mm/year wear in vitro

Bibliography

1. Crowninshield RD, Muratoglu OK. Implant Wear Symposium 2007 Engineering Work Group. How have new sterilization techniques and new forms of polyethylene influenced wear in total joint replacement? J Am Acad Orthop Surg. 2008;16 Suppl 1:S80–5.
2. Digas G, Kärrholm J, Thanner J, Malchau H, Herberts P. The Otto Aufranc Award. Highly cross-linked polyethylene in total hip arthroplasty: randomized evaluation of penetration rate in cemented and uncemented sockets using radiostereometric analysis. Clin Orthop Relat Res. 2004;(429): 6–16.
3. D'Lima DD, Hermida JC, Chen PC, Colwell Jr CW. Polyethylene cross-linking by two different methods reduces acetabular liner wear in a hip joint wear simulator. J Orthop Res. 2003;21(5):761–6.
4. Engh CA, Sychterz CJ, Engh Jr CA. Conventional ultra-high molecular weight polyethylene: a gold standard of sorts. Instr Course Lect. 2005;54: 183–7.
5. Engh Jr CA, Hopper Jr RH, Huynh C, Ho H, Sritulanondha S, Engh CA Sr. A prospective, randomized study of cross-linked and non-cross-linked polyethylene for total hip arthroplasty at 10-year follow-up. J Arthroplasty. 2012;27(8 Suppl):2–7.e1.
6. Hopper Jr RH, Young AM, Orishimo KF, Engh Jr CA. Effect of terminal sterilization with gas plasma or gamma radiation on wear of polyethylene liners. J Bone Joint Surg Am. 2003;85-A(3):464–8. Kurtz SM.

7. Lachiewicz PF, Geyer MR. The use of highly cross-linked polyethylene in total knee arthroplasty. J Am Acad Orthop Surg. 2011;19(3):143–51.
8. Li S, Burstein AH. Ultra-high molecular weight polyethylene. The material and its use in total joint implants. J Bone Joint Surg Am. 1994;76(7):1080–90.
9. McCalden RW, MacDonald SJ, Rorabeck CH, Bourne RB, Chess DG, Charron KD. Wear rate of highly cross-linked polyethylene in total hip arthroplasty. A randomized controlled trial. J Bone Joint Surg Am. 2009;91(4):773–82.
10. Micheli BR, Wannomae KK, Lozynsky AJ, Christensen SD, Muratoglu OK. Knee simulator wear of vitamin E stabilized irradiated ultrahigh molecular weight polyethylene. J Arthroplasty. 2012;27(1):95–104.
11. Muratoglu OK, Evans M, Edidin AA. Advances in the processing, sterilization, and crosslinking of ultra-high molecular weight polyethylene for total joint arthroplasty. Biomaterials. 1999;20(18):1659–88.
12. Muratoglu OK, Merrill EW, Bragdon CR, O'Connor D, Hoeffel D, Burroughs B, Jasty M, Harris WH. Effect of radiation, heat, and aging on in vitro wear resistance of polyethylene. Clin Orthop Relat Res. 2003;(417):253–62.
13. Sychterz CJ, Orishimo KF, Engh CA. Sterilization and polyethylene wear: clinical studies to support laboratory data. J Bone Joint Surg Am. 2004; 86-A(5):1017–22.

7 Revision Total Knee Arthroplasty

Matthew P. Abdel

Take-Home Message

- The most common indications for revision total knee arthroplasty (TKA) include infection, patellofemoral issues, aseptic loosening, osteolytic wear, arthrofibrosis, and instability (flexion, varus, or valgus).
- Infection must be ruled out before proceeding with revision TKA:
- ESR, CRP, and aspiration (*WBC count above 1,700 cells/μL and/or neutrophil count >65 % is suspicious for infection*).
- Management of the extensor mechanism during revision TKA is essential, with virtually *no drawbacks to a quadriceps snip*.

Indications for Revision

- Septic – should be evaluated using serum ESR and CRP, as well as a synovial fluid aspiration:
  - *Aspiration results of WBC >1,700 cells/μL, neutrophil count >65 % is suspicious for infection.*
  - *Sinus tract* communicating with the joint is an infection despite aspiration results.

- Aseptic:
  - Patellofemoral issues/extensor mechanism complications (poor patellar tracking, overstuffing of the patellofemoral joint, patellar fracture, incompetent extensor mechanism)
  - Abnormal joint line problems (e.g., instability)
  - Component loosening
  - Osteolytic wear:
    - Gamma irradiated polyethylene in air has most rapid wear rates.
    - Wear may be accelerated by third body wear.
  - Instability (most commonly midflexion instability, coronal plane instability, and flexion instability)
  - Periprosthetic fracture
  - Arthrofibrosis
  - Patellar clunk:
    - In *posterior-stabilized (PS)* total knee arthroplasties (TKAs), especially with *older designs*
    - Typically occurs at 30–45° flexion
    - Pain and audible clunk associated with the entrapment of hypertrophied nodule (scar) at the proximal pole of the patella in the box

Assessment

- History
  - Risk factors for infection: *previous infection*, draining wound, recent dental work, recent systemic infection (e.g., urosepsis), or prior revision procedure.
  - Query most recent antibiotic use.
  - Neurogenic pain such as radiculopathy (numbness, tingling into the foot).
  - Symptoms:
    - *Pain with weight bearing → mechanical etiology*
    - *Night pain and/or pain at rest → infection or tumor*
- Physical examination:
  - Appearance of wound (often difficult to differentiate aseptic versus septic etiology, unless persistent draining sinus present).
  - Effusion – good predictor of mechanical problem if the aspiration is normal:
    - Hemarthrosis can be a sign of midflexion instability.
  - Range of motion (ROM) – a stiff knee in a patient with previously good motion is suspicious for infection.
  - Ligamentous stability in both coronal and sagittal planes.
- Laboratory analysis:
  - ESR

- CRP – most specific systemic test
- CBC with differential
- Aspiration:
  - Obtain if infectious laboratories (ESR, CRP) are abnormal.
  - Send aspiration for cell count with differential and cultures (aerobic, anaerobic, fungal, AFB, gram stain).
  - WBC count above 1,700 cells/μL and/or neutrophil count >65 % is suspicious for infection.
  - Gram stain is a poor test, though often used.
  - Systemic WBC count does not correlate with periprosthetic joint infection.
  - Other possible tests to rule out infection include urinary dipstick test for strong presence of leukocyte esterase.

Imaging

- Radiographs:
  - *AP pelvis* (evaluate if hip joint may be source of pain)
  - *Full-le*ngth standing hip-to-ankle radiograph to evaluate alignment
  - Standing AP radiograph of both knees
  - Lateral radiograph of affected knee
  - Patellar views of both knees (i.e., merchant view)
  - *Prior radiographs*:
    - Pre-index surgical intervention radiographs
    - Immediate radiograph after primary procedure
    - Helps to confirm loosening, wear, and osteolysis
- Computerized tomography (CT)
  - Useful to determine extent of bone loss and osteolysis (usually underestimated by radiographs)
  - Allows for accurate assessment of component position (particularly *femoral and tibial component rotation*)

Goals of Revision TKA

- Remove components with minimal bone loss.
- Restore bony deficiencies and metaphysis with either allograft or tantalum metal or cement (if small contained defects).
- Restore joint line.
- Balance knee ligaments.
- Obtain stable and rigid fixation of revision implants.

Prosthesis Selection

- Unconstrained posterior cruciate ligament (PCL)-retaining TKA:
  - Rarely utilized during revision TKA
  - May be used when converting a unicompartmental knee arthroplasty or a high tibial osteotomy to a total knee arthroplasty
- Unconstrained PS TKA:
  - Utilize if *lateral collateral ligament (LCL) and medial collateral ligament (MCL) are functional* and there is no varus or valgus instability, respectively.
- Constrained PS TKA without a hinge:
  - *Wider and higher* central post assists with varus and valgus instability *if LCL and MCL are deficient*, respectively.
  - May assist with flexion instability given taller post.
- Constrained hinged TKA with rotating platform (RP):
  - Most constrained option
  - Constrained in the sagittal and coronal planes
  - Allows polyethylene to rotate, reducing forces at the bone-prosthesis interface
  - Indications:
    - MCL or LCL deficiency with global instability
    - Flexion gap instability, often in the setting of prosthetic knee dislocation
    - Posttraumatic TKA with compromised ligaments
    - Multiply revised TKA with compromised ligaments
    - Hyperextension instability (or recurvatum) seen in neurogenic patients
    - Oncologic reconstruction
    - In conjunction with extensor mechanism allograft
    - Deficient extensor mechanism
- Stemmed implants are always required for revision knee arthroplasty given the improved results over nonstemmed components:
  - Hybrid technique – cement around the metaphysis and the junction of the stem and keel of the component, but also use a press fit stem.
  - Fully cemented – difficult to remove if acutely infected.

Anderson Orthopedic Research Institute (AORI) Classification of Bone Defects

- Type 1: Minor femoral or tibial defects with intact metaphyseal bone, not compromising the stability of a revision component

- Type 2: Damaged metaphyseal bone that is typically cancellous in nature and requires reconstruction (cement fill, prosthetic augment, or bone graft) to provide stability of the revision component:
  - A: Defects in one femoral condyle or one tibial plateau
  - B: Defects in both femoral condyles or both tibial plateaus
- Type 3: Segmental deficiencies compromising a major portion of either femoral condyles or tibial plateaus, occasionally associated with collateral or patellar ligament detachment

Surgical Treatment

- Surgical exposure:
  - Large incision: Clean the medial and lateral gutters, and safely mobilize the extensor mechanism.
  - Advanced techniques in the setting of a tight extensor mechanism with difficult exposure:
    - Quadricep snip: *no difference in outcome.*
    - V-Y turndown: high incidence of extensor lag.
    - Tibial tubercle osteotomy (TTO): can be used in the setting of a fully cemented stemmed TKA to gain access to the metaphysis for cement removal; complications include nonunion, hardware prominence.
- Removal of implants:
  - The goal is minimal bone loss.
  - Lateral release may help expose lateral aspect of tibial baseplate.
  - Establish joint line:
    - 1.5–2 cm above head of fibula.
    - 3 cm distal to the medial epicondyle.
    - 1 cm from the superior pole of the patella to the proximal most portion of femoral component flange in extension.
    - Utilize contralateral knee x-rays to assess patellar height on the femur, distance from the inferior pole of the patella to joint line, or the distance from the adductor tubercle to the joint line.
- Balance flexion/extension gaps
- Balance medial and lateral gaps/ligamentous stability.
- Address patellofemoral tracking:
  - Keep current patella unless infection case or etiology of maltracking.
  - Patellar thickness should be *>12 mm* to avoid fracture.
- Salvage options:
  - Arthrodesis
  - Amputation

Complications

- Wound complications
- Infection
- Stiffness
- Extensor mechanism disruption
- Pain
- Neurovascular injury

Bibliography

1. Leopold SS, McStay C, et al. Primary repair of intraoperative disruption of the medial collateral ligament during total knee arthroplasty. J Bone Joint Surg Am. 2001;83A(1):86–91.
2. Meftah M, Ranawat AS, et al. All-polyethylene tibial implant in young, active patients a concise follow-up, 10 to 18 years. J Arthroplasty. 2012;27(1):10–4.
3. Meneghini RM, Lewallen DG, et al. Use of porous tantalum metaphyseal cones for severe tibial bone loss during revision total knee replacement. J Bone Joint Surg Am. 2008;90(1):78–84.
4. Meneghini RM, Lewallen DG, et al. Use of porous tantalum metaphyseal cones for severe tibial bone loss during revision total knee replacement. J Bone Joint Surg-Am. 2009;91A:131–8.
5. Swanik CB, Lephart SM, et al. Proprioception, kinesthesia, and balance after total knee arthroplasty with cruciate-retaining and posterior stabilized prostheses. J Bone Joint Surg-Am. 2004;86A(2):328–34.
6. Varela-Egocheaga JR, Suarez-Suarez MA, et al. Minimally invasive subvastus approach: improving the results of total knee arthroplasty: a prospective, randomized trial. Clin Orthop Rel Res. 468(5):1200–8.

8 Unicompartmental Osteoarthritis: Options for Management

Rachel M. Frank

Take-Home Message

- Osteoarthritis (OA) affecting either the medial or lateral compartment only (or patellofemoral compartment only), with medial compartment OA > lateral compartment OA.
- Etiology can vary, with predisposing factors including malalignment (varus leading to medial compartment OA, valgus leading to lateral compartment OA), prior meniscectomy, and prior articular cartilage injury; risk factors such as prior arthroscopy and prior ACL tear are controversial.
- Nonoperative options include weight loss, injections, and bracing; surgical options include cartilage/meniscal restoration, realignment, UKA, and TKA.

Definitions

- OA affecting either the medial or lateral compartment only; medial > lateral
- Can be primary (intrinsic) or secondary (trauma, infection, congenital)

Etiology

- Malalignment → varus leading to medial compartment OA, valgus leading to lateral compartment OA
- Prior articular cartilage injury
- Prior partial, subtotal, or total meniscectomy
- Prior ACL injury or prior knee arthroscopy (controversial)

Pathophysiology

- Changes in articular cartilage → increased water content, increased IL-1 content, increased matrix metalloproteinase (plasmin, stromelysin) levels, increased chondrocyte activity and proliferation, decreased proteoglycan quantity, and decreased collagen quantity and stiffness
- Changes in subchondral bone → increased thickness, osteophyte development, osteochondral junction breakdown, cyst formation, and microfracture formation
- Changes confined to medial or lateral compartment

Radiography

- Standard AP, lateral, merchant views + the Rosenberg view (45° flexion PA view).
- Bilateral long-leg standing axis films to assess alignment.
- Unilateral findings OA → joint space narrowing, osteophytes, subchondral sclerosis, and subchondral cysts.
- MRI can be helpful in documenting status of ACL, but not necessary.

Treatment

- Nonoperative:
  - Weight loss
  - Injections → corticosteroid ± hyaluronic acid
  - Unloader bracing → attempts to unload affected compartment, effectiveness controversial; compliance is an issue.
- Operative:
  - Articular cartilage ± meniscus restorative procedures:
    - Strict indications → isolated full-thickness chondral defects and/or meniscal deficiency:
      - Not for diffuse unicompartmental or bi-/tricompartmental OA
    - Must consider concomitant pathologies including malalignment and ligamentous instability → staged versus concurrent procedures
    - Salvage procedure(s)
  - Osteotomy:
    - The goal is to realign mechanical axis to unload affected compartment:
      - High tibial osteotomy typical for varus malalignment
      - Distal femoral osteotomy typical for valgus malalignment
    - Open or closed wedge
    - Strict recovery/compliance required with NWB regimen
    - Good-excellent 10+ year outcomes:
      - No difference in osteotomy patients post-TKA versus primary TKA patients
  - Unicompartmental knee arthroplasty (UKA):
    - Typically reserved for older (>60 years), nonobese (weight <82 kg), and lower-demand patients; however, indications are evolving.
    - Strictly contraindicated in inflammatory arthritis, fixed varus deformity >10°, fixed valgus deformity >5°; flexion contracture >10°, grade IV patellofemoral articular cartilage disease:
      - ACL deficiency absolute contraindication to mobile-bearing UKA and fixed-bearing lateral UKA:
        - Controversial in fixed-bearing medial UKA
    - Compared to TKA → faster recovery, less EBL, less soft tissue morbidity, and less expensive.
    - Preserves "normal" knee kinematics given retention of ACL and PCL.
  - Total knee arthroplasty (TKA):

- Preferred in cases with severe unicompartmental OA + mild-moderate arthritic changes in opposite compartment and/or patellofemoral compartment
- Advantageous in larger patients and ACL-deficient patients
- Potential longer survivorship in TKA versus UKA

Treatment Algorithm

- Attempt nonoperative management first as described above
- Surgical intervention for patients that remain symptomatic
  - Main indications → pain relief + improve function
- Obese patients → weight loss first
- Young, athletic patients with high-demand, high-activity levels → osteotomy
  - Cartilage/meniscus restoration if appropriate
- Active patients with low-moderate activity levels → UKA
- Active patients with diffuse arthritic changes in either opposite compartment or patellofemoral compartment → TKA

Complications

- Main complication from UKA → tibial stress fracture (after pain-free interval)

Bibliography

1. Choong PF, Dowsey MM. Update in surgery for osteoarthritis of the knee. Int J Rheum Dis. 2011;14:167–74.
2. Fu D, Li G, Chen K, Zhao Y, Hua Y, Cai Z. Comparison of high tibial osteotomy and unicompartmental knee arthroplasty in the treatment of unicompartmental osteoarthritis: a meta-analysis. J Arthroplasty. 2013;28:759–65.
3. Johnstone SF, Tranovich MJ, Vyas D, Wright VJ. Unicompartmental arthritis in the aging athlete: osteotomy and beyond. Curr Rev Musculoskelet Med. 2013;6:264–72.
4. Lombardi Jr AV, Berend KR, Berend ME, et al. Current controversies in partial knee arthroplasty. Instr Course Lect. 2012;61:347–81.
5. Lyons MC, MacDonald SJ, Somerville LE, Naudie DD, McCalden RW. Unicompartmental versus total knee arthroplasty database analysis: is there a winner? Clin Orthop Relat Res. 2012;470:84–90.
6. Schroer WC, Barnes CL, Diesfeld P, et al. The Oxford unicompartmental knee fails at a high rate in a high-volume knee practice. Clin Orthop Relat Res. 2013;471: 3533–9.

9 Spontaneous Osteonecrosis of the Knee (SONK)

Rachel M. Frank and Michael B. Cross

Take-Home Message

- SONK presents with a *sudden* onset of *severe* knee pain and by definition is an osteonecrosis lesion without clear etiology that can lead to osteoarthritis and subsequent knee surgery.
- Most common in *middle-aged and elderly females*, most often in the *medial femoral condyle*.
- *MRI* is the most helpful to make the diagnosis.
- Mainstay of treatment is *nonoperative* with *protected weight bearing*, though surgical intervention is sometimes warranted.

Definitions

Spontaneous osteonecrosis of the knee (SONK) – sudden onset subchondral insufficiency fracture often without a known etiology that is most commonly found in the medial femoral condyle

Etiology

- Unclear in most cases
- Important to differentiate from other diagnoses, including *osteochondritis dissecans* (more common in *lateral femoral condyle* in *younger* patients), *transient osteoporosis* (more common in *young to middle-aged men*), and occult fractures
- Can occur *following arthroscopy* of the knee

Pathophysiology

- Not well understood
- Likely component of *localized vascular insufficiency* causing necrosis of the subchondral bone, which ultimately leads to disruption of the nutrition and structural support of the overlying articular cartilage

Radiography

- AP, lateral, and merchant views of the knee with weight-bearing *flexion views.*
- Radiographs initially are likely to be normal or with minimal changes early in the disease process.

- *MRI* is the most helpful in diagnosis and in determining the extent of the disease.
  - The absence of focal epiphyseal contour depression and absence of lines of low signal intensity deep in condyle are good prognostic factors for benign disease course.
  - MRI can rule out other soft tissue injuries including meniscal and/or ligamentous pathology.
  - MRI can also be used to follow nonoperative treatment course to determine resolution of disease process.

Classification
None described

Treatment

- Nonoperative:
  - NSAIDs
  - Pain relievers, including narcotics for a short-term basis
  - Activity modification
  - *Protected weight bearing for up to 6–8 weeks*
  - Physical therapy to strengthen core and quadriceps
  - Possible role for vitamin D and bisphosphonate therapy
- Operative:
  - *Avoid arthroscopy*
  - Osteotomy to correct malalignment
  - Unicompartmental or total knee arthroplasty if nonoperative treatment fails

Bibliography

1. Breer S, Oheim R, Krause M, Marshall RP, Amling M, Barvencik F. Spontaneous osteonecrosis of the knee (SONK). Knee Surg Sports Traumatol Arthrosc. 2013;21(2):340–5.
2. Jureus J, Lindstrand A, Geijer M, Robertsson O, Tagil M. The natural course of spontaneous osteonecrosis of the knee (SPONK). Acta Orthop. 2013;84:410–4.
3. Pape D, Seil R, Fritsch E, Rupp S, Kohn D. Prevalence of spontaneous osteonecrosis of the medial femoral condyle in elderly patients. Knee Surg Sports Traumatol Arthrosc. 2002;10(4):233–40.
4. Uribe JW. Spontaneous osteonecrosis of the knee (SONK) developing as a possible consequence of the use of radiofrequency is misleading and illogical. Arthroscopy. 2004;20(8):895; author reply 895–6.
5. Yates PJ, Calder JD, Stranks GJ, Conn KS, Peppercorn D, Thomas NP. Early MRI diagnosis and non-surgical management of spontaneous osteonecrosis of the knee. Knee. 2007;14(2):112–6.

10 Common Complications After TKA

Brandon J. Erickson and Michael Hellman

Take-Home Message

- Extensor tendon injury:
  - Patellar tendon rupture: 0.22–2.5 %.
  - Quad tendon rupture: 0.1 %.
  - Concomitant patella fracture can occur as well.
  - When surgically correcting these, you must address malrotation.
  - If patient needs reoperation for this, outcomes are poor (23 % required reoperation after extensor mechanism repair).
- Patellofemoral joint issues:
  - Soft tissue impingement (patellar clunk syndrome) – synovial/scar tissue or Hoffa's fat pad impinges between patellar and femoral components; treat conservatively but if this fails, perform arthroscopic debridement.
  - Instability/dislocation – most common reason for repeat surgery after TKA.
  - Component wear – often in obese patients secondary to increased forces across joint.
  - Fracture – often spontaneous and asymptomatic; older implant designs with single peg had increased risk of fracture and loosening.
  - Implant loosening – 0.06 to 4.8 %; often asymptomatic; lateral release increases risk as does obesity.
- Periprosthetic fracture:
  - The most common area is the supracondylar region of femur above a well-fixed TKA:

    Often treated with ORIF if implant is stable
  - Tibia fractures are less common:

    Often associated with implant loosening
  - 0.3–2.5 % of patients who get TKA will sustain a periprosthetic fracture:

    Patella: 0.33–5.2 %
  - Where the fracture occurs/implant stability will dictate treatment:

    Above a well-fixed implant – treat with fixed-angled, locked, percutaneous plate

    If implant is loose – revision TKA to long-stem prosthesis

    With significant bone loss – revision TKA to distal femoral replacement tumor prosthesis

Definitions

- PFJ: patellofemoral joint
- MPFL: medial patellofemoral ligament

Etiology

- Extensor tendon injury:
  - Risk factors: obese patients, revision cases, difficult exposure, preoperative flexion contracture/angular deformity, quadriceps release (quadsnip), diabetes, and kidney malfunction
- Patellofemoral joint issues:
  - Soft tissue impingement (patellar clunk syndrome) – synovial/scar tissue or Hoffa's fat pad impinges between patellar and femoral components; can cause mechanical symptoms of locking/catching/popping and pain.
  - Instability/dislocation – from patient factors, errors in surgical technique, or implant design flaws.
  - Component wear – obesity increases stress across PFJ, leading to faster wear of polyethylene, as does increased deep knee bending.
  - Fracture – often spontaneous and asymptomatic; older implant designs with single peg had increased risk of fracture and loosening secondary to stress riser created by large peg.
  - Implant loosening – 0.06–4.8 %; often asymptomatic; obesity increases risk by 6.3 times, lateral release increases risk by 3.8 times, an elevated joint line increases the risk 2.2 times, and flexion beyond 100° increases the risk by 2.1 times the normal.
- Periprosthetic fracture:
  - Trauma, often low energy, in elderly patients secondary to osteoporosis, disuse osteopenia, and stress shielding around implant (transition from implant to native bone is a stress riser).
  - Patella fracture can be secondary to excessive or inadequate bone resection at the time of the TKA; improper alignment increases risk for patella fracture:
    - Medial parapatellar approach compromises patella vascularity (if combined with lateral release, vascularity is significantly damaged).

Pathophysiology

- Extensor tendon injury:
  - Often follows trauma
  - Can also be an eccentric load on tendon
- Patellofemoral joint issues:
  - Instability/dislocation:

    - Patient risk factors: severe patellofemoral degeneration, significant preoperative valgus malalignment, and patellar subluxation
    - Technique errors: patella alta, leaving limb in significant valgus, uneven patellar resection or lateral placement of button, increased internal rotation of tibial/femoral components, and medial translation of femoral component
    - Design flaws: shallow/narrow trochlear groove

- Periprosthetic fracture:
  - Patient risk factors:
    - Rheumatoid arthritis, osteolysis, osteoporotic bone, and steroid use
  - Technique-specific risk factors:
    - Notching the anterior femoral cortex
- Beware of bipartite patella (accessory ossification center) – not a fracture:
  - Superolateral aspect of patella, often bilateral

Radiography

- AP/lat/merchant views of knee – evaluate patellar height (lateral) for quad/patellar tendon rupture and resting position of patella (merchant).
- CT scan to determine component stability and malpositioning, especially in patellofemoral instability.
- MRI rarely necessary.

Classification

- Lewis and Rorabeck (periprosthetic femur fracture around TKA):
  - Type I – non-displaced, component stable
  - Type II – displaced, component stable
  - Type III – displaced or non-displaced, component loose or failing
- Felix and associates (periprosthetic tibia fracture):
  - Type I – fracture at tibial plateau.
  - Type II – adjacent to prosthetic stem.
  - Type III – distal to prosthetic stem.
  - Type IV – involving the tibial tubercle.
  - Each type is further classified as A, B, and C:
    - A – fracture around well-fixed implant
    - B – fracture around radiographically loose implant
    - C – Intraoperative fracture

- Goldberg (periprosthetic patella fracture):
  - I – fractures not involving implant/cement composite or quad mechanism
  - II – fractures disrupting the quad mechanism or implant fixation
  - IIIA – fracture of inferior pole w/ patella tendon rupture
  - IIIB – fracture of inferior pole, non-displaced, intact patella tendon
  - IV – lateral fracture-dislocation (shear fracture)

Treatment

- Extensor tendon injury:
  - Quad injury can be treated conservatively if patient maintains the ability to extend knee to 20° and is low demand:
    - Immobilize in extension.
    - If this fails or patient is unable to straighten leg, operative intervention with suture repair will be needed:
      - Use the Scuderi (quad flap) turndown technique.
  - Patellar tendon injury:
    - Poor outcomes (up to 75 % failure rate with suture repair).
    - Often require graft augmentation (Achilles allograft, semitendinosus autograft) to aid suture repair.
    - Soft tissue coverage can be an issue – medial gastrocnemius flap can help tale tension off the skin.
  - Periprosthetic fracture:
    - Non-displaced:
      - Can consider cast immobilization with NWB and close radiographic follow-up
    - Displaced femoral fracture with well-fixed prosthesis:
      - Consider retrograde IM nail if prosthesis is cruciate-retaining TKA:
        - Posterior-stabilized design does not allow access to canal.
      - Often treated with fixed-angled, locked, percutaneous plate.
    - Displaced tibial fracture with loose prosthesis:
      - Revision arthroplasty with longer stem.
      - If implant is stable, consider ORIF.
    - External fixators are not frequently used because of risk of pin-site infections.
  - Patellofemoral joint:

- Patella fracture:
  - Conservative – if component is not loose and patient can extend to 20°, this is a viable option.
  - Operative intervention (CRIF or component revision) if patient has significant loss of extension or component is loose.
  - In non-resurfaced patella: ORIF – cannulated screws alone or tension band construct via cerclage wires, suture, cannulated screws/wires or sutures:
    - Biomechanically, cannulated screws with tension band construct fail at the highest loads.
  - Patellectomy (only if not repairable):
    - You will lose the benefit of the patella which is to increase the moment arm of the extensor mechanism by moving the attachment point for the quadriceps away from the center of rotation of the knee (basically the pt will be weaker in extension by approximately 50 % without their patella).
  - Loosening:
    - Only treat if patient has pain and mechanical symptoms or implant has become dislodged.
  - Instability/dislocation:
    - Conservative – IT band stretching and vastus medialis strengthening, patellar stabilization brace
    - Operative – if conservative measures fail:
      - Lateral release – although risks increasing overall instability.
      - Vastus medialis advancement of medial soft tissue imbrication.
      - Tibial tubercle osteotomy – either medialization or anteromedialization.
      - Last resort is component revision.
  - Patella clunk syndrome:
      - Start conservative with strengthening of quads, massage, and ultrasound.
      - If this fails, perform arthroscopic debridement.

Complications

- Periprosthetic fractures:
  - Malalignment (usually valgus deformity with hyperextension)
- Repeated subluxation or possible frank dislocation:
  - Often associated with MPFL rupture

- PF joint:
  - Refracture
  - Malunion or nonunion
  - Component loosening
  - Continued instability

Bibliography

1. Dobbs RE, Hanssen AD, Lewallen DG, Pagnano MW. Quadriceps tendon rupture after total knee arthroplasty. Prevalence, complications, and outcomes. J Bone Joint Surg Am Vol. 2005;87(1):37–45.
2. Hendrix MR, Ackroyd CE, Lonner JH. Revision patellofemoral arthroplasty: three- to seven-year follow-up. J Arthroplasty. 2008;23(7):977–83.
3. Ilan DI, Tejwani N, Keschner M, Leibman M. Quadriceps tendon rupture. J Am Acad Orthop Surg. 2003;11(3):192–200.
4. Lustig S, Magnussen RA, Dahm DL, Parker D. Patellofemoral arthroplasty, where are we today? Knee Surg Sports Traumatol Arthrosc. 2012;20(7):1216–26.
5. Rosenberg AG. Management of extensor mechanism rupture after TKA. J Bone Joint Surgery Br Vol. 2012;94(11 Suppl A):116–9.
6. Ruchholtz S, Tomas J, Gebhard F, Larsen MS. Periprosthetic fractures around the knee-the best way of treatment. Eur Orthop Traumatol. 2013;4(2): 93–102.
7. Saidi K, Ben-Lulu O, Tsuji M, Safir O, Gross AE, Backstein D. Supracondylar periprosthetic fractures of the knee in the elderly patients: a comparison of treatment using allograft-implant composites, standard revision components, distal femoral replacement prosthesis. J Arthroplasty. 2014;29:110–4.

11 Deep Venous Thrombosis, Venous Thromboembolism (Prevention and Treatment)

Rachel M. Frank and Michael B. Cross

Take-Home Message

- *Prevention* of symptomatic venous thromboembolism is essential, but one must outweigh risk of bleeding versus risk of pulmonary embolism for each individual patient.
- The AAOS recommends the use of *pharmacologic and/or mechanical devices* for VTE prophylaxis in patients undergoing elective TKA/THA; however, there are *no consensus pharmacologic* agent recommendations.
- Proximal DVTs require treatment; however, the necessity of treatment for DVTs distal to the trifurcation is unclear.
- Early diagnosis and treatment is the key to survival in patients with PE.

Definitions

- *Virchow's triad → endothelial injury, hypercoagulable state, venous stasis*
- VTE → venous thromboembolic event, which encompasses the disease spectrum of both DVT and PE

Etiology/Risk Factors

- Risk factors for VTE (Table 1):

Table 1 Risk factors for DVT/PE

Genetic		Protein S deficiency
		Factor V Leiden mutation (Arg506Gln mutation)
		Prothrombin gene mutation (G20210A mutation)
		Protein C deficiency
		Antithrombin III deficiency
		Heparin cofactor II deficiency
		Plasminogen deficiency
		Factor XII deficiency
		Dysfibrinogenemia
		Increased factor VIII activity
		Increased factor XI activity
		Primary hyperhomocysteinemia

Acquired	Traumatic	Acute trauma
		Surgery within the last 3 months
		Especially major abdominal, pelvic, and orthopedic surgery
	Lifestyle	Obesity
		Cigarette smoking
		Increasing age
		Travel (e.g., air) lasting longer than 4 h within the last 2 months
		Prolonged immobilization
	Medical	Prior history of VTE
		Malignancy
		Hypertension
		Stroke with paresis/paralysis of the extremity
		Secondary hyperhomocysteinemia
		Antiphospholipid syndromes (e.g., SLE)
		Congestive heart failure
		Myocardial infarction
		Myeloproliferative disorders (e.g., polycythemia vera, essential thrombocythemia)
		Nephrotic syndrome
		Inflammatory bowel disease
		Sickle cell anemia
		Marked leukocytosis in acute leukemia
		Chronic kidney disease
		Hematopoietic stem cell transplantation
		Pregnancy and puerperium
	Medication related	Oral contraceptive
		Hormonal replacement
		Heparin-induced thrombocytopenia

- Factors specifically associated with increased risk of DVT:
  - Polytrauma
  - Hip fracture or pelvic fracture requiring prolonged immobilization or bed rest
  - Elective TKA/THA:
    - *Elective TKA 2–3× greater rate than elective THA*
- Factors specifically associated with increased risk of PE:
  - Hip fracture or pelvic trauma
  - Elective TKA/THA:
    - Occurs more frequently with *cement pressurization* of femoral canal
    - In general, during THA, DVTs occur most frequently during *femoral preparation*:
      - *Intraoperative heparin* can be used to prevent DVT during femoral preparation.
      - *Neuraxial anesthesia* also reduces risk of VTE.

Pathophysiology

- During surgical dissection, blood vessel intimal injury can be sustained:
  - In an attempt to form a clot to prevent excessive bleeding:
    - Vessel contraction
    - Collagen release
    - Tissue thromboplastin (tissue factor) release → extrinsic coagulation pathway
      - Activates factor VII → activates factor X → converts prothrombin to thrombin
        - Converts fibrinogen to *fibrin* → induces clot formation
- Venous stasis → clot formation

Diagnostic Modalities

- Physical examination
  - DVT → calf pain, low-grade fevers, and erythema and swelling in the lower extremity; *Homans' sign* not specific
  - PE → pleuritic chest pain, dyspnea, tachypnea, tachycardia, and fever
- Imaging
  - DVT → venous duplex ultrasound more sensitive and specific for DVTs *proximal to trifurcation* compared to distal, helical CT with contrast (when PE is being evaluated)
  - PE → CXR (often negative), V/Q scan (rare), *helical chest CT with contrast (most commonly used)*, pulmonary angiography (gold standard but rarely used)
- EKG → tachycardia, nonspecific ST-T wave changes; "classic" finding of S1-Q3-T3 is nonspecific.
- ABG on room air → typically reveals hypoxemia, hypocapnia, and respiratory alkalosis

Prophylaxis

- Mechanical prophylaxis
  - Compressive stocking
  - Pneumatic compression devices → recommended by AAOS across all risk groups:
    - Increase venous return
    - Increase endothelial-derived fibrinolysis
    - Decrease venous compliance
    - Decrease venous stasis
- Chemical prophylaxis
  - Multiple possible agents:

  - Warfarin → limits *vitamin K metabolism* by inhibition of vit K 2,3 epoxide reductase, limiting production of *clotting factors II, VII, IX, and X*
    - Also *limits* production of *protein C and protein S*
      - *Temporary prothrombotic effect*
    - Reversed by *vitamin K, fresh frozen plasma (FFP)*
    - *Half-life of single dose → 2–5 days*
  - Aspirin → acts on *platelets* and inhibits production of prostaglandins and thromboxanes via irreversible inactivation of cyclooxygenase *(COX) enzyme;* remains active for *7–10 days*
  - Low molecular weight heparin (enoxaparin, dalteparin) → enhances *inhibition of Xa*:
    - Reversed by *protamine*
    - Not associated with heparin-induced thrombocytopenia (HIT)
    - Half-life approximately 4.5 h, duration in plasma approximately 12 h
  - Unfractionated heparin → enhances *ATIII inhibition of IIa and Xa*:
    - Reversed by *protamine.*
    - Risk of heparin-induced thrombocytopenia (HIT) → typically thrombocytopenia 5–12 days into therapy.
    - Half-life is 1–2 h but is dose dependent.
  - *Fondaparinux (Arixtra)* → factor *Xa inhibitor*:
    - Increased bleeding complications given that there is *no reversal agent.*
    - *Half-life is 15–20 h and may last for 2–3 days.*

- *Inferior vena cava filter*
  - Preoperatively placed in patients with known DVT or who are at high risk for DVT
  - Preoperatively placed in patients who *cannot tolerate chemical prophylaxis due to high risk of bleeding*

Treatment Considerations

- Prevention of symptomatic venous thromboembolism is essential but must *outweigh risk of bleeding* versus *risk of pulmonary embolism.*
- Risk factors for major bleeding:
  - History of bleeding disorder
  - History of recent GI bleed
  - History of recent hemorrhagic stroke
- Risk factors for pulmonary embolism:
  - History of hypercoagulable state
  - Previous PE

Treatment Options for DVT and PE

- *Proximal DVT:* intravenous *heparin* (until warfarin therapeutic) + *warfarin*; another option is *therapeutic Lovenox* if warfarin cannot be tolerated:
  - Distal DVT treatment (below knee) → controversial if warrants treatment.
  - Duration of treatment is variable, typically *3–6 months*.
- *PE: IV heparin + warfarin*:
  - Duration of treatment is variable, typically 3–6 months.
  - Occasionally thrombolytics are warranted in emergent situations.
  - Surgical removal (embolectomy) of the clot if PE life threatening.

AAOS 2011 Clinical Practice Guidelines

- Recommend *against* routine postoperative Doppler.
- Recommend *for* work-up of potential previous VTE events.
- Recommend *for* work-up of known bleeding disorders or active liver disease.
- Recommend *for* cessation of antiplatelet agents before TKA/THA (usually 7 days).
- Recommend *for* use of pharmacologic and/or mechanical devices for VTE prophylaxis:
  - Unable to recommend specific agents
  - Unable to recommend duration of prophylaxis
- Patients with previous VTE should receive mechanical and pharmacologic prophylaxis.
- Patients with known bleeding disorder should receive mechanical prophylaxis.
- Recommend *for* early mobilization following TKA/THA.
- Recommend neuraxial anesthesia to help limit blood loss.
- Unable to recommend for or against IVC filters.

Bibliography

1. Barrack RL. Current guidelines for total joint VTE prophylaxis: dawn of a new day. J Bone Joint Surg Br. 2012;94:3–7.
2. Cross MB, Boettner F. Pathophysiology of venous thromboembolic disease. Sem Arthroplasty. 2009;20(4):210–6.
3. Falck-Ytter Y, Francis CW, Johanson NA, et al. Prevention of VTE in orthopedic surgery patients: Antithrombotic Therapy and Prevention of Thrombosis, 9th ed: American College of Chest Physicians Evidence-Based Clinical Practice Guidelines. Chest. 2012;141:e278S–325S.
4. Guyatt GH, Eikelboom JW, Gould MK, et al. Approach to outcome measurement in the prevention of thrombosis in surgical and medical patients: Antithrombotic Therapy and Prevention of Thrombosis, 9th ed: American

College of Chest Physicians Evidence-Based Clinical Practice Guidelines. Chest. 2012;141:e185S–94S.
5. He ML, Xiao ZM, Lei M, Li TS, Wu H, Liao J. Continuous passive motion for preventing venous thromboembolism after total knee arthroplasty. Cochrane Database Syst Rev 2012;(1):CD008207.
6. Kakkos SK, Warwick D, Nicolaides AN, Stansby GP, Tsolakis IA. Combined (mechanical and pharmacological) modalities for the prevention of venous thromboembolism in joint replacement surgery. J Bone Joint Surg Br. 2012;94:729–34.
7. Mont MA, Jacobs JJ. AAOS clinical practice guideline: preventing venous thromboembolic disease in patients undergoing elective hip and knee arthroplasty. J Am Acad Orthop Surg. 2011;19:777–8.
8. Raphael IJ, Tischler EH, Huang R, Rothman RH, Hozack WJ, Parvizi J. Aspirin: an alternative for pulmonary embolism prophylaxis after arthroplasty? Clin Orthop Relat Res. 2014;472:482–8.
9. Zhang H, Chen J, Chen F, Que W. The effect of tranexamic acid on blood loss and use of blood products in total knee arthroplasty: a meta-analysis. Knee Surg Sports Traumatol Arthrosc. 2012;20:1742–52.

12 Perioperative Management of the Rheumatoid Arthritis Patient

Nicolas M. Fort, Natalie L. Zusman, and Michael B. Cross

Take-Home Message

- Rheumatoid arthritis (RA) patients should be evaluated for cardiovascular/pulmonary disease, cervical spine involvement, and cricoarytenoid arthritis, in addition to the usual perioperative evaluation.
- RA patients with prolonged use of glucocorticoids may have suppression of the HPA-axis and require stress dose steroids in the perioperative period.
- Methotrexate and hydroxychloroquine can be continued in the perioperative period.
- Discontinue agents that can cause leukopenia such as cyclophosphamide, azathioprine, and sulfasalazine at least 1 day prior to surgery.
- Discontinue biologic disease-modifying antirheumatic drugs (DMARD) for 1–2 treatment cycles; resume postoperatively once wound healing is complete.

Background

- Patients with RA should receive the same preoperative cardiovascular, pulmonary, and other risk assessment as other patients.
- Additional considerations:
  - Coordinate care with rheumatologist.
  - Assess:
    - Level of immune suppression
    - Hypercoagulable states
    - Status of rheumatologic disease
    - Steriod use

Perioperative Evaluation and Management

- Cardiovascular disease:
  - RA is associated with a 60 % increase risk of cardiovascular death as compared to the general population.
- Pulmonary disease:
  - Variety of pulmonary diseases:
    - Fibrosis, bronchiolitis, and pleuritis
- Cervical spine disease:
  - C1/C2 instability, atlantoaxial impaction, and subaxial disease:
    - Risk factors associated with instability include glucocorticoid use, seropositivity, nodular disease, and erosive peripheral joint disease.
  - *Obtain C-spine flexion/extension views to detect subluxation.*
- Cricoarytenoid joint disease:
  - Prevalence: up to 75 % of patients affected.
  - May lead to *difficulty with intubation.*
  - Physical symptoms include hoarseness, sore throat, dysphagia, odynophagia, pain with speech, and radiation of pain to ears.
  - Consider in patients with postoperative respiratory difficulty.
  - Assess with direct laryngoscopy.
- Anemia:
  - Common in patients with RA.
  - Postoperative blood transfusions often required in large joint arthroplasty.
  - Consider preoperative autologous blood donation.

- Neutropenia:
  - Common in patients with Felty's syndrome
  - Usually no intervention is required
  - Extremely low counts can be treated with G-CSF
- Laboratory testing:
  - Urinalysis, bone morphogenetic protein, complete blood count, and coagulation panel.
  - Vitamin D deficiency associated with suboptimal outcomes in patients undergoing total joint arthroplasty.
  - Exclude asymptomatic urinary tract infection.

General Preoperative Management

- Preoperative physical therapy:
  - Associated with better physical function at 12 weeks
- Weight reduction:
  - Reduce stress on joints
  - Possible increased incidence of infection in obese patients following total joint arthroplasty
- Thrombosis risk:
  - Incidence of 1 %.
  - Patients with RA have a reduced relative risk for venous thromboembolism as compared to patients with OA.

Perioperative Antirheumatic Medication Management

- Glucocorticoids:
  - Prolonged use can *suppress HPA-axis*.
  - Usefulness of ACTH stimulation testing unclear.
  - Supplementation of glucocorticoids may be necessary in perioperative period:
    - Patients on low dose (*<7.5 mg/day prednisone*) or any dose for less than 3 weeks:
      - Give usual daily dose (no need for stress dose steroids).
    - Patients on intermediate doses (*7.5–20 mg/day*):
      - Data suggest overuse of stress dose steroids.
      - Individualize steroid use based on chronicity of treatment, stress of surgery, and infection risk.

- Patients on chronic moderate- to high-dose therapy *(>20 mg/day prednisone or >3 weeks)*:
  - Assume secondary adrenal suppression.
  - Treat with stress dose steroids.

- Methotrexate:
  - Concern that immune modulating effect may increase risk of infection.
  - Most prospective and retrospective studies suggest *MTX can be continued without impairing wound healing or increasing risk of infection.*
  - Little evidence to suggest stopping MTX perioperatively improved wound healing or decreased incidence of infection.
- Leflunomide:
  - May impair wound healing; studies are contradictory.
  - *Consider holding in patients where large wounds are anticipated.*
  - Long half-life (approximately 2 weeks).
  - Resume 3 days post-op.
- Cyclophosphamide, azathioprine, sulfasalazine:
  - All may cause neutropenia.
  - Discontinue on day of surgery.
- Hydroxychloroquine:
  - Continue in perioperative period.
  - One study showed increased risk of post-op infection in association.
  - *Long half-life and persists in tissues, therefore impractical to discontinue.*
- Biologic agents:
  - Interfere with TNF-alpha IL-1, IL-6, T cell costimulation, or deplete B lymphocytes.
  - Little evidence regarding the optimal use in perioperative period.
  - Generally, discontinue and restart once wound healing has completed:
    - TNF-alpha inhibitors:
      - *Infection is a known complication of therapy.*
      - Hold in the perioperative period, at least 1–2 treatment cycles.
      - Restart after wound healing has progressed to suture or staple removal.
      - Half-lives of drugs vary.
    - B cell-depleting agents (rituximab):
      - Prolonged B cell depletion with treatment
      - Associated with increased risk of pulmonary infection

- No published data regarding surgical complications
- Elective surgery: await return of B cells (CD 19+)
- *Not a contraindication to non-elective surgery*
- Recommend discussion with rheumatologist

• IL-1 receptor antagonist (anakinra):

- Insufficient data to guide use
- Infection rate similar to those patients receiving placebo

• T cell costimulation (abatacept):

- No trials assessing perioperative safety.
- Recommend discussion with rheumatologist:

  • NSAIDs

    - *Stop three half-lives prior to surgery.*
    - Aspirin should be discontinued 1 week prior to surgery.

Bibliography

1. Chmell MJ, Scott RD. Total knee arthroplasty in patients with rheumatoid arthritis. An overview. Clin Orthop Relat Res. 1999;366:54–60.
2. Cooke TD. A scientific basis for surgery in rheumatoid arthritis. Clin Orthop Relat Res. 1986;208:20–4.
3. Donahue KE, Gartlehner G, Jonas DE, et al. Systematic review: comparative effectiveness and harms of disease-modifying medications for rheumatoid arthritis. Ann Intern Med. 2008;148:124.
4. Goodman SM. Rheumatoid arthritis: preoperative evaluation for total hip and total knee replacement surgery. J Clin Rheumatol. 2013;19(4):187–92.
5. Goodman SM, Mackenzie CR. Cardiovascular risk in the rheumatic disease patient undergoing orthopedic surgery. Curr Rheumatol Rep. 2013;15(9):354.
6. Halla JT, Hardin JG, Vitek J, et al. Involvement of the cervical spine in rheumatoid arthritis. Arthritis Rheum. 1989;32:652–34.
7. Jain A, Stein BE, Skolasky RL, et al. Total joint arthroplasty in patients with rheumatoid arthritis: a United States experience from 1992 – 2005. J Arthroplasty. 2012;27(6):881–8.
8. Nelissen RG. The impact of total joint replacement in rheumatoid arthritis. Best Pract Clin Rheumatol. 2003;17:5.
9. Ravi B, Croxford R, Hollands S, et al. Increased risk of complications following total joint arthroplasty in patients with rheumatoid arthritis. Arthritis Rheum. 2014;66(2):254–96.
10. So AK, Varisco PA, Kemkes-Matthew B, et al. Arthritis is linked to local and systemic activation of coagulation and fibrinolysis pathways. J Throm Haemost. 2003;1:2510–5.

11. Somayaji R, Barnabe C, Martin L. Risk factors for infection following total joint arthroplasty in rheumatoid arthritis. Open Rheumatol J. 2013;7:119–24.
12. Stundner O, Danninger T, Chiu YA, et al. Rheumatoid arthritis vs osteoarthritis in patients receiving total knee arthroplasty: perioperative outcomes. JBJS. 2014;29(2):308–13.
13. Unger AS, Inglis AE, Ranawat CS, Johnason NA. Total hip arthroplasty in rheumatoid arthritis: a long term follow-up study. J Arthroplasty. 1987;2(3): 191–7.

Part IX
Foot and Ankle Surgery

Anish R. Kadakia

General Principles

Anish R. Kadakia, Paul J. Switaj, Bryant S. Ho, Mohammed Alshouli, Daniel Fuchs, and George Ochengele

1 Biomechanics

Take-Home Message

- The complex bony and ligamentous anatomy of the foot and ankle allows multiple foot positions and motion in three axes of rotation.
- Transverse tarsal joints provide both flexibility and stability to the hindfoot and midfoot.
- The midfoot is an important bridge between hindfoot and forefoot and is stabilized by longitudinal and transverse arches.
- The gait cycle is composed of a stance and swing phase, the mechanics of which are influenced by important soft-tissue contributions.

Ankle Biomechanics

Ankle joint: articulation between tibial plafond, medial malleolus, lateral malleolus, and talus.

- Mortise widens and ankle is more stable in dorsiflexion due to shape of talar dome.
- Responsible for most sagittal plane motion of foot and ankle: dorsiflexion (10–23°) and plantarflexion (23–48°). Secondary motion rotation and inversion and eversion.
- Medial deltoid ligament complex is the main stabilizer of the ankle during stance. Functions to resist lateral translation and valgus forces, i.e., talar tilt.
- Lateral ankle ligaments function as a restraint to varus forces.

A.R. Kadakia, MD (✉) • P.J. Switaj • B.S. Ho • M. Alshouli • D. Fuchs • G. Ochengele
Department of Orthopedic Surgery, Northwestern University – Feinberg School of Medicine, Northwestern Memorial Hospital, Chicago, IL, USA
e-mail: Kadak259@gmail.com; paul.switaj@gmail.com; bryant.s.ho@gmail.com; mtshouli@gmail.com; dfuchs0011@gmail.com; gochenjele@gmail.com

C. Mauffrey, D.J. Hak (eds.), *Passport for the Orthopedic Boards and FRCS Examination*, DOI 10.1007/978-2-8178-0475-0_38

Distal tibiofibular joint: consists of distal fibula (medial convex surface) and incisura fibularis of distal tibia (lateral concave surface).

- Fibula rotates within the incisura (~2°) during normal gait.
- Along with syndesmotic ligaments, provides stability against lateral talar translation.

Hindfoot Biomechanics

Subtalar joint: articulation between talus and calcaneus.

- Functions in eversion and inversion.
- Limited eversion accommodation contributes to disability derived from even a mild cavovarus foot deformity.

Transverse tarsal joint (Chopart): articulation between talus and navicular (TN) and between calcaneus and cuboid (CC).

- Important for providing stability to the hindfoot and midfoot to produce rigid lever at toe-off.
- During heel strike, these joints are supple and parallel to adapt to uneven ground, then during toe-off become divergent and lock, providing stiffness to the foot.
- Failure of the posterior tibial tendon to lock the transverse tarsal joints is the biomechanical etiology for lack of a heel rise in patients with posterior tibial tendon dysfunction.

Midfoot and Forefoot Biomechanics

Midfoot: consists of intercuneiform joints, naviculocuneiform joint, and tarsalmetatarsal joints (TMT).

- Midfoot functions in adduction and abduction.
- Provides important bridge between hindfoot and forefoot and both flexibility and stability for normal gait.
- TMT joint complex (Lisfranc joint) divided into medial, middle, and lateral columns.
  - Lateral column has most sagittal mobility and allows for flexibility during necessary for walking on uneven ground.
  - Middle column is least mobile and allows for rigidity during push-off.
  - Medial column experiences the most force while in stance.
- The foot has longitudinal and transverse arches → stabilized by bony architecture, ligaments, and muscle forces.
  - The plantar ligaments are thicker and stronger than the dorsal ligaments.
  - The interosseous ligaments are the primary stabilizer of the longitudinal arch. The plantar fascia is a secondary stabilizer.
  - The specialized architecture of the Lisfranc joint complex imparts a bony "keystone" effect which stabilizes the transverse arch. The Lisfranc ligament (from medial cuneiform to base of the 2nd MT) is the largest and strongest of the ligaments which stabilize the Lisfranc joint.

Forefoot: consists of all structures distal to TMT joints.

- First metatarsal is the widest and the shortest and bears 50 % of weight during gait.
- Second metatarsal experiences more stress than the other lesser metatarsals (commonly involved in stress fractures).
- Lesser toes are balanced by the extrinsic muscles (EDL, FDL), intrinsic muscles (interossei, lumbricals), and passive restraints (plantar plate, extensor hood, joint capsule, collateral ligaments).
- Loss of intrinsic function predictably leads to claw toes.

Foot Positions Versus Foot Motions

Foot positions are defined in a manner different from foot motions → they are varus/valgus (hindfoot), abduction/adduction (midfoot), and equinus/calcaneus (ankle).

Foot motions are in three axes of rotation (Table 1).

Gait Cycle

- One gait cycle, or "stride," is measured from heel strike to heel strike.
- Ground reaction forces are approximately 1.5 times body weight during walking and 3–4 times body weight during running.

Stance phase: 62 % of gait cycle. Heel strike to toe-off

- Heel strike:
  - Hindfoot valgus, forefoot abduction, dorsiflexion of ankle.
  - Anterior tibialis contracts eccentrically to control rate at which foot strikes the ground.
  - Quadriceps contract to stabilize knee.
  - Hindfoot unlocked/everted for energy absorption.
- Foot flat: Single-limb support
  - Gastrocnemius-soleus complex contracts eccentrically.
  - Knee extends, hip extensors under concentric contraction.
  - Hindfoot unlocked/everted for ground accommodation.

Table 1 Description of foot motion in three axes of rotation

Plane of motion	Motion
Sagittal (X-axis)	Dorsiflexion/plantar flexion
Frontal (coronal) (Z-axis)	Inversion/eversion
Transverse (Y-axis)	Forefoot/midfoot: adduction/abduction
	Ankle/hindfoot: internal rotation/external rotation
Tri-planar motion	Supination: adduction, inversion, plantar flexion
	Pronation: abduction, eversion, dorsiflexion

Swing phase: 38 % of gait cycle. Toe-off to heel strike

- Toe-off:
  - Hindfoot varus, forefoot adduction, plantarflexion of ankle.
  - Hip flexors contract. Gastrocnemius-soleus complex contracts concentrically.
  - Plantar fascia tightens, longitudinal arch is accentuated (windlass mechanism), and transverse tarsal joint locks → allows foot to convert from flexible shock absorber to rigid propellant.
- Mid-swing: Foot clearance
  - Ankle dorsiflexors contract concentrically.
  - Loss of function results in steppage gait.
- Terminal swing: Hamstring muscles decelerate forward motion of thigh.

Bibliography

1. Chambers HG, Sutherland DH. A practical guide to gait analysis. J Am Acad Orthop Surg. 2002;10:222–31.
2. Dicharry J. Kinematics and kinetics of gait: from lab to clinic. Clin Sports Med. 2010;29:347–64.
3. Irwin TA, Kadakia AR. Miller review of orthopedics. 6th ed. Philadelphia: Elsevier Publications; 2012.
4. Rodgers MM. Dynamic biomechanics of the normal foot and ankle during walking and running. Phys Ther. 1988;68:1822–30.

2 Ankle Arthroscopy

Take-Home Message

- Indications for arthroscopy include treatment of OCLT, debridement of osteophytes and synovitis, removal of loose bodies, and cartilage debridement for ankle fusions.
- Joint distraction, correct instrumentation, and systematic arthroscopic approach are vital to successful surgical procedure.
- Arthroscopic portal options include anterolateral, anteromedial, posterolateral, and posteromedial and require a systematic approach for a thorough procedure.
- Superficial peroneal nerve is most at risk from iatrogenic injury.

Relevant Anatomy

- Tibiotalar joint: comprised of the ankle mortise superiorly and talar dome inferiorly (Fig. 1).

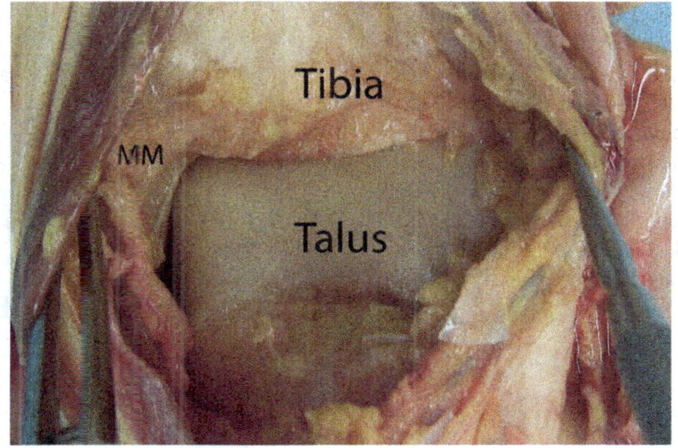

Fig. 1 Anatomic dissection of the anterior aspect of the ankle. The anterior aspect of the distal tibia, medial malleolus, and the talus are visualized

- Distal tibiofibular joint: convex surface of medial fibular articulates with incisura fibularis. Syndesmotic ligaments include anterior inferior tibiofibular ligament, posterior inferior tibiofibular ligament, interosseous tibiofibular ligaments, and interosseous membrane.
- Deltoid ligament complex: deep and superficial deltoid → to resist lateral talar translation and valgus.
- Lateral ankle ligaments: anterior talofibular (ATFL), calcaneofibular (CFL), posterior talofibular (PTFL) → to resist varus forces.
- Anterior neurovascular structures: superficial peroneal nerve (SPN), saphenous nerve, anterior tibial artery, vein, and deep peroneal nerve (DPN) (Fig. 2).
- Posterior neurovascular structures: sural nerve, tibial nerve, posterior tibial artery and vein.

Surgical Indications

- Osteochondral lesions – chronic (debridement with microfracture) or acute (fixation of bony component)
- Debridement of synovitis
- Ankle impingement – excision of soft tissue and tibial/talar osteophytes
- Removal of loose bodies
- Cartilage debridement in conjunction with ankle fusion

Perioperative Considerations

- Thorough history and physical examination provide a differential diagnosis and guide acquisition of appropriate imaging studies.
- Positioning: supine, bump under ipsilateral pelvis to achieve neutral foot rotation. Flex hip and knee to allow distraction and relax gastrocnemius tension.
- Use noninvasive distraction methods in a sterile fashion to access tibiotalar articular surface (Fig. 3). Anterior ankle arthroscopy for impingement and synovitis without distraction minimizes risk to the deep neurovascular structures and articular cartilage as the ankle can be dorsiflexed during the procedure.
- 2.7 mm 30-degree angle arthroscope is suitable in most cases. Small joint instruments are useful, in addition to 3.5 mm shaver, 4.0 mm round burr, and microfracture awl.

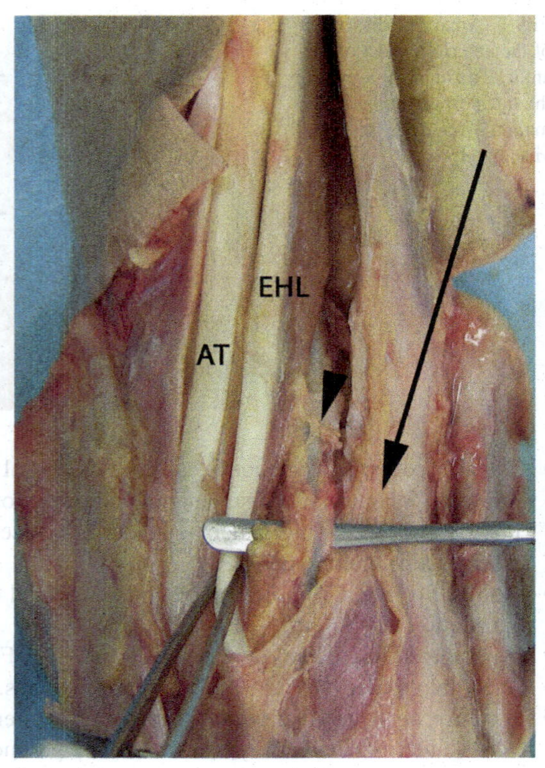

Fig. 2 Anterior tibial artery, vein, and deep peroneal nerve (*arrowhead*). The bundle lies deep the EHL at the level of the ankle and visualizing of the structures requires retraction of the tendon. The superficial peroneal nerve is also seen distally; it has been transected proximally (*arrow*)

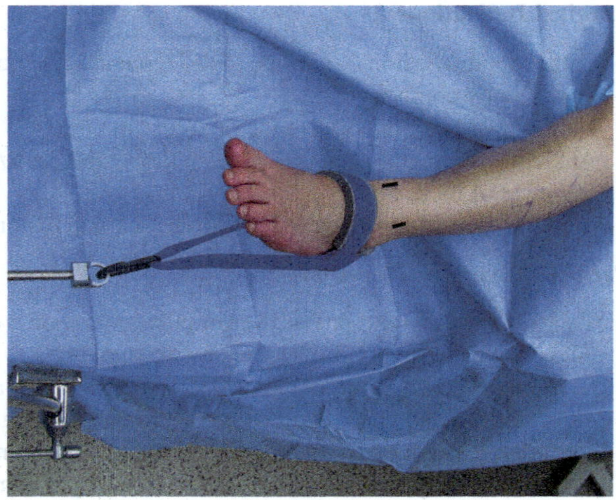

Fig. 3 Patient positioning and noninvasive ankle distractor. Ipsilateral flexion of the thigh elevates the ankle to allow for posterior portal placement and stabilizes the proximal leg to allow for ankle distraction. The anteromedial and anterolateral portals have been marked in this case (*black lines*)

Portal Placement

Many arthroscopic portals have been described to access the ankle, but anteromedial and anterolateral remain the staple.

- Anteromedial: primary viewing portal. Established first. Make portal 2.5 mm medial to tibialis anterior tendon directly at level of joint. Incise skin; bluntly dissect to joint capsule. Enter joint with trochar and cannula; introduce arthroscope and distend joint.
- Anterolateral: primary working portal. Create once arthroscope is introduced and joint is distracted. Make portal at level of joint line, just lateral to peroneus tertius tendon. Incise skin sharply; bluntly dissect carefully to protect the superficial peroneal nerve.
- Posterolateral: Make portal just lateral to Achilles tendon, 2 cm superior to the distal tip of the lateral malleolus. Incise skin; bluntly dissect to capsule. Direct trochar slightly medially, toward 1st and 2nd interdigital webspace. Portal is at the level of the posterior process of the talus.
- Posteromedial: rarely indicated given proximity to the posterior neurovascular bundle (posterior tibial artery, vein, tibial nerve). Incision just medial to the Achilles tendon above 2 cm superior to distal tip of lateral malleolus. Enter joint capsule under direct visualization from the posterolateral portal. All instruments must remain lateral to the FHL tendon.

Diagnostic Arthroscopy

- Begins in anterior aspect of joint. Inspect for synovitis, loose bodies, and osteophytes.
- Visualize articular surfaces of tibiotalar joint. Probe gently for softening to assess for an OCLT (Fig. 4).

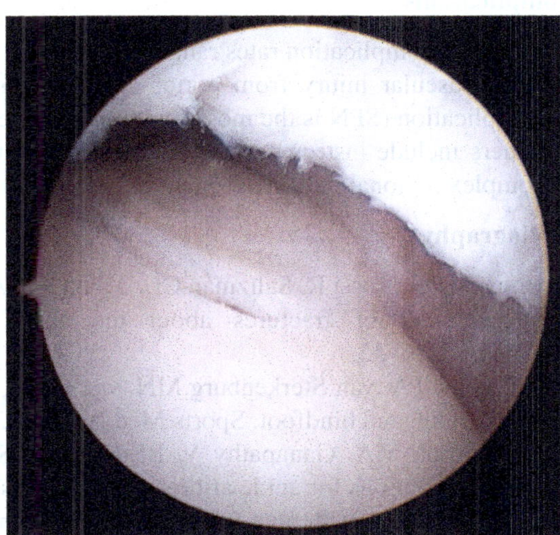

Fig. 4 Osteochondral lesion of the talus with fissuring of the articular surface

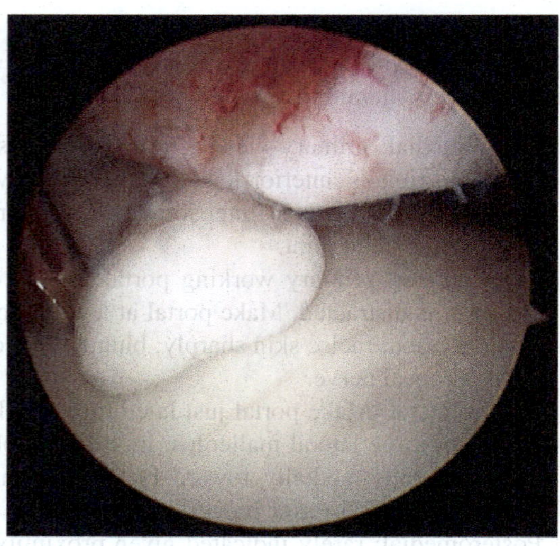

Fig. 5 Loose body noted in the anterior aspect of the ankle joint. These commonly reside in the posterior ankle capsule. Use of the shaver to provide suction can "pull" the loose bodies into the shaver and allow for removal

- View the lateral gutter, between the lateral talar dome and fibula, both from the anterior ankle and within the tibiotalar articulation. Inspect inferior aspect of syndesmosis.
- View the medial gutter, between the medial talar dome and medial malleolus in a similar fashion.
- May view the posterior aspect of joint by rotating the arthroscope appropriately, but some pathology may necessitate a posterior portal due to curvature of talar dome.
- Loose bodies commonly reside posteriorly, so a thorough inspection of the posterior aspect is essential (Fig. 5).

Complications

- Reported complication rates range from 3 to 17 %.
- Neurovascular injury from portal placement is the most commonly reported complication (SPN is the most commonly injured).
- Others include instrument failure, damage to articular cartilage, infection, and complex regional pain syndrome.

Bibliography

1. Bonasia DE, Rossi R, Saltzman CL, Amendola A. The role of arthroscopy in the management of fractures about the ankle. J Am Acad Orthop Surg. 2011;19:226–35.
2. de Leeuw PA, van Sterkenburg MN, van Dijk CN. Arthroscopy and endoscopy of the ankle and hindfoot. Sports Med Arthrosc. 2009;17:175–84.
3. Glazebrook MA, Ganapathy V, Bridge MA, Stone JW, Allard JP. Evidence-based indications for ankle arthroscopy. Arthroscopy. 2009;25:1478–90.
4. van Dijk CN, van Bergen CJ. Advancements in ankle arthroscopy. J Am Acad Orthop Surg. 2008;16:635–46.

3 Ankle Arthrodesis

Take-Home Message

- Ankle arthrodesis is indicated for the patient with recalcitrant arthritic ankle pain.
- The most common etiology of ankle arthritis is posttraumatic.
- Surgical techniques can involve arthroscopic or open procedures and rely on adequate joint preparation for bony union.
- The results from ankle arthrodesis are excellent overall but with time will result in adjacent joint arthritis; the most common is the subtalar joint.
- Position of the arthrodesis in neutral dorsiflexion, 5° of valgus, and slight external rotation is critical to maximize function and minimize adjacent joint stress.

Introduction

- Nonoperative treatment of symptomatic ankle arthritis includes the use of shoe inserts or shoe modifications (SACH heel with rocker bottom), anti-inflammatory medications, and intra-articular injections (corticosteroid or hyaluronate) and use of either an ankle-foot orthosis or a rigid lace-up leather brace (Arizona type).
- The use of a walking cast has been suggested as a trial device to evaluate patient acceptance and degree of pain relief prior to arthrodesis.

Surgical Indications

- Persistent ankle arthritic pain that is functionally debilitating to the patient and is not relieved by nonoperative treatment methods.
- Etiology: most commonly posttraumatic arthritis (cause of more than 70 % of ankle arthritis).
- Other causes of painful arthritis include postinfectious, chronic instability, inflammatory arthropathy, neuropathic arthropathy, primary osteoarthritis, failed total ankle arthroplasty, and avascular necrosis.

Perioperative Considerations

- Need weight-bearing standing anteroposterior, lateral, and mortise views to assess radiographic changes in the joint, arthritis in the subtalar joints, and bony alignment (Fig. 6).
- Patient needs to be compliant with postoperative weight-bearing status and should be counseled on smoking cessation.

Surgical Techniques

Arthroscopic arthrodesis: typically for patients with little or no deformity of the ankle and good bone stock and density. Fixation can only be performed with screws.

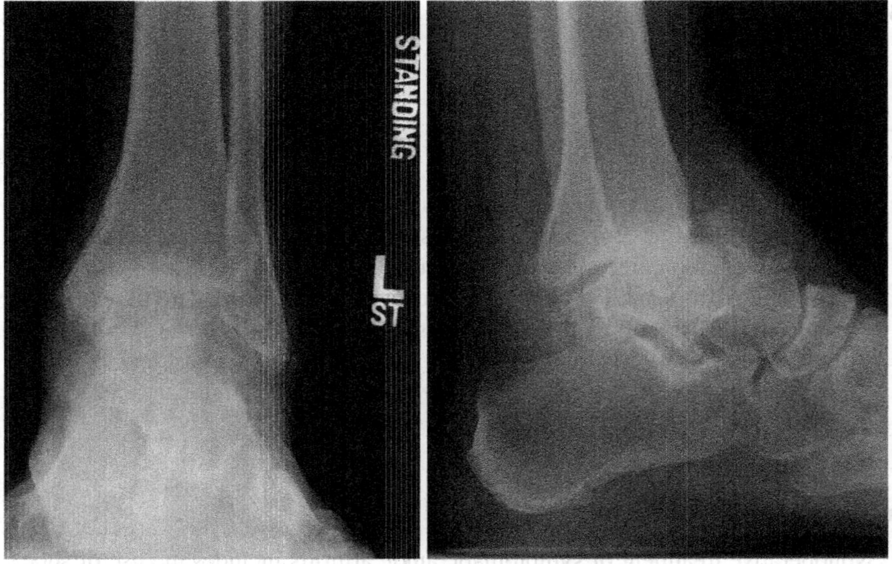

Fig. 6 AP and lateral WB views of a patient with end-stage ankle arthritis. Note the significant anterior subluxation of the talus on the lateral radiograph which must be addressed intraoperatively

Open arthrodesis: particularly useful for patients with severe ankle joint deformity. Better visualization of joint, correction of deformity, and allows use of plate fixation.

- Approaches: Options include lateral exposure where the fibula is either resected or osteotomized and replaced or an anterior approach (between the tibialis anterior and the extensor hallucis longus tendons), and least commonly performed is the posterior approach (in setting of compromised tissues).
- After achieving operative exposure of the joint to be fused → remove remaining cartilage and subchondral bone from the arthritis joint surfaces (Fig. 7).
- Obtain good bony apposition and reduction with compression of the joint surfaces.
- Then use rigid internal fixation (multiple 6.5 mm screws or a plate and screw construct) or external fixation for preexisting septic joint and those with severe osteopenia. Both isolated screw and plate and screw constructs have demonstrated a similarly high union rate that approaches 95–100 % with modern techniques (Fig. 8).

Optimal position of ankle joint: neutral dorsiflexion, 5–10° of external rotation, 5° hindfoot valgus (in order to keep hindfoot unlocked for accommodative hindfoot motion) (Fig. 9).

Tibiotalocalcaneal arthrodesis: can be performed with retrograde nail or a plate for concomitant subtalar and tibiotalar arthrodesis. Use of screws in isolation for a TTC fusion has demonstrated a higher nonunion rate compared to the other constructs.

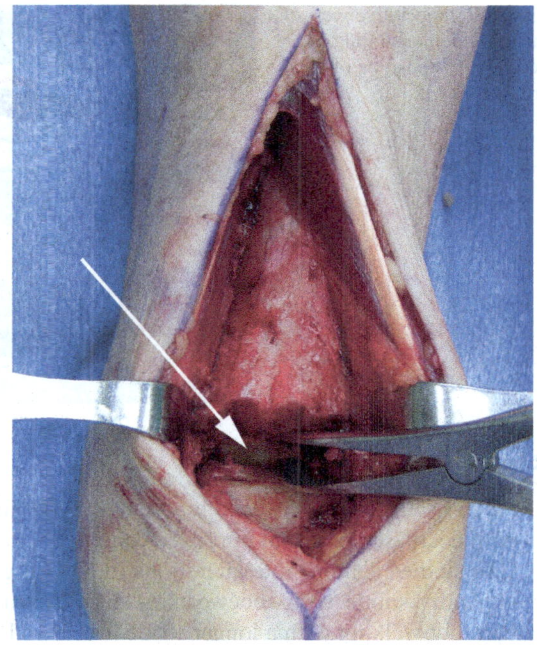

Fig. 7 The use of a lamina spreader allows visualization of the tibial articular surface (*arrow*) and facilitates cartilage removal and bony preparation. Alternating the lamina spreader medially and laterally will provide access to the entire joint

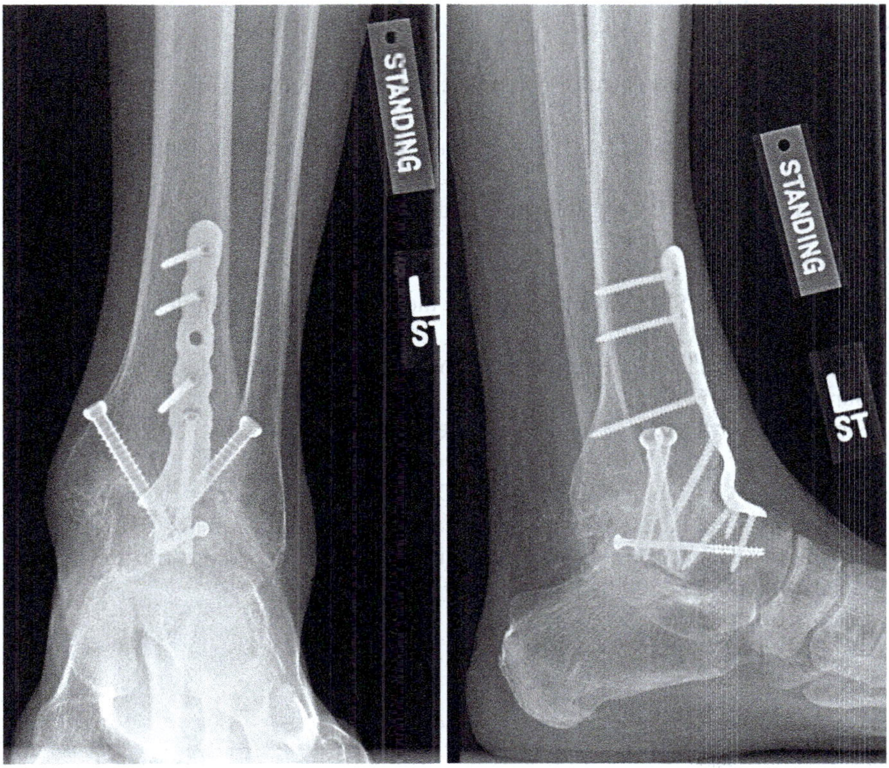

Fig. 8 AP and lateral WB views of a patient who is 1 year s/p an open ankle arthrodesis. Note the neutral position of the ankle with bony union at the tibiotalar joint

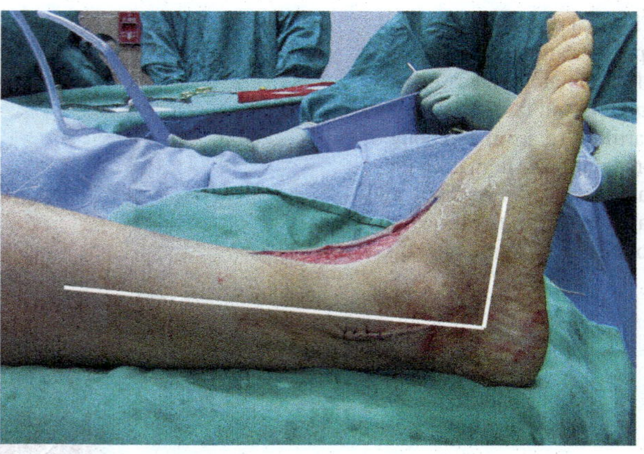

Fig. 9 Intraoperative view of the ankle demonstrating a neutral (90°) position of the arthrodesis

Results

- Patient satisfaction has been reported as 90 % following successful arthrodesis, with decreased pain and improved function.
- Gait studies demonstrate alterations in normal gait, but these changes are often clinically subtle with shoewear. A clear contrast has been demonstrated with barefoot walking with a longer stride length and decreased velocity compared to the normal population and total ankle arthroplasty.

Complications

- Adjacent joint arthritis (most common): usually considered an expected sequel of the subtalar joint
- Nonunion: rates range from 0 to 5 % in a recent meta-analysis to 40 %, elevated in tobacco users
- Malunion, wound healing, infection, and nerve injury

Bibliography

1. Ahmad J, Raikin SM. Ankle arthrodesis: the simple and the complex. Foot Ankle Clin. 2008;13:381–400, viii.
2. Nihal A, Gellman RE, Embil JM, Trepman E. Ankle arthrodesis. Foot Ankle Surg. 2008;14:1–10.
3. Stone JW. Arthroscopic ankle arthrodesis. Foot Ankle Clin. 2006;11:361–8, vi–vii.
4. Thevendran G, Younger A, Pinney S. Current concepts review: risk factors for nonunions in foot and ankle arthrodeses. Foot Ankle Int. 2012;33:1031–40.
5. Thordarson DB. Fusion in posttraumatic foot and ankle reconstruction. J Am Acad Orthop Surg. 2004;12:322–33.

Hindfoot

Anish R. Kadakia, Paul J. Switaj, Bryant S. Ho, Mohammed Alshouli, Daniel Fuchs, and George Ochengele

1 Arthritis

> **Take-Home Message**
> - Post-traumatic arthritis is the most common etiology.
> - Classified based on etiology.
> - Nonoperative management (Arizona brace or AFO) is the first-line treatment strategy.
> - Arthrodesis is indicated when nonoperative management is not effective to control pain and disability. No role for arthroplasty in the hindfoot.

Definition

- Inflammation and degenerative disease of the hindfoot articulations that includes the talonavicular, subtalar, and calcaneocuboid joints.

Etiology

- Post-traumatic arthritis is the most common cause. Mechanical degeneration of the articular surface as a result of post-traumatic articular injury, incongruity, or collapse (Fig. 1).
- Osteoarthritis is the second most common and is commonly associated with a deformity (pes planus secondary PTTD or cavus).
- Others include inflammatory arthropathy, osteonecrosis, gout, or rarely septic arthritis.

A.R. Kadakia (✉) • P.J. Switaj • B.S. Ho • M. Alshouli • D. Fuchs • G. Ochengele
Department of Orthopedic Surgery, Northwestern University – Feinberg School of Medicine, Northwestern Memorial Hospital, Chicago, IL, USA
e-mail: Kadak259@gmail.com; paul.switaj@gmail.com; bryant.s.ho@gmail.com; mtshouli@gmail.com; dfuchs0011@gmail.com; gochenjele@gmail.com

C. Mauffrey, D.J. Hak (eds.), *Passport for the Orthopedic Boards and FRCS Examination*, DOI 10.1007/978-2-8178-0475-0_39

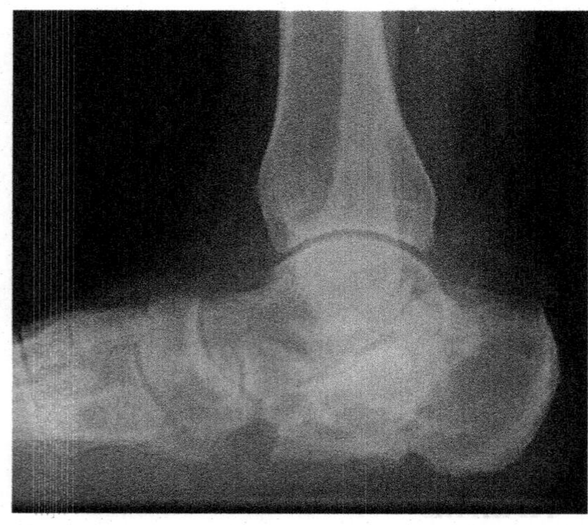

Fig. 1 Nonoperatively treated calcaneus fracture with resultant post-traumatic arthritis. Note the loss of height and obvious articular incongruity and joint space narrowing. The patient had no anterior ankle impingement or pain and was treated with an in situ subtalar arthrodesis

Pathophysiology

- Post-traumatic articular incongruity leads to abnormal joint contact forces and loading, resulting in mechanical wear.
- Deformity/instability can also lead to joint subluxation, decreased contact area, and increased contact pressure.
  - Post-traumatic deformity, end-stage posterior tibialis tendon disorder (PTTD), tarsal coalitions, and cavovarus are commonly associated.
- Inflammatory processes such RA lead to articular cartilage destruction and wear.
- Abnormal purine metabolism results in precipitation and deposition of monosodium urate crystals in joint spaces, resulting to severe inflammatory response.

Radiography

- Weight-bearing x-ray (AP, lateral, and oblique views) of the hindfoot
  - Joint space narrowing or loss (Fig. 2)
  - Subchondral sclerosis/cysts
  - Osteophytes and bony erosions
  - Hindfoot malalignment and deformity (Fig. 3)
    Computed tomography (CT) scan
  - In the setting of deformity, the obliquity if plain radiographs prevent appropriate visualization of the joints. CT is critical in these cases to accurately determine the presence of articular erosion.

Classification

Based on Etiology

- Mechanical (post-traumatic)
- Degenerative (osteoarthritis)

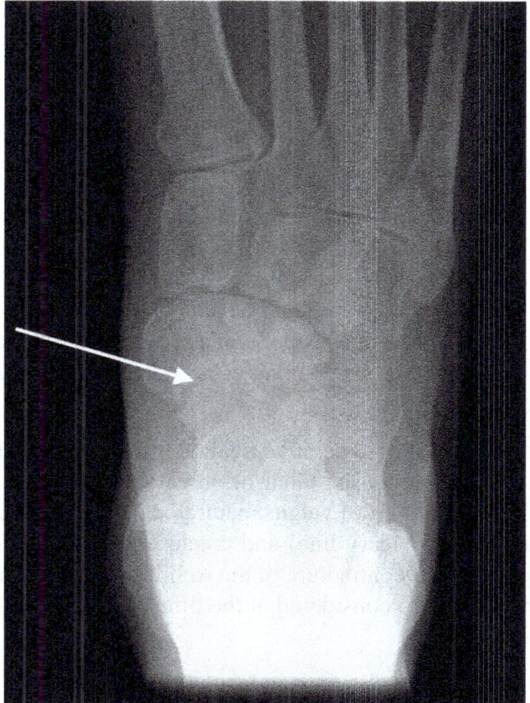

Fig. 2 Joint space narrowing in a patient who has isolated talonavicular (*arrow*) arthritis

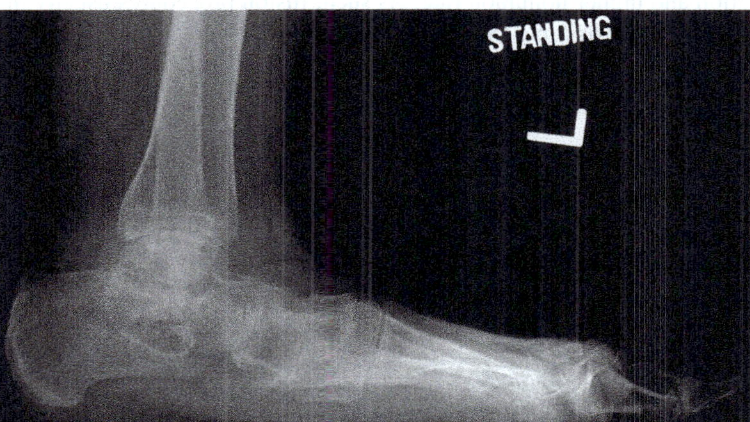

Fig. 3 The severe malalignment of the hindfoot precludes visualization of the hindfoot joints in particular the subtalar joint in patients with a pes planus deformity. In these cases, this may be misinterpreted as subtalar DJD. A CT is appropriate in these cases to determine viability of the joints to determine if the patient is a candidate for joint salvage or requires an arthrodesis

- Inflammatory (rheumatoid, seronegative spondyloarthropathy)
- Metabolic (gout, pseudogout (chondrocalcinosis))
- Neuropathic

Treatment

Nonoperative

- Nonsteroidal anti-inflammatory drugs (NSAIDs)
- Activity modification (avoidance of impact and uneven ground)
- Bracing such as an ankle-foot orthosis (AFO) or rigid lace up brace such as Arizona brace with an associated rocker bottom shoe modification
- Corticosteroid/anesthetic injections: both diagnostic and therapeutic
- Treatment of underlying causes such as gout, RA

Operative

Failure of nonoperative treatment with persistent pain and disability is an indication for arthrodesis. Goal of surgery is to obtain a solid fusion and position the hindfoot in 0–5° of valgus, neutral abduction/adduction, congruent talus-first metatarsal axis (Meary line) and create a plantigrade foot (Fig. 4). In many patients a concomitant contracture of the Achilles tendon is present, and an Achilles lengthening should be considered at the time of arthrodesis if a fixed equinus contracture is present.

- Single joint fusion is indicated for isolated joint arthritis. However, isolated joint fusions, especially TN (TN > ST > CC), are associated to severe hindfoot motion limitation and higher nonunion rate. As such, fusion procedures usually involve ST and TN fusion or triple (ST, TN, and CC) fusion (Fig. 5).

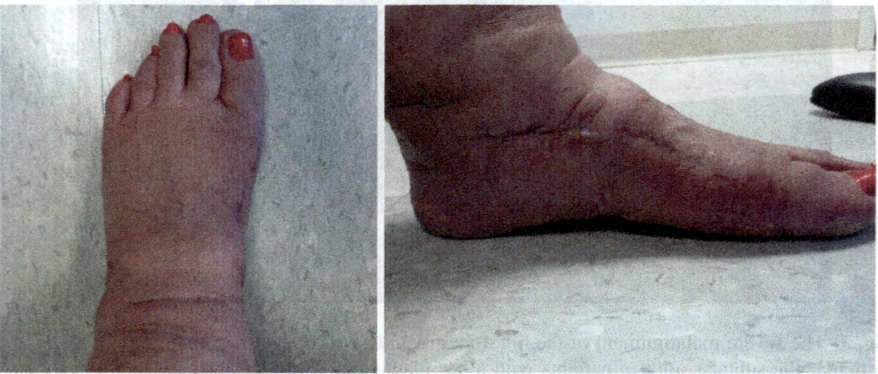

Fig. 4 Postoperative clinical appearance of a patient s/p subtalar and talonavicular arthrodesis for a severe pes planus deformity. Note the neutral adduction/abduction and restoration of the longitudinal arch

- In the setting of stage 3 PTTD, a TN and ST fusion without violation of the CC joint may be employed. In many cases additional midfoot correction is required to obtain a plantigrade foot (Fig. 6)
- A triple arthrodesis is an effective strategy to treat pan hindfoot arthritis and deformity and is typically required for any congenital deformity.
- Subtalar bone block arthrodesis is an effective option to treat post-traumatic arthritis secondary to a calcaneus fracture with loss of height. This operation is only indicated if the patient has ankle impingement (pain or limited dorsiflexion). The higher risk of nonunion and technical difficulty is why this should not be performed if the patient is asymptomatic in the ankle.
- Tibiotalocalcaneal (TTC) fusion is an option for subtalar arthritis with associated tibiotalar arthritis or if there is a concern for bone stock and fixation as may seen in neuroarthropathy or sever osteonecrosis.

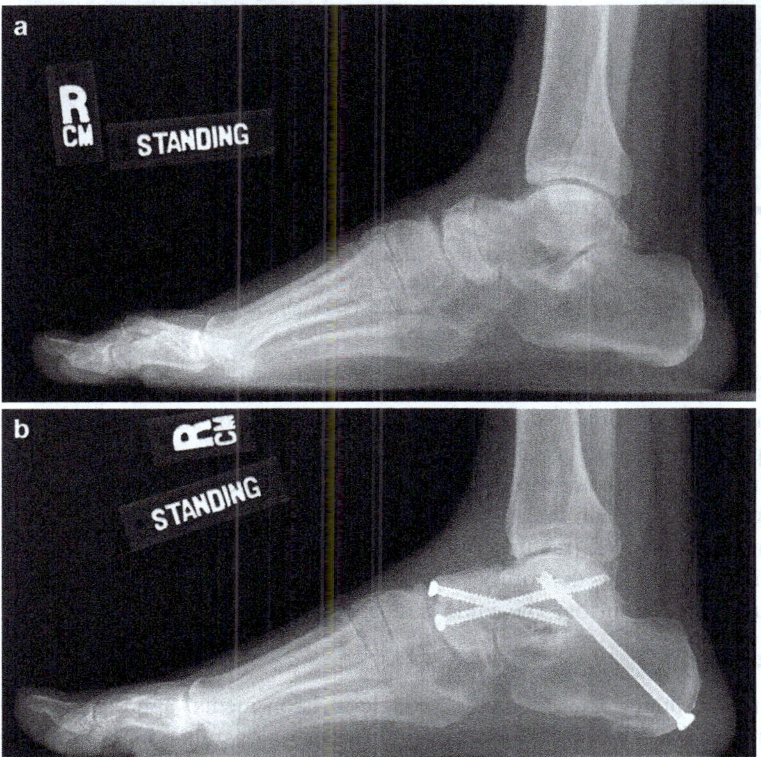

Fig. 5 Attempted isolated TN fusion that resulted in a nonunion (**a**) that was successfully revised with a combined TN and ST fusion (**b**)

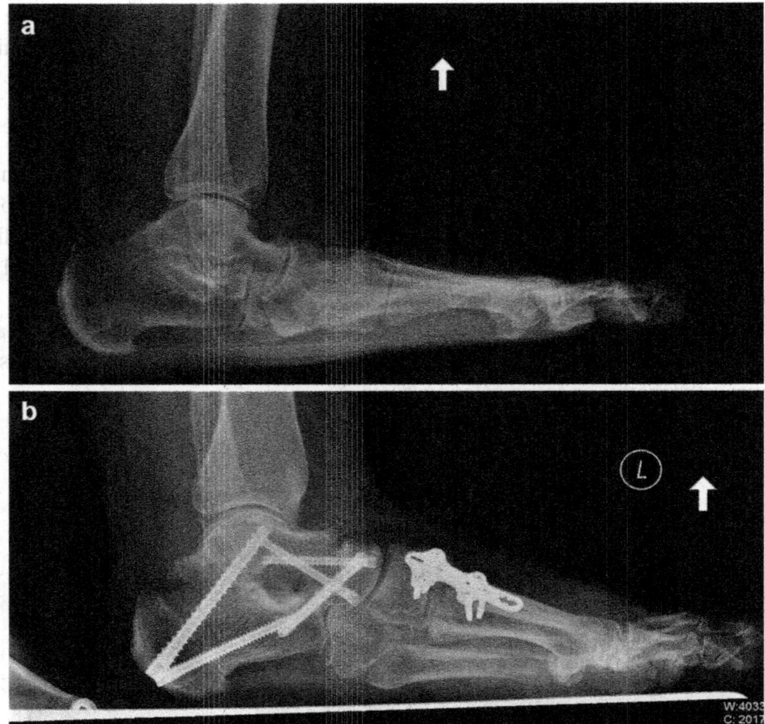

Fig. 6 The radiographic appearance of the patient in Fig. 4 with collapse of the medial arch and subtalar DJD noted on CT (**a**). Postoperative radiograph demonstrating restoration of the arch and additional 1 TMT fusion that was required to create a plantigrade foot (**b**)

Complications

- Wound complications: Higher in a lateral approach for subtalar joint in severe pes planus deformity and bone block arthrodesis s/p calcaneus fractures.
- Nonunion risk factors: prior ankle arthrodesis, isolated TN fusion, and smoking
- Malunion: Resultant malposition of foot and abnormal joint loading. Post-traumatic talar neck fractures with varus require a triple arthrodesis to prevent persistent cavovarus deformity.
- Adjacent joint arthritis: The ankle is most common.

Bibliography

1. Anand P, Nunley JA, DeOrio JK. Single-incision medial approach for double arthrodesis of hindfoot in posterior tibialis tendon dysfunction. Foot Ankle Int. 2013;34(3):338–44.
2. Herscovici D, Sammarco GJ, Sammarco VJ, Scaduto JM. Pantalar arthrodesis for post-traumatic arthritis and diabetic neuroarthropathy of the ankle and hind-foot. Foot Ankle Int. 2011;32(6):581–8.

3. Radnay CS, Clare MP, Sanders RW. Subtalar fusion after displaced intra-articular calcaneal fractures: does initial operative treatment matter? J Bone Joint Surg Am. 2009;91(3):541–6.
4. Rammelt S, Zwipp H. Corrective arthrodeses and osteotomies for post-traumatic hindfoot malalignment: indications, techniques, results. Int Orthop. 2013;37(9):1707–17.
5. Rammelt S, Pyrc J, Agren PH, Hartsock LA, Cronier P, Friscia DA, et al. Tibiotalocalcaneal fusion using the hindfoot arthrodesis nail: a multicenter study. Foot Ankle Int. 2013;34(9):1245–55.

2 Ankle Instability

Take-Home Message

- The lateral ligamentous complex is most commonly involved (ATFL > CFL > PTFL).
- Nonoperative management is the first-line treatment for all acute injuries → therapy (peroneal strengthening and proprioception) and functional bracing.
- Surgical reconstruction indicated for persistent instability → Anatomic repair is most appropriate first-line treatment (Brostrom-Gould).
- Concomitant hindfoot varus may require lateral slide/closing wedge calcaneal osteotomy.

Introduction

- Acute injuries → Traumatic injury to the lateral ligamentous complex presenting with pain, swelling, and ecchymosis.
- Chronic instability → Repeated episodes of "giving way" or recurrent ankle sprains without significant trauma.
- These symptoms can be debilitating to athletes, and recurrent ankle sprains are felt to be an etiologic factor for ankle arthritis.

Etiology

- Injury and incompetence of the ligamentous structures (most commonly laterally)
- Certain factors put patient at risk for ankle instability:
  - Mechanical: varus hindfoot alignment, generalized ligamentous laxity
  - Functional: muscle weakness (peroneal tendons), impaired proprioception, and impaired neuromuscular control
- Suggested mechanism of injury → inverted, plantar flexed foot with an internally rotated hindfoot, and an externally rotated leg

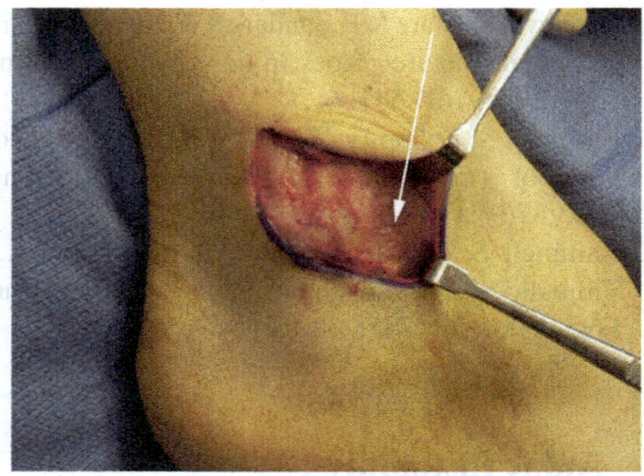

Fig. 7 Intraoperative photograph of the ATFL (*white arrow*)

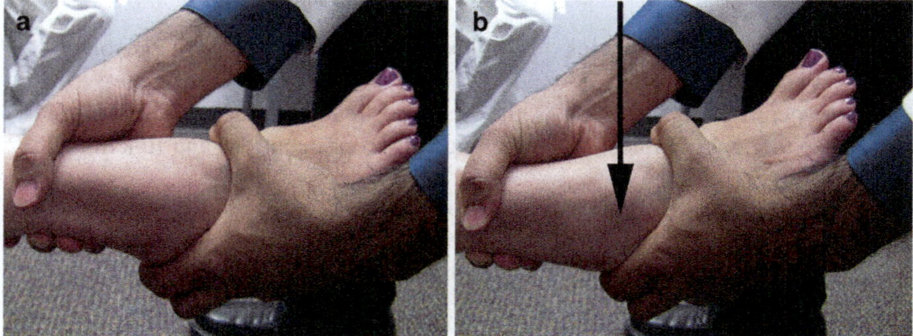

Fig. 8 To perform the anterior drawer test, ne hand stabilizes the anterior distal tibia, while the other is cupped around the posterior calcaneus (**a**). The heel is translated anteriorly with respect to the tibia, and any subluxation should be noted (**b**). Note the sulcus that is created over the anterolateral ankle with an unstable ankle (*arrow*)

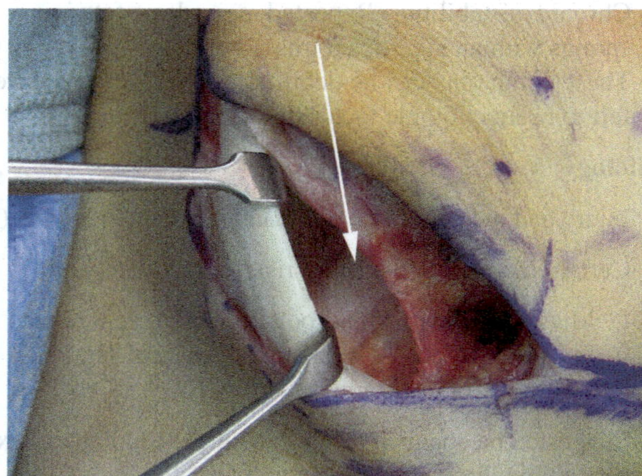

Fig. 9 Intraoperative photograph of the CFL (*white arrow*). Note how the fibers become taught with dorsiflexion of the ankle

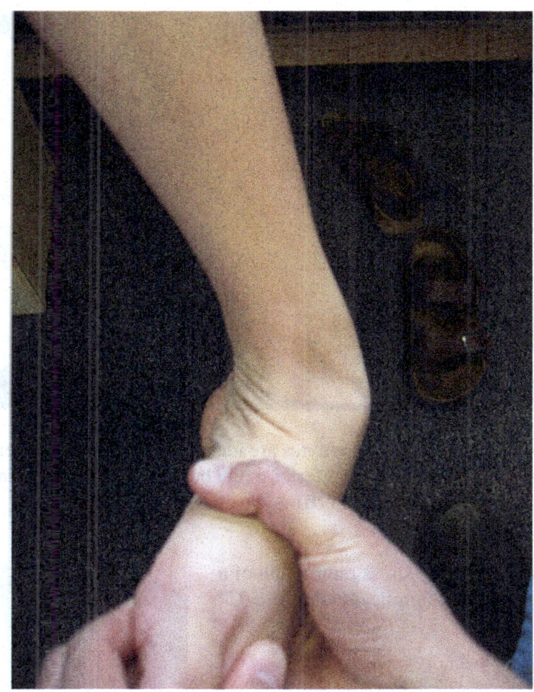

Fig. 10 Inversion stress test in a patient with severe laxity of the CFL

- Can lead to chronic instability

Pathophysiology

Ankle Joint Stability

- Lateral ligamentous structures: most commonly involved (medial side rarely injured). Always compare to contralateral lower extremity.
  - Anterior talofibular ligament (ATFL) (Fig. 7) → most commonly injured → once injured, causes stress on the remaining ligaments; tested by anterior drawer test (Fig. 8). Also assessed with inversion in plantarflexion.
  - Calcaneofibular ligament (CFL) (Fig. 9) → second most commonly injured; tested by talar tilt stress (inversion test) in dorsiflexion (Fig. 10)
  - Posterior talofibular ligament (PTFL)
- Can check joint hyperlaxity by calculating the Beighton score. Signs of ligamentous laxity should be evaluated using the Beighton scoring system. Out of a possible nine points, four points indicates a generalized ligamentous laxity.
  - 5th finger metacarpophalangeal joint extension past 90° (bilateral, 2 points)
  - Thumb to volar forearm (bilateral, 2 points)
  - Hyperextension of the elbow (bilateral, 2 points)
  - Hyperextension of the knee (bilateral, 2 points)
  - Hands flat on floor with forward trunk flexion (1 point)

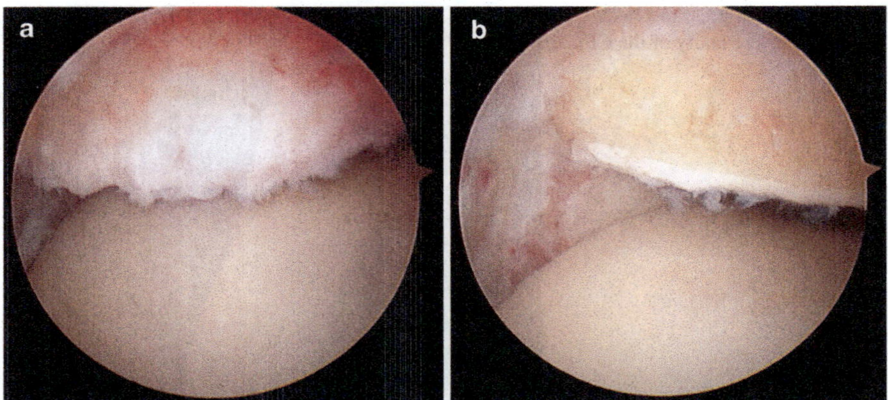

Fig. 11 Anterior osteophytes are identified by their prominence relative to the remaining tibia and by the lack of cartilage inferior to the bone (**a**). After excision of the osteophyte, the normal articular surface is easily seen (**b**)

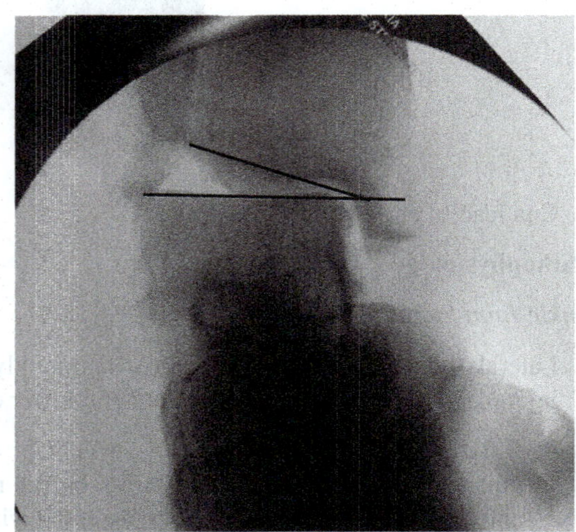

Fig. 12 Varus stress radiograph of a patient with significant talar tilt >15°

Radiography

- Standard weight-bearing anteroposterior, lateral, and mortise views to assess avulsion fractures, arthritis, or osteochondral lesions. A common finding is anterior tibial osteophytes in patient with chronic instability; this must be addressed at the time of surgical intervention (Fig. 11).
- Anterior drawer stress x-ray and talar tilt views are helpful in cases of suspected ankle instability. Absolute values for normal talar tilt vary widely; however, the talar tilt is less the 15° in 95 % of patients (Fig. 12).
- MRI → Not required to make the diagnosis of an acute injury. May consider to evaluate for OCLT or syndesmotic injury if appropriate clinical suspicion is

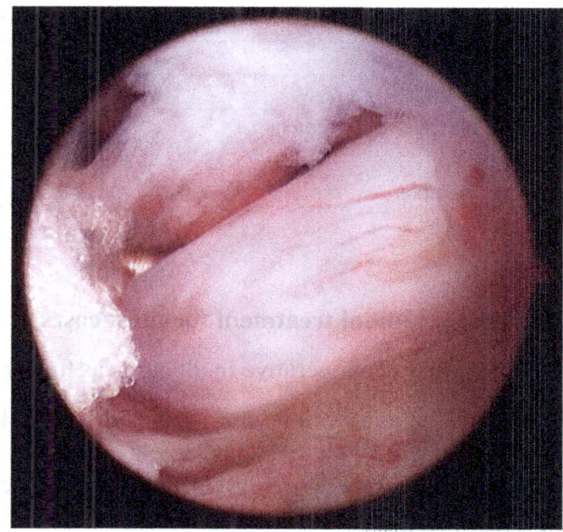

Fig. 13 Large adhesion in a patient that obliterates the anterolateral aspect of the ankle

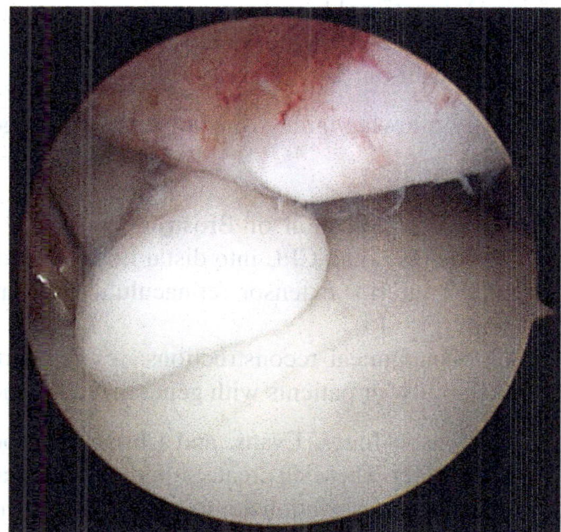

Fig. 14 Loose bodies can be the source of instability in patients who have functional instability without any mechanical laxity. Arthroscopic excision of the loose body is critical in order to relieve the symptoms

given. Recommended in the setting of chronic instability with ankle pain to evaluate for intra-articular pathology (OCLT, loose body, anterior tibial osteophyte, synovitis) given the high incidence of concomitant intra-articular pathology (Figs. 13 and 14).

Classification

- Malliaropoulos classification of acute ankle sprains (Table 1)
- There is no relevant classification for chronic instability.

Table 1 Malliaropoulos classification of acute ankle sprains

Grade	I	II	III
Injured structures	Partial	ATFL	ATFL and CFL
Decrease in range of movement	<5	5–10	>10
Edema	up to 0.5 cm	0.5–2 cm	> 2 cm
Stress radiographs	Normal	Normal	>3 mm laxity

Treatment

Nonoperative: **initial treatment for most cases**

- Acute injury (nonoperative in all cases as first-line treatment)
  - Rest, immobilization, and protected weight bearing immediately, then early mobilization with functional bracing and early rehabilitation (peroneal strengthening and proprioception). Demonstrated superior to cast immobilization
- Chronic instability
  - Physical therapy (including peroneal strengthening and proprioceptive training), functional bracing
  - Orthotic treatment for cavovarus deformity (lateral heel wedge, decreased arch, well-out for first metatarsal)

Operative: following failure of nonoperative management with persistent instability

- Two methods:
  - Gould modification of Brostrom (anatomic repair) → Imbrication of elongated ATFL and CFL into distal fibula. Additional reinforcement with a flap of the inferior extensor retinaculum that improves stability of the subtalar joint (Fig. 15).
  - Non-anatomical reconstructions: reserved for revision cases, long-standing instability, or patients with generalized ligamentous laxity.
    - Watson-Jones, Evans, and Chrisman-Snook: all involve peroneus brevis transfer. These all create significant subtalar stiffness and less restriction of anterior translation compared to an anatomic reconstruction.
    - Autograft or allograft reconstructions have been utilized for revision cases or for patients with ligamentous laxity as these can be placed into a more anatomic position (Fig. 16).
- Arthroscopic exam: controversial, high percentage of intra-articular pathology found, but unknown clinical benefit proven. Consider if MRI demonstrates intra-articular pathology.

Complications

- Recurrence (especially with hindfoot malalignment that is uncorrected)
- Persistent pain
- Post-traumatic osteoarthritis (associated with significant long term instability)

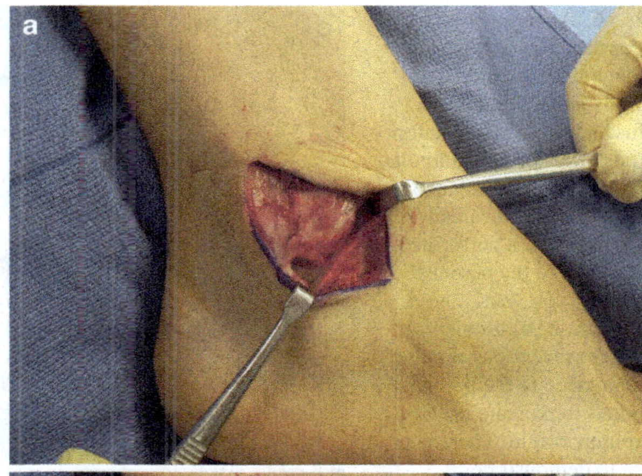

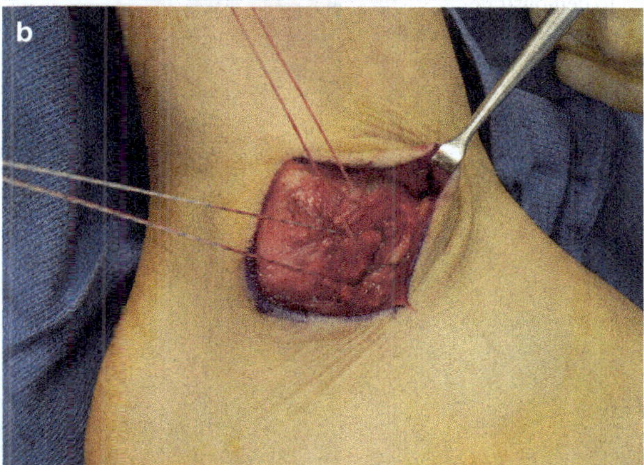

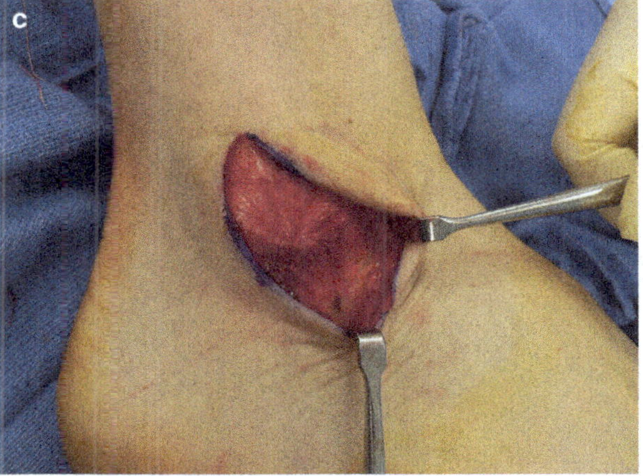

Fig. 15 Brostrom anatomic reconstruction for lateral ankle instability. The ATFL and CFL are incised from the fibular origin (**a**). Utilizing suture anchors in this case the ligaments are imbricated (**b**). Final appearance of the ligaments shows them taut (**c**)

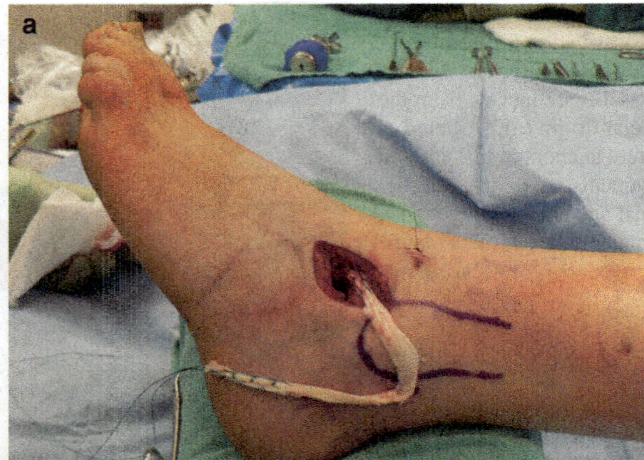

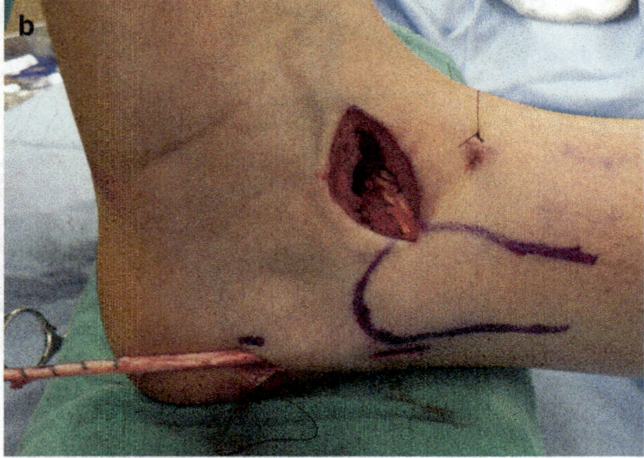

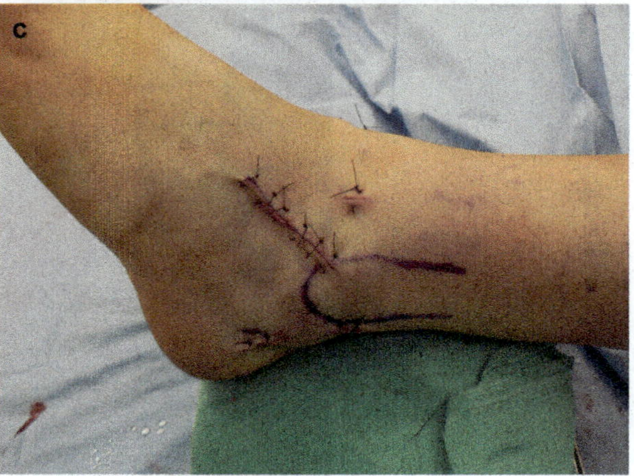

Fig. 16 Anatomic allograft reconstruction of the lateral collateral ligaments. The graft is fixated within the talus and routed from anterior to posterior through a fibular drill hole (**a**). Subcutaneous passage to the calcaneal insertion is then performed superficial to the peroneal tendons to prevent subluxation (**b**). Some authors prevent passing the tendon deep to the peroneal tendons to recreate the CFL's anatomic origin. There is no data to demonstrate superiority of one technique over the other. Final appearance of the reconstructed ankle (**c**)

Bibliography

1. de Vries JS, Krips R, Sierevelt IN, Blankevoort L. Interventions for treating chronic ankle instability. Cochrane Database Syst Rev. 2006;(4):CD004124.
2. DiGiovanni CW, Brodsky A. Current concepts: lateral ankle instability. Foot Ankle Int. 2006;27:854–66.
3. Ferkel RD, Chams RN. Chronic lateral instability: arthroscopic findings and long-term results. Foot Ankle. 2007;28:24–31.
4. Maffulli N, Ferran NA. Management of acute and chronic ankle instability. J Am Acad Orthop Surg. 2008;16:608–15.

3 Talar Osteochondral Defects

Take-Home Message

- Lateral OCLT are usually of traumatic etiology, smaller, more shallow and more symptomatic than medial lesions. However, lateral lesions have superior surgical outcome.
- Persistent ankle pain after acute sprain → obtain MRI to rule OCLT.
- Lateral lesions have less potential for spontaneous resolution.
- Choice of operative treatment is dependent on lesion size.
- Arthroscopic verse open procedure has comparative results.

Definition

- Osteochondral lesions of the talar dome is a cause of ankle pain and disability. Presenting symptoms includes pain, swelling, and mechanical symptoms such as catching and locking. Up to 10 % are bilateral.

Etiology

- Acute trauma
- Repetitive microtrauma

Pathophysiology

- Osteochondral lesions of the talar dome may result from acute trauma or repetitive microtrauma. Pathophysiology differs based on lesion location. Recent data has demonstrated that both medial and lateral OCLT are found most common in the central talar dome in the sagittal plane.
- Lateral talar dome
  - Tends to be traumatic etiology, typically inversion or inversion-dorsiflexion mechanism
  - Lesions usually smaller, more shallow and more symptomatic than medial lesions (Fig. 17)
  - Superior surgical results

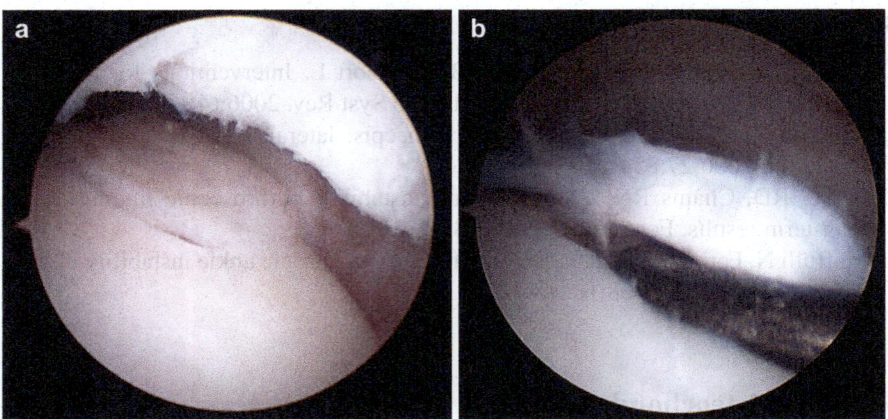

Fig. 17 Arthroscopic view of a lateral talar osteochondral defect. (**a, b**) Note the shallow nature of the defect with the clear detached articular surface (**a, b**)

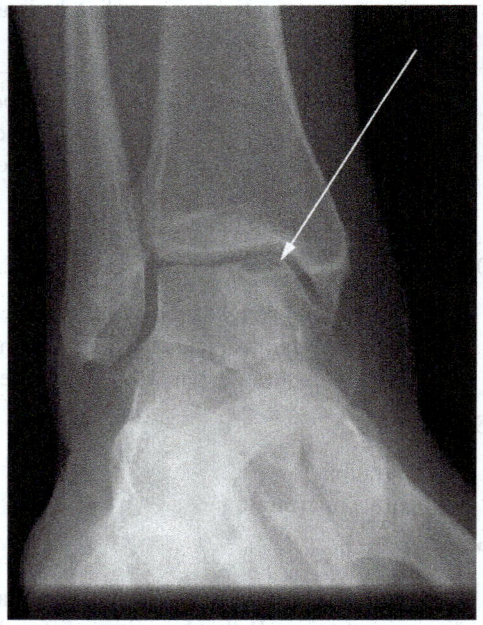

Fig. 18 Ankle radiograph demonstrating an obvious lucency of the medial talar dome (*arrow*) consistent with an OCLT

- Medial talar dome
  - Tends to be atraumatic etiology
  - Lesions usually larger and deeper than lateral lesions

Radiography

- Ankle x-ray
  - Maybe normal or subtle radiolucency, articular surface irregularity, or subchondral bone fragmentation (Fig. 18)

- CT/MRI
  - Further evaluate lesions apparent on x-ray or for persistent ankle pain after trauma such ankle sprain/fracture despite appropriate management (Fig. 19)
  - Helpful for classification of lesions

Classification

- The Berndt and Harty radiographic staging classification (Table 2)
- The Ferkel and Sgaglione CT staging classification (Table 3)
- The Hepple and associates MRI staging classification (Table 4)
- Arthroscopic evaluation is the reliable means of determining lesion size and the intactness of articular surface of lesions.

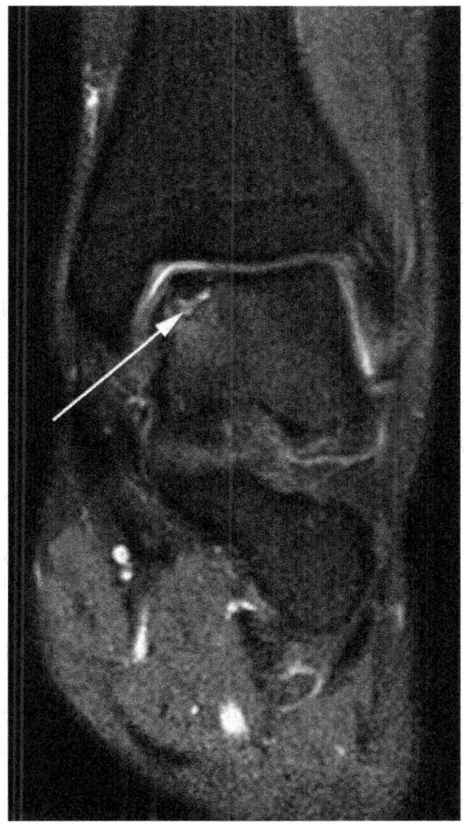

Fig. 19 MRI demonstrating a medial OCLT with fluid inferior to articular surface (*arrow*) that denotes instability of the lesion

Table 2 The Berndt and harty radiographic staging classification of OCLT

Stage 1	Small area of subchondral compression/depression
Stage 2	Partial fragment detachment
Stage 3	Complete fragment detachment, non-displaced
Stage 4	Complete fragment detachment, displaced

Table 3 The Ferkel and Sgaglione CT staging classification of OCLT

Stage 1	Cystic lesion within talar dome with an intact roof in all views
Stage 2a	Cystic lesion with communication to talar dome surface
Stage 2b	Open articular surface lesion with overlying non-displaced fragment
Stage 3	Non-displaced lesion with lucency
Stage 4	Displaced fragment

Table 4 The Hepple and Associates MRI staging classification of OCLT

Stage 1	Articular cartilage
Stage 2a	Cartilage injury with underlying fracture with surrounding bone edema
Stage 2b	Cartilage injury with underlying fracture without surrounding bone edema
Stage 3	Detached but non-displaced fragment
Stage 4	Displaced fragment
Stage 5	Subchondral cyst formation

Treatment

Nonoperative

- Indication: Non-displaced fragment. No proven risk of DJD with nonoperative management.
- Short leg cast immobilization
- Restricted weight bearing

Operative

- Indication: displaced fragment in the acute setting. Persistent pain or mechanical symptoms in the chronic setting.
- Treatment choice is based on size of lesion.
- Results of arthroscopic verse open procedures are comparable.
- Lesion with intact cartilage cap: retrograde drilling ± bone grafting.
- Lesion < 1.5 cm^2: debridement and microfracture/drilling (Figs. 20 and 21)
- Lesion > 1.5 cm^2 cm with displaced cartilage cap: joint restorative procedures – osteochondral autograft, chondrocyte implantation, or osteochondral allograft
- Lesions >3 cm^2: osteochondral allograft (Fig. 22).

Complications

- Nonunion of autograft/allograft
- Persistent pain
- Tibiotalar arthritis

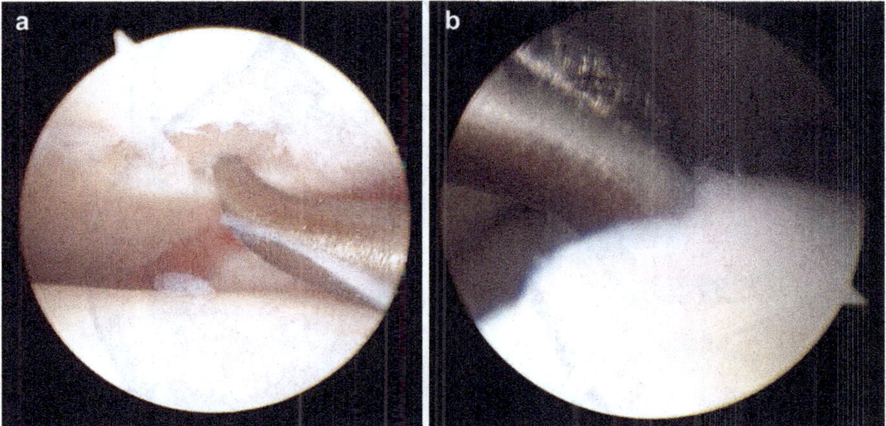

Fig. 20 Microfracture technique of a tibial (**a**) and talar (**b**) osteochondral lesion

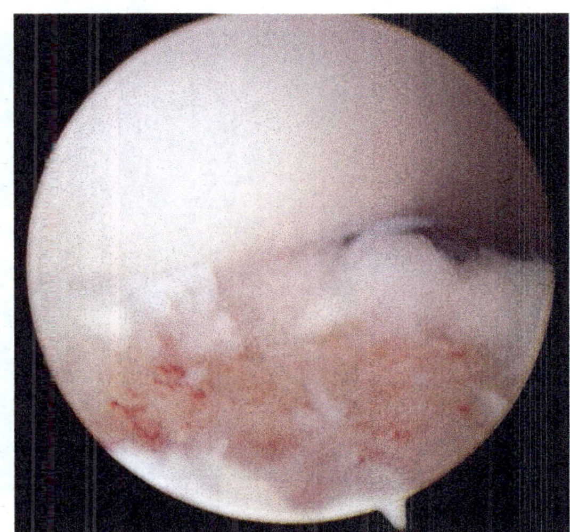

Fig. 21 Final appearance of a talar osteochondral defect following microfracture. Note the blood that is emanating from the microfracture holes made in the talus

Bibliography

1. Choi WJ, Park KK, Kim BS, Lee JW. Osteochondral lesion of the talus: is there a critical defect size for poor outcome? Am J Sports Med. 2009;37:1974–80.
2. Choi WJ, Kim BS, Lee JW. Osteochondral lesion of the talus: could age be an indication for arthroscopic treatment? Am J Sports Med. 2012;40:419–24.
3. Cuttica DJ, Smith WB, Hyer CF, et al. Osteochondral lesions of the talus: predictors of clinical outcome. Foot Ankle Int. 2011;32(11):1045–51.
4. Orr JD, Dawson LK, Garcia EJ, Kirk KL. Incidence of osteochondral lesions of the talus in the United States military. Foot Ankle Int. 2011;32:948–54.
5. Ventura A, Terzaghi C, Legnani C, Borgo C. Treatment of post-traumatic osteochondral lesions of the talus: a four-step approach. Knee Surg Sports Traumatol Arthrosc. 2012;21:1245–50.

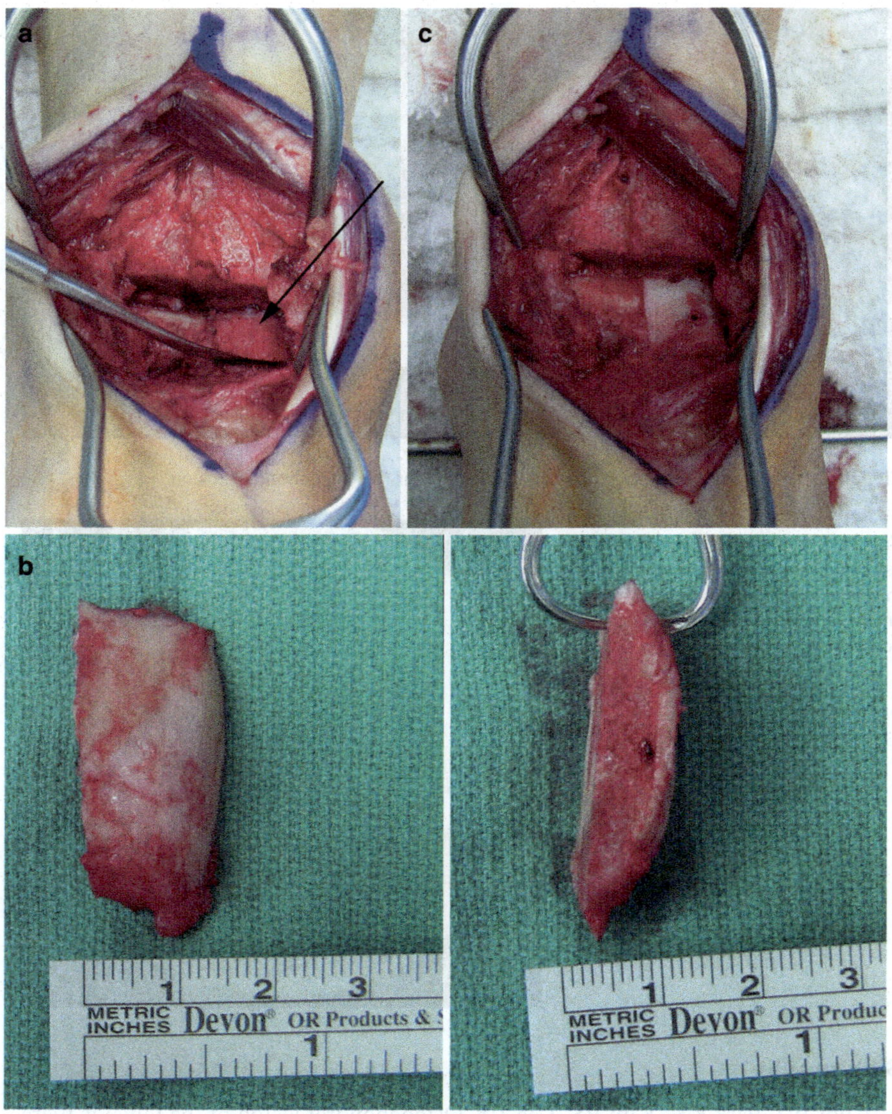

Fig. 22 Large (>3 cm^2) osteochondral defect (*arrow*) that was approached via an anterior ankle arthrotomy (**a**). The entire ½ of the articular surface was abnormal (**b**). Given the large surface area involved an allograft reconstruction (**c**) was performed

4 Heel Pain

Take-Home Message

- Plantar fasciitis is the most common cause, present classically with "start-up" pain in the AM that improves after the first few steps.
- Location of pain provides diagnostic clue.
  - Inferior heel pain ->plantar fasciitis
  - Medial heel pain→Baxter's neuritis (Lateral plantar nerve compression)
  - Posterior heel pain→retrocalcaneal bursitis, Haglund's deformity, insertional and Achilles tendinitis/tendinosis
  - Pain with lateral and medial compression→calcaneal stress fracture
- Nonoperative management is the first treatment. Plantar fascia-specific stretch is most important for PF.

Definition Heel pain is a common foot problem that causes significant discomfort and disability. The differential diagnosis for heel pain is broad and includes plantar fasciitis, calcaneal stress fracture, calcaneal apophysitis (Sever disease), central heel pain (fat pad atrophy, fat pad contusion), and nerve entrapment (tarsal tunnel syndrome, entrapment of the first branch of the lateral plantar nerve) and posterior heel pain (retrocalcaneal bursitis, Haglund's deformity, insertional Achilles tendinitis/tendinosis).

Etiology

- Repetitive microtrauma (stress fracture, Baxter's neuritis in runners)
- Inflammatory
- Degenerative
- Drug induced (fluoroquinolone use with Achilles pathology)

Pathophysiology Etiology is multifactorial, as such presentation and pathophysiology unique to each disease process.

Plantar Fasciitis

- Most common cause of heel pain. Affects both sedentary and active.
- Presents classically as "start-up" plantar medial heel pain and preference for toe walking for first few steps and improvement with progressive walking
- Repetitive microtrauma to plantar fascia→microtears and inflammatory response→reparative response
- Other risk factors: obesity, pes planus, pes cavus, gastrocnemius contracture, and excessive femoral anteversion increase the traction load at the origin of the plantar fascia during weight bearing
- About 50 % have heel spurs, however not cause of heel pain.

Calcaneal Stress Fracture

- Heel absorbs about 110 % of body weight during walking and 200 % during running.
- Repetitive loading of the calcaneus results in fatigue fractures. Common in active individual and military recruits.
- Risk factors: female, female athlete triad, hormonal deficiency, and osteopenia

Calcaneal Apophysitis (Sever Disease)

- Common cause of heel pain in pediatric population
- Overuse injury of calcaneal apophysis
- Natural history: self-limiting, resolves with closure of the apophysis

Central Heel Pain (Fat Pad Atrophy, Fat Pad Contusion)

- The heel pad provides significant shock absorber function to the hindfoot.
- Fat pad atrophy can result from inflammatory disease process, corticosteroid injection, trauma, and advanced age.
- Fat pad contusion from trauma can present as central heel pain.

Nerve Entrapment

- Entrapment of the First Branch of the Lateral Plantar Nerve (Baxter's Neuritis)

  The first branch of the lateral plantar nerve is a mixed (sensory and motor) nerve. Compression of this nerve occurs between the deep fascia of the abductor hallucis and inferomedial margin of the quadratus plantae.

  Common in running athletes and presents as plantar medial heel pain that mimic plantar fasciitis

  Tarsal tunnel syndrome can have similar presentation; however, symptoms originate more proximal and tend to involve entire foot and not just heel.

Posterior Heel Pain

Retrocalcaneal bursitis and Haglund's deformity

- Inflammation of retrocalcaneal bursa (lies between anterior surface of Achilles tendon and the posterosuperior calcaneus tuberosity).
- Haglund's deformity: enlargement of the calcaneal posterosuperior tuberosity

Insertional Achilles tendinitis/tendinosis

- Inflammatory changes at the tendon insertion site from repetitive microtrauma
- Progressive bony metaplasia and prominence at the calcaneal insertion

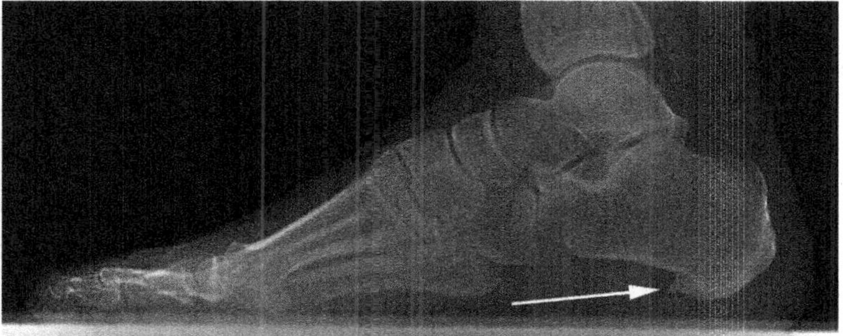

Fig. 23 Inferior plantar spur (*arrow*) commonly seen in patients with plantar fasciitis

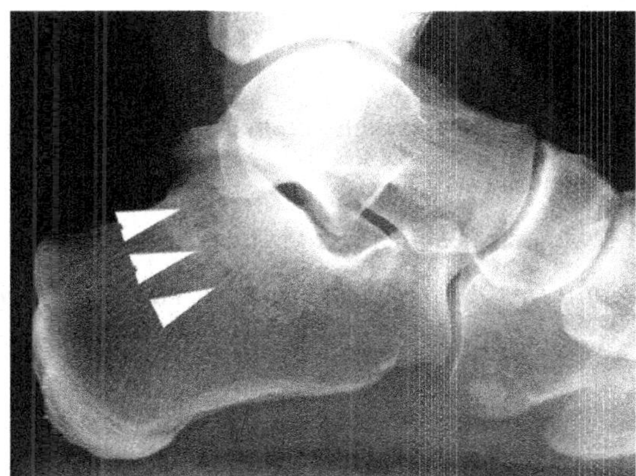

Fig. 24 Lateral radiograph of a calcaneal stress fracture. Note the linear and vertically oriented increased density in the calcaneus (*arrowheads*). The finding is subtle but more easily identified as the normal lines of stress are oriented from the tuberosity towards the posterior facet, with the fracture line crossing multiple normal lines of stress

Radiography

Plantar Fasciitis

- Weight-bearing x-ray
  - Usually normal
  - Heel spurs (Fig. 23)

Calcaneal Stress Fracture

- Heel x-ray: Initially normal, but few weeks after onset of symptoms, radio-dense line becomes apparent (Fig. 24).
- MRI: fracture apparent in setting of normal x-ray (Fig. 25)

Calcaneal Apophysitis (Sever Disease)

- Heel x-ray
  - Apophyseal sclerosis not specific finding
  - Apophyseal fragmentation more specific finding

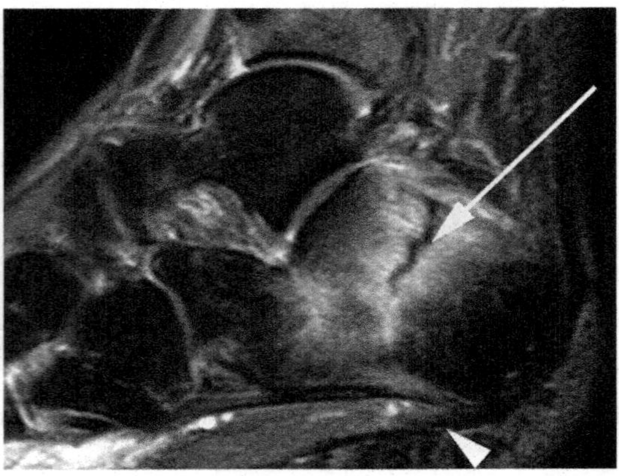

Fig. 25 Sagittal STIR image of a calcaneal stress fracture. Note the hypointense signal (*arrow*) delineating the fracture line with adjacent bony edema (high signal)

- MRI
  - Apophyseal inflammation, rule out other diagnosis
- Bone scan
  - Apophyseal increased uptake

Central Heel Pain (Fat Pad Atrophy, Fat Pad Contusion)

- Weight-bearing x-ray
  - Heel spurs
  - Rule out other pathology

Baxter's Neuritis

- EMG/NCV: increased motor latency of the abductor digiti quinti
- MRI: fatty atrophy of abductor digiti quinti or space-occupying lesion

Retrocalcaneal Bursitis and Haglund's Deformity

- Foot x-ray: Haglund's deformity on lateral view

Insertional Achilles Tendinitis/Tendinosis

- Lateral Heel x-ray: bone spur, intratendinous calcification/ossification (Fig. 26)
- Ultrasound/MRI: evaluate tendon degeneration

Treatment

Plantar Fasciitis

- Nonoperative
  - Plantar fascia-specific and heel cord stretching protocol
  - NSAIDs, low impact activity, physical therapy
  - Orthotics: Night splints, heel cushion inserts
  - Corticosteroid injection if failed non-op

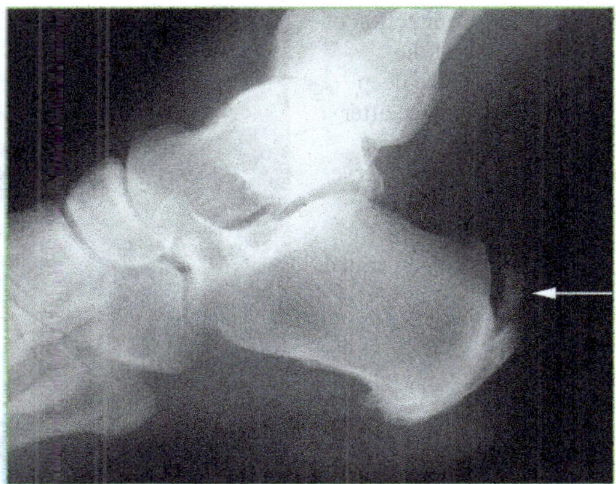

Fig. 26 Lateral radiograph of a patient with insertional calcific Achilles tendinosis. A large posterior heel spur is diagnostic (*white arrow*)

  - High-energy extracorporal shock wave therapy and PRP have demonstrated efficacy in some trials compared to standard non-op treatment in the short term. Cannot be recommended over standard non-op management at this time.

- Operative
  - Plantar fascia release. Release only medial ½. Baxter's nerve release for concomitant Baxter's neuritis symptoms
  - Gastrocnemius recession instead of a PF release if contracture is present

Calcaneal Stress Fracture

- Rest/activity modification and protected weight bearing
- Cushioned heel orthotics

Calcaneal Apophysitis (Sever Disease)

- Rest/activity modification and heel cord stretching
- Brief immobilization with short leg cast for persistent pain
- Cushioned heel orthotics

Central Heel Pain (Fat Pad Atrophy, Fat Pad Contusion)

- Cushioned heel cups

Baxter's Neuritis

- NSAIDs, cessation of aggravating activity, heel cord stretching
- Orthotics: cushioned heel inserts, correct for any underlying deformity.
- Operative
  - Surgical release and decompression of Baxter's nerve, deep fascia of the abductor hallucis must be released (Fig. 27).
  - Medial ½ plantar fascia release for concomitant plantar fasciitis symptoms

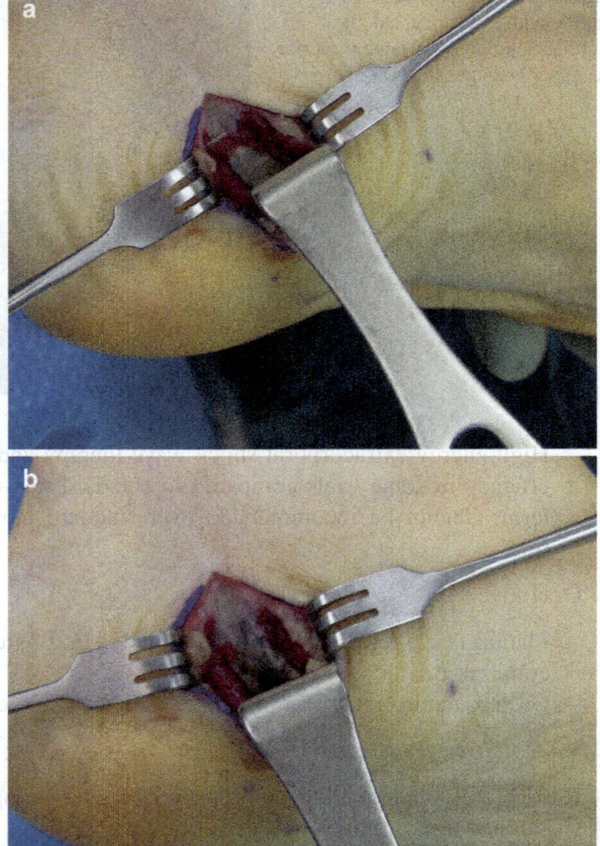

Fig. 27 Inferior retraction of the muscle belly of the abductor exposes the deep fascia (**a**). Appearance after incision of the deep fascia (**b**). The lateral plantar nerve lies directly superior to the deep fascia, and careful dissection must be performed

Retrocalcaneal Bursitis and Haglund's Deformity

Nonoperative

- NSAIDs
- Shoe modification (open or low back shoes) or padding to minimize mechanical irritation
- Corticosteroid injection of the bursa, avoid tendon injection → risk of rupture

Operative

- Retrocalcaneal bursectomy and resection of Haglund's deformity
- <50 % release of Achilles tendon mandates repair with anchors to calcaneus.

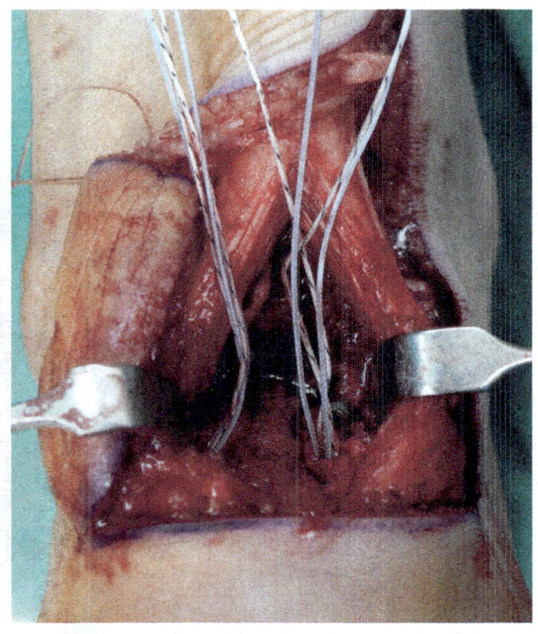

Fig. 28 Intraoperative photograph of a patient who had insertional Achilles tendinosis. After debridement of the diseased tissue and Haglund's deformity, more than 50 % of the Achilles was detached. Repair with suture anchors is important in preventing postoperative rupture

Insertional and Non-Insertional Achilles Tendinitis/Tendinosis

Nonoperative

- NSAIDs, activity modification (limit impact, push-off).
- Heel cord stretching and therapy with eccentric training (most critical).
- Shoe modification or padding to minimize mechanical irritation or small heel lift.
- Avoid corticosteroid injection → risk of rupture.

Operative

- Tendon and prominent bone debridement with repair to bone with anchors (Fig. 28).
- Tendon augmentation with FHL, FHL transfer if > 50 % tendon debrided (Fig. 29)

Complications

Plantar Fasciitis

- Fat pad atrophy from corticosteroid injection
- Longitudinal arch collapse and chronic foot pain from excessive plantar fascia release
- Injury to the lateral plantar nerve

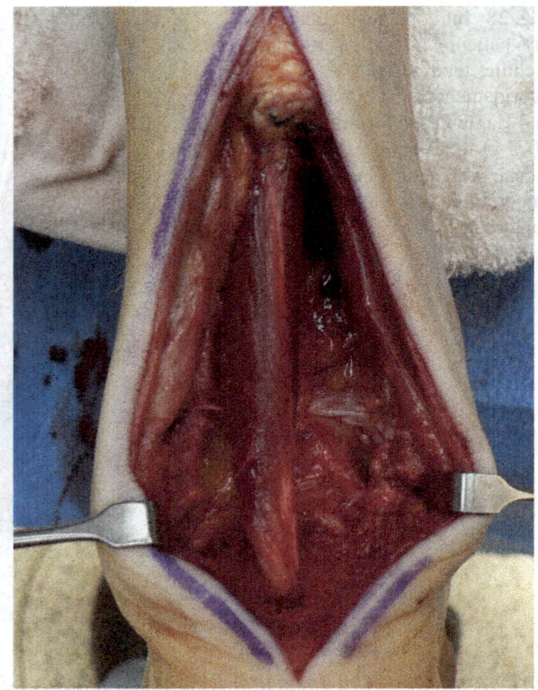

Fig. 29 Intraoperative photograph of a FHL transfer in a patient who had a severe insertional Achilles tendinosis. After resection of the nonviable tissue, the FHL was transferred through a drill hole in the calcaneus and fixed with an interference screw

Baxter's Neuritis

- Inadequate decompression
- Injury to the lateral plantar nerve

Retrocalcaneal Bursitis and Haglund's Deformity

- Achilles tendon rupture from corticosteroid injection or excessive debridement

Insertional Achilles Tendinitis/Tendinosis

- Achilles tendon rupture from corticosteroid injection or excessive debridement

Bibliography

1. DiGiovanni BF, Moore AM, Zlotnicki JP, Pinney SJ. Preferred management of recalcitrant plantar fasciitis among orthopaedic foot and ankle surgeons. Foot Ankle Int. 2012;33(6):507–12.
2. Garrett TR, Neibert PJ. The effectiveness of a gastrocnemius-soleus stretching program as a therapeutic treatment of plantar fasciitis. J Sport Rehabil. 2013;22(4):308–12.
3. Ngo KT, Del Toro DR. Electrodiagnostic findings and surgical outcome in isolated first branch lateral plantar neuropathy: a case series with literature review. Arch Phys Med Rehabil. 2010;91(12):1948–51.

4. Schon LC, Glennon TP, Baxter DE. Heel pain syndrome: electrodiagnostic support for nerve entrapment. Foot Ankle. 1993;14(3):129–35.
5. Schon LC, Shores JL, Faro FD, Vora AM, Camire LM, Guyton GP. Flexor hallucis longus tendon transfer in treatment of Achilles tendinosis. J Bone Joint Surg Am. 2013;95(1):54–60.
6. Sinnaeve F, Vandeputte G. Clinical outcome of surgical intervention for recalcitrant infero-medial heel pain. Acta Orthop Belg. 2008;74(4):483–8.
7. Wiegerinck JI, Kerkhoffs GM, van Sterkenburg MN, Sierevelt IN, van Dijk CN. Treatment for insertional Achilles tendinopathy: a systematic review. Knee Surg Sports Traumatol Arthrosc. 2013;21(6):1345–55.

Midfoot

Anish R. Kadakia, Paul J. Switaj, Bryant S. Ho, Mohammed Alshouli, Daniel Fuchs, and George Ochengele

1 Arthritis

> **Take-Home Message**
> - Primary osteoarthritis most common.
> - Nonoperative management with a carbon fiber plate and midfoot rocker shoe modification is the first-line treatment strategy.
> - Operative management consists of a tarsometatarsal arthrodesis with realignment in the cases of midfoot deformity (RA and chronic Lisfranc).
> - Arthrodesis of medial and middle columns is effective and does not significantly adversely affect foot function.
> - Arthrodesis of lateral column adversely alters foot function as it alters ground accommodation. Therefore, interpositional arthroplasty (tendon, implant, collagen matrix) has been advocated as an alternative treatment instead of arthrodesis for the 4th and 5th TMT joints.

Introduction

- Arthritis of the midfoot is a significant cause of pain and disability. Midfoot articulations include naviculocuneiform (NC) and tarsometatarsal (TMT) joints.

A.R. Kadakia, MD (✉) • P.J. Switaj • B.S. Ho • M. Alshouli • D. Fuchs • G. Ochengele
Department of Orthopedic Surgery, Northwestern University – Feinberg School of Medicine, Northwestern Memorial Hospital, Chicago, IL, USA
e-mail: Kadak259@gmail.com; paul.switaj@gmail.com; bryant.s.ho@gmail.com; mtshouli@gmail.com; dfuchs0011@gmail.com; gochenjele@gmail.com

C. Mauffrey, D.J. Hak (eds.), *Passport for the Orthopedic Boards and FRCS Examination*, DOI 10.1007/978-2-8178-0475-0_40

Etiology

- Primary osteoarthritis is the most common cause of hindfoot arthritis.
- Posttraumatic arthritis is second.
- Inflammatory.

Pathophysiology

- The middle column has limited motion but is exposed to large forces.
- Abnormally high forces through the midfoot lead to the incompetence of supporting soft tissue structures → joint subluxation → increased contact pressure → degeneration.
- Inflammatory processes and posterior tibialis tendon dysfunction (PTTD) can lead to midfoot collapse and arthritis.
- Gastrocnemius contracture will increase forces across the midfoot possibly accelerating the disease.

Radiography

- AP (1st, 2nd, 3rd, and N-C joints), oblique (3rd, 4th, and 5th TMT joints), and lateral WB radiographs:
  - Joint-space narrowing or loss (The lateral view may reveal joint-space narrowing not appreciated on the AP or oblique radiographs (Fig. 1))
  - Subchondral sclerosis/cysts
  - Osteophytes and bony erosions – best seen on lateral view
  - Disruption of Meary's line (loss of colinearity between talus and 1st MT) with apex deformity at midfoot and longitudinal arch collapse on lateral view
  - Forefoot abduction deformity. Critical to differentiate from PTTD flatfoot deformity where TN in abduction > TMT (Fig. 2)

Treatment

Nonoperative

- A stiff carbon fiber plate inserted underneath the insole of the shoe or a rocker-bottom shoe will offload stress on the midfoot during gait and may relieve mild degenerative symptoms.
- Rigid deformity should be managed with accommodative, not corrective orthotics that support and offload the deformity.
- Corticosteroid/anesthetic injections: both diagnostic (determine symptomatic joints) and therapeutic

Operative

Indication is failure of nonoperative with persistent pain and disability. Arthrodesis is the treatment of choice. Goal of surgery is to obtain solid fusion and restoration of normal foot alignment.

- Medial and middle column arthrodesis ensuring a normal anatomic alignment. Residual deformity will predictably result in a poor outcome (Fig. 3).

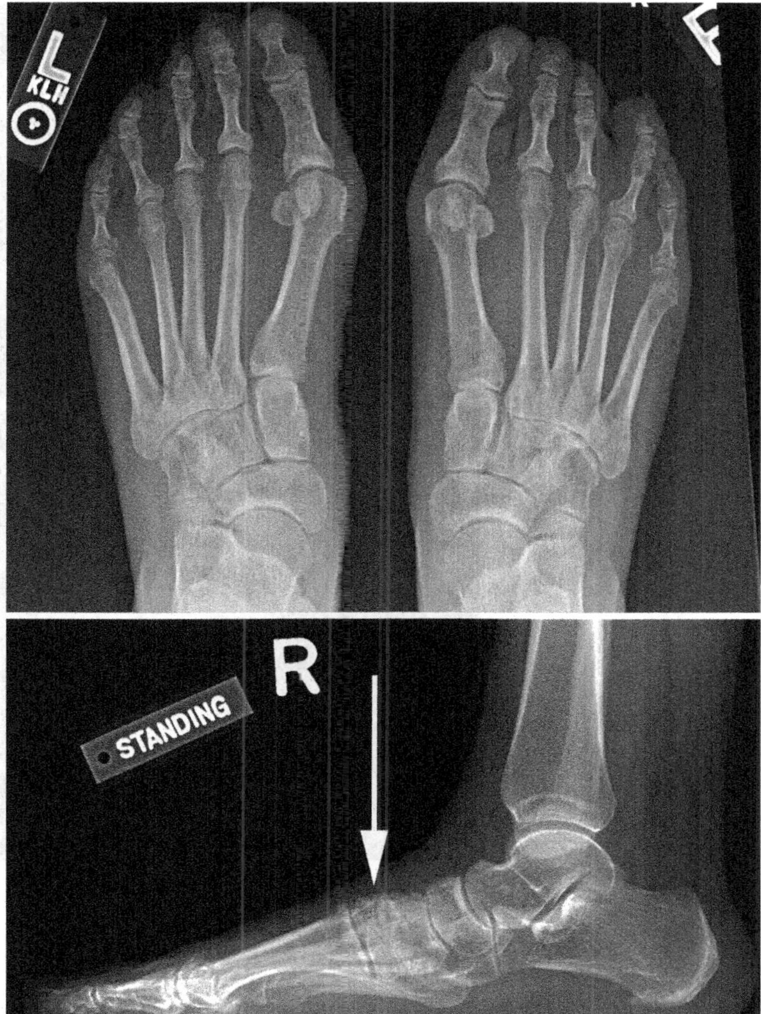

Fig. 1 Patient with midfoot arthritis primarily at the middle column. Note the subtle asymmetric narrowing on the AP radiograph. The presence of 2nd TMT degeneration is clearly seen on the lateral radiograph (*arrow*)

- Interpositional arthroplasty (motion sparring) of lateral column is preferred for symptomatic 4th and 5th TMT arthritis given the biomechanical advantage. However, no significant data is present to support motion-sparing procedures over arthrodesis.
- A simultaneous gastrocnemius recession and/or hindfoot osteotomy might be required to restore normal foot alignment (Fig. 4).

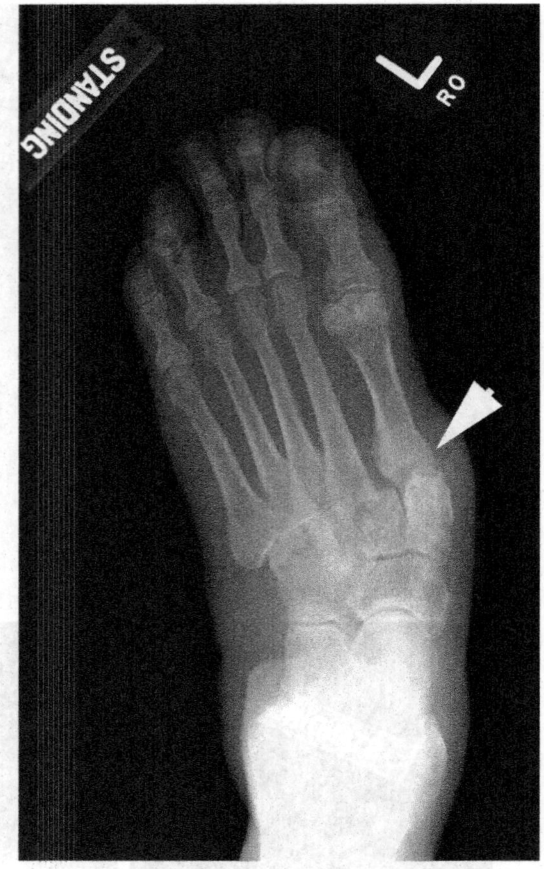

Fig. 2 AP WB radiograph demonstrating abduction deformity of the foot that is clearly focused at the TMT joints (*arrowhead*). Note the minimal amount of TN joint subluxation despite the severe deformity, indicating this is a midfoot driven flatfoot and not related to PTTD

Complications

- Nonunion/malunion
- Wound complications

Bibliography

1. Nemec SA, Habbu RA, Anderson JG, Bohay DR. Outcomes following midfoot arthrodesis for primary arthritis. Foot Ankle Int. 2011;32(4):355–61.
2. Patel A, Rao S, Nawoczenski D, Flemister AS, DiGiovanni B, Baumhauer JF. Midfoot arthritis. J Am Acad Orthop Surg. 2010;18(7):417–25.
3. Russell DF, Ferdinand RD. Review of the evidence: surgical management of 4th and 5th tarsometatarsal joint osteoarthritis. Foot Ankle Surg. 2013;19(4):207–11.
4. Verhoeven N, Vandeputte G. Midfoot arthritis: diagnosis and treatment. Foot Ankle Surg. 2012;18(4):255–62.
5. Zonno AJ, Myerson MS. Surgical correction of midfoot arthritis with and without deformity. Foot Ankle Clin. 2011;16(1):35–47.

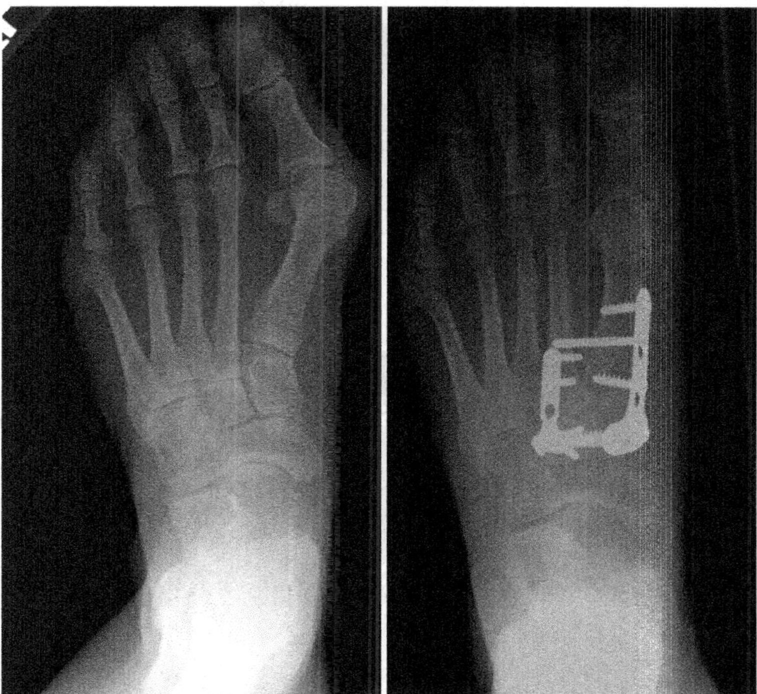

Fig. 3 A Lapidus and 2nd TMT arthrodesis was performed in this patient who presented with complaints of hallux valgus and midfoot pain with radiographic evidence of midfoot DJD. The patient had osteopenic bone and therefore plate fixation was chosen

2 Kohler's Disease

Take-Home Message

- Pediatric avascular necrosis of the navicular of unknown etiology.
- Boys preferentially affected.
- 25 % can be bilateral.
- Usually self-limiting with favorable prognosis, surgery is not indicated.
- Immobilization with short leg walking cast is indicated for activity-related symptoms.
- Immobilization decreases duration of symptoms.

Definition

- Avascular necrosis of the navicular bone of unclear etiology. Occurs in pediatric population. Patients usually present with pain (dorsomedial), swelling, and warmth/redness and limp.
- However, some patients are asymptomatic.

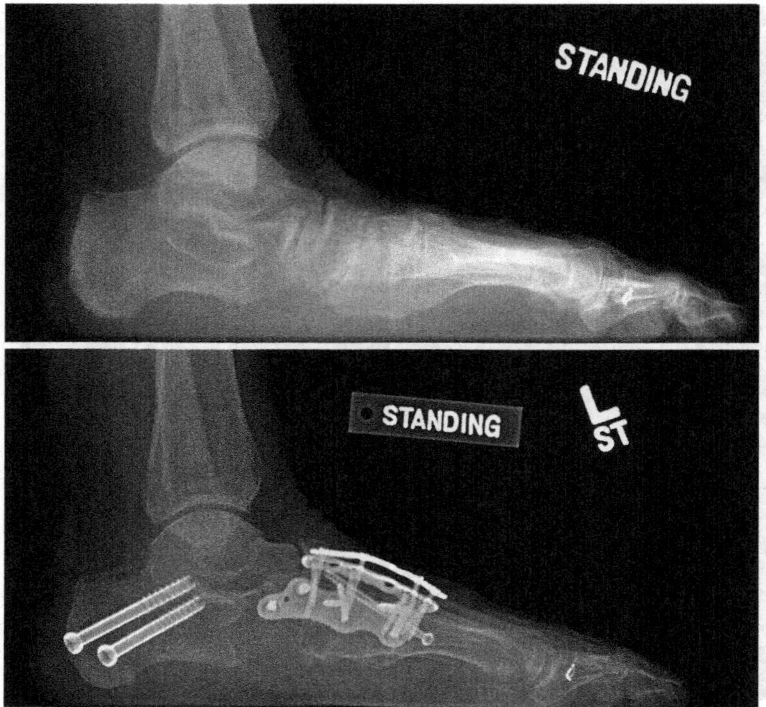

Fig. 4 Extended midfoot arthrodesis with concomitant medial slide calcaneal osteotomy was required in this patient who presented with midfoot arthritis and secondary hindfoot valgus deformity. Note the restoration of the longitudinal arch in the postoperative radiograph

- More common in boys (up 80 % of cases).
- 25 % of cases are bilateral.

Etiology

- Unknown

Pathophysiology

- Blood supply: the central 1/3 of the navicular is a watershed area → avascular necrosis
- Late ossification → predisposition to injury and mechanical compression

Radiography

- Foot X-ray
  - Active disease: sclerosis, fragmentation, and flattening of navicular
  - Post resolution: bone remodeling and reconstitution, asymptomatic deformity can persist

Treatment

- Usually self-limiting with good prognosis. Symptoms usually associated with activities.

Nonoperative

- NSAIDs, activity modification (eliminate impact)
- Shoe insert orthotics (accommodative)
- Immobilization with short leg walking cast
  - Indication: activity-related pain and failure of above modalities

Operative

- No indication for surgery

Complications

- Very good prognosis without post-resolution sequela. Deformity is usually asymptomatic.

Bibliography

1. Borges JL, Guille JT, Bowen JR. Köhler's bone disease of the tarsal navicular. J Pediatr Orthop. 1995;15(5):596–8.
2. DiGiovanni CW, Patel A, Calfee R, Nickisch F. Osteonecrosis in the foot. J Am Acad Orthop Surg. 2007;15(4):208–17.
3. Tsirikos AI, Riddle EC, Kruse R. Bilateral Köhler's disease in identical twins. Clin Orthop Relat Res. 2003;409:195–8.

3 Sinus Tarsi Syndrome

Take-Home Message

- Sinus tarsi syndrome presents as lateral heel pain that is relieved by local anesthetic injection into sinus tarsi and associated with feeling of instability.
- Highly associated with ankle inversion injuries.
- MRI and arthroscopy reveal inflammatory changes and partial ligamentous tear.
- Nonoperative management is the first-line treatment: serial local anesthetic/corticosteroid injections are effective.
- Favorable results for both arthroscopic and open excision and debridement.

Definition

- Sinus tarsal syndrome (STS) is a clinical entity that represents local pain in the lateral heel over sinus tarsi – located between the talus and the calcaneus.
  - Pain that is relieved by local anesthetics/corticosteroid injection.
  - Associated with hindfoot instability.
- Canalis tarsi syndrome is a variant of STS → medial side pain

Etiology

- Anatomy: The sinus tarsi is an anatomic space → bounded by inferior talus, the superior aspect of the calcaneus, posterior subtalar facet, and the calcaneonavicular joint anteriorly.
  - Medially continuous with the tarsal canal
  - Space filled with fat and contains vessels and ligaments
- The true etiology of STS is unknown, although several theories have been postulated → posttraumatic fibrosis, synovial hyperplasia, hemosiderin deposition, inflammatory response, compression of herniated synovial membrane, and proprioceptive disorder.
- There is high association with previous ankle inversion/supination injuries and independent of lateral ankle ligament complex rupture or osteochondral lesion.

Pathophysiology

- Similar to the etiology, the pathophysiology of STS is poorly understood.
- Related to posttraumatic ligamentous injury, inflammatory changes, and instability.

Radiography

X-Ray

Normal in most cases. Stress radiography may demonstrate instability of the subtalar joint, although this is difficult to demonstrate. Clinical laxity to varus stress with a normal stress X-ray of the ankle is suggestive of subtalar instability.

Subtalar Arthrogram

- Demonstrates a saclike anterior bulge of the capsule

MRI

- Visualize ligament tears, synovial thickening, and fibrosis. Loss of sinus tarsi fat is a useful objective finding.

Classification

- There is no classification for this entity

Treatment

Nonoperative

- NSAIDs, ankle/hindfoot bracing, physical therapy (peroneal strengthening and proprioception to minimize instability)
- Serial local anesthetics/corticosteroid injections
  - Reports of complete resolution

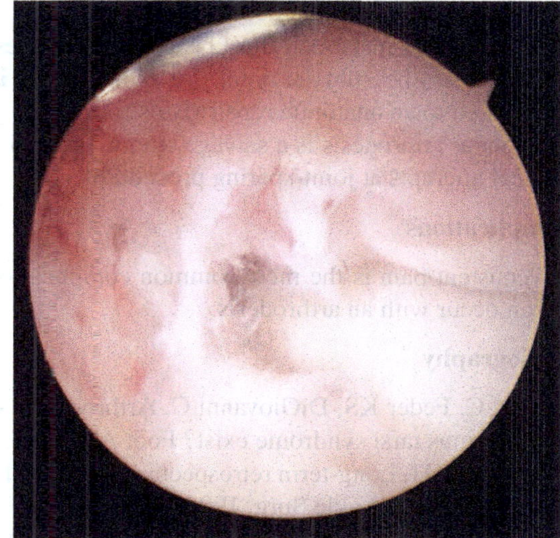

Fig. 5 Subtalar arthroscopy demonstrated synovitis and soft tissue impingement in a patient with sinus tarsi syndrome

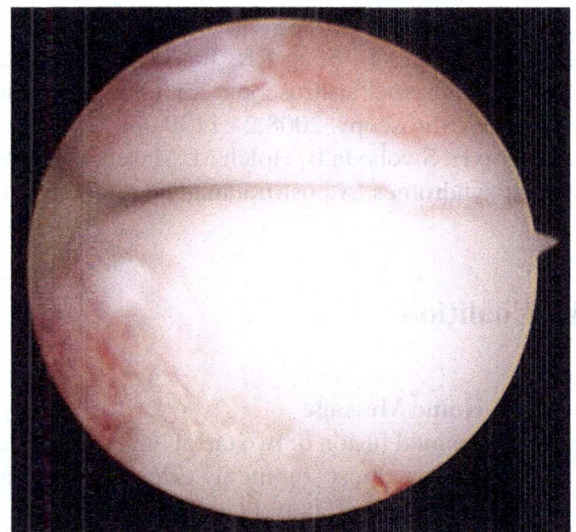

Fig. 6 Post-debridement of the same patient demonstrating removal of the offending tissue that theoretically allows impingement free motion of the subtalar joint and mechanical excision of the offending synovitis

Operative

- Arthroscopy
  - In a level IV study, arthroscopy identified pathologies in the subtalar joints of patients with STS → including partial tear of Interosseous talocalcaneal ligament (ITCL), cervical ligament (CL), synovitis, arthrofibrosis, and soft tissue impingement (Fig. 5).
    - Treatment of these pathologies led to improved pain and function.
    - Treatment included synovectomy and debridement (Fig. 6).

- Open surgical excision/debridement.
- Concomitant instability must be addressed if present. Reconstructive procedures that cross the subtalar joint are indicated to improve subtalar instability as opposed to an anatomic repair (Brostrom).
- Subtalar arthrodesis is a salvage operation in patients who have failed prior surgical attempts at joint-sparing procedures.

Complications

- Persistent pain is the most common complication with debridement. Nonunion can occur with an arthrodesis.

Bibliography

1. Frey C, Feder KS, DiGiovanni C. Arthroscopic evaluation of the subtalar joint: does sinus tarsi syndrome exist? Foot Ankle Int. 1999;20:185–91.
2. Kuwada GT. Long-term retrospective analysis of the treatment of sinus tarsi syndrome. J Foot Ankle Surg. 1994;33:28–9.
3. Lee KB, Bai LB, Park JG, Song EK, Lee JJ. Efficacy of MRI versus arthroscopy for evaluation of sinus tarsi syndrome. Foot Ankle Int. 2008;29: 1111–6.
4. Lee KB, Bai LB, Song EK, Jung ST, Kong IK. Subtalar arthroscopy for sinus Tarsi syndrome: arthroscopic findings and clinical outcomes of 33 consecutive cases. Arthroscopy. 2008;24:1130–4.
5. Zwipp H, Swoboda B, Holch M, Maschek HJ, Reichelt S. Sinus tarsi and canalis tarsi syndromes. A post-traumatic entity. Unfallchirurg. 1991;94:608–13.

4 Coalition

Take-Home Message

- Congenital fusion of two tarsal bones which could be fibrous, cartilaginous, or osseous (most commonly calcaneonavicular (CN) > talocalcaneal).
- Can lead to rigid flatfoot deformity → spastic peroneal flatfoot.
- Onset of symptoms corresponds with timing of ossification of coalition.
- Can be a cause of recurrent ankle sprains.
- Nonoperative management for asymptomatic – accommodative orthotics.
- Operative management – surgical resection with interposition (tendon or bone wax) for CN or talocalcaneal (<50 % involved). Triple arthrodesis for revision (CN) or subtalar fusion (>50 % talocalcaneal or revision)

Definition

- Tarsal coalition is a congenital abnormal union of two tarsal bones at variable levels
- Leads to rigid flatfoot deformity → peroneal spastic flatfoot

Etiology

- Presumed lack of differentiation of mesenchymal tissue, resulting in failure of normal joint articulation.
- Genetic predisposition

Pathophysiology

- Abnormal tissue bridge between two tarsal bones
  - Fibrous coalition
  - Cartilaginous coalition
  - Osseous coalition
- Two most common areas involved are → calcaneonavicular > talocalcaneal
- Onset of symptoms corresponds with timing ossification of coalition, calcaneonavicular (8–12), and talocalcaneal (12–16).
  - Sinus tarsi, medial hindfoot, and peroneal tendons
  - Persistent pain following ankle sprain
- Rigid flatfoot deformity: restricted subtalar motion results in
  - The subtalar joint lacks the ability to invert and create a normal longitudinal arch. The chopart joints are forced to develop in an abducted position with a pes planus deformity.
  - The peroneal tendons develop in a shortened fashion which accounts for the "spasm" that is felt with attempted inversion.
  - Subtalar arthrosis (late finding)

Radiography

- AP, lateral (standing), 45-degree oblique, and Harris axial X-ray views
  - 45-degree oblique view → calcaneonavicular (Fig. 7)
  - Lateral view
    - Calcaneonavicular → elongated anterior process of calcaneus ("anteater sign")
    - Talocalcaneal → talar beaking (Fig. 8)
  - Harris heel view → talocalcaneal → irregular middle facet joint
- CT scan
  - Better characterize size and extent of coalition

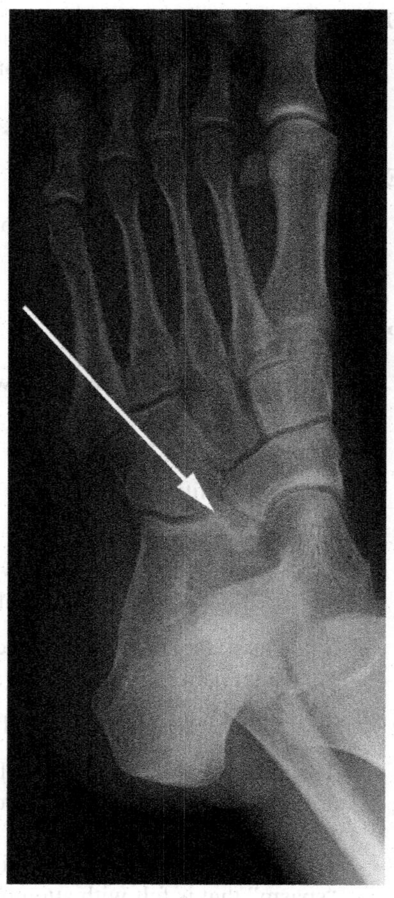

Fig. 7 Oblique radiograph of a patient with a fibrous calcaneonavicular coalition. The anteater sign is evidenced by the elongated anterior process with the associated flattening (*arrow*)

- MRI
  - Evaluate fibrous or cartilaginous coalition (Fig. 9)

Classification

On the basis of anatomic location

- Talocalcaneal
  - Anterior facet
  - Middle facet (most common)
  - Posterior facet

On the basis of completeness of ossification

- Synostosis: completely ossified bar, associated with fibular hemimelia and proximal focal femur deficiency and Apert syndrome.
- Synchondrosis: partially cartilaginous bar.
- Syndesmosis: fibrous bar.

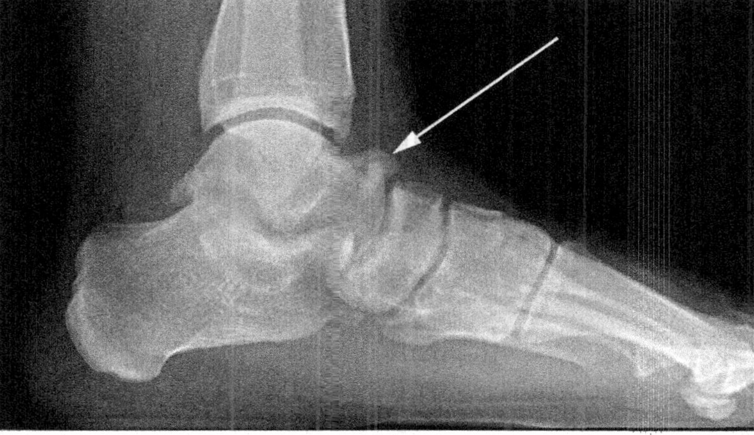

Fig. 8 Lateral radiograph demonstrating talar beaking (*arrow*) in a patient with a talocalcaneal coalition. The prominence is directed superior and distal

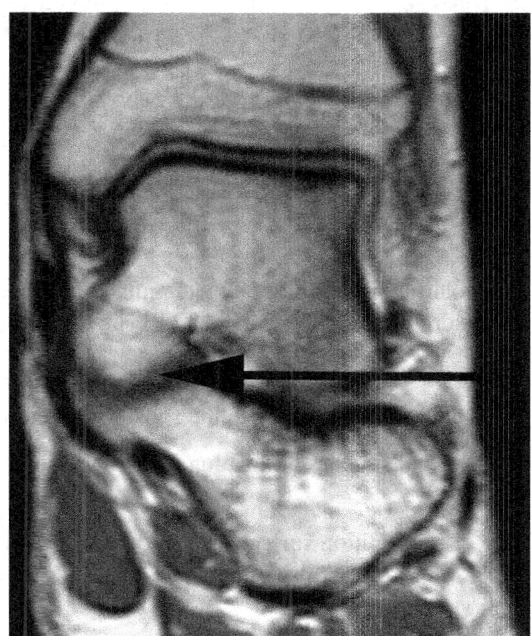

Fig. 9 Coronal T1 MRI of a nonosseous talocalcaneal coalition (*arrow*). There is a lack of bony continuity that distinguishes this from an osseous coalition. The middle facet is irregular with a very thin fibrous bridge present

Treatment Most coalitions are asymptomatic.

Nonoperative

- Observation for asymptomatic
- Short leg walking cast immobilization
- Accommodative full length orthotic

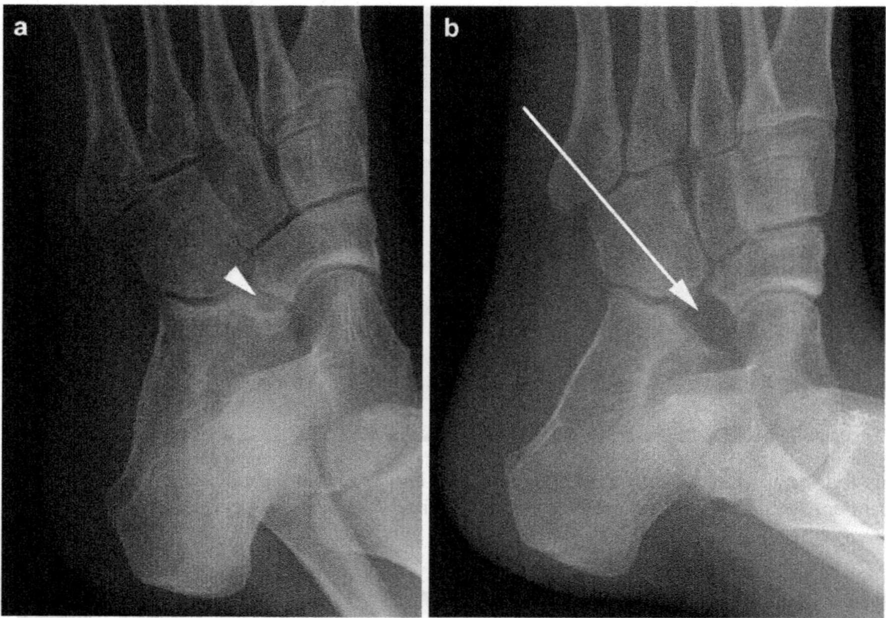

Fig. 10 Preoperative appearance (**a**) of a CN coalition (*arrowhead*) and the appropriate postoperative appearance after resection (**b**). Note how the resection removes a block of bone from the coalition which should create a square defect (*arrow*)

Operative

- Calcaneonavicular
  - Coalition resection of a rectangular 1 cm block (Fig. 10)
  - Interposition: bone wax or EDB (increases risk of wound complications)
- Talocalcaneal
  - Coalition resection with interposition (bone wax or split FHL)
    - Gold standard indication is lacking.
      - <50 % involvement of middle facet
      - Coalition surface area <50 % of the surface area of the posterior facet
      - <16° of valgus
  - Subtalar arthrodesis
    - >50 % involvement, subtalar arthrosis, and revision (Fig. 11)
- Triple arthrodesis
  - Any coalition with multiple joint arthrosis, revision, or severe hindfoot valgus or abduction

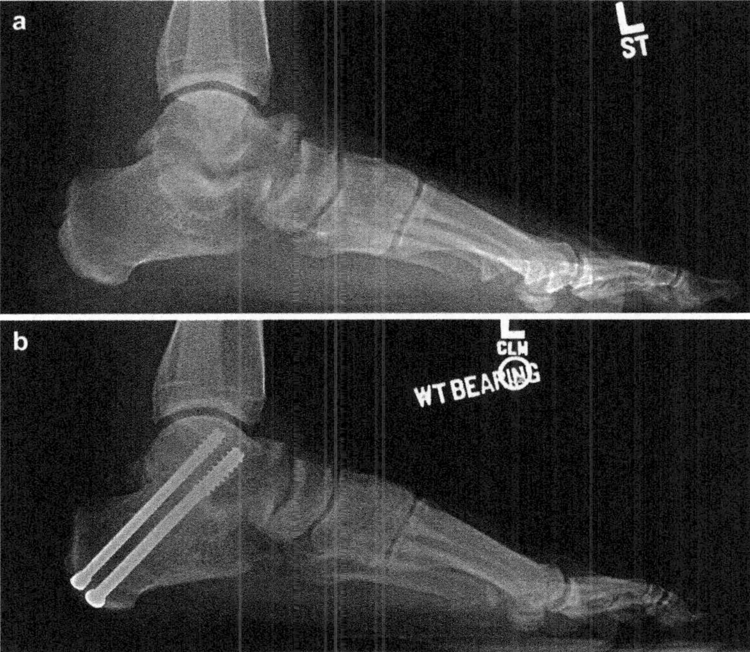

Fig. 11 Preoperative lateral radiograph (**a**) of a talocalcaneal coalition with associated talar beaking. Postoperative lateral radiograph (**b**) following coalition resection, subtalar arthrodesis, and excision of the talar beaking

Complications

- Hindfoot joint arthritis
- Persistent pain and deformity

Bibliography

1. Cass AD, Camasta CA. A review of tarsal coalition and pes planovalgus: clinical examination, diagnostic imaging, and surgical planning. J Foot Ankle Surg. 2010;49(3):274–93. doi:10.1053/j.jfas.2010.02.003.
2. Lemley F, Berlet G, Hill K, Philbin T, Isaac B, Lee T. Current concepts review: Tarsal coalition. Foot Ankle Int. 2006;27(12):1163–9.
3. Thorpe SW, Wukich DK. Tarsal coalitions in the adult population: does treatment differ from the adolescent? Foot Ankle Clin. 2012;17(2):195–204. doi:10.1016/j.fcl.2012.03.004.
4. Zaw H, Calder JD. Tarsal coalitions. Foot Ankle Clin. 2010;15(2):349–64. doi:10.1016/j.fcl.2010.02.003.

Forefoot

Anish R. Kadakia, Paul J. Switaj, Bryant S. Ho, Mohammed Alshouli, Daniel Fuchs, and George Ochengele

1 Hallux Rigidus

Take-Home Message

- Pain and stiffness of the first metatarsophalangeal (MTP) joint consistent with degenerative disease of the first MTP.
- Nonsurgical management should be attempted first, with the goal of avoiding painful first MTP joint dorsiflexion – Morton's extension carbon fiber plate.
- Surgery is determined based on radiographic and physical exam findings. Cheilectomy – >50 % joint preservation or negative grind test. Arthrodesis – <50 % joint preservation with a positive grind test or total joint obliteration or deformity (associated hallux valgus or varus).

Definition

- Functional limitation of motion of the first metatarsophalangeal joint in adults due to degenerative arthritis often associated with dorsal osteophyte

A.R. Kadakia (✉) • P.J. Switaj • B.S. Ho • M. Alshouli
D. Fuchs • G. Ochengele
Department of Orthopedic Surgery,
Northwestern University – Feinberg School of Medicine,
Northwestern Memorial Hospital, Chicago, IL, USA
e-mail: Kadak259@gmail.com; paul.switaj@gmail.com; bryant.s.ho@gmail.com; mtshouli@gmail.com; dfuchs0011@gmail.com; gochenjele@gmail.com

C. Mauffrey, D.J. Hak (eds.), *Passport for the Orthopedic Boards and FRCS Examination*, DOI 10.1007/978-2-8178-0475-0_41

Etiology

- Idiopathic arthritis
- *Extrinsic causes*
  - Post-traumatic arthritis: intra-articular fractures, repetitive dorsiflexion-compression injuries, and hyperdorsiflexion injury
  - Improper shoe wear: high-heeled shoes, pointed-toe shoes, and shoes with small or short toe boxes
- *Intrinsic causes*
  - Secondary to inflammatory arthropathies

Pathophysiology

- Change in the first MTP joint biomechanics leads to displacement of the instant centers of motion to an eccentric position on the first metatarsal head and higher plantar pressures.
- Contracted flexor hallucis longus (FHL) may increase plantar pressures and MTP joint force.
- Clinical presentation
  - Pain with shoe wear secondary to pressure over dorsal osteophyte
  - Limited range of motion (limited ability to wear heels)
  - Pain with activity

Radiography

- Weight-bearing anteroposterior, lateral, and oblique views → Look for narrowing of the joint space, osteophytes at the lateral and dorsal surface of the joint, flattened first metatarsal head, and subchondral cysts (Fig. 1).
- MRI scan: look for osteochondral injury in the setting of normal X-rays.

Classification Coughlin clinical-radiographic classification of hallux rigidus (Table 1)

Treatment Algorithm *Nonoperative*: short period of rest followed by activity modifications, NSAIDS, intra-articular steroid injections, shoe modification (rigid sole). Orthotic = Morton's extension carbon fiber plate
Operative (Table 2)

- Simplified
  - Cheilectomy: some preservation of joint space without pain in the central range of motion (Grades 1–3) (Fig. 2)
  - Fusion for deformity, pain with grind at central range of motion (grade 4), 100 % joint space loss, no motion (Figs. 3 and 4)

Complications

- Persistent pain
- Recurrence of osteophyte formation

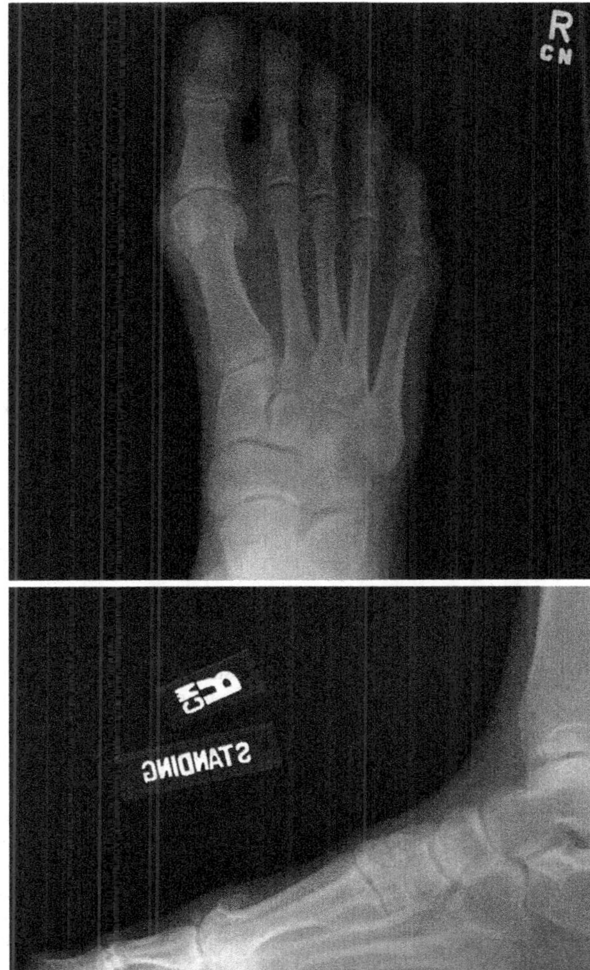

Fig. 1 AP and lateral view of a patient with hallux rigidus. Note the narrowing of the joint space on the AP with the common findings of a dorsal osteophyte on the metatarsal head with a loose body within the first MTP. Hallux rigidus is most easily identified on the lateral radiograph

- Progression of joint degeneration requiring additional surgery
- Iatrogenic hallux valgus or varus deformity
- Nonunion or malunion (ideal position – neutral rotation, slight hallux valgus, and dorsiflexion parallel to the floor. Best done with a flat plate intraoperatively to simulate the final clinical position. Superior to absolute values secondary to anatomic variability)

Bibliography

1. Coughlin MJ, Shurnas PS. Hallux rigidus. Grading and long-term results of operative treatment. J Bone Joint Surg Am Vol. 2003;85-A:2072–88.
2. Deland JT, Williams BR. Surgical management of hallux rigidus. J Am Acad Orthop Surg. 2012;20:347–58.

Table 1 Coughlin clinical-radiographic classification of hallux rigidus

Grade	Dorsiflexion	Radiographic findings	Clinical findings
0	40–60° and/or 10–20 % loss compared with normal side	Normal	No pain; stiffness, loss of motion
1	30–40° and/or 20–50 % loss compared with normal side	Dorsal osteophytes; minimal joint-space narrowing, periarticular sclerosis, flattening of metatarsal head	Pain at extremes of dorsiflexion and/or plantar flexion
2	10–30° and/or 50–75 % loss compared with normal side	Dorsal, lateral, and possibly medial osteophytes; flattened appearance to metatarsal head, ¼ or less of dorsal joint space involved on lateral radiograph, mild-to-moderate joint-space narrowing and sclerosis; sesamoids not usually involved	Moderate-to-severe pain and stiffness; pain occurs just before maximum dorsiflexion/plantar flexion on examination
3	=10° and/or 75–100 % loss compared with normal side. There is notable loss of metatarsophalangeal plantar flexion	Substantial joint space narrowing, periarticular cystic changes, more than 1/4 of dorsal joint space involved on lateral radiograph, sesamoids enlarged and/or cystic and/or irregular	Constant pain and stiffness at extremes of range of motion but not at mid-range
4	Same as in Grade 3	Same as in Grade 3	Definite pain at mid-range of passive motion

Table 2 Operative algorithm for hallux rigidus

Grade	Operative
0	Arthroscopic or open débridement, drilling, or grafting of metatarsal head OCD (if present)
1	Cheilectomy
2	Cheilectomy
3	Cheilectomy
4	MTP joint arthrodesis

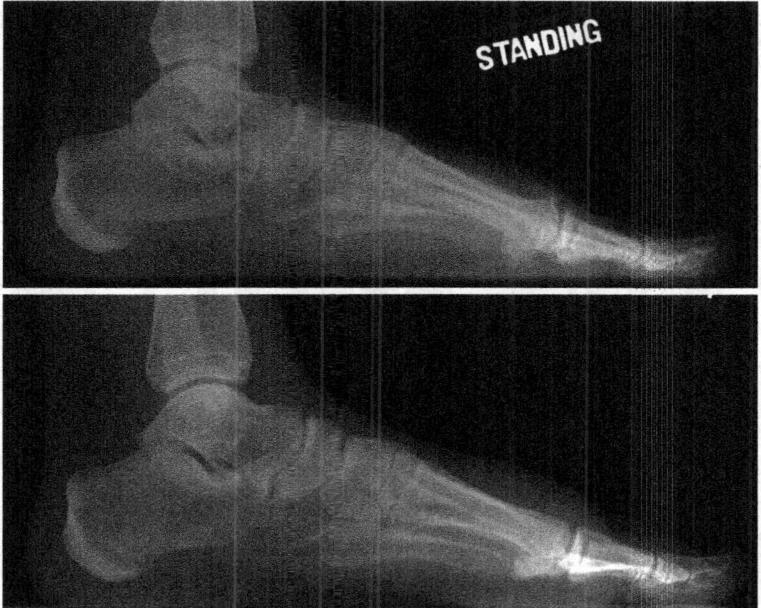

Fig. 2 Preoperative appearance of the dorsal osteophyte (*top radiograph*) and the postoperative appearance (*bottom radiograph*) following a cheilectomy. No more than 30 % of the metatarsal head should be resected to prevent iatrogenic instability

3. Seibert NR, Kadakia AR. Surgical management of hallux rigidus: cheilectomy and osteotomy (phalanx and metatarsal). Foot Ankle Clin. 2009;14:9–22.
4. Simpson GA, Hembree WC, Miller SD, Hyer CF, Berlet GC. Surgical strategies: hallux rigidus surgical techniques. Foot Ankle Int. 2011;32:1175–86.

2 Hallux Valgus

Take-Home Message

- Hallux valgus is defined as a lateral deviation of the great toe with medial deviation of the first metatarsal.
- DJD of the first MTP requires arthrodesis.
- Hypermobility of first TMT requires Lapidus (first TMT arthrodesis).
- Increased DMAA required redirectional osteotomy of distal metatarsal, in addition to other required osteotomies to correct the IMA.
- Increased HVI requires an Akin osteotomy (medial closing wedge of phalanx).

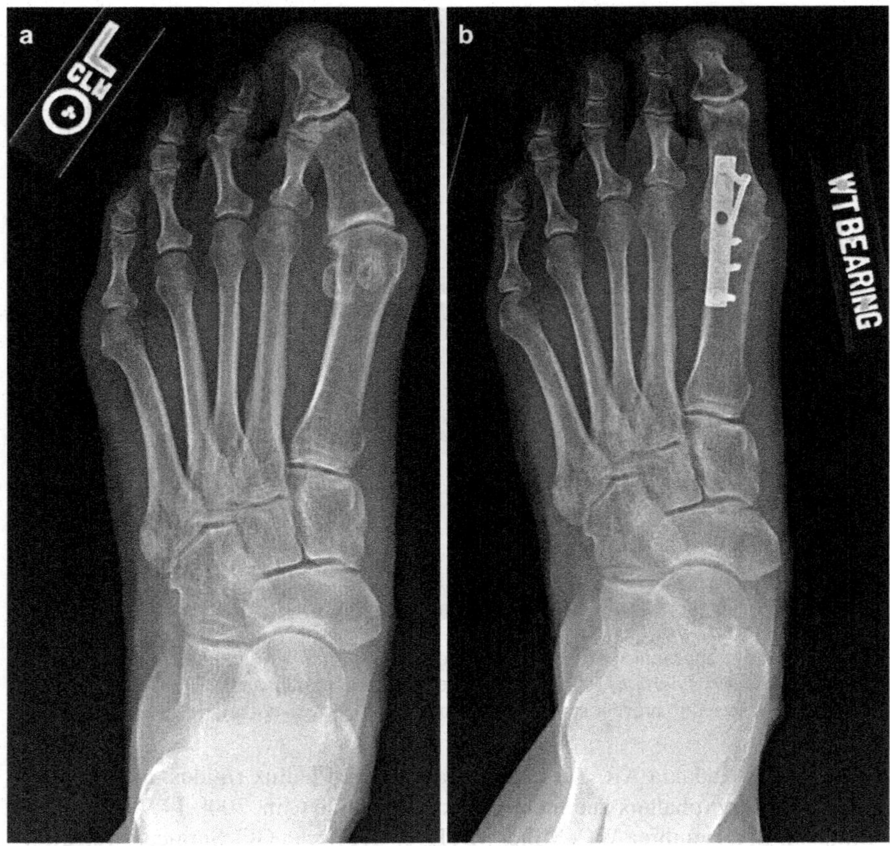

Fig. 3 Patient presented with hallux valgus and hallux rigidus (**a**). Correction of both deformities is best corrected with an arthrodesis (**b**) as an isolated cheilectomy or osteotomy to correct the hallux valgus will not be successful

Definition Hallux valgus is defined as a lateral deviation of the great toe with medial deviation of the first metatarsal (Fig. 5).

Etiology Related to multiple factors and more common in females

Extrinsic Causes

Improper shoe wear (high-heeled shoes, pointed-toe shoes, and shoes with narrow toe boxes)

Intrinsic Causes

- Genetic predisposition, ligamentous laxity, and predisposing anatomy (convex metatarsal head, pes planus) are contributory.
- Inflammatory arthropathies (rheumatoid arthritis), metabolic bone disorders (gout), neuromuscular disorders (cerebral palsy, stroke)

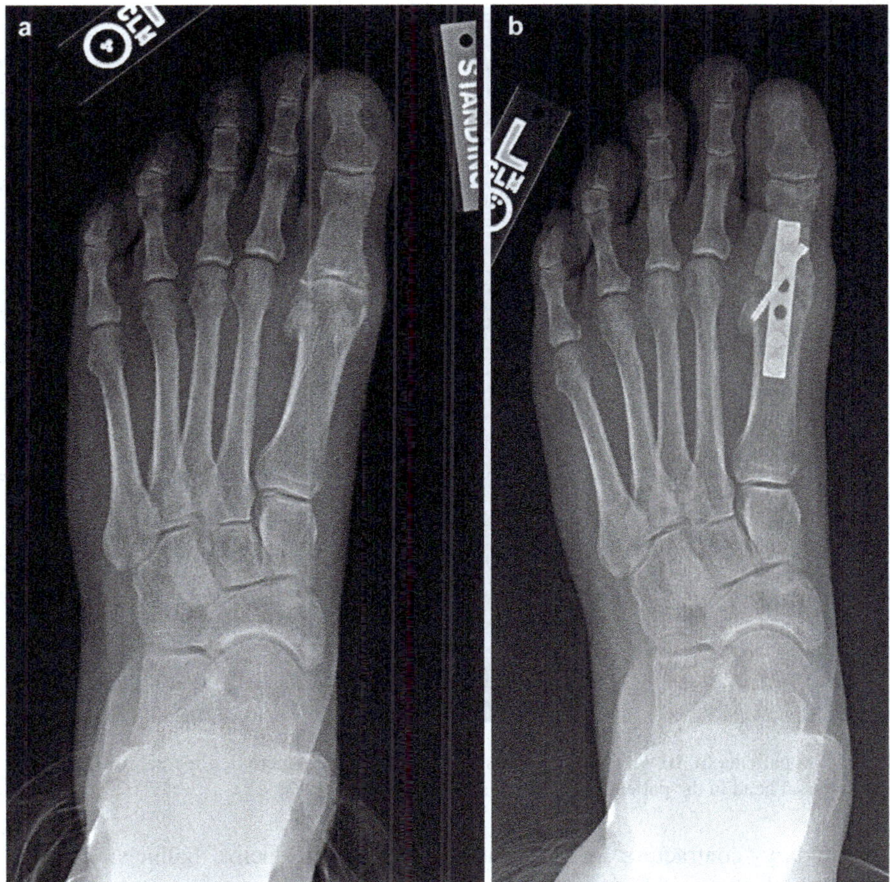

Fig. 4 Patient with grade 4 hallux rigidus (**a**) (>50 % joint space loss with central grind). This is best treated with an arthrodesis (**b**)

Pathoanatomy

- Medial capsular attenuation.
- Proximal phalanx drifts laterally, leading to the following conditions:
  - Plantar-lateral migration of abductor hallucis; change in position causes the muscle to plantar flex and pronate the phalanx.
  - Stretching of the extensor hood of the extensor hallucis longus.
  - Lateral deviation of the extensor hallucis longus and flexor hallucis longus (FHL), causing a muscular imbalance and deforming force for valgus progression and pronation of the great toe.
- The first metatarsal head moves medially off the sesamoids, increasing the intermetatarsal angle (IMA).

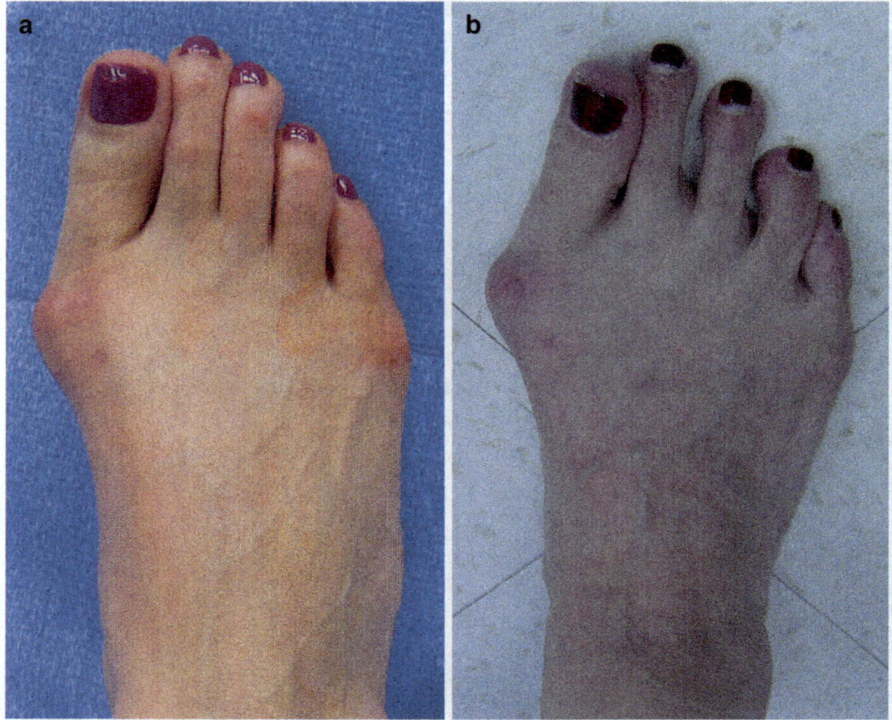

Fig. 5 Two patients (**a**, **b**) with hallux valgus deformity. Note the increased medial deviation of the metatarsal head in the patient with a more severe deformity (**b**)

- Secondary contracture of the lateral capsule, adductor hallucis, lateral metatarsal-sesamoid ligament, and intermetatarsal ligament.

Radiography

- Multiple measurements can be obtained from standard radiographs that guide treatment options
  - Hallux valgus angle (HVA): angle formed by a line along the first metatarsal shaft and a line along the shaft of proximal phalanx (Fig. 6)
    - Normal <15°
  - First to second intermetatarsal angle (IMA): angle formed by a line along the first metatarsal shaft and a line along the second metatarsal shaft (Fig. 7)
    - Normal <9°
  - Hallux valgus interphalangeus (HVI) angle: angle formed by a line along the shaft of proximal phalanx and a line along the shaft of distal phalanx (Fig. 8)

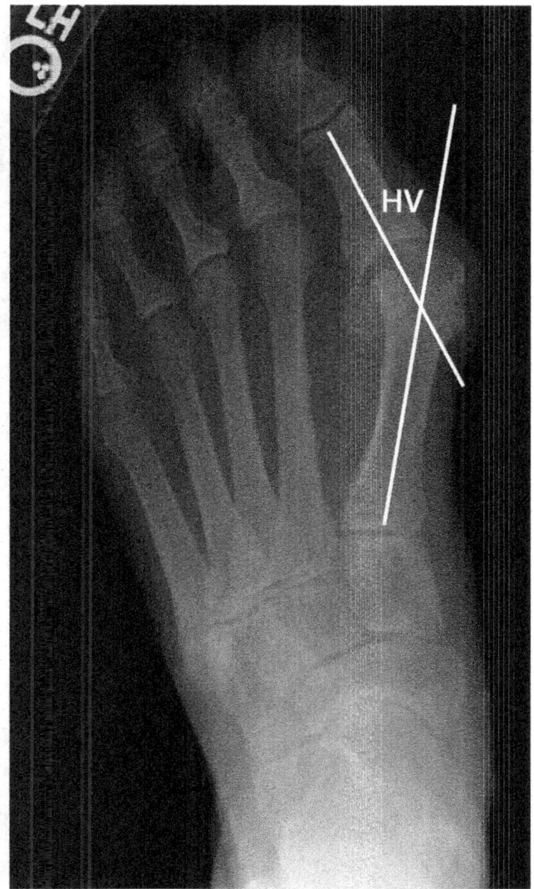

Fig. 6 AP radiograph denoting the hallux valgus angle. The acute angle (*HV*) formed by a line parallel to the first metatarsal shaft and a line parallel to the proximal phalangeal shaft is measured

    - Normal <10°
    - Associated with a congruent deformity

  - Distal metatarsal articular angle (DMAA): angle formed by a line along the articular surface of the first metatarsal and a line perpendicular to the axis of the first metatarsal

    - Normal <10°
    - Associated with a congruent deformity

Classification

- There is no specific classification for hallux valgus that is routinely utilized. Specific recommendations are based upon the degree of deformity, which is discussed below.

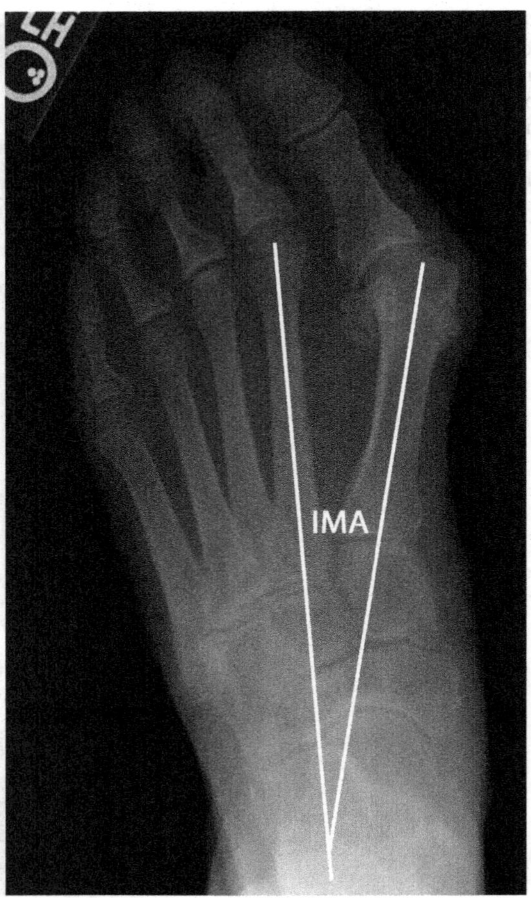

Fig. 7 AP radiograph denoting the intermetatarsal angle. The acute angle (*IMA*) formed by a line parallel to the first metatarsal shaft and the second metatarsal shaft is measured

- The use of the term congruency has been utilized and is a source of confusion
  - Congruency is determined by comparing the line connecting the medial and lateral edge of the first metatarsal head articular surface with the similar line for the proximal phalanx, and when these lines are parallel, the joint is congruent; otherwise, it is incongruent (Fig. 9).
  - The implication is that the patient has an intrinsic deformity of either an increased DMAA or HVI. These can be present with an incongruent deformity as well, and therefore each radiograph must be carefully reviewed.

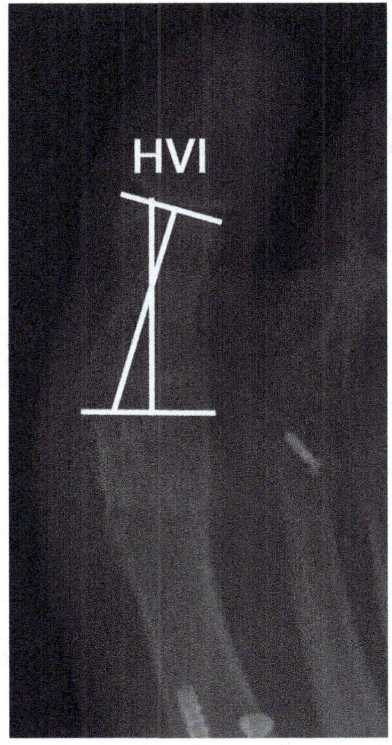

Fig. 8 AP radiograph of the proximal phalanx denoting the hallux valgus interphalangeus angle. A *line* is drawn parallel to the proximal and distal articular surfaces. Perpendicular lines are drawn relative to these lines. The acute angle (*HVI*) formed by the perpendiculars is measured

Treatment

Nonoperative

NSAIDS for associated bursitis, shoe modifications (wide toe box, flat sole), orthotics (arch support in flat foot and metatarsal pad for second metatarsalgia), toe spacers if flexible deformity. These will not correct the deformity.

Operative

Algorithmic approach to identifying the appropriate surgical intervention. Rigid deformity, pain within the first MTP joint, inflammatory arthropathy, or radiographic evidence of arthritis requires the first MTP arthrodesis (Fig. 10).

All patients should undergo a soft tissue release with all associated osteotomies and the first TMT arthrodesis (Lapidus).

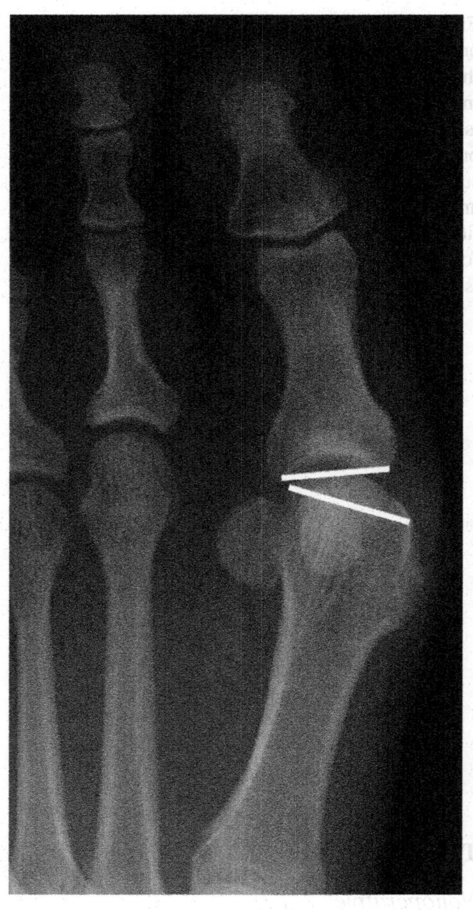

Fig. 9 This patient has an incongruent deformity noted by the lack of parallelism between the articular surface of the metatarsal and the proximal phalanx

IMA is ≤13° and HVA is ≤40°

- Distal metatarsal osteotomy (chevron) (Fig. 11)
- Distal soft tissue release
- Medial eminence resection and capsular repair

IMA is >13° or HVA is >40°

- Proximal metatarsal osteotomy
- Distal soft tissue release
- Medial eminence resection and capsular repair

Instability of the First TMT/Joint Laxity

- Lapidus (fusion of the first TMT joint) (Fig. 12)
- Soft tissue release
- Medial eminence resection and capsular repair

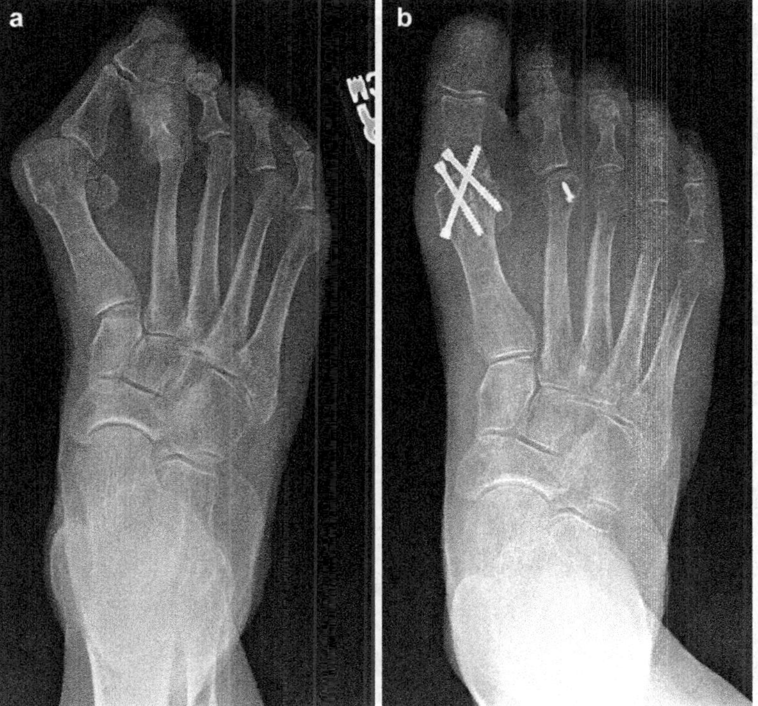

Fig. 10 This patient has a significant hallux valgus deformity with hallux rigidus and pain within the first MTP joint. (**a**) Correction of both the IMA and HVA is easily achieved with an arthrodesis without the need for additional metatarsal osteotomy (**b**)

Increased DMAA (>10°)

- Distal medial closed-wedge metatarsal osteotomy in addition to what is required based on the angular measurements.
  - IMA is ≤13°, and HVA is ≤40°
    - Distal biplanar closed-wedge metatarsal osteotomy.
    - Translate and redirect the metatarsal head simultaneously.
  - IMA is >13° HVA is >40°
    - Proximal metatarsal osteotomy and distal medial closed-wedge metatarsal osteotomy (Fig. 13)
  - Instability of the first TMT/joint laxity
    - Lapidus and distal medial closed-wedge metatarsal osteotomy

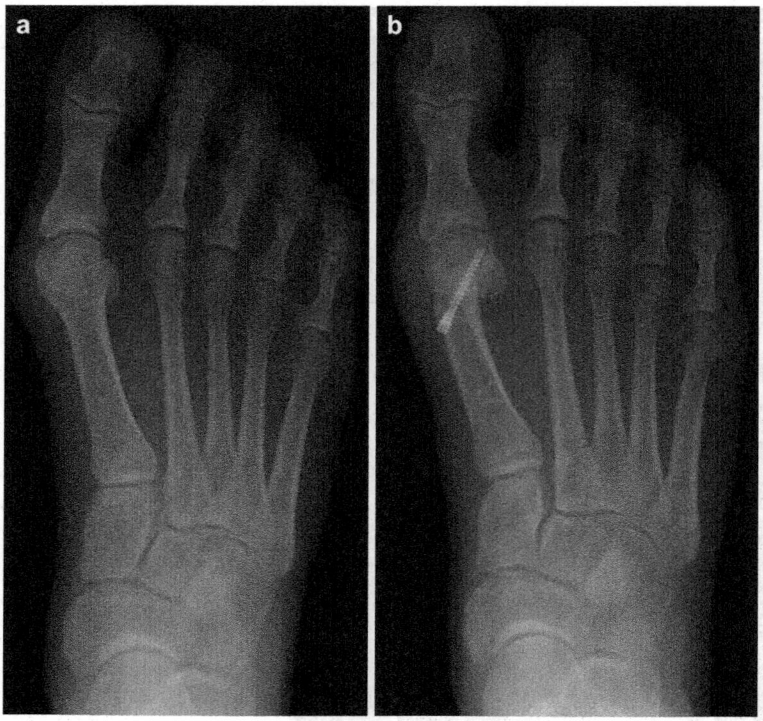

Fig. 11 In patients with a HVA ≤40 and an IMA ≤13 (**a**), a distal osteotomy with soft tissue correction is the most appropriate procedure (**b**)

Hallux valgus interphalangeus

- Akin osteotomy can be done in isolation if no other deformity present.
- Commonly performed in addition to other procedures.

Complications

- Avascular necrosis (AVN)
  - Distal metatarsal osteotomy and lateral soft tissue release may be performed simultaneously without increased risk of AVN.
- Recurrence
  - Can occur with any procedure – highly associated with:
    - Under correction of the IMA
    - Isolated soft tissue reconstruction (modified McBride)
    - Isolated resection of the medial eminence
- Dorsal malunion
  - Results in transfer metatarsalgia – highly associated with:

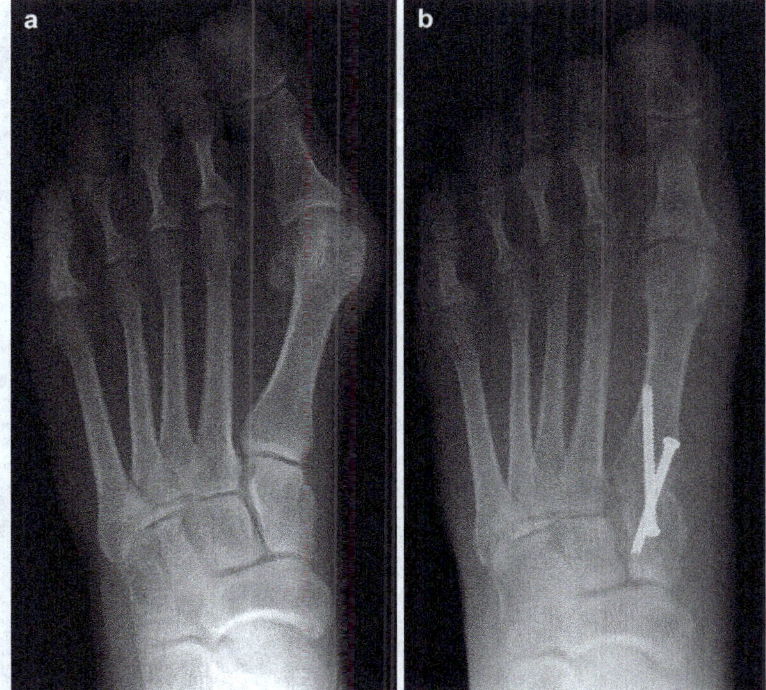

Fig. 12 Regardless of preoperative deformity (**a**), in a patient with hypermobility, a Lapidus procedure is required (**b**)

- Lapidus (first TMT fusion)
- Proximal crescentic osteotomy

- Hallux Varus (Fig. 14)

– Resection of the fibular sesamoid (original McBride)
– Over-resection of the medial eminence
– Excessive lateral release
– Overcorrection of the IMA

Bibliography

1. Coughlin MJ, Jones CP. Hallux valgus: demographics, etiology, and radiographic assessment. Foot Ankle Int. 2007;28(7):759–77.
2. Ellington JK, Myerson MS, Coetzee JC, Stone RM. The use of the Lapidus procedure for recurrent hallux valgus. Foot Ankle Int. 2011;32(7):674–80.
3. Perera AM, Mason L, Stephens MM. The pathogenesis of hallux valgus. J Bone Joint Surg Am. 2011;93(17):1650–61.
4. Smith BW, Coughlin MJ. Treatment of hallux valgus with increased distal metatarsal articular angle: use of double and triple osteotomies. Foot Ankle Clin. 2009;14(3):369–82.

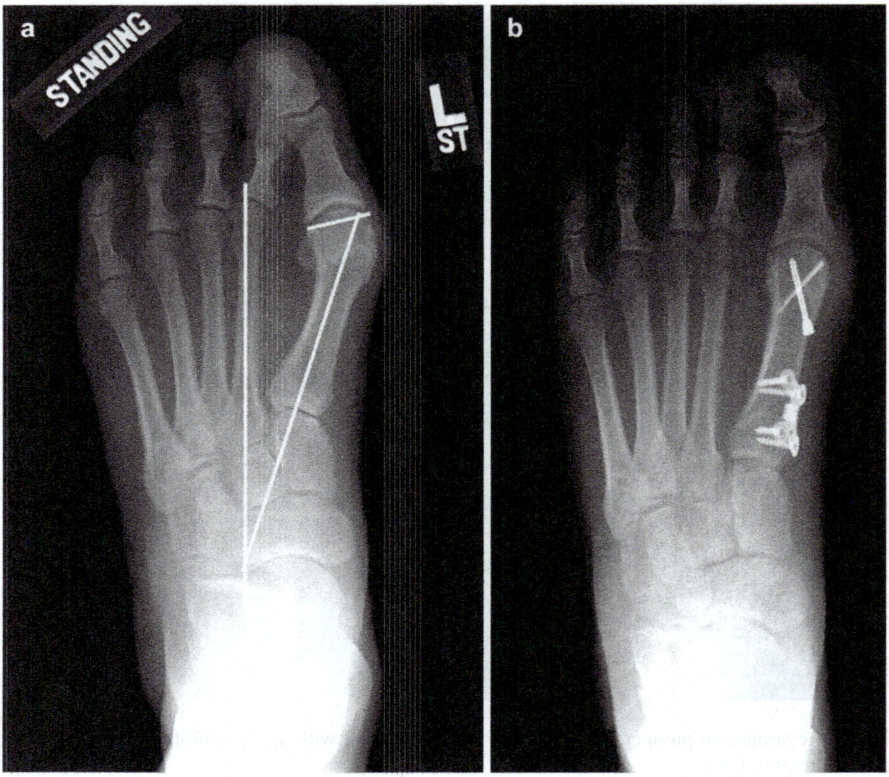

Fig. 13 In this patient with an IMA >13 and an increased DMAA >10 (**a**), a double osteotomy is required (**b**). A proximal osteotomy in addition to a distal closing wedge osteotomy fully corrects the deformity

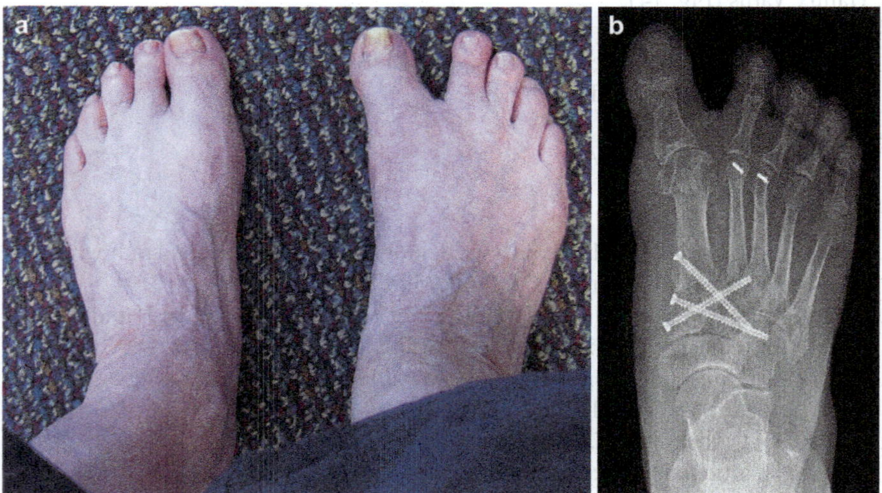

Fig. 14 In this patient with clinical hallux varus (**a**), the etiology is the overcorrection of the IM angle with excessive lateral release (**b**)

3 Interdigital Neuroma

Take-Home Message

- Classically, a patient with a symptomatic interdigital neuroma complains of pain located on the plantar aspect of the foot at or distal to the metatarsal heads. The pain is described as burning, often with radiation to the toes.
- Adjacent or multiple neuroma is an uncommon diagnosis and should alert the surgeon to the possibility of alternate diagnoses.
- Excision of neuroma from either a dorsal (higher rate of missed neuroma) or plantar (higher rate of painful scar) approach is the surgical treatment of choice.

Definition

- A neuralgia of the interdigital nerve in the forefoot due to entrapment of the nerve near the distal edge of the transverse intermetatarsal ligament

Etiology

Extrinsic Causes

- Mass effect from soft tissues
- Extrinsic mechanical stresses → improper shoe wear (high-heeled shoes, pointed-toe shoes, and shoes with small or short toe boxes) – result in compression and tensile stress on the nerve (from dorsiflexion)

Intrinsic Causes

- Ischemic changes to the perineural tissue
- Repetitive microtrauma affecting the nerve
- Traditionally, it was thought that both the medial and lateral plantar nerves send branches to the third web space, creating a larger nerve that was predisposed to increased microtrauma. However, the incidence of a communicating branch to the third web space was noted at 27 %, decreasing support of the anatomic theory.

Pathophysiology

- Histologic analysis has revealed that the nerve is affected distal to the intermetatarsal ligament.
- Fusiform swelling of the nerve has generated the term *neuroma*.
- Chronic entrapment leads to sclerosis and edema of the endoneurium, thickening of the perineurium, deposition of eosinophilic material, and demyelination of nerve fibers distal to the ligament.
- The culmination of this pathologic process is an increased diameter of the affected nerve through intrasubstance hypertrophy and swelling.

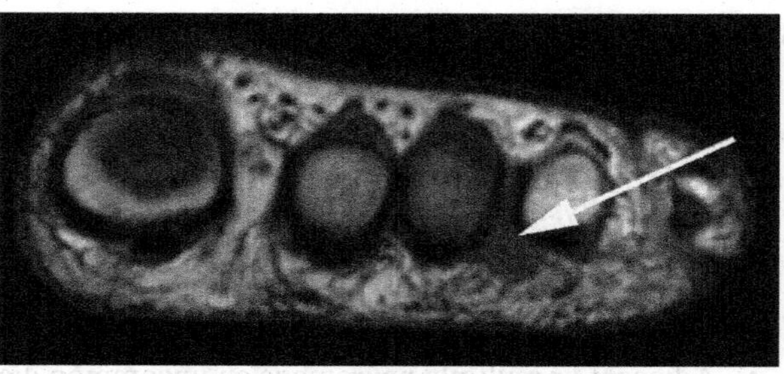

Fig. 15 Coronal T1 image of a Morton's neuroma (*arrow*). Note that the neuroma is pear shaped and is plantar to the intermetatarsal ligament

Radiography

- Three views of weight bearing of the foot should be performed to rule out any pathologic process of the metatarsophalangeal joint.
- Ultrasonography has demonstrated a high sensitivity with a variable specificity in the diagnosis of a neuroma and, however, is not required to make the diagnosis.
- Currently, an MRI scan may detect aberrant pathology such as a cyst or ganglion; however, it may show thickening of the nerve (Fig. 15). The routine use of MRI to identify a neuroma is not indicated given the difficulty of interpreting the clinical value of the findings.
- In general, the diagnosis is usually made without the use of ultrasound or MRI and should only be considered with rare clinical presentations.

Diagnostic Tests

- Lidocaine injection test: lidocaine is injected approximately 2 cm proximal to the metatarsal head, below the intermetatarsal ligament → resolution of symptoms confirms the diagnosis.
- Mulder's test: squeeze the transverse arch of the foot and apply pressure between the interdigital space; a positive test will result in a click, as well as pain in the plantar surface of the involved interspace with paresthesias radiating into the affected toes.

Treatment

Nonoperative: shoe modification (soft shoe with wide toe box and firm sole that provides metatarsal support), modification of daily activity, NSAIDS, corticosteroid injection

Operative: indicated after failure of nonoperative treatment

- Excision of the neuroma can be carried out through the dorsal or plantar approach to the web space. Isolated intermetatarsal ligament release is not appropriate.
  - Dorsal approach requires sectioning of the transverse metatarsal ligament (Fig. 16). However, this approach may result in failure to excise the neuroma in 5 % of cases (Fig. 17).
  - Plantar approach spares the intermetatarsal ligament and is noted to universally achieve nerve resection, however, results in a painful plantar scar in 5 % of patients.
- Successful in 75–90 % of cases

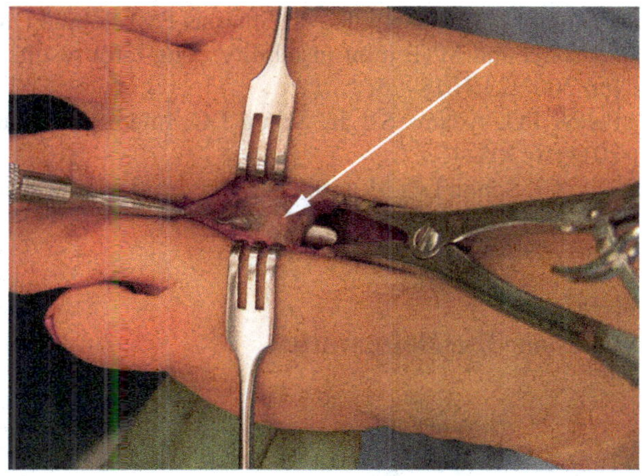

Fig. 16 The intermetatarsal ligament (*arrow*) must be incised with the use of a dorsal approach in order to visualize the neuroma

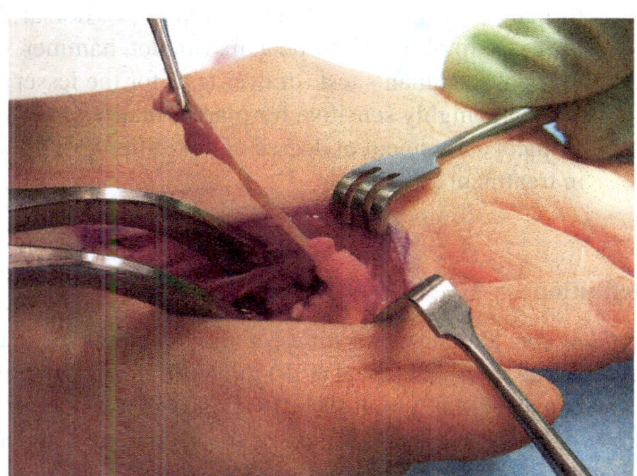

Fig. 17 The digital nerve has been transected proximally and elevated out of the wound. Adequate proximal resection must be performed in order to prevent recurrence. Surgical pathology confirmed the diagnosis of neuroma

Complications

- Painful plantar scars or plantar keratosis with surgical plantar approach
- Regeneration or formation of stump neuroma
- Residual tenderness and/or numbness
- Infection, plantar fat atrophy (related to steroid injections)
- Digital ischemia if adjacent vascular structures injured

Bibliography

1. Akermark C, Crone H, Saartok T, Zuber Z. Plantar versus dorsal incision in the treatment of primary intermetatarsal Morton's neuroma. Foot Ankle Int. 2008;29(2):136–41.
2. Coughlin MJ, Pinsonneault T. Operative treatment of interdigital neuroma. A long-term follow-up study. J Bone Joint Surg Am Vol. 2001;83-A:1321–8.

3. Coughlin MJ, Schenck RC Jr, Shurnas PS, Bloome DM. Concurrent interdigital neuroma and MTP joint instability: long-term results of treatment. Foot Ankle Int. 2002;23:1018–25.
4. Peters PG, Adams SB Jr, Schon LC. Interdigital neuralgia. Foot Ankle Clin. 2011;16:305–15.
5. Title CI, Schon LC. Morton neuroma: primary and secondary neurectomy. J Am Acad Orthop Surg. 2008;16:550–7.

4 Lesser Toe Deformities

Take-Home Message

- Lesser toe deformities can present with pain, contractures, and callosities formation at the plantar MTP (claw toes), dorsal PIP (hammer and claw toes), or tip of the distal phalanx (mallet, hammer, or claw toes).
- Vertical Lachman's test (drawer test) for the lesser MTP joints that results in pain is highly sensitive for plantar plate rupture.
- Clinical assessment of degree of flexibility (flexible or fixed) is the key role in treatment.

Definition

- *Claw toe*: flexion deformities of the distal interphalangeal (DIP) joint and the proximal interphalangeal (PIP) joint with fixed hyperextension at the metatarsophalangeal (MTP) joint (Fig. 18).
- *Mallet toe*: flexion deformity at the DIP joint with the PIP and MTP joints in neutral position.
- *Hammer toe*: flexion of the PIP joint with flexion or extension of the DIP. With weight bearing, the MTP joint will appear extended; however, this should correct with as the foot is elevated from the ground. The MTP extension is secondary to the flexion deformity of the PIP joint (Fig. 19).
- *Crossover toe:* Defined by rupture of the plantar plate with associated attenuation of the lateral collateral ligament. This results in multiplanar instability of the toe with the end-stage deformity of the second toe (most common) overlapping the great toe (Fig. 20).

Etiology and Pathophysiology

- Lesser toe deformities occur much more commonly in women (up to 5:1 ratio), thought to be secondary to high fashion shoe wear which constricts the forefoot and maintains the MTP joints in hyperextension.
  - A hammer deformity most commonly involves the second toe due to its relative length compared to the remainder of the lesser toes. A short toe box will cause the second toe to buckle and extend at the MTP joint.

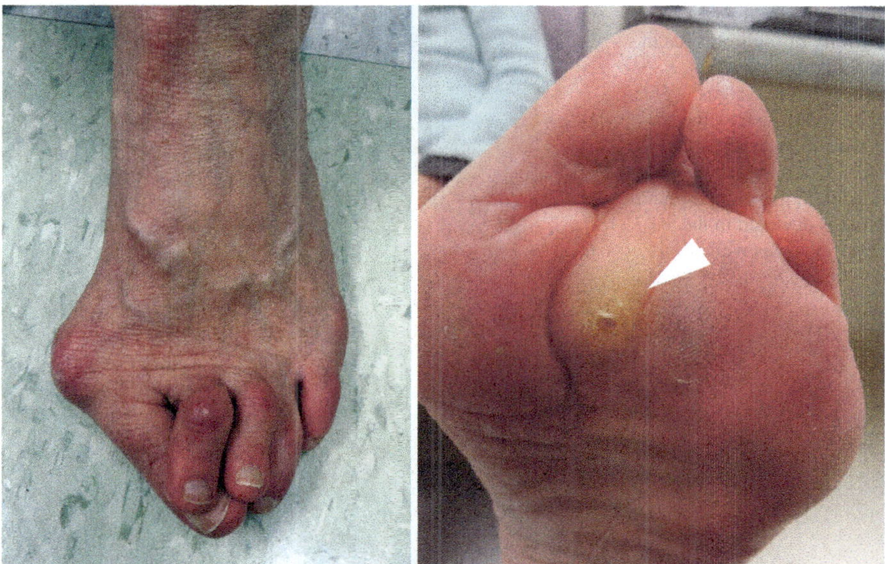

Fig. 18 Dorsal and plantar view of a patient with severe claw toes affecting primarily the second and third toes. Note the severe callus (*arrowhead*) on the plantar aspect of the second and third metatarsal heads

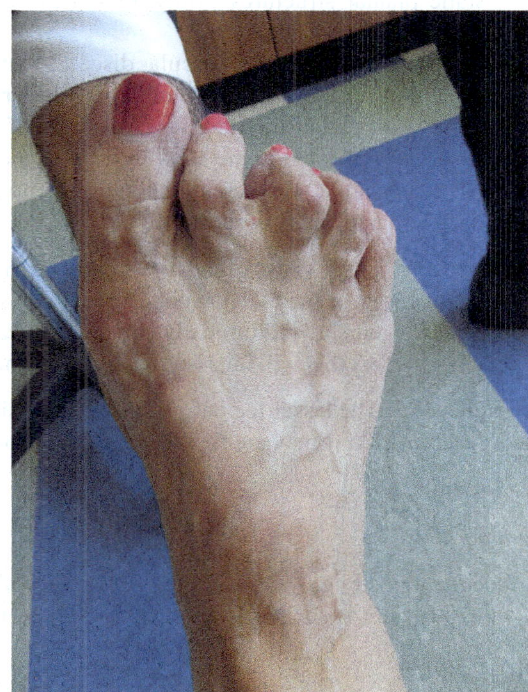

Fig. 19 Hammertoe deformity of the toes two through five in a patient. As opposed to claw toes, the MTP extension resolves with removing the foot off the floor

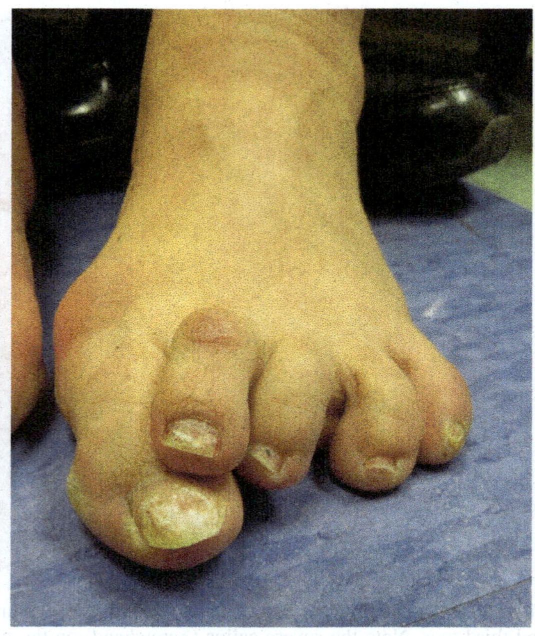

Fig. 20 Crossover toe deformity of multiple toes in a patient who has long-standing hallux valgus deformity. Note how the toe has deformity in multiple planes. Not only is it extended in the sagittal plane, the toe is deviated in the coronal plane as well

- Chronic positioning of the MTP joint in hyperextension will attenuate the static plantar structures, which underlies both claw toes and crossover toe deformities.
- Cavus deformity, neuromuscular diseases that affect the balance of the extrinsic and intrinsic musculature inflammatory arthropathies that lead to attenuation of soft tissue structures and instability of the MTP joint, and trauma have all been implicated in the etiology of claw toes.
- Claw toes are a noted complication of compartment syndrome involving the deep compartments of the foot.

Radiography Three views of the foot weight bearing should be performed to identify if dislocations of the metatarsophalangeal joints have occurred as this will alter surgical management. Additionally, in chronic cases, the presence of arthrosis should be noted as this will alter surgical management as well.

Classification The lesser toe deformities are classified as detailed above, but critically differentiated if they are flexible (reducible) or fixed (irreducible).

Treatment

Nonoperative

- Adequate padding, shoe wear modifications with an adequate shoe box to provide sufficient space for the toes and silicone toe caps to protect the toes are useful.

- Orthotic management may be accomplished by simple (i.e., metatarsal pads) or custom orthotics to include a metatarsal bar and well-outs for the affected metatarsal heads.

Operative

Persistent pain despite shoe wear modification or significant pressure sores, creating an at-risk environment for an ulcer, or history of ulceration secondary to shoe wear

- General principles: flexible ->soft tissue reconstruction. Fixed ->bone procedures required
- Mallet Toe
  - Flexible – flexor tenotomy at DIP
  - Fixed – DIP arthroplasty/fusion
- Hammer Toe
  - Flexible – flexor tenotomy at PIP or flexor to extensor tendon transfer (if mild MTP extension noted)
  - Fixed – PIP arthroplasty or arthrodesis (Fig. 21)
- Claw Toe
  - Flexible – flexor to extensor tendon transfer
  - Fixed – PIP arthroplasty or arthrodesis with associated MTP capsulotomy and extensor lengthening
    - Dislocated or unstable MTP joint
      - Requires shortening osteotomy of the metatarsal
- Crossover Toe
  - Flexible
    - Direct repair of the plantar plate has demonstrated clinical success and directly corrects the pathology.
    - Alternate options include flexor to extensor tendon transfer or transfer of the EHB deep to the intermetatarsal ligament.
  - Fixed
    - Metatarsal shortening osteotomy to reduce the MTP with associated soft tissue correction detailed above

Complications

- Recurrence of the deformity
- Floating toe (noted with a Weil osteotomy)
- Interdigital joint Instability
- Loss of active motion of the affected toe (occurs commonly secondary to the altered tendon function from tenotomies or bony shortening)

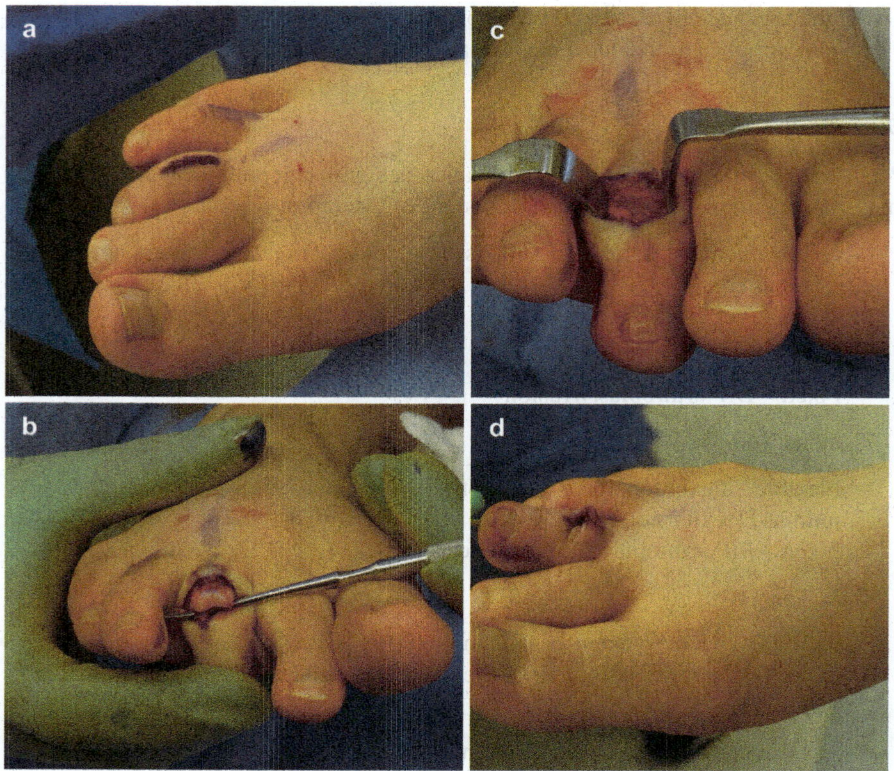

Fig. 21 PIP arthroplasty for a patient with a rigid hammer toe deformity of the fourth (**a**). Exposure of the distal aspect of the proximal phalanx (**b**) is followed by resection of the distal 3–4 mm of the phalanx (**c**) to allow the rigid deformity to correct (**d**). Pinning is performed to stabilize the toe for 4 weeks

Bibliography

1. Chadwick C, Saxby TS. Hammertoes/Clawtoes: metatarsophalangeal joint correction. Foot Ankle Clin. 2011;16(4):559–71.
2. Ellis SJ, Young E, Endo Y, Do H, Deland JT. Correction of multiplanar deformity of the second toe with metatarsophalangeal release and extensor brevis reconstruction. Foot Ankle Int. 2013;34(6):792–9.
3. Kwon JY, De Asla RJ. The use of flexor to extensor transfers for the correction of the flexible hammer toe deformity. Foot Ankle Clin. 2011;16(4):573–82.
4. Shirzad K, Kiesau CD, DeOrio JK, Parekh SG. Lesser toe deformities. J Am Acad Orthop Surg. 2011;19:505–14.
5. Smith BW, Coughlin MJ. Disorders of the lesser toes. Sports Med Arthrosc Rev. 2009;17:167–74.

5 Freiberg's Disease

Take-Home Message

- Incompetence of the first ray (elevation or shortening) may be a causal factor and must be addressed when treating the second ray.
- Aggressive early conservative management may prevent late-stage arthritis by minimizing further extrinsic trauma to the metatarsal head.
- Surgical management: If no arthritis, then dorsal closing wedge osteotomy of the second metatarsal. If arthritis is present, then an MTP arthroplasty with interposition versus metatarsal head excision.

Definition Osteochondrosis of unknown origin that occurs in the metatarsal head, most commonly affects the second and, however, can also affect the third and fourth. Most commonly occurs in second decade of life and in women

Etiology *Primarily Unknown*

Extrinsic causes: repetitive microtrauma of the subchondral bone secondary to impact activity (running, sports, high-heeled shoes). Increased load transfer during gait secondary to an iatrogenically elevated, short, or unstable first metatarsal most commonly occurs following correction of hallux valgus.

Intrinsic causes: avascular necrosis, inflammatory arthropathies, predisposing anatomy (relatively long second metatarsal compared to the first), corticosteroids

Pathophysiology

A disruption in the blood supply due to mechanical or inflammatory process leading to eventual infarction and weakening of the bony architecture with concomitant disruption of articular surface. Persistent trauma leads to collapse of the weakened metatarsal head that progresses to arthrosis as the cartilage degenerates.

Pain within the affected MTP with swelling, thickening, and decreased range of motion.

Radiography Weight-bearing anteroposterior, lateral, and oblique views are required.

Common findings in Freiberg's disease include:

Resorption of the central metatarsal bone adjacent to the articular surface with flattening of the metatarsal head (Fig. 22)

Osteochondral loose bodies

Joint space narrowing in late-stage disease with associated osteophyte formation along with collapse of the articular surface (Fig. 23)

MRI scan: Low T1 and variable T2 fat sat in the subchondral bone of the metatarsal head with flattening

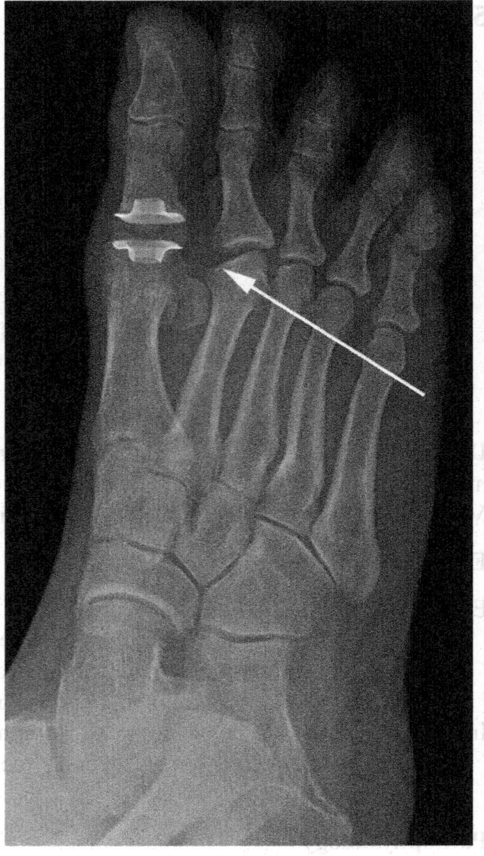

Fig. 22 Note the flattening of the metatarsal head that is commonly seen with Freiberg's disease (*arrow*). This patient had a prior silicone arthroplasty of the great toe and developed Freiberg's disease secondary to overload from an incompetent first ray

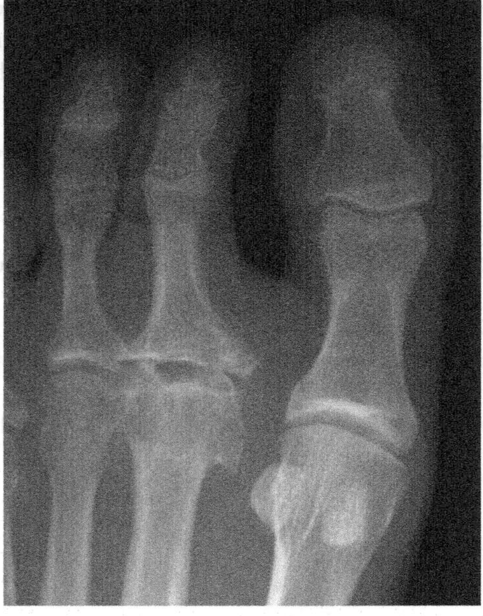

Fig. 23 Focused AP view of the forefoot demonstrating the natural history and long-term sequela of untreated Freiberg's. Note the significant subchondral cysts and osteophyte formation indicating OA

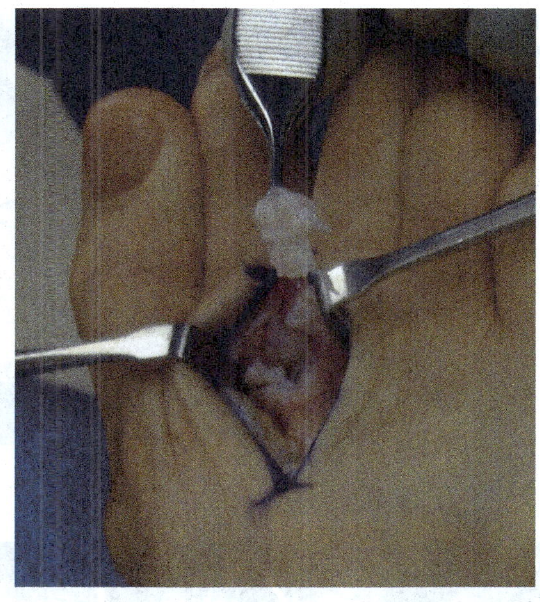

Fig. 24 Loose body removal in a patient who requires a dorsal closing wedge osteotomy

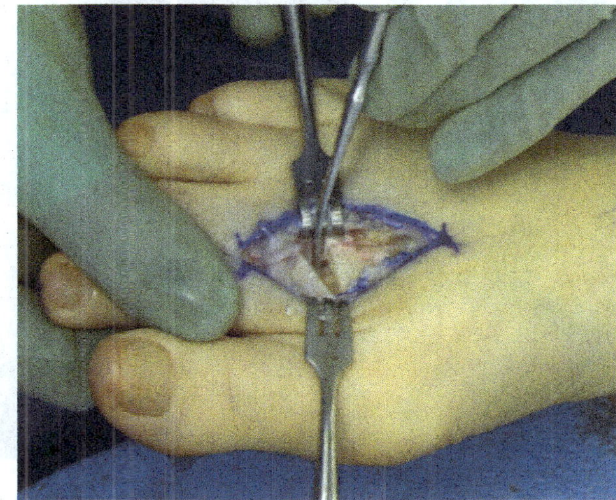

Fig. 25 A freer is placed in the osteotomy demonstrating the amount of bone that was resected. Note the dorsal to plantar direction of the osteotomy. The intact plantar cartilage will be rotated dorsally and recreate the dorsal articular surface

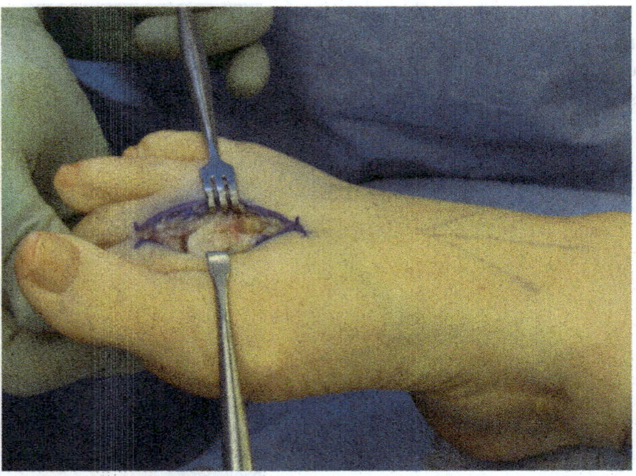

Fig. 26 Final appearance of the osteotomy after closure. Note the intact plantar cartilage now clearly present dorsally

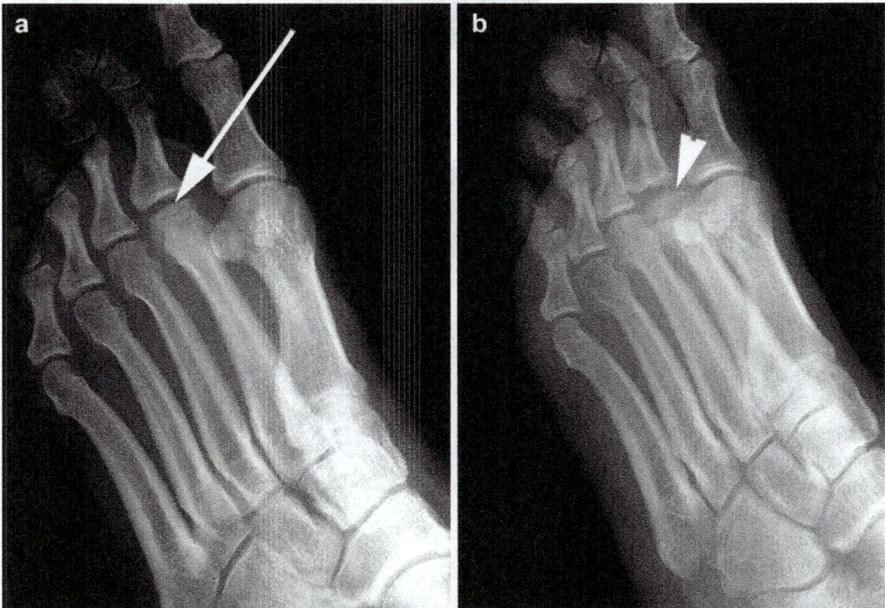

Fig. 27 Radiograph of a patient with Freiberg's disease (**a**) with the characteristic flattening of the metatarsal head (*arrow*) treated with a dorsal closing wedge osteotomy (**b**). Note how the contour of the metatarsal head has been recreated (*arrowhead*)

Classification

Smillie radiographic classification of the metatarsal head appearance	
Stage I	Fracture of the epiphysis
Stage II	Subsidence of the central portion (altered head contour)
Stage III	Central reabsorption
Stage IV	Loose body separation
Stage V	Flattening, deformity, arthritis of the metatarsal head

Treatment

	Nonoperative	Operative
Clinical indication	Early stage of disease/low demand in late stage	Failed conservative treatment and/or advanced stage of disease
Options	(a) Activity modifications (elimination of impact) (b) Protected weight bearing in a short CAM walker or short leg cast with toe extensions with crutches (c) NSAIDS (d) Shoe modifications (wide toe box, extra depth, flat rigid sole) (e) Full-length semirigid orthosis with metatarsal bar or pad	1. Early – synovitis: simple débridement and loose body removal (Fig. 24) 2. Late – joint collapse without arthritis: metatarsal dorsal closing wedge osteotomy with resection of nonviable bone and cartilage (Figs. 25, 26, and 27) 3. Late – arthritis: resection arthroplasty or interpositional arthroplasty. If severe and low demand, metatarsal head excision can be considered 4. *In all cases:* correction of the biomechanics of the foot must be performed (restore WB of the first metatarsal and/or shorten second metatarsal as indicated)

Complications

- Progression of joint degeneration
- Transfer metatarsalgia
- Limited ROM with extension contracture

Bibliography

1. Carmont MR, Rees RJ, Blundell CM. Current concepts review: Freiberg's disease. Foot Ankle Int. 2009;30(2):167–76.
2. DiGiovanni CW, Patel A, Calfee R, Nickisch F. Osteonecrosis in the foot. J Am Acad Orthop Surg. 2007;15(4):208–17.
3. Ozkan Y, Oztürk A, Ozdemir R, Aykut S, Yalçin N. Interpositional arthroplasty with extensor digitorum brevis tendon in Freiberg's disease: a new surgical technique. Foot Ankle Int. 2008;29(5):488–92.

6 Sesamoids

Take-Home Message

- Turf toe is a complex injury to the sesamoid complex and plantar plate of the 1st MTP joint. Return to play requires 60° of painless dorsiflexion.
- The most effective treatment for pain secondary to the sesamoid is isolated sesamoid resection.
- Tibial > fibular

Definition The sesamoids are embedded within the tendons of flexor hallucis brevis. They are connected to each other by the intersesamoid ligament, and each sesamoid has an associated ligament inserting onto its respective side of the metatarsal head. The sesamoids function to increase the mechanical force of the flexor hallucis brevis (FHB) in addition to absorption forces to the great toe during weight bearing.

Etiology and Pathophysiology

- Trauma: stress fracture and acute fracture (hyperextension and axial loading of the metatarsophalangeal joint)
- Sesamoiditis: mechanical (repetitive trauma, cavus foot) or inflammatory disorders (infection, autoimmune disease)

Radiography

- Non-weight-bearing anteroposterior and lateral foot views
- Oblique views: a lateral 40° oblique view (for assessment of the fibular sesamoid) (Fig. 28) and a medial 40° oblique radiograph (for assessment of the tibial sesamoid)
- An axial view of the first metatarsophalangeal joint → may identify fractures in the sagittal plane not visible on the AP radiograph (Fig. 29)
- Bone scan: nonspecific as noted to be increased in 26–29 % of normal individuals
- CT scan: able to reveal irregular fracture margins in acute or early stress fractures
- MRI: marrow edema noted in stress fractures. Avascular necrosis (lack of signal intensity) (Fig. 30). Very useful in the setting of turf toe to identify the presence of articular injury, complete tear of the plantar plate (Fig. 31).

Classification

Turf Toe

- Grade 1: strain of the capsule without loss of continuity. Normal range of motion with ability to bear weight
- Grade 2: partial tear of the capsule. Limited and painful range of motion
- Grade 3: complete tear with loss of continuity of the plantar plate and capsule or associated sesamoid fracture. Inability to bear weight, limited range of motion, severe swelling, and ecchymosis

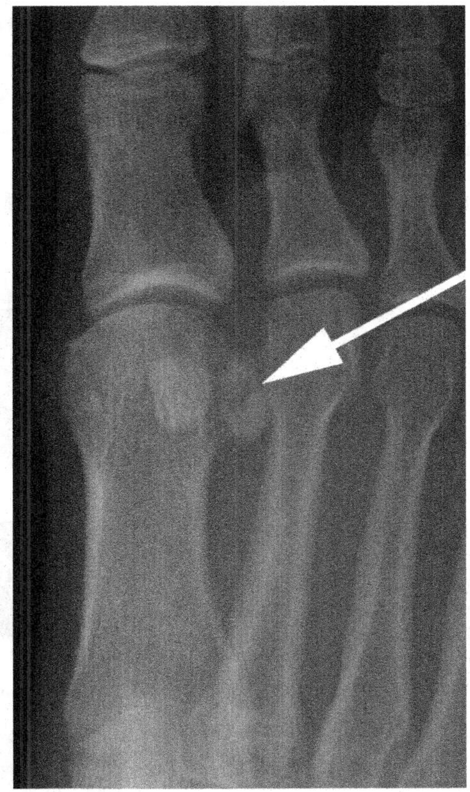

Fig. 28 Oblique view of the foot demonstrating a linear lucency within the fibular sesamoid (*arrow*). This is consistent with an acute fracture and not a bipartite sesamoid. The fibular sesamoid is rarely bipartite in isolation, and the irregular line is consistent with a fracture

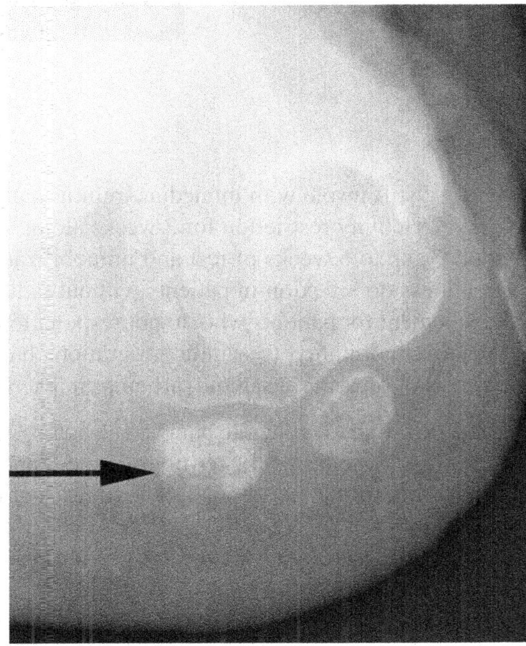

Fig. 29 Sesamoid views allow visualization of the metatarsal-sesamoid articulation. This view clearly demonstrates sclerosis (*arrow*), flattening, arthritis, and fracture

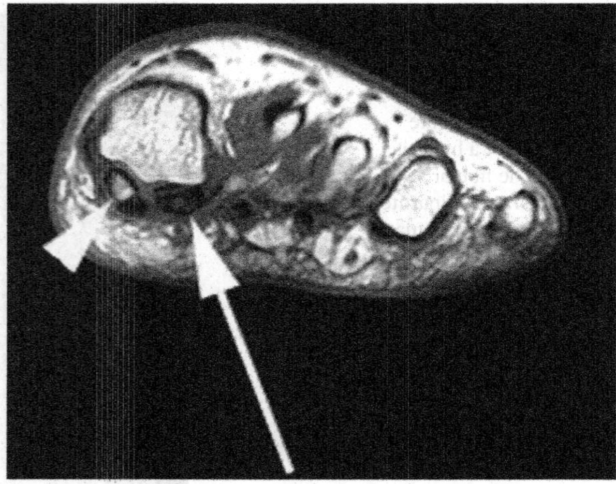

Fig. 30 Coronal T1 image of a patient with osteochondritis of the fibular sesamoid. Osteochondritis will appear as dark (*arrow*), in contrast to the normal bone that appears bright on T1 imaging (*arrowhead*)

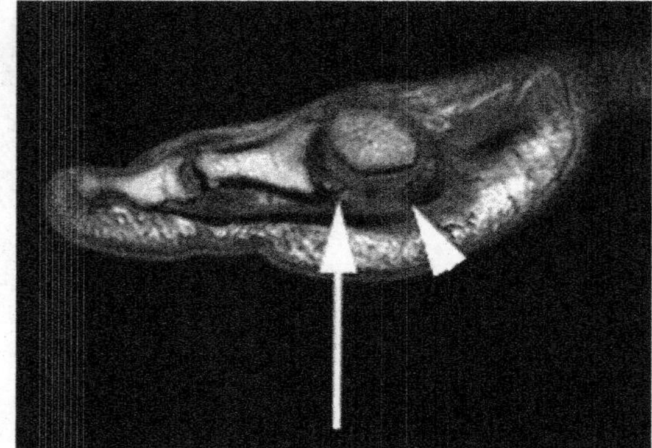

Fig. 31 Sagittal T1 image of an acute grade 3 turf toe injury. Note the disruption of the distal attachment of the plantar plate (*arrow*) with proximal retraction of the sesamoids (*arrowhead*)

Treatment

Turf Toe

- Grade 1: stiff insole with immediate return to play
- Grade 2: activity restriction for 2 weeks along with a stiff insole
- Grade 3: up to 6 weeks of rest and immobilization with return to play after 60° of painless dorsiflexion in patients without radiographic abnormality. Operative management for patients who do not respond to the above protocol or any radiographic abnormality (sesamoid migration, hallux valgus, sesamoid fracture, diastasis of bipartite sesamoid, articular impaction)

Sesamoiditis: mild to moderate pain can be controlled with anti-inflammatory medication, a stiff-soled or rocker-bottom shoe, and a dancer's pad (C-shaped pad with a relief for the sesamoids). Severe cases or fracture are treated with a CAM walker for 6 weeks followed by use of a dancer's pad and activity restriction until resolution of pain. Shoe wear modification (avoidance of high-heeled shoes) is also required.

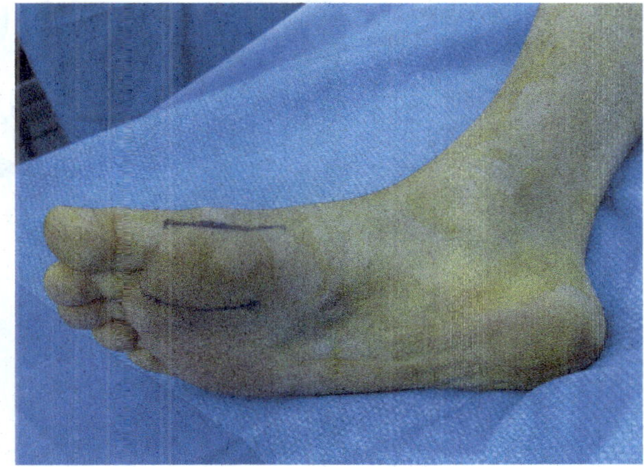

Fig. 32 Plantar medial and plantar lateral incisions for repair of a Grade 3 turf toe injury

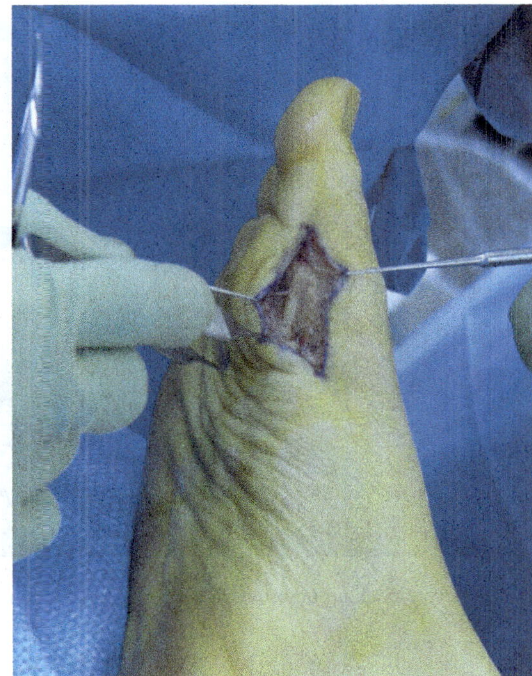

Fig. 33 Plantar medial approach to the tibial sesamoid must be undertaken carefully to avoid injury to the plantar medial digital nerve (pictured)

Operative

Turf Toe

- Dual incision technique to repair the plantar plate (Fig. 32). Avoid damage to plantar medial digital nerve (tibial sesamoid) and plantar lateral digital nerve (fibular sesamoid) (Fig. 33). Repair plantar plate directly or via bony tunnel through the distal aspect of the sesamoid (Fig. 34).

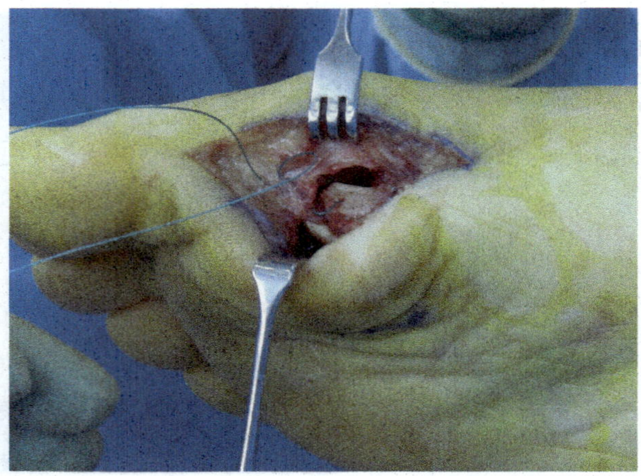

Fig. 34 Bone tunnel made within the distal aspect of the tibial sesamoid to allow fixation to the proximal aspect of the remaining plantar plate

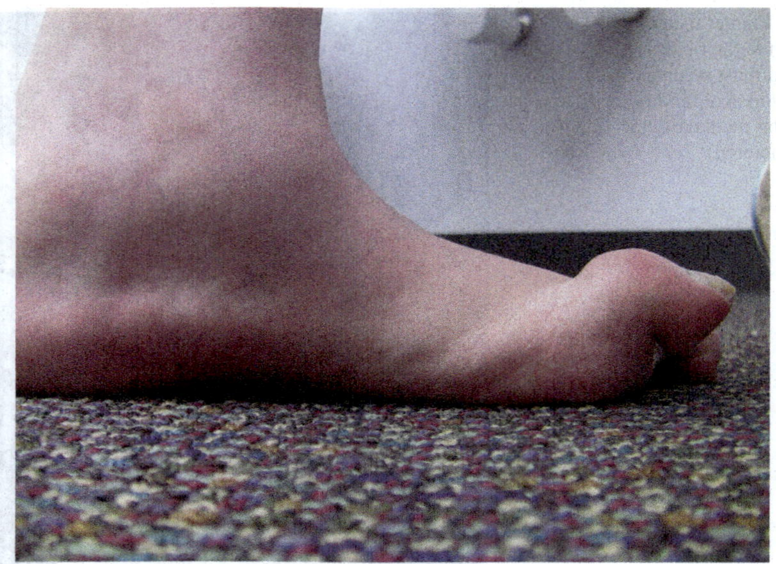

Fig. 35 Severe cock-up deformity occurred after excision of both the medial and lateral tibial sesamoids

Chronic sesamoid pain (sesamoiditis, AVN, fracture).

- Complete or partial sesamoidectomy. Partial sesamoidectomy for a proximal or distal pole fracture. Repair of the FHB is critical to prevent complications of a coronal plane deformity. Ninety percent of patients will be able to return to pre-injury level of activity.

- Curettage and grafting of long-standing symptomatic nonunion has been described and, however, has not been proven to be superior to excision and is not the most reliable procedure.
- Excision of both the tibial and fibular sesamoid is not routinely performed secondary to the known complication of cock-up toe.

Complications

- Cock-up deformity: increased incidence after excision of both sesamoids (Fig. 35)
- Hallux valgus: related to excision of the tibial sesamoid
- Hallux varus: related to excision of the fibular sesamoid
- Chronic pain and neuroma formation at the surgical incision site with the plantar approach to the sesamoids

Bibliography

1. Anderson RB. Turf toe injuries of the hallux metatarsophalangeal joint. Tech Foot Ankle Surg. 2002;1:102–11.
2. Cohen BE. Hallux sesamoid disorders. Foot Ankle Clin. 2009;14:91–104.
3. Kadakia AR, Molloy A. Current concepts review: traumatic disorders of the first metatarsophalangeal joint and sesamoid complex. Foot Ankle Int. 2011;32: 834–9.
4. McCormick JJ, Anderson RB. The great toe: failed turf toe, chronic turf toe, and complicated sesamoid injuries. Foot Ankle Clin. 2009;14:135–50.

Generalized Conditions

Anish R. Kadakia, Paul J. Switaj, Bryant S. Ho, Mohammed Alshouli, Daniel Fuchs, and George Ochengele

1 Neuropathic Foot

Take-Home Message

- The neuropathic foot is most commonly a sequela of diabetes but can also result from upper motor neuron (UMN) lesions and hereditary motor-sensory neuropathies (HSMN).
- Surgical treatment of UMN disorders often include Achilles lengthening, tibialis anterior transfer, and toe flexor release.
- Surgical treatment of HSMN requires a thorough evaluation into what drives the pes cavovarus deformity and its flexibility.

Definition

- Mechanical changes in the foot which develop as a result of a disturbance in the normal sensory and motor innervation of joints.

Etiology

- Diabetic neuropathy: most common cause of neuropathic foot (see chapters Paediatric hip conditions and Paediatric feet conditions).
- Sequelae of upper motor neuron (UMN) disorders: most commonly secondary to traumatic brain injury, stroke, and spinal cord injury.

A.R. Kadakia (✉) • P.J. Switaj • B.S. Ho • M. Alshouli • D. Fuchs • G. Ochengele
Department of Orthopedic Surgery, Northwestern University – Feinberg School of Medicine, Northwestern Memorial Hospital, Chicago, IL, USA
e-mail: Kadak259@gmail.com; paul.switaj@gmail.com; bryant.s.ho@gmail.com; mtshouli@gmail.com; dfuchs0011@gmail.com; gochenjele@gmail.com

C. Mauffrey, D.J. Hak (eds.), *Passport for the Orthopedic Boards and FRCS Examination*, DOI 10.1007/978-2-8178-0475-0_42

- Hereditary motor-sensory neuropathies (HMSN): inherited progressive peripheral neuropathy (e.g., Charcot-Marie-Tooth disease). Specific etiology depends on the particular variant. For CMT it is autosomal dominant with a duplication of chromosome 17.
- Can also be caused by chemotherapeutic agents and certain infectious diseases such as HIV.

Pathophysiology

- Diabetic neuropathy (see chapters Paediatric hip conditions and Paediatric feet conditions):
- Upper motor neuron disorders:
  - Disruption of UMN pathways can lead to paralysis, muscle imbalance, and acquired spasticity, which ultimately may cause deformity.
  - Secondary problems are contractures, calluses, pressure sores, joint subluxation, hygiene issues, shoe-wear difficulties, and dissatisfaction with personal experience.
  - The most common deformity is equinovarus caused by overactivity of gastrocnemius-soleus complex and relative overactive tibialis anterior.
- HMSN, depends on the specific type:
  - For CMT the basis is an abnormal myelin sheath protein.
  - Leads to motor imbalance and bilateral → first ray is plantarflexed due to relative unopposed pull of peroneus longus → forefoot cavus and compensatory hindfoot varus → symmetric pes cavovarus deformity (Fig. 1).
  - Intrinsic wasting → overpull of extrinsic musculature → claw toe deformity (Fig. 2).
  - Variable sensory deficits → can lead to recurrent ulceration, infection, and arthropathy.
  - Forefoot-driven hindfoot varus: deformity corrects with Coleman block test. Concomitant intrinsic hindfoot varus: deformity does not correct.

Treatment
Diabetic Neuropathy **(see chapters Paediatric hip conditions and Paediatric feet conditions):**
UMN disorders:

Nonoperative Care

- Physical therapy, stretching, maintenance of joint range of motion. Other modalities include splinting, serial casting, oral muscle relaxants, phenol and lidocaine nerve blocks, and botulinum type A toxin.
- Phenol block have proven history with longer-lasting effect and are less expensive than botulinum toxin. However, botulinum toxin is easy to deliver since it needs only an injection into the muscle belly rather than precise injection around nerve.

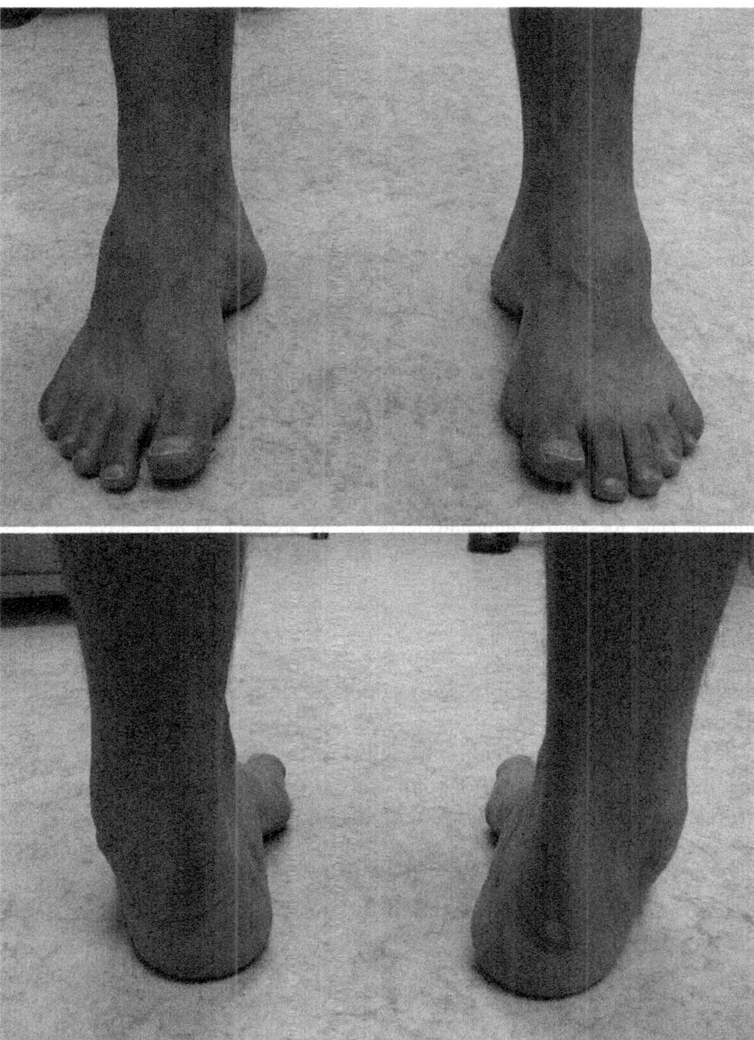

Fig. 1 *Anterior view* of a patient with HSMN with bilateral cavus feet. Note the ability to see the heel from this view with the elevated arches. The *posterior view* clearly demonstrates the varus of the hindfoot

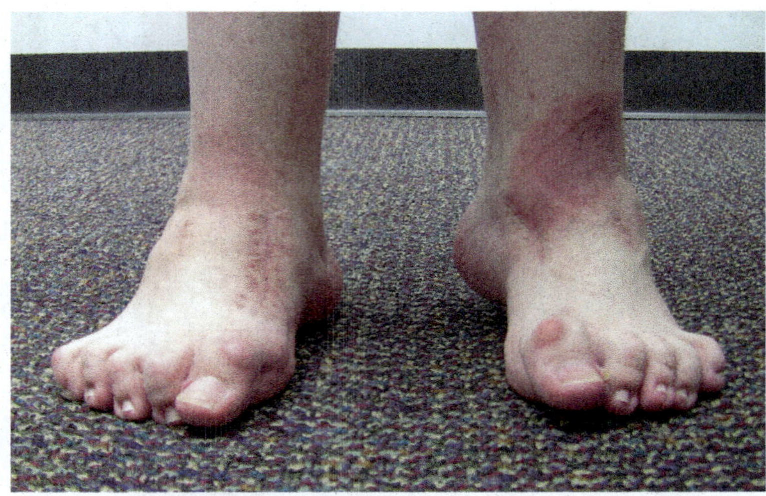

Fig. 2 Multiple claw toes and significantly claw hallux are seen in more advanced stages of HSMN. Claw hallux and claw toes in young patients should always increase the suspicion of a neurologic disorder

Surgical Treatment

- Address equinus deformity with open Z-lengthening or percutaneous lengthening.
- Varus deformity addressed with split anterior tibialis tendon transfer (SPLATT) to lateral cuneiform or cuboid or total anterior tibialis tendon transfer to lateral cuneiform. Release of toe flexors often required.

Hereditary motor-sensory neuropathies (HMSN)

Flexible Deformity (hindfoot can be passively manipulated):
Nonsurgical management:

- Not currently recommended given progressive pattern of disease
- Surgical management:
- Forefoot driven: closing wedge dorsiflexion osteotomy of first metatarsal (Fig. 3), release of plantar fascia, transfer of peroneus longus into peroneus brevis at level of distal fibula.
- Hindfoot driven: in addition to abovementioned procedures, include lateral calcaneal slide and/or closing wedge osteotomy (Fig. 4).
- Clawed hallux can be surgically treated with Jones procedure (arthrodesis of interphalangeal joint and transfer of EHL to the first metatarsal).
- Consider posterior tibial tendon transfer to dorsum (lateral cuneiform) or lengthening of the tendon to restore balance.

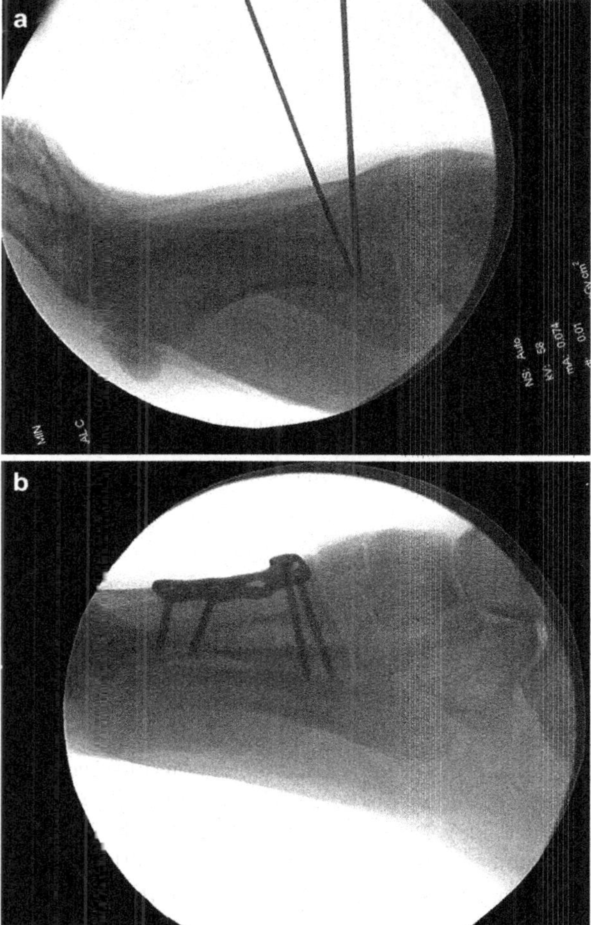

Fig. 3 Dorsiflexion osteotomy to correct the plantarflexed first ray is performed by marking the osteotomy with two K-wires (**a**). Following resection of the wedge, the osteotomy is closed and fixated with resultant elevation of the first ray (**b**)

Fixed Deformity (hindfoot cannot be passively manipulated):
Nonsurgical management:

- Attempted with locked-ankle, short-leg ankle-foot orthosis with a lateral T-strap.
- Rocker sole can improve gait and decrease energy expenditure.

Surgical management:

- Triple arthrodesis usually required for hindfoot correction. Posterior tibialis tendon transfer through the interosseous membrane can correct equinus contracture and dorsiflexion weakness.
- Must address imbalance of tendon forces even in the setting of an arthrodesis to prevent recurrence.
- Dorsiflexion osteotomy of first metatarsal, release of plantar fascia.
- Forefoot correction is performed according to the guidelines outlined previously.

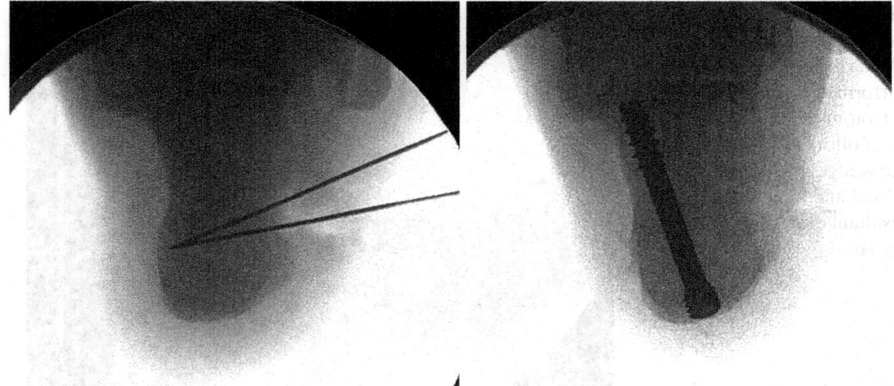

Fig. 4 Lateral closing wedge osteotomy of the calcaneus in a patient who had concomitant intrinsic hindfoot varus (failure to correct with Coleman block). This is performed in addition correction of the plantarflexed first ray and is not a substitute for a dorsiflexion osteotomy of the first metatarsal

Bibliography

1. Botte MJ, Bruffey JD, Copp SN, Colwell CW. Surgical reconstruction of acquired spastic foot and ankle deformity. Foot Ankle Clin. 2000;5:381–416.
2. Piazza S, Ricci G, Caldarazzo Ienco E, et al. Pes cavus and hereditary neuropathies: when a relationship should be suspected. J Orthop Traumatol. 2010;11:195–201.
3. Roy DR, Al-Sayyad MJ. Complications of surgery of the foot and ankle in hereditary neurologic disorders. Clin Orthop Relat Res. 2001:181–7.
4. Schenone A, Nobbio L, Monti Bragadin M, Ursino G, Grandis M. Inherited neuropathies. Curr Treat Opt Neurol. 2011;391(13):160–79.
5. van der Ven A, Chapman CB, Bowker JH. Charcot neuroarthropathy of the foot and ankle. J Am Acad Orthop Surg. 2009;17:562–71.

2 Rheumatoid Foot

Take-Home Message

- Rheumatoid arthritis is a chronic autoimmune disease that results in polyarthropathy that commonly involves the forefoot.
- Typical deformity includes dorsal and valgus toe deviation, claw toe deformity, and pes planovalgus.
- Conservative treatment involves proper shoe and orthotic wear and immune-modulating drugs under the direction of a rheumatologist.
- Surgical treatment of the forefoot includes first MTP arthrodesis, lesser MT head resections, osteoclasis of interphalangeal joints, and extensor brevis tenotomy, while midfoot or triple arthrodesis is needed for pes planovalgus deformity in the rheumatoid foot.

Definition

- Chronic, symmetrical polyarthropathy that most commonly presents in the third and fourth decades and is more prevalent in women

Etiology

- Autoimmune disease with a genetic predisposition
- Cell-mediated immune response against soft tissues, cartilage, and bone

Pathophysiology

- ESR, CRP will be elevated, and RF titers positive (most commonly IgM).
- Chronic synovitis leads to ligament and capsular laxity and cartilage and bony erosion.
- Forefoot involvement very common:
  - Complaints of forefoot swelling, poorly defined pain, and eventually deformity.
  - Incompetence of joint capsules and lateral ligaments causes toes to subluxate or dislocate dorsally and deviate into valgus (Fig. 5).
  - Contracture of the intrinsic musculature exacerbates claw toe deformity.
  - Plantar fat pad migrates distally and atrophies, causing metatarsalgia and forming keratoses.
  - As lesser toes deviate, hallux valgus occurs, and transfer metatarsalgia worsens (Fig. 6).
- Midfoot and hindfoot less commonly and less severely involved:
  - Midfoot/hindfoot arthrosis often results in pes planovalgus deformity that can be midfoot driven (tarsometatarsal joints are subluxated with a congruent hindfoot) or hindfoot driven (transverse tarsal and subtalar joint is subluxated with normal midfoot).
- Tibiotalar joint is also commonly involved and may be caused by chronic subtalar joint malalignment.

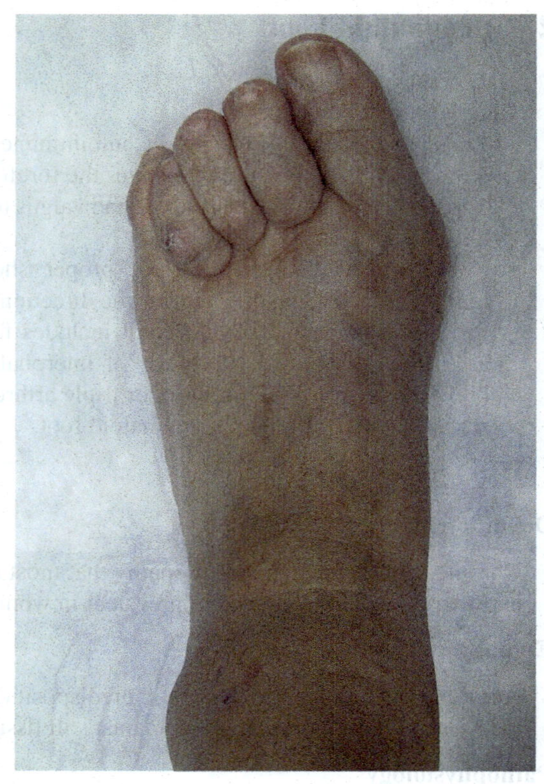

Fig. 5 Clinical photograph of a patient with RA with swelling of the digits and characteristic valgus deviation of all digits with claw toes

Radiography

- Can have significant midfoot and hindfoot arthrosis (talonavicular joint is characteristic)
- Typically has diffuse osteopenia, symmetrical joint space narrowing, and lack of osteophyte formation (which easily differentiates RA from osteoarthritis) (Fig. 7)

Treatment

- Vasculitis and soft tissue fragility is common, requiring diligent care of the soft tissues regardless of treatment.

Conservative

- Rest, NSAIDs, immune-modulating drugs under the direction of rheumatologists, toe taping, orthoses, careful use of corticosteroid injections to help symptoms related to synovitis, and patient education

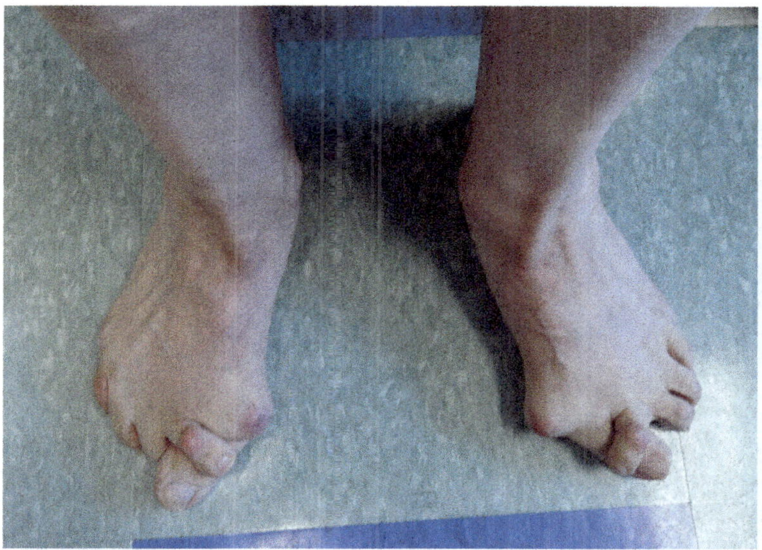

Fig. 6 In severe cases, the joint laxity that occurs results in significant hallux valgus with overlap of the second toe over the first

Surgical

- Should discuss use of immune-mediating pharmacologic therapies with rheumatologist prior to surgery → while most medications can be continued (prednisone, methotrexate, plaquenil), the newer biologic agents (such as TNF inhibitors) should be discontinued.
- "Rheumatoid forefoot reconstruction" for deformity correction:
  - First MTP arthrodesis, lesser metatarsal head resection with pinning of lesser MTP joints, closed osteoclasis of interphalangeal joints versus PIP arthroplasty (silicone arthroplasty not recommended) through the use of three dorsal incisions. Extensor brevis tenotomy and Z-lengthening of extensor longus tendons may be necessary (Fig. 8).
- Pes planovalgus: Midfoot driven, realignment midfoot arthrodesis. Hindfoot-driven and fixed deformity, triple arthrodesis
- Tibiotalar arthrosis: Ankle arthrodesis is treatment of choice, ankle arthroplasty emerging as more reliable technique (though it is associated with increased risk of wound complications).

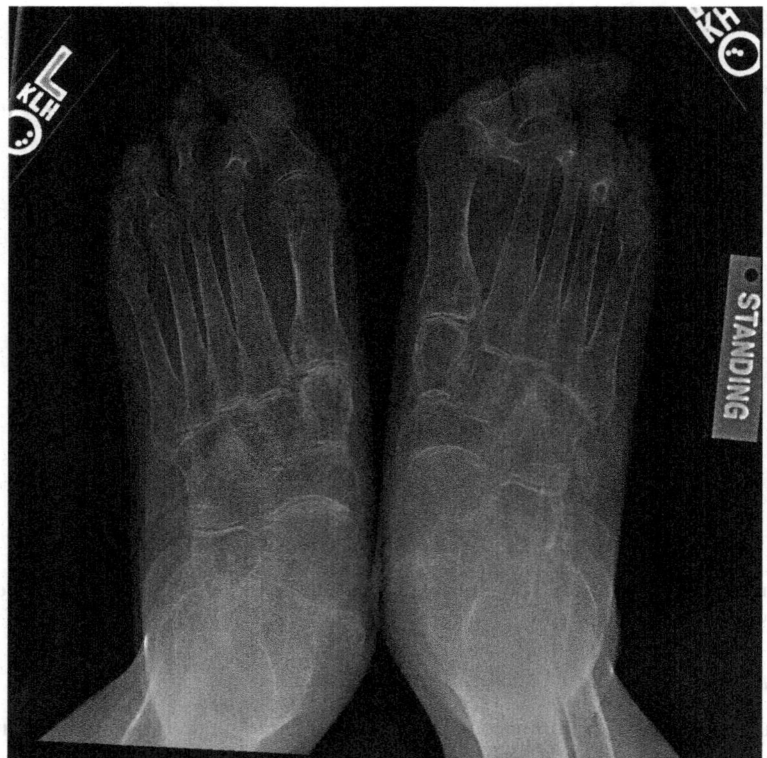

Fig. 7 Typical radiographic appearance of a patient with RA. Note the multiple joint involvement with symmetric joint space narrowing, osteopenia without osteophyte formation with associated pes planus deformity. The typical dislocation of the lesser MTP joints can be noted as well

Complications

- Wound complications common following surgical treatment.
- Current literature controversial whether patients on immunosuppressive therapies have significantly increased infection rates.
- Late recurrence of deformity has been reported and some consideration for joint sparing lesser toe surgery has been considered. However, no long-term data to support joint sparing treatment to date.

Bibliography

1. Aronow MS, Hakim-Zargar M. Management of hindfoot disease in rheumatoid arthritis. Foot Ankle Clin. 2007;12:455–74, vi.
2. Goodman SM, Paget S. Perioperative drug safety in patients with rheumatoid arthritis. Rheum Dis Clin North Am. 2012;38:747–59.

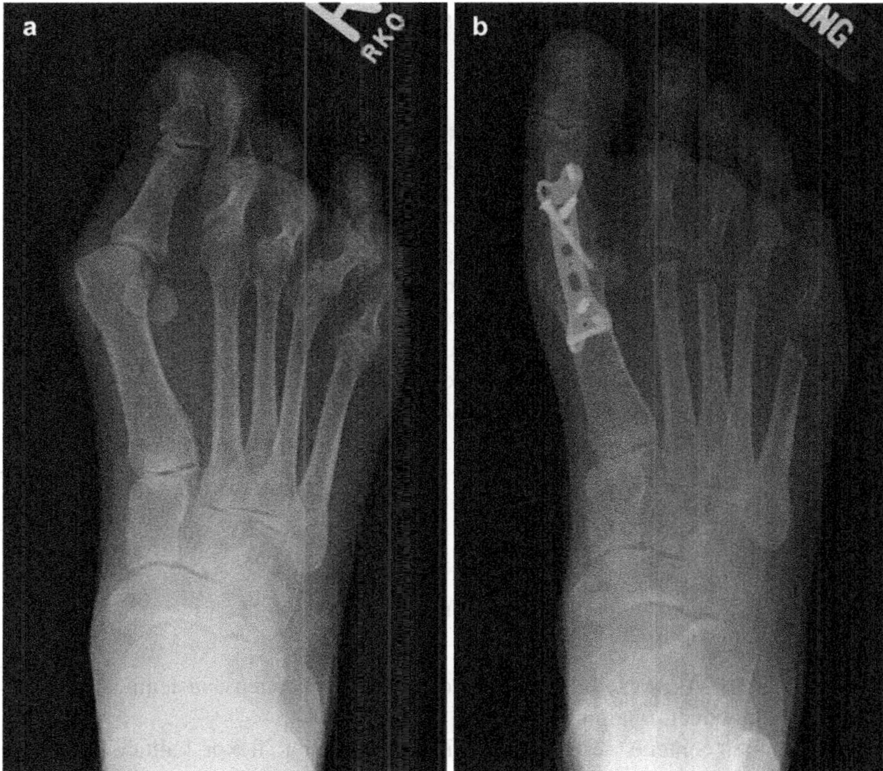

Fig. 8 Preoperative AP radiograph (**a**) of a patient with RA with clinical hallux valgus with subluxation of the lesser MTP joints. Post-op AP radiograph (**b**) demonstrating excellent alignment following first MTP arthrodesis with metatarsal head resection of joints 2–5 and osteoclysis of the PIP joints. Interposition of the extensors into the potential space created may decrease risk of late subluxation

3. Jeng C, Campbell J. Current concepts review: the rheumatoid forefoot. Foot Ankle Int. 2008;29:959–68.
4. Loveday DT, Jackson GE, Geary NP. The rheumatoid foot and ankle: current evidence. Foot Ankle Surg. 2012;18:94–102.
5. Sammarco VJ. Ankle arthrodesis in rheumatoid arthritis: techniques, results, and complications. Foot Ankle Clin. 2007;12:475–95, vii.

3 Nerve Entrapment Syndromes

Take-Home Message

- Nerve entrapment related to space-occupying mass is more likely to improve with surgical treatment than nerve entrapment without a related mass.
- The first branch of lateral plantar nerve compression between the fascia of abductor hallucis and quadratus plantae is the most common cause of nerve-related heel pain, common in running athlete.
- Superficial peroneal nerve entrapment related to chronic ankle instability and peroneal muscle herniation through fascial defect.
- Nerve entrapment syndromes most commonly cause neuropraxia type of nerve injury with nerve contusion and focal demyelination of axon sheath.

Definition

Nerve Entrapment

- Localized pressure causing nerve dysfunction.
- Tarsal tunnel syndrome → tibial nerve:
  - Boundaries – flexor retinaculum (medial); talus, calcaneus, sustentaculum tali (lateral); abductor hallucis (inferior)
  - Additional contents – tendons of tibialis posterior, flexor hallucis longus, flexor digitorum longus, posterior tibial artery, venae comitantes, numerous septa
- First branch of lateral plantar nerve (Baxter's nerve)
- Anterior tarsal tunnel syndrome → deep peroneal nerve
  - Boundaries – inferior extensor retinaculum (anterior), tibia and talus (posterior)
  - Additional contents – dorsalis pedis artery
- Superficial peroneal nerve.
- See Table 1 for symptoms and physical exam findings.

Etiology

- External compression from adjacent structures – tenosynovitis, engorged or varicose veins.
- Space-occupying mass – synovial or ganglion cyst, pigmented villonodular synovitis, nerve sheath tumors, lipomas (Fig. 9).
- Systemic disease can cause compression indirectly due to inflammatory edema – diabetes mellitus, rheumatoid arthritis.
- See Table 2 for nerve-specific etiologies.

Table 1 Nerve entrapment symptoms and physical exam findings

	Symptoms	Physical exam findings
Tarsal tunnel syndrome	Burning sensation of plantar foot, medial ankle	Positive Tinel and nerve compression tests
	Plantar foot numbness variable	Pain with dorsiflexion-eversion
	Worse with prolonged standing, walking, running	Diminished two-point discrimination
		Wasting of intrinsic musculature
		Hindfoot valgus, pes planus
First branch of lateral plantar nerve	Chronic heel pain, pain at plantar medial foot, may radiate laterally	Maximal point of tenderness at site of compression by fascia of abductor hallucis and quadratus plantae
	Symptoms similar to plantar fasciitis	
	Symptoms without weight bearing	Wasting of abductor digiti quinti
	No numbness – nerve has no sensory innervation	
Anterior tarsal tunnel syndrome	Burning pain in dorsal first webspace	Positive Tinel sign
	Vague dorsal foot pain	Diminished two-point discrimination
	Worse at night with foot in plantarflexion	Forced ankle plantarflexion reproduces symptoms
	Worse with shallow, laced shoes	Weak great toe extension
Superficial peroneal nerve	Pain and paresthesias radiating to dorsum of foot	Positive Tinel sign
	Numbness is variable	Diminished two-point discrimination
	Symptoms increase with activity	Palpable fascial defect and peroneal herniation
	May feel a bulge at lateral leg – area of muscle herniation	Forced plantarflexion and inversion reproduces symptoms
		Signs of ankle instability

Pathophysiology

- Pressure on nerve causes ischemia and neuroma formation.
- Neuroma contains bundled disorganized nerve endings within collagenous mass.
- Can result in loss of sensory and motor function.
- Pain and paresthesia replace normal sensation.

Radiography

- Weight-bearing radiographs of the foot and ankle
  - Detect bony abnormality causing or contributing to nerve entrapment.
  - Evaluate alignment of foot and ankle.
  - Rule out other source of symptoms.
- MRI – if concern for space-occupying mass
- EMG and NCV – can help confirm diagnosis but variable sensitivity

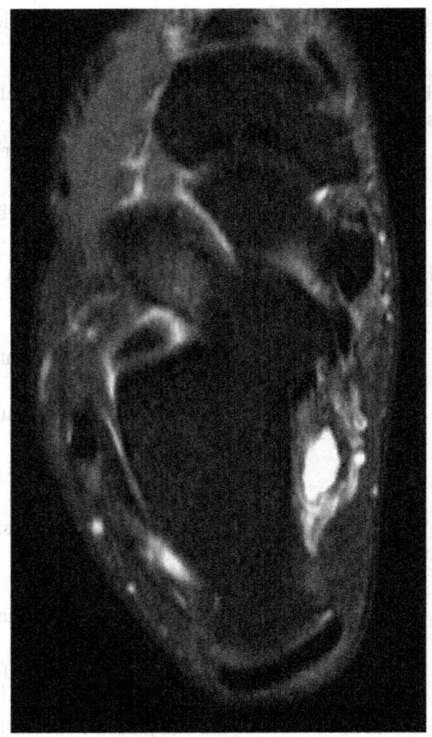

Fig. 9 Axial T2 fat-saturated image of a patient with tarsal tunnel syndrome that was noted to have a ganglion within the tarsal tunnel that required excision in addition to decompression of the nerve

Table 2 Nerve entrapment etiology

	Etiology
Tarsal tunnel syndrome	Increased nerve tension from hindfoot valgus and pes planus
	Fracture of sustentaculum tali, medial tubercle of posterior process of talus
	Accessory muscle
First branch of lateral plantar nerve	Compression between fascia of abductor hallucis and quadratus plantae
	Lateral plantar nerve injury can occur from insertion of intramedullary nail for tibiotalocalcaneal fusion
Anterior tarsal tunnel syndrome	Anterior osteophytes of tibiotalar or talonavicular joints
	Tightly laced shoes
Superficial peroneal nerve	Chronic ankle instability
	Herniation of peroneal musculature through fascial defect
	Iatrogenic injury

Classification

Seddon Classification

- Neuropraxia – nerve contusion, focal demyelination of axon sheath, no Wallerian degeneration, good prognosis
  - Most common resulting injury following nerve entrapment:
- Axonotmesis – axon and myelin sheath disruption, Wallerian degeneration, endoneurium intact
- Neurotmesis – complete disruption of nerve including endoneurium, Wallerian degeneration

Treatment

Nonoperative: first line unless a space-occupying mass is present

- Activity modification
- Medications
  - Nonnarcotic analgesics
  - Centrally acting anticonvulsants
  - Tricyclic antidepressants, selective serotonin reuptake inhibitors
  - Topically applied compounds – include local anesthetic, anti-inflammatory medication, capsaicin
- Physical and occupational therapy
- Injection of local anesthetic with or without corticosteroid medication
  - Useful for diagnosis

Operative: indicated after 3–6 months of unsuccessful conservative treatment

- Complete nerve decompression (Fig. 10)

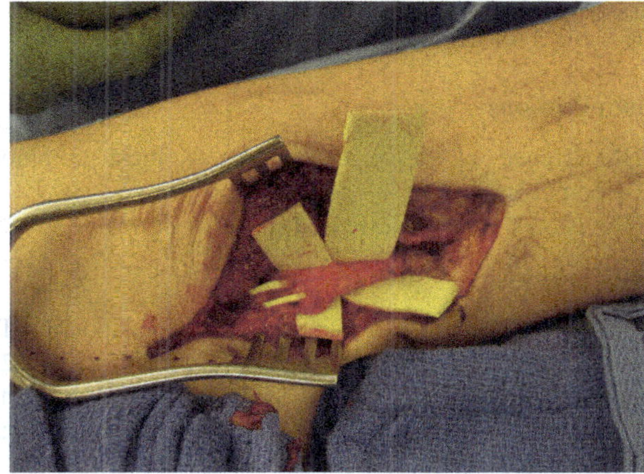

Fig. 10 Intraoperative photograph demonstrating an appropriate incision with decompression of the tibial nerve and the requisite branches. Note release of the abductor hallucis in the distal aspect of the incision, ensuring that both the medial and lateral plantar branches are adequately released

Table 3 Nerve entrapment treatment options

	Nonoperative	Operative
Tarsal tunnel syndrome	Medial heel and sole wedge if hindfoot valgus and pes planus	Identify nerve proximally
		Release deep investing fascia proximally, flexor retinaculum, deep and superficial fascia of the abductor hallucis
	Short period of immobilization with cast or boot	Assure that all branches – medial calcaneal, lateral plantar, medial plantar – are decompressed
		Release all septa
First branch of lateral plantar nerve	Heel pad	Release superficial and deep abductor hallucis fascia
	Arch support if pes planus	Remove heel spur if present
		Release part of plantar fascia if appears pathologic
Anterior tarsal tunnel syndrome	Night splint	Incise inferior extensor retinaculum
	Shoe tongue padding	Decompress both medial and lateral branch of nerve (divide 1 cm proximal to ankle joint)
		Excise bone spur if present
Superficial peroneal nerve	Lateral shoe wedge	Identify nerve distally and trace proximally to level that it pierces crural fascia (10–12 cm proximal to tip of lateral malleolus)
	Ankle brace	Partial fasciotomy
	Physical therapy for peroneal strengthening and proprioception	Test for residual tethering with intraoperative plantarflexion
		Correct concurrent ankle instability

- Removal of space-occupying mass if present:
  - Greater rate of surgical success if nerve compression secondary to space-occupying lesion

See Table 3 for nerve-specific treatment information.

Complications

- Recurrence of nerve entrapment – most commonly due to incomplete decompression
- Revision surgery – decreased success rate

Bibliography

1. Ahmad M, Tsang K, Mackenney PJ, Adedapo AO. Tarsal tunnel syndrome: a literature review. Foot Ankle Surg. 2012;18(3):149–52.
2. Donovan A, Rosenberg ZS, Cavalcanti CF. MR imaging of entrapment neuropathies of the lower extremity. RadioGraphics. 2010;30(4):1001–19. PubMed PMID: 20631365.

3. Flanigan RM, DiGiovanni BF. Peripheral nerve entrapments of the lower leg, ankle, and foot. Foot Ankle Clin. 2011;16(2):255–74.
4. Hirose CB, McGarvey WC. Peripheral nerve entrapments. Foot Ankle Clin. 2004;9(2):255–69.
5. Kennedy JG, Baxter DE. Nerve disorders in dancers. Clin Sports Med. 2008;27(2):329–34.

4 Pes Planus

Take-Home Message

- Adult-acquired flatfoot secondary to dysfunction of the posterior tibial tendon is the most common cause of pes planus in adults.
- Correct flexible deformity with corrective osteotomy (medial slide calcaneal osteotomy) + soft tissue reconstruction (FDL tendon transfer).
- Correct fixed deformity with arthrodesis (triple arthrodesis).
- Correct forefoot varus/supination with Cotton osteotomy (dorsal opening wedge osteotomy medial cuneiform).

Definition

Pes Planus (Flat Foot)

- Loss of medial longitudinal arch.
- Hindfoot valgus (Fig. 11) with forefoot abduction (Fig. 12).
- Fixed supination of the forefoot occurs with long-standing disease (Fig. 13).

Etiology

Congenital (Flexible) Pes Planus

- Ligamentous laxity.
- Normal development of infants/children or normal adult variant.
- In many cases is asymptomatic and does not require treatment. May additionally suffer degeneration of the posterior tibial tendon during adulthood.

Acquired Pes Planus

- Insufficiency of the posterior tibial tendon with subsequent strain on the static medial stabilizers of the hindfoot. Asymmetric deformity in contrast to congenital pes planus.

Pathophysiology

Congenital Pes Planus

- Ligamentous laxity, hindfoot valgus, forefoot abduction
- Normal strength and integrity of the posterior tibial tendon

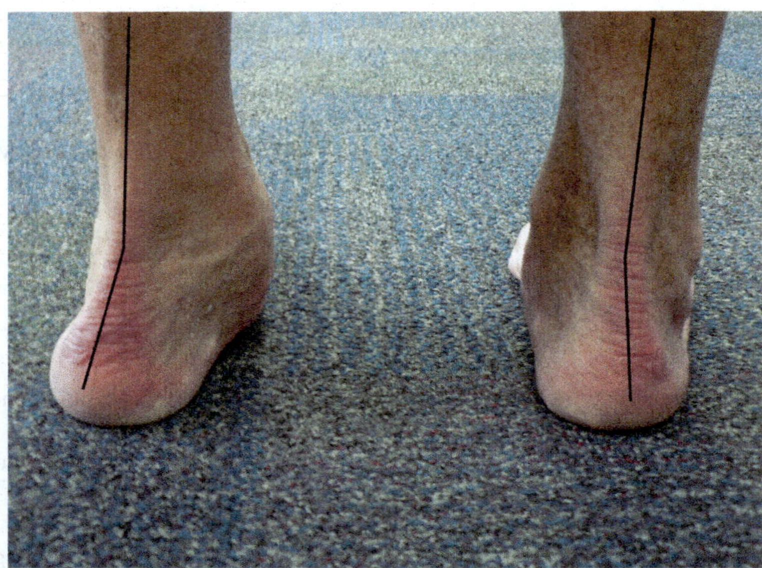

Fig. 11 The left hindfoot has significant hindfoot valgus compared to the right. This is indicative of failure of the ligamentous support of the hindfoot that occurs in stage II, III, and IV PTTD. Simple debridement of the tendon will fail once the hindfoot is in valgus

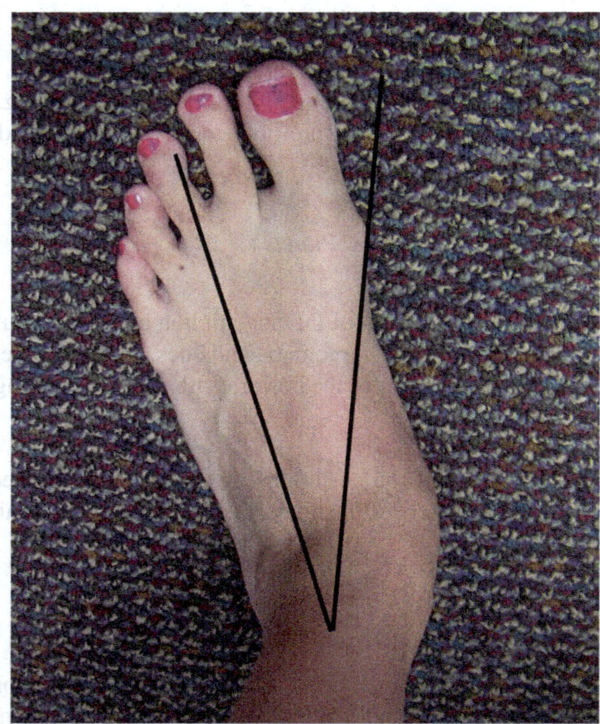

Fig. 12 The axis of the forefoot deviates into abduction relative to the axis of the hindfoot in patient with late-stage PTTD

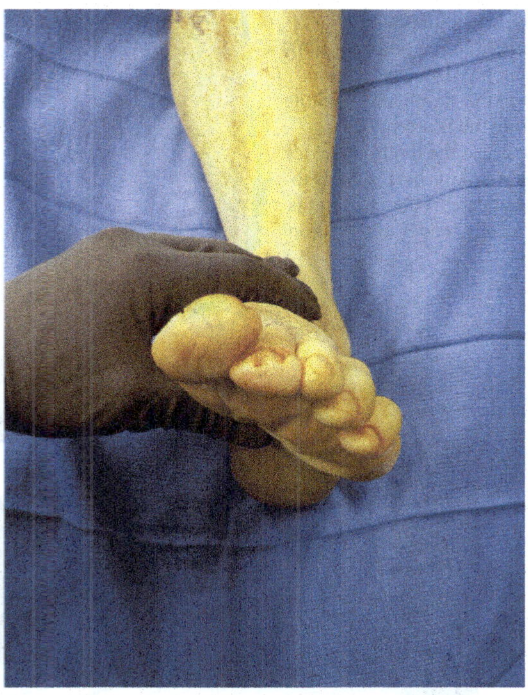

Fig. 13 Patient with fixed forefoot varus after correction of the hindfoot deformity

Acquired Pes Planus

1. Posterior tibial tendon (PTT) insufficiency – inability to perform a single-limb heel rise with associated pain and swelling (Fig. 14).
2. Loss of dynamic arch support.
3. Arch attenuation (spring ligament > talocalcaneal interosseous ligament > deltoid ligament).
4. Results in increased hindfoot valgus and forefoot abduction. More long-standing deformity results in fixed forefoot supination/varus.
5. Rigid deformity may occur with long-standing disease or arthritis.
6. Strain across the deltoid ligament may result in ankle valgus with persistent asymmetric ankle joint pressure, placing the joint at risk for ankle arthritis.

Radiography

Weight-Bearing AP/Lateral Foot/Ankle

- Talo-first metatarsal angle on AP (normal =0) – increased angle associated with flatfoot deformity.
- Talo-first metatarsal angle on lateral (normal =0) – negative angle (directed plantarward) associated with flatfoot deformity (Fig. 15).
- Talar head uncoverage – the amount of uncoverage (lack of apposition of the navicular) may direct surgical intervention (Fig. 16):
  - >50 % uncovering indicative to perform lateral column lengthening

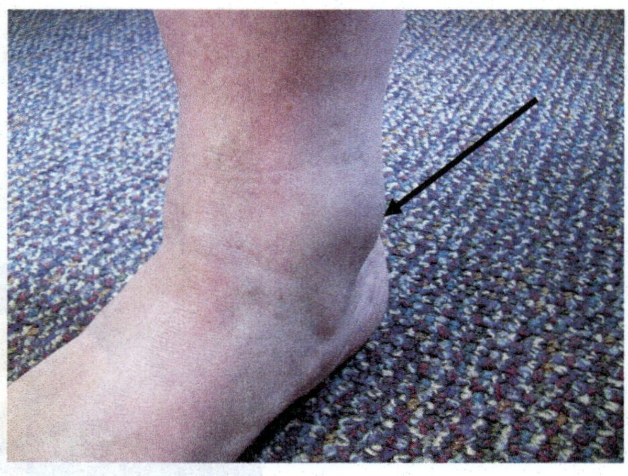

Fig. 14 Patient with complaints of posterior tibial tendon (PTT) dysfunction. Note the significant swelling along the posteromedial aspect of the hindfoot (*black arrow*). This corresponds to the course of the PTT and is typically tender to palpation

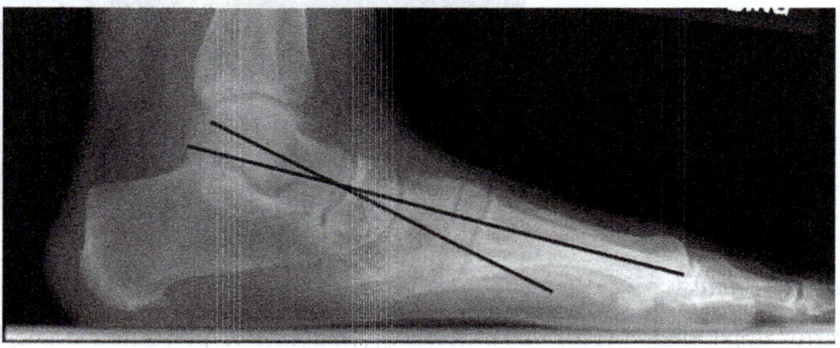

Fig. 15 Lateral weight-bearing radiograph of a patient with posterior tibial tendon dysfunction. Note the plantarflexed position of the talus relative to the first metatarsal

- Look for evidence of degenerative changes of the hindfoot – requires triple arthrodesis. Midfoot arthritis may be present and requires realignment midfoot fusion in addition to hindfoot correction.

AP/Lateral/Mortise Ankle

- Evaluate for valgus talar tilt, ankle arthritis

Ultrasound/MRI – not routinely utilized in the decision making process

Classification

- Truro classification: posterior tibial tendon dysfunction (Table 4)
- Nonoperative management for all stage II is best treated with an articulated AFO and physical therapy focused on strengthening of PTT. Stage III/IV is treated with a rigid AFO or Arizona brace.

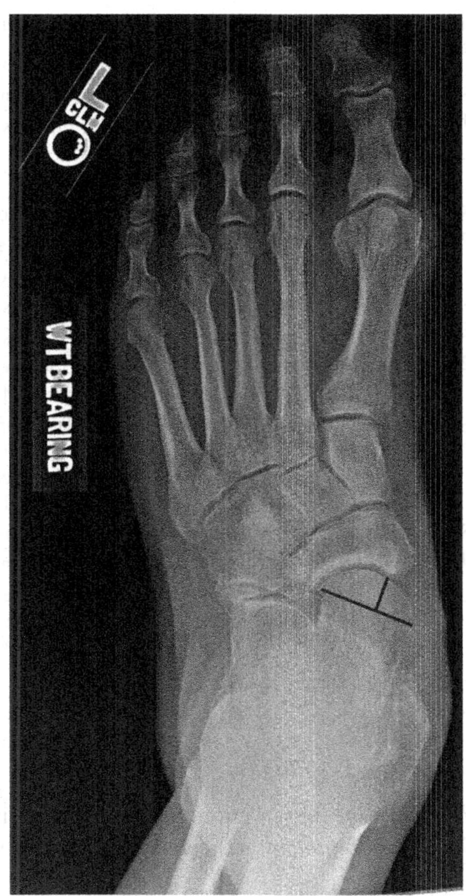

Fig. 16 AP weight-bearing radiograph of the foot in a patient with stage IIB PTTD. The navicular is laterally subluxated, resulting in greater than 30 % uncovering of the talar head

Table 4 Truro classification: Posterior tibial tendon dysfunction

Stage 1	No deformity
	Tenosynovitis
Stage 2A	Flexible hindfoot valgus
	Normal forefoot
Stage 2B/C	Flexible hindfoot valgus
	Forefoot varus >15° or fixed forefoot varus
Stage 3	Rigid hindfoot valgus
	Rigid forefoot abduction
Stage 4	Deltoid insufficiency (ankle valgus) or ankle arthritis

Table 5 Posterior tibial tendon dysfunction treatment options

	Nonoperative treatment	Operative treatment
Stage 1	Immobilization (CAM Walker)	Tenosynovectomy
	Orthotics (medial wedge and arch support) (Fig. 17)	Equinus correction (GSR/TAL)
	PT	
Stage 2A	Orthotics (articulated AFO with focused PT to strengthening PTT)	FDL transfer (Fig. 18) +
		Medial slide calcaneus osteotomy (Fig. 19)
		Lateral column lengthening (>50 % uncoverage)
		Equinus correction (GSR/TAL)
Stage 2B	Orthotics (articulated AFO with focused PT to strengthening PTT)	As per stage 2A
		Cotton osteotomy (stable first TMT) (Fig. 20) vs. first TMT fusion – arthritis or instability (Fig. 21)
Stage 3	Orthotics (AFO, Arizona brace)	Triple arthrodesis (subtalar, talonavicular, calcaneocuboid) (Fig. 22) (Some current consideration to perform isolated talonavicular and subtalar arthrodesis)
Stage 4	Orthotics (AFO, Arizona brace)	Rigid ankle: tibiotalocalcaneal arthrodesis or
		Pantalar fusion (Fig. 23)
		Flexible non-arthritic ankle: may consider deltoid reconstruction (Fig. 24) + triple arthrodesis with medial slide calcaneal osteotomy

Treatment

Congenital Pes Planus

Nonoperative: observation, heel cord stretching, orthotics (arch support)
Operative treatment: indicated for failure of nonoperative treatment

- Gastrocnemius recession (GSR) or tendo-Achilles lengthening (TAL) if equinus contracture
- Calcaneus osteotomy:
  - Calcaneal lengthening osteotomy (Evans)
  - Medial calcaneal slide osteotomy, medial cuneiform plantar closing wedge osteotomy, cuboid opening wedge osteotomy (triple C)

Acquired Pes Planus

Treatment (Table 5)

Complications

- Nonunion of arthrodesis
- Failure to achieve satisfactory correction of deformity
- Failure to achieve pain relief – 10 %

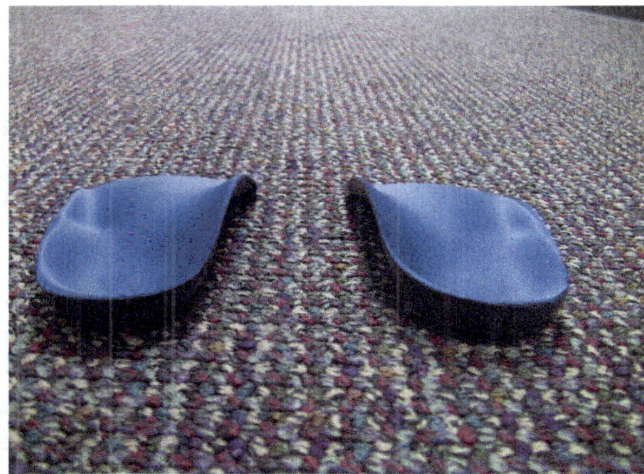

Fig. 17 Standard 3/4 length orthotic. Note the longitudinal arch support. Custom orthotics are useful if the patient has a severe deformity that would not be amenable to over the counter orthotics – however, custom orthotics are 10–20 times more expensive

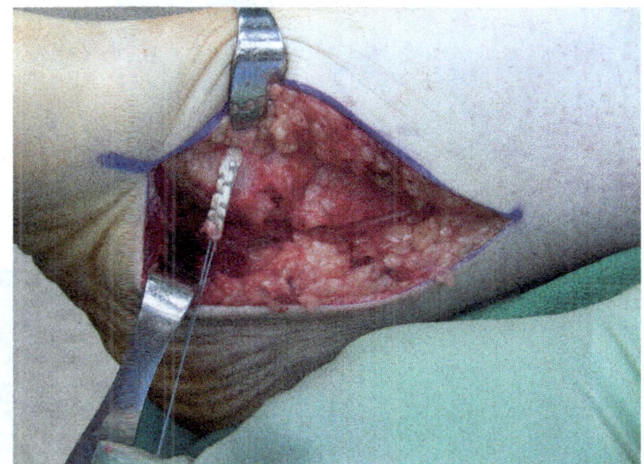

Fig. 18 Use of the FDL is the most common tendon transfer to recreate the function of the posterior tibial tendon. The tendon is placed through a drill hole in the navicular and routed from plantar to dorsal

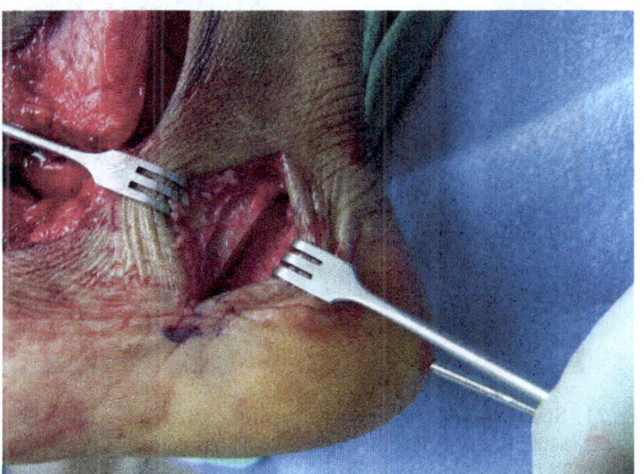

Fig. 19 Note the medial translation of the calcaneal tuberosity. A 1 cm shift is sufficient

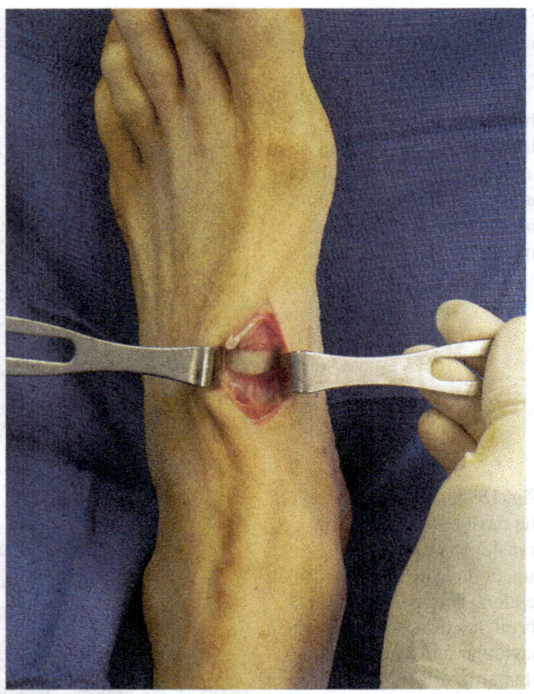

Fig. 20 Plantarflexion osteotomy of the medial cuneiform is commonly used to correct the fixed forefoot varus. Use of allograft to achieve the correction is demonstrated here

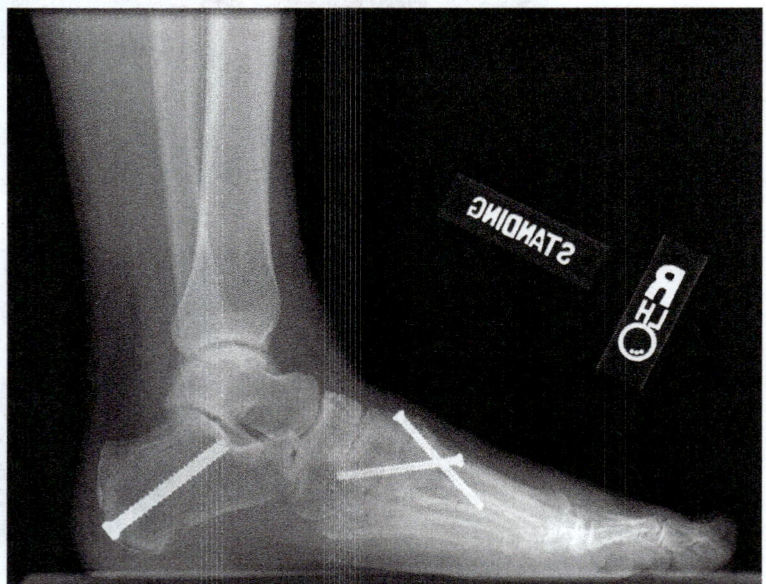

Fig. 21 Stabilization of the first tarsometatarsal (TMT) joint is critical in flatfoot reconstruction if there is instability of that joint. After joint preparation – the first MTP is dorsiflexed – which forces the first TMT joint to plantarflex secondary to the windlass mechanism. Fixation is typically performed with cross screws

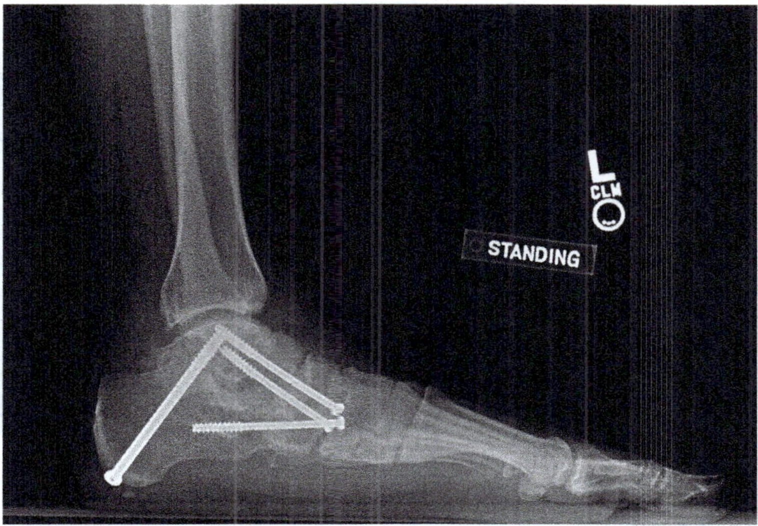

Fig. 22 Lateral radiograph of a patient who underwent a triple arthrodesis for a fixed hindfoot valgus deformity – stage III

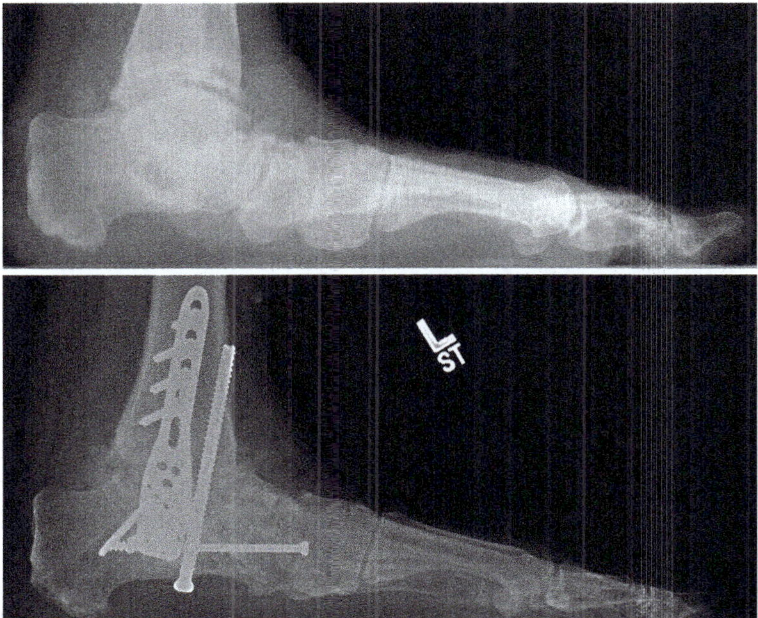

Fig. 23 Lateral radiograph of a patient with stage IV PTTD with ankle arthritis. A pantalar fusion is the gold standard in this case. Performing an ankle replacement and triple arthrodesis is possible – however, there are no long-term results of ankle replacements in this setting

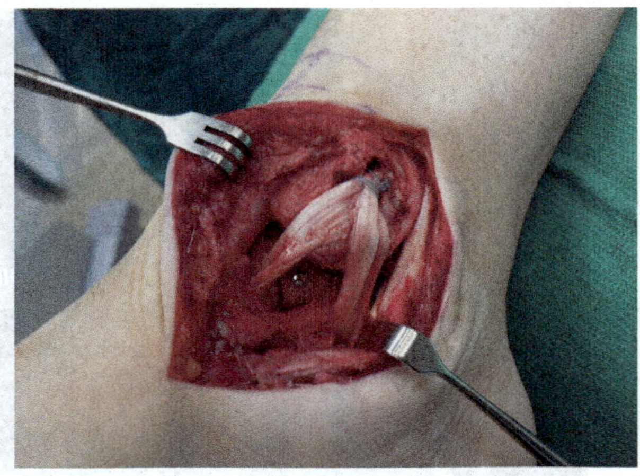

Fig. 24 Allograft reconstruction of the deltoid ligament can be performed in a patient with stage IV PTTD with ankle valgus without evidence of arthritis. Concomitant correction of the hindfoot deformity is required

Bibliography

1. Ahmad J, Pedowitz D. Management of the rigid arthritic flatfoot in adults: triple arthrodesis. Foot Ankle Clin. 2012;17(2):309–22.
2. Kulig K, Reischl SF, Pomrantz AB, Burnfield JM, Mais-Requejo S, Thordarson DB, Smith RW. Nonsurgical management of posterior tibial tendon dysfunction with orthoses and resistive exercise: a randomized controlled trial. Phys Ther. 2009;89(1):26–37.
3. Schuh R, Gruber F, Wanivenhaus A, Hartig N, Windhager R, Trnka HJ. Flexor digitorum longus transfer and medial displacement calcaneal osteotomy for the treatment of stage II posterior tibial tendon dysfunction: kinematic and functional results of fifty one feet. Int Orthop. 2013;37(9):1815–20.
4. Smith JT, Bluman EM. Update on stage IV acquired adult flatfoot disorder: when the deltoid ligament becomes dysfunctional. Foot Ankle Clin. 2012;17(2):351–60.

5 Pes Cavus

Take-Home Message

- Primarily progressive, eventually rigid deformity from prolonged muscle imbalance.
- Etiology primarily neurologic.
- Rigid deformities should be treated with corrective osteotomies as well as tendon transfers to remove deforming forces.

Definition Cavovarus:

- Hindfoot varus, forefoot pronation

Etiology

- Neurologic
  - Hereditary motor and sensory neuropathies – Charcot-Marie-Tooth (typically bilateral disease)
  - Cerebral palsy
  - Stroke
  - Spinal cord lesions (typically unilateral disease)
- Traumatic
  - Compartment syndrome
  - Talar neck malunion
  - Peroneal nerve injury
- Residual clubfoot
- Idiopathic

Pathophysiology

- Muscle imbalance
  - Strong peroneus longus (PL) and posterior tibialis (PT)
  - Weak peroneal brevis (PB) and anterior tibialis (AT)
- Posttraumatic
  - Deep posterior compartment contractures (PT, FDL)
- Prolonged deformity leads to plantar fascia contraction; flexible deformity becomes rigid.

Radiography Weight-bearing AP/lateral foot/ankle, calcaneus axial

- Hindfoot varus
- First MT plantarflexion

Classification Coleman block test – block under lateral forefoot

- If hindfoot corrects – flexible hindfoot deformity, forefoot driven
- If hindfoot does not correct – rigid hindfoot deformity rigid ± forefoot deformity

Treatment

Nonoperative

- Orthotics – lateral wedge, depression for first ray
- Ankle-foot orthosis with varus correction for rigid deformities

Table 6 Cavovarus surgical treatment options

Coleman block test finding	
Flexible hindfoot	PT/PL tendon transfer + plantar fascia release + tendo-Achilles lengthening (TAL) ±1st metatarsal (MT) dorsiflexion osteotomy
Rigid hindfoot	Above procedures + calcaneal osteotomy (lateral slide vs. closing wedge)
Hindfoot/midfoot arthritis or severe deformities	Triple arthrodesis + PT/PL tendon transfer

Operative (Table 6)

Complications

- Nonunion of arthrodesis
- Recurrence of deformity
- Wound breakdown/infection

Bibliography

1. Krause FG, Wing KJ, Younger AS. Neuromuscular issues in cavovarus foot. Foot Ankle Clin. 2008;13:243–58, vi.
2. Ryssman DB, Myerson MS. Tendon transfers for the adult flexible cavovarus foot. Foot Ankle Clin. 2011;16:435–50.
3. Ward CM, Dolan LA, Bennett DL, Morcuende JA, Cooper RR. Long-term results of reconstruction for treatment of a flexible cavovarus foot in Charcot-Marie-Tooth disease. J Bone Joint Surg Am Vol. 2008;90:2631–42.
4. Younger AS, Hansen ST, Jr. Adult cavovarus foot. J Am Acad Orthop Surg. 2005;13:302–15.
5. Zide JR, Myerson MS. Arthrodesis for the cavus foot: when, where, and how? Foot Ankle Clin. 2013;18:755–67.

6 Tendinopathies

Take-Home Message

- Tendinosis is a chronic noninflammatory degeneration and should not be confused with tendonitis, an acute inflammatory disease.
- Nonoperative treatment should focus on eccentric strengthening.
- Operative intervention should focus on removing diseased tendon with appropriate tendon transfers if >50 % of operative tendon is removed.

Definition

- Tendonitis – inflammation of the tendon
- Tendinosis – chronic damage to tendons with microscopic analysis showing tissue necrosis and mucoid degeneration

Etiology

- Anterior tibial (AT) – tendonitis from overuse, partial/complete rupture from trauma. May present as a mass along the anterior ankle (pseudotumor) (Fig. 25).
- Flexor hallucis longus (FHL) – tendonitis from overuse (ballet dancers) or impingement/stenosis along posterior ankle. Prolonged symptoms can lead to partial rupture.
- Peroneal tendons
  - Subluxation/dislocation from forced eversion/dorsiflexion ->disruption of superior peroneal retinaculum (Fig. 26)
  - Tendon tears caused by degeneration from tendon subluxation/dislocation, ankle sprains, ankle instability

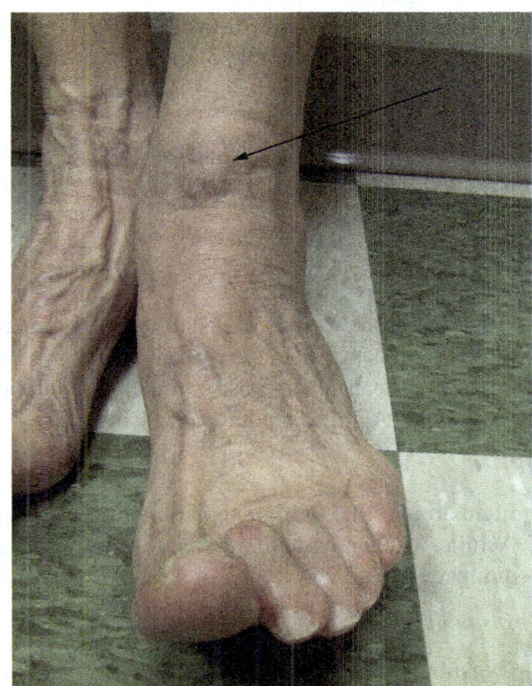

Fig. 25 Patient with a chronic anterior tibial tendon rupture. Note the extensor recruitment and the stump of the anterior tibial tendon (*arrow*) at the level of the ankle. This patient presented for evaluation of ankle mass

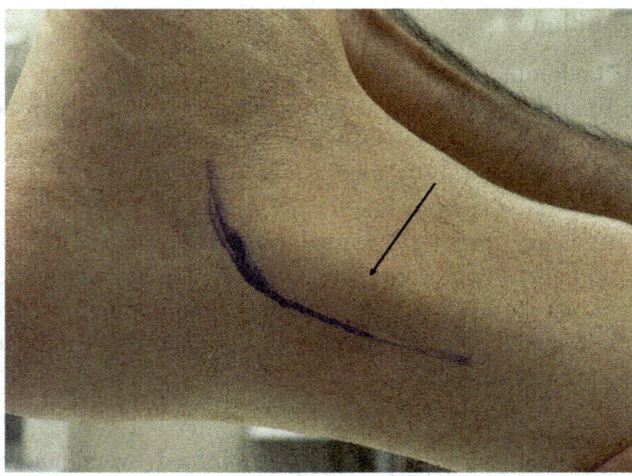

Fig. 26 Subluxation of the peroneal tendons (*arrow*). Note the tendons are displaced anterior to the posterior border of the fibula (*line*)

- Achilles
  - Insertional tendinopathy – tendinosis (cause unknown)
  - Non-insertional tendinopathy – inflammation of peritenon alone from overuse, fluoroquinolone antibiotics, mechanical imbalance
  - Rupture – "weekend warrior," sudden active plantarflexion against resistance or forced dorsiflexion in plantarflexed foot

Pathophysiology

- Tendinosis degenerative changes → collagen fiber disorientation; hypocellularity; patchy necrosis, calcification; minimal inflammatory cells

Radiography

AP/Lateral Radiographs of the Foot/Ankle

- Fracture of lateral ridge of distal fibula (peroneal subluxation/dislocation)
- Fracture of os peroneum (peroneal longus rupture)
- Superior calcaneal tuberosity bone spur and calcification at Achilles insertion (insertional Achilles tendinopathy) (Fig. 27)

MRI

- Fluid around FHL – high-signal intensity surrounding the tendon (Fig. 28)
- Achilles thickening with intermediate intrasubstance signal (non-insertional tendinopathy) (Fig. 29)

Ultrasound

- Dynamic exam peroneal subluxation/dislocation

Classification Ogden classification of superficial peroneal retinaculum (SPR) tears (Table 7)

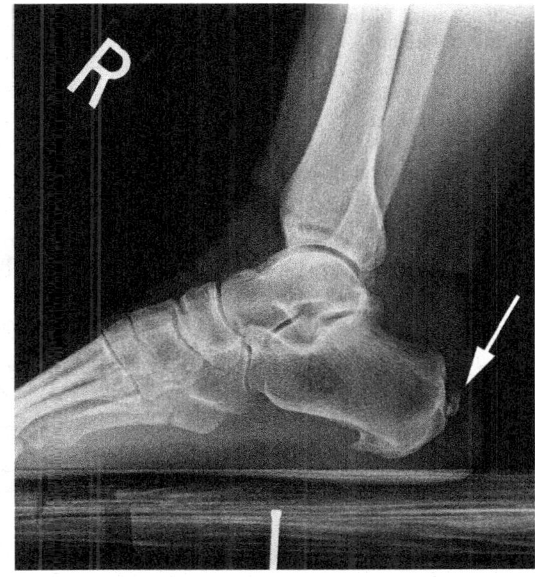

Fig. 27 Lateral radiograph demonstrating calcification of the Achilles tendon at the insertion (*arrow*)

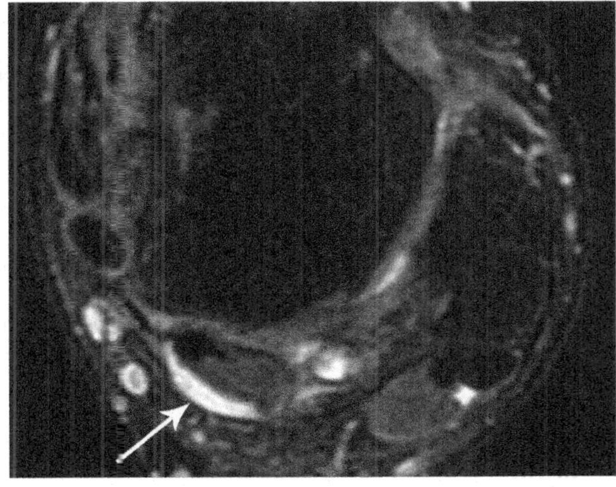

Fig. 28 Axial T2 image consistent with synovitis of the flexor hallucis longus. Note the increased signal intensity (*arrow*) surrounding the tendon

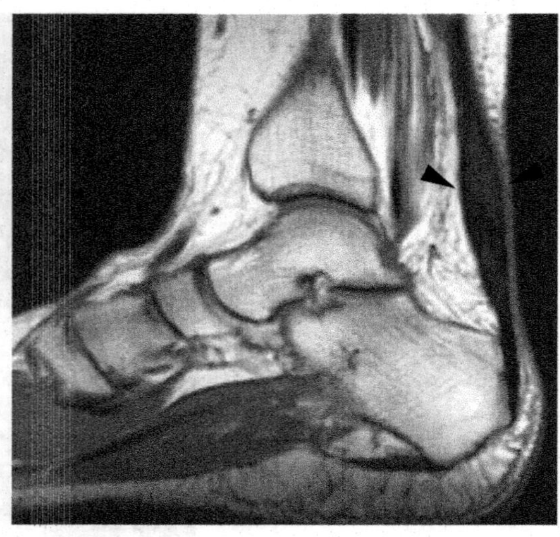

Fig. 29 Sagittal T1 imaging of a patient with non-insertional Achilles tendinosis. Note the thickening of the tendon (*arrowheads*) and the intermediate-signal intensity within the tendon consistent with degeneration

Table 7 Ogden classification of Superficial Peroneal Retinaculum (SPR) tears

Grade 1	SPR partially elevated off fibula
Grade 2	SPR separated from cartilofibrous ridge lateral malleolus, subluxation between SPR and ridge
Grade 3	Cortical avulsion SPR off fibula, subluxation under fracture
Grade 4	SPR avulsed from calcaneus

Table 8 Anterior tibialis and FHL treatment options

	Nonoperative	Operative
Anterior tibialis	NSAIDs, CAM boot or walking cast	Acute rupture – primary repair
		Chronic rupture – reconstruction with interpositional graft
Flexor hallucis longus	Activity modification	Tenosynovectomy, fibro-osseous tunnel release

Treatment

Treatment of anterior tibialis, flexor hallucis longus disorders (Table 8)
Treatment of peroneal tendon disorders (Table 9)
Treatment of Achilles tendon disorders (Table 10)

Complications

- Wound breakdown/infection
- Tendon re-rupture

Bibliography

1. Cerrato RA, Myerson MS. Peroneal tendon tears, surgical management and its complications. Foot Ankle Clin. 2009;14:299–312.
2. Heckman DS, Gluck GS, Parekh SG. Tendon disorders of the foot and ankle, part 1: peroneal tendon disorders. Am J Sports Med. 2009;37:614–25.

Table 9 Peroneal tendon treatment options

	Nonoperative	Operative
Peroneal tendon subluxation/dislocation	Cast immobilization, protected weight bearing 6 weeks (acute injuries in reduced position)	Reconstruction SPR, fibular groove deepening
Peroneal tendon tear	NSAIDs, activity modification, physical therapy, lace-up ankle brace	<50 % diseased tendon – tenosynovectomy, debridement, tendon repair ± groove deepening
		> 50% diseased tendon or complete rupture 1 tendon – excision and tenodesis
		>50% diseased tendon or complete rupture 2 tendons – FHL transfer to fifth metatarsal (MT)
		Hindfoot varus – lateral closing wedge calcaneus osteotomy (Dwyer)

Table 10 Achilles tendon treatment options

	Nonoperative	Operative
Achilles insertional tendinopathy	Activity/shoe modification, heel lifts, stretching, physical therapy (eccentric strengthening), silicone sleeves/pads, NO corticosteroid injections	Debridement degenerative tendon, resection prominent superior calcaneal tuberosity, excision retrocalcaneal bursa
		If >50 % tendon detached, reattach insertion with suture anchors
		If >50 % tendon excised, FHL transfer
Achilles non-insertional tendinopathy	Activity modification, heel lifts, physical therapy (eccentric strengthening), shock-wave therapy	Mild disease – percutaneous tenotomies
		Moderate disease – debridement, tendon tubularization
		If >50 % tendon excised, FHL transfer
Achilles rupture	Acute – bracing/cast in equinus with early functional rehabilitation (no difference in re-rupture rate)	Acute – direct repair (improved satisfaction in age <45)
	Chronic – AFO	Chronic – VY advancement ± FHL transfer

3. Heckman DS, Gluck GS, Parekh SG. Tendon disorders of the foot and ankle, part 2: achilles tendon disorders. Am J Sports Med. 2009;37:1223–34.
4. Jones DC. Tendon disorders of the foot and ankle. J Am Acad Orthop Surg. 1993;1:87–94.
5. Reddy SS, Pedowitz DI, Parekh SG, Omar IM, Wapner KL. Surgical treatment for chronic disease and disorders of the achilles tendon. J Am Acad Orthop Surg. 2009;17:3–14.

7 Diabetic Foot

Take-Home Message

- The diabetic foot is at a constant risk for recurrent ulcerations, especially due to neuropathy and peripheral vascular disease.
- Ulcer classification is essential to set a treatment strategy and determine prognosis.
- Treatment in the setting of infection should include culture-directed therapy and a thorough understanding of the different levels of amputations.

Introduction

- Diagnosis of foot ulcerations results in the greatest rate of hospital admissions in diabetics, as well as lower extremity amputations.

Pathophysiology

- Diabetic neuropathy:
  - Sensation: sensory loss begins in stocking distribution and progressive proximally. Ninety percent of patients who cannot feel the 5.07 monofilament have lost protective sensation to their feet and are at risk for ulceration.
  - Autonomic neuropathy: abnormal sweating mechanism leads to a dry foot → vulnerable to fissuring cracks → portals for infection.
  - Motor neuropathy: most commonly involves the common peroneal nerve → resultant loss of tibialis anterior function and foot drop; small intrinsic musculature also affected → claw toes and subsequent toe-tip ulcerations.
- Hypomobility syndrome:
  - Decreased range of motion in joints from excessive glycosylation of soft tissues
- Peripheral vascular disease:
  - Occurs in 60–70 % of patients who have diabetes for over 10 years, involving both large and small vessels.
  - Noninvasive vascular examination should be performed when pulses not palpable (normal waveform is triphasic); ankle brachial index of 0.45 is minimum for healing and greater than 1.3 is consistent with calcification of vessels.
  - Minimum toe pressures for healing: 40 mmHg.
  - Transcutaneous oxygen measurements of the toes greater than 40 mmHg have been found to be predictive of healing.

Table 11 Wagner grading system for diabetic foot infections

Grade	Depth of ulcer
0	Skin intact with bony deformity that leads to “at risk” foot
1	Localized superficial ulcer without tendon or bone involvement
2	Deep ulcer with exposed tendon or joint capsule
3	Extensive ulcer with exposed bone/osteomyelitis or abscess
4	Partial gangrene
5	Extensive gangrene

Table 12 Brodsky grading system: Based on ischemia

Grade	
A	Normal vascularity
B	Ischemia without gangrene
C	Partial gangrene
D	Complete gangrene

- Immune system impairment:
  - Poor cellular defenses, altered chemotaxis of white blood cells, and poor cytotoxic environment (due to hyperglycemia) to fight bacteria lead to difficulty in fighting off infection.
- Metabolic deficiency:
  - Total protein less than 6.0, WBC count less than 1,500, and albumin levels less than 2.5 result in poor healing potential.

Radiography

- Routine radiographic series of the foot and ankle should be obtained to determine the extent of bone loss and deformity. Findings can be difficult to interpret in the setting of neuroarthropathy. Bony desctruction directly over an open ulcer is highly suspicious for osteomyelitis.
- MRI can be obtained is an abscess is suspected.
- MRI has high false-positive rate in the diagnosis of osteomyelitis, particularly with concurrent Charcot arthropathy.
- WBC-labeled scan or dual-image Tc/In scan is more sensitive and specific for osteomyelitis than isolated technetium scan.

Classification Wagner classification based on depth of ulcer (Table 11)
Brodsky classification: based on ischemia (Table 12)

Table 13 Diabetic ulcer management based on the Wagner Grading system

Grade	Treatment
0	Extra-depth shoe and pressure relief insoles
1	In office debridement, shoe modification or total contact cast if no infection
2/3	Operative debridement of all exposed bone/tendon and nonviable tissue. Dressing changes and total contact casting once wound bed is healthy
4/5	Local vs. larger amputation

Treatment

Ultimate goal is an ulcer-free, functional, plantigrade foot that can fit within a brace or shoe (Table 13).

- The Therapeutic Shoe Bill allocated money for neuropathic patients to purchase extra-depth shoes and total contact inserts (3 per year) for ulcer prevention.
- Workup should include noninvasive vascular studies and surgical revascularization if indicated and metabolic assessment with delay in surgery if possible until nutritional status is improved.
- Additional treatment includes:
  - Tendo-Achilles lengthening to offload the midfoot/forefoot if recurrent ulcerations with equinus deformity.
  - Ostectomy of bony prominences (stable deformity) or fusion if instability present.
  - Toe deformities often require joint resection or amputation.
- Diabetic foot infections are polymicrobial:
  - Should not perform superficial wound culture → deep cultures provide most accurate results.
  - Treat infections with initial broad-spectrum antibiotic coverage once surgical cultures obtained, and adjust once sensitivity returns.
  - Abscesses require surgical drainage and antibiotics.
  - Osteomyelitis is treated with antibiotics and usually surgical debridement.
- Amputation as needed at different levels with appropriate tendon transfers:
  - Transmetatarsal → lowest energy expenditure, no tendon transfer needed
  - Lisfranc → requires a transfer of peroneals to cuboid to prevent varus; Achilles lengthening
  - Chopart → requires transfer anterior tibialis to talus to prevent equinus; Achilles lengthening
  - Syme's → next lowest energy expenditure (superior to Lisfranc and Chopart with regard to amount of energy needed to ambulate)
  - Transtibial → superior results with postoperative casting for 3–5 days with conversion to rigid removal dressing

Bibliography

1. Anakwenze OA, Milby AH, Gans I, Stern JJ, Levin LS, Wapner KL. Foot and ankle infections: diagnosis and management. J Am Acad Orthop Surg. 2012;20:684–93.
2. Arad Y, Fonseca V, Peters A, Vinik A. Beyond the monofilament for the insensate diabetic foot: a systematic review of randomized trials to prevent the occurrence of plantar foot ulcers in patients with diabetes. Diabetes Care. 2011;34:1041–6.
3. Lipsky BA. Medical treatment of diabetic foot infections. Clin Infect Dis. 2004;39 Suppl 2:S104–14.
4. Robinson AH, Pasapula C, Brodsky JW. Surgical aspects of the diabetic foot. J Bone Joint Surg Br Vol. 2009;91:1–7.
5. Wukich DK, Armstrong DG, Attinger CE, et al. Inpatient management of diabetic foot disorders: a clinical guide. Diabetes Care. 2013;36:2862–71.

8 Charcot Arthropathy

Take-Home Message

- Charcot arthropathy is a limb-threatening destructive process that occurs in patients with sensory, motor, and autonomic neuropathy associated with medical diseases such as diabetes mellitus.
- The Eichenholtz classification describes the evolution of the condition through time, whereas the Brodsky classification is defined by location.
- Initial treatment consists of prompt immobilization and non-weight bearing but may warrant arthrodesis or amputation with long-standing deformity.

Definition

- Chronic, progressive, noninfectious destructive process affecting bone architecture and joint alignment in people lacking protective sensation (Fig. 30)

Etiology

- In developed world, diabetic neuropathy is the most frequent cause of Charcot arthropathy.
- Other possibilities are alcoholism, leprosy, tabes dorsalis, myelomeningocele, and congenital insensitivity to pain.
- Often challenge is determining whether there is superimposed osteomyelitis.

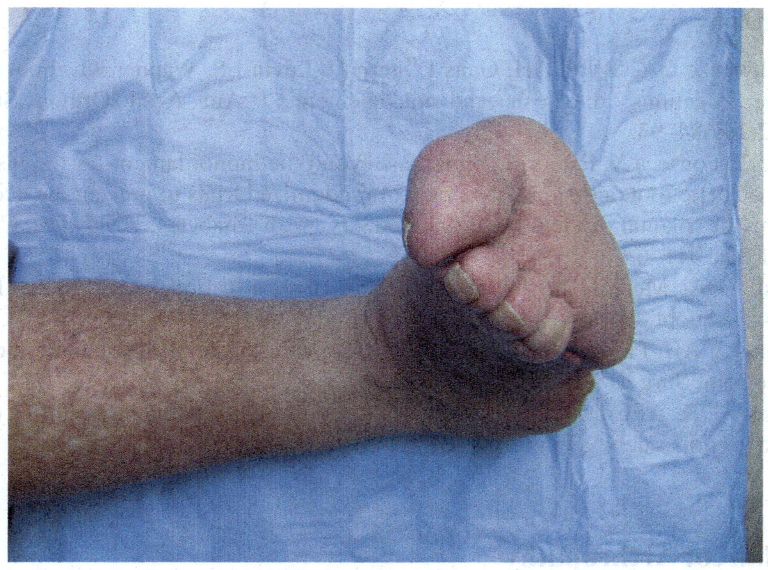

Fig. 30 Varus deformity of the ankle and hindfoot is a common deformity seen in Charcot. The deformity can be severe with some patient presenting with callous or ulcer over the fibula as it now contacts the ground

Pathophysiology Two traditional theories:

- Neurotraumatic: exaggerated overuse injury where insensate joints that cannot adopt normal protective mechanisms are subjected to repetitive microtrauma
- Neurovascular destruction: autonomic dysfunction leads to increased blood flow, resulting in osteoclast stimulation, bone resorption, and weakening

Likely results from a combination of these processes → the development of abnormal bone with no ability to protect the joint results in gradual bone fracture and subluxation of the joint (Fig. 31).

Radiography

- Radiographic appearance dependent on what stage the disease is in (see below).
- The hallmark deformity associated with this condition is midfoot collapse, described as a "rocker bottom" foot (Fig. 32).
- Technetium bone scan may be positive in all stages. Indium WBC scan may be negative for neuropathic joints and positive for osteomyelitis.
- Difficult to differentiate infection from Charcot based on MRI, although MRI allows detection of subtle changes in early stages of Charcot arthropathy.

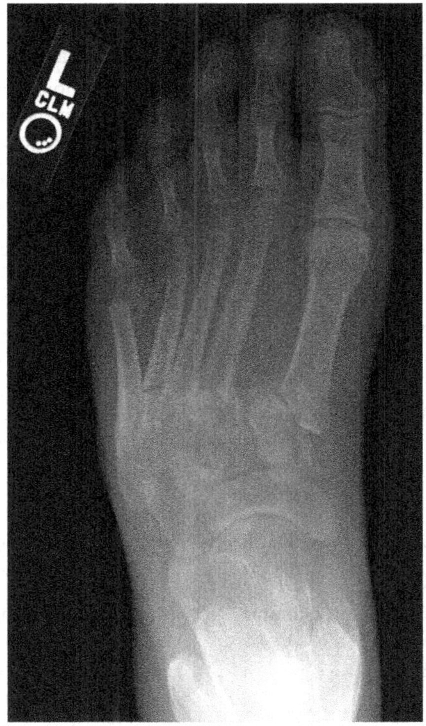

Fig. 31 AP radiograph of a patient with midfoot Charcot in Eichenholtz stage 1. The patient had 2 weeks of swelling without significant trauma. Note the fractures and dislocations through the tarsometatarsal joints

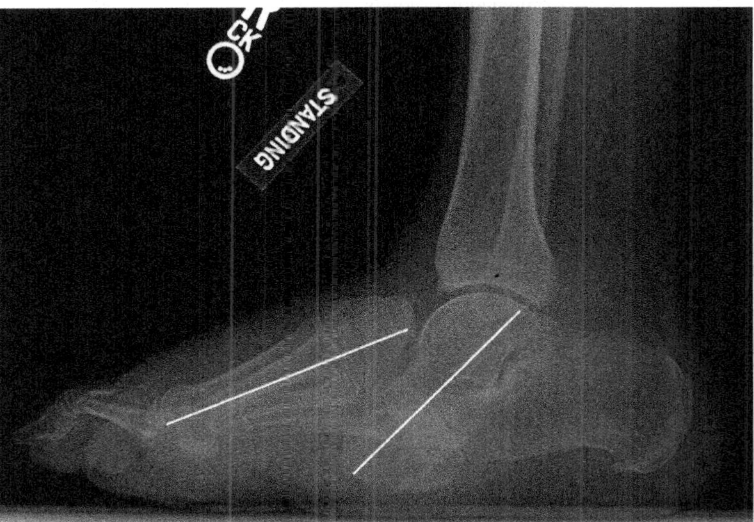

Fig. 32 Rocker bottom deformity in a patient with hindfoot Charcot. Note the severe plantarflexed position of the talus relative to the forefoot and the break through the talonavicular and metatarso-cuboid joint. Plantar prominence of the cuboid risks ulceration in this patient

Table 14 Modified Eichenholtz stages for neuroarthropathy

Stage	Clinical manifestations	Radiographs
0: Pre-fragmentation	Acute inflammation, swelling, erythema with dependent rubor; confused with infection. Lack of systemic symptoms. Pain may not always be present	Normal or regional bone demineralization
1: Fragmentation (dissolution)	Acute inflammation, swelling, erythema, warmth (typically >2.0 °C in the affected foot). May have ligamentous laxity	Osseous periarticular fragmentation, joint subluxation/dislocation
2: Coalescence	Decreased local swelling, erythema, and warmth	Absorption of fine bone debris, early bone healing and periosteal new bone formation
3: Resolution	Resolved inflammation, more stable but often deformed	Consolidation and remodeling of fracture fragments, joint arthrosis, osteophytes

Table 15 Modified Brodsky classification for neuroarthropathy

Type	Location
Type 1 (most common – about 60 %)	Tarsometatarsal and naviculocuneiform joints (leads to fixed rocker bottom deformity)
Type 2	Subtalar, talonavicular, or calcaneocuboid joints (unstable, requires long periods of immobilization)
Type 3	Tibiotalar joint (late varus or valgus deformity produces ulceration and osteomyelitis of malleoli)
Type 4	Combination of joints
Type 5	Only within the forefoot

Classification Modified Eichenholtz stages: related to the degree of warmth, swelling, and erythema. Continuum from resorption and fragmentation to bone formation and consolidation that takes 6–18 months (Table 14).
Modified Brodsky classification: based on anatomic location (Table 15)

Treatment

- The goal is to achieve stage 3 (resolution) while maintaining alignment and ambulatory status and minimizing soft tissue breakdown.

Initial

- Frequent follow-up with serial radiographs and patient education on diabetic foot care.
- Immobilization and non-weight bearing → best with serial total contact casting (the aim is to achieve homogenous pressure distribution in plantar arch through gait); can transition to custom brace (AFO or Charcot restraint orthosis walker (CROW) boot) once swelling and warmth subsides.
- Some studies use bisphosphonates to help reduce osteoclastic resorption and increase the osteoblastic redeposition of bone.

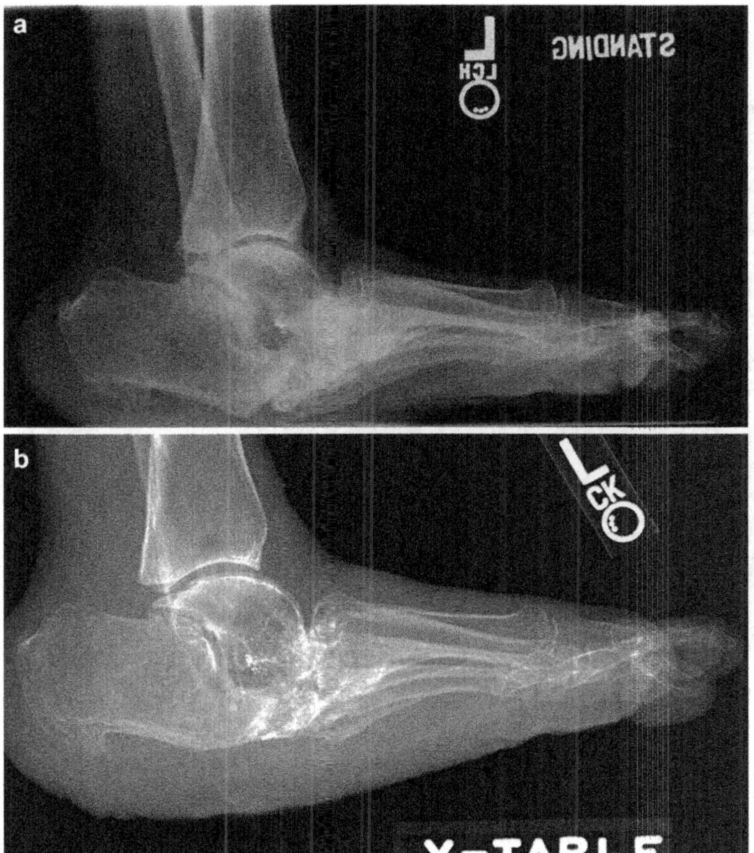

Fig. 33 Patient with a rocker bottom deformity with a large plantar prominence (**a**). The patient is in the consolidated phase and therefore exostectomy can be performed (**b**). The exostectomy removes the offending prominence, but does not correct the malalignment of the joints

Surgical

- Stable deformity with recurrent ulcers secondary to prominence → exostectomy (Fig. 33)
- Unstable/un-braceable deformity → arthrodesis with internal or external fixation (Fig. 34)
- Tendo-Achilles lengthening almost universally required
- Amputation as salvage procedure (Fig. 35)

Complications

- High complication rate (up to 70 %)
- Infection, hardware malposition, recurrent ulceration, fracture

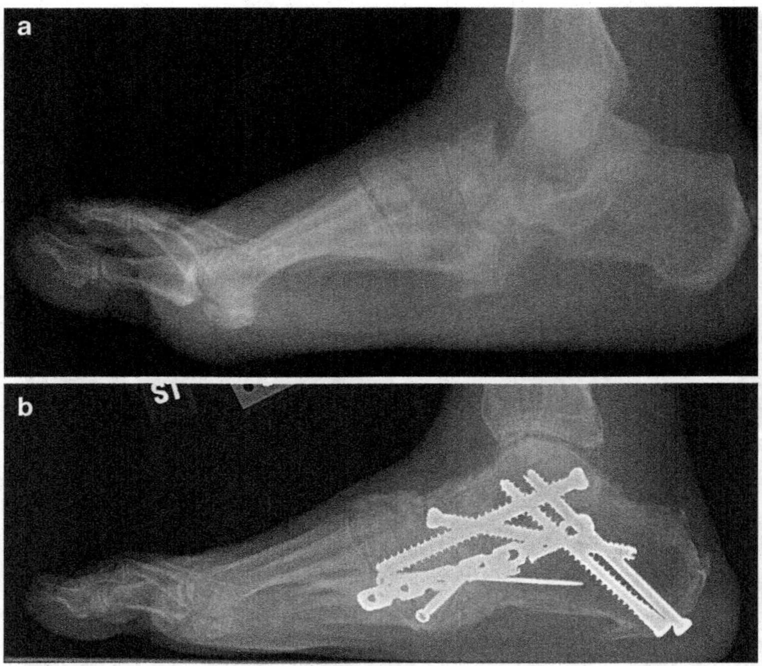

Fig. 34 Patient with hindfoot Charcot and rocker bottom deformity (**a**) treated with an extended hindfoot arthrodesis (**b**)

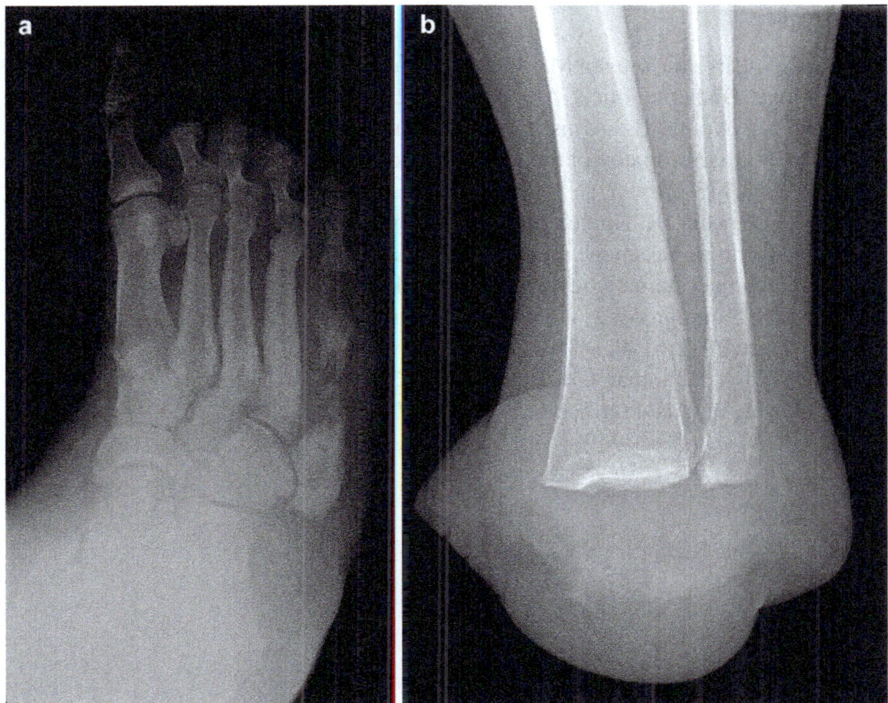

Fig. 35 AP radiograph of patient with poorly treated diabetic neuropathy with osteomyelitis of the fifth metatarsal (**a**). Reconstructive surgery was not possible and a Syme's amputation was performed (**b**)

Bibliography

1. Kaynak G, Birsel O, Guven MF, Ogut T. An overview of the Charcot foot pathophysiology. Diabetic Foot & Ankle 2013;4:21117.
2. Lowery NJ, Woods JB, Armstrong DG, Wukich DK. Surgical management of Charcot neuroarthropathy of the foot and ankle: a systematic review. Foot Ankle Int. 2012;33:113–21.
3. Milne TE, Rogers JR, Kinnear EM, et al. Developing an evidence-based clinical pathway for the assessment, diagnosis and management of acute Charcot Neuro-Arthropathy: a systematic review. J Foot Ankle Res. 2013;6:30.
4. Pinzur MS, Sammarco VJ, Wukich DK. Charcot foot: a surgical algorithm. Instr Course Lect. 2012;61:423–38.
5. van der Ven A, Chapman CB, Bowker JH. Charcot neuroarthropathy of the foot and ankle. J Am Acad Orthop Surg. 2009;17:562–71.

Part X
Amputation and Prosthetics

Katherine Payne and Jessica Pruente

Amputation and Prosthetics of the Lower Extremity

Katherine Payne and Jessica Pruente

1 Amputation: Lower Extremity

Take-Home Message

- Amputation is a reconstructive procedure which serves as a means to return the patient to a more functional status
- Syme amputation is the most common level of amputation in the foot and provides an excellent weight-bearing surface as well as a long lever arm.
- Ideal length of transtibial amputation is the meeting point of the upper third and middle third of the tibia.
- Ambulation requires increased levels of energy consumption.

Definition

Major amputation: any amputation performed above the level of the ankle.

Etiology/Epidemiology

97 % of all amputations involve the lower limb.
130,000 lower limb amputations annually in the United States.

- 82 % dysvascular
- 16 % trauma
- <1 % malignancy
- <1 % congenital

K. Payne, MD (✉)
Department of PMNR, University of Colorado, Aurora, CO, USA
e-mail: Katherine.payne@ucdenver.edu

J. Pruente, MD
Department of PMNR, University of Colorado Hospital, Aurora, Colorado, USA
e-mail: Jessica.pruente@ucdenver.edu

C. Mauffrey, D.J. Hak (eds.), *Passport for the Orthopedic Boards and FRCS Examination*, DOI 10.1007/978-2-8178-0475-0_43

Long-term survival after vascular amputation 69 % at 1 year, 35–45 % at 5 years

Goals of Amputation

Removal of diseased, damaged, or dysfunctional portion of limb
Wound healing
Reconstruction of the residual limb
Restore maximal functional independence

Classification

Principles of Limb Length

- Longer lever arm provides better mechanical advantage for muscle function.
- More proximal level almost always less energy efficient.
- Avoid limb length discrepancies; anticipate space required by prosthetic joint/ terminal device.

Levels of Amputation

Partial toe amputation, toe disarticulation, and metatarsal ray resection – preserves length of foot and provides mechanical advantage.

Partial foot

- Transmetatarsal amputation – preserves attachment of dorsiflexors and plantar flexors
- Lisfranc amputation (tarsometatarsal junction) – can develop significant equinovarus deformity
- Chopart amputation (through transverse tarsal joints, preserves talus and calcaneus) – can develop significant equinovarus deformity

Ankle disarticulation (Syme) – attachment of distal heel pad to end of tibia. Maintains length of limb and provides excellent weight-bearing surface.

Transtibial amputation (below knee, BKA) – ideal limb length is meeting point of upper and middle thirds of tibia; provides better flap at expense of length of lever arm.

- Too long: longer than distal 2/5 of tibia creates difficult skin and soft tissue management.
- Too short: proximal to tibial tubercle; lose knee extension.

Boyd amputation – ankle disarticulation with calcaneotibial arthrodesis

Knee disarticulation – long lever arm with excellent end-bearing but challenging to fit with prosthesis

Transfemoral amputation (above knee, AKA) – standard level 35–60 % of femur. Difficult to fit with prosthesis if very short (just below lesser trochanter)

Hip disarticulation – removal of entire lower limb by transection through hip joint

Hemipelvectomy – removal of entire lower limb and ilium. Bear weight on abdominal viscera

Treatment: Lower Limb Prostheses

Appropriate Candidate

Majority of patients benefit from prosthetic, even if only for transfers.
Trial warranted in all willing patients
Exceptions: dementia, severe contracture, and high risk of breakdown

Timing

Immediate postoperative prosthesis (IPOP) may be used in transtibial amputees.
Limited evidence to support benefit, limited weight bearing allowed and concern for possible wound dehiscence and infection.
3–6 weeks after amputation: Early fitting custom prosthesis, edema resolved, and shaping cylindrical, full weight bearing allowed
3–9 months after amputation: Definitive or custom prosthesis, allows for complete limb healing, edema resolution. Decreased wound problems but increase risk of contracture, deconditioning, and pressure ulcers

Prosthetic Training

How to don and doff prosthesis
Care of skin and prosthetic components
Safe use in transfers
Ambulation with appropriate assistive device
Community ambulation and activities

Prosthesis Construction

Socket: Goal is to achieve total contact with residual limb, helps decrease edema, increase proprioception, and increase weight-bearing surface.

Suspension: Method to hold prosthesis to the residual limb.

- Common Systems: Anatomic Shape of Limb, Liner, Sleeve, and Suction
- Socks – ply refers to thickness of socks, used to compensate for volume changes and ensure good prosthetic fit.

Pylon

- Endoskeletal – inner pylon covered with soft foam cover, easy to adjust components, angles, length; lighter weight.
- Exoskeletal – strength through outer lamination, durable, and hard to adjust

Feet

- Solid ankle, cushion-heel (SACH) – no ankle motion in any direction; the cushioned heel allows for simulated plantar flexion during loading response.
- Single axis – motion in sagittal plane, mostly plantar flexion, provides knee extension moment, improved ambulation down inclines.
- Multi-Axis – 3 planes of motion plantar/dorsiflexion, inversion/eversion, and transverse plane.

- Dynamic response – use "energy storing" material, decrease energy expenditure. Indicated in variable cadence ambulation, better for high-level activities.

Knee

- Outside hinges: no resistance of flexion/extension, often used in knee disarticulation to equalize femur length
- Manual Locking: most stable; lock into full extension throughout gait cycle, switch to allow flexion during sitting
- Single axis: bends freely during swing phase, no inherent stability. Requires fixed slow cadence
- Stance control: weight-activated braking mechanism prevents further flexion when weight bearing; must shift weight onto opposite leg to flex the knee. Allows for momentary stability and stumble recovery, but disrupts gait pattern and requires slow cadence.
- Polycentric: multiple axes provide single center of rotation located posteriorly and proximally; allows shortening during swing phase
- Fluid controlled: incorporates pneumatic or hydraulic unit, provides smoother gait and allows for changes in cadence
- Microprocessor controlled: measure knee angle and force to determine phase of gait and speed, automatically adjusts resistance to fluid flow in hydraulic joint to control rate of flexion. Offers most normal gait pattern, can provide specialized resistances to facilitate activities (e.g., bent-knee stance for golfing)

Transtibial Amputation

Pressure-tolerant areas – pretibial/gastrocnemius musculature, medial tibial flare, fibular shaft, and patellar tendon

Pressure-sensitive areas – patella, hamstring tendons, fibular head, femoral epicondyles, tibial shaft, distal tibia, and distal fibula

Socket

- Patellar tendon bearing (PTB): positions socket to load pressure-tolerant areas and offload sensitive areas
- Total surface bearing (TSB): use total limb contact, evenly distribute forces, often used with gel interface
- Hydrostatic: similar to TSB design, attempt to resist translation of bony anatomy within soft tissue

Suspension

- Fork strap with waist belt – Bulky, poor cosmesis, used for maximum security and other techniques not viable, e.g., obese patients.
- Sleeve – elastic material (neoprene, latex, silicone), stretched over prosthesis that is held in place by compression of sleeve against outer wall. Some provide vacuum seal to enhance suspension.
- Supracondylar – compression of med/lat dimension above the femoral condyles, may be used with suprapatellar wedging as well.

- Gel liner suspension – gel liner combined with pin-locking mechanism; creates suction environment between limb and liner.
- Suction – one way valve at distal end of socket to allow air exit.
- Vacuum suspension – Gel liner with sealing sleeve, valve at distal end to remove air.

Knee disarticulation/supracondylar amputation – not commonly used, problems with suspension, cosmesis, and wound healing. Indicated in pediatric population to preserve the growth plate

Transfemoral Amputation

Socket

- Quadrilateral – 4 walls to support femur, abductor, adductor, allow gluteal muscle function
- Ischial containment – provide bony lock of ischium into prosthetic socket. Better medial/lateral stability, better adduction. Most commonly used design

Suspension

- Suction: most secure, better prosthesis control
- Gel liner: good for volume fluctuations
- Belt: either primary or auxiliary suspension, worn around pelvis for improved support, can be combined with any suspension system

Pylon

- May contain a positional rotator between socket and knee – aids in dressing and donning sock/shoe. Need 10 cm from skin to ideal knee center with rotator, 7.5 cm without.

Prosthetic Prescription

Requires designation of K level – measurement of the capacity or potential of the patient to accomplish expected post-rehabilitation daily function

K0: does not have ability or potential to ambulate of transfer, prosthesis does not enhance quality of life
K1: transfer of ambulate on level surface at fixed cadence
K2: ambulate on uneven surfaces
K3: ambulate with variable cadence
K4: ambulation that exceeds basic ambulation skills (high impact, high stress, or high energy levels; e.g., child, active adult, athlete)

Energy Requirements of Prosthetic Gait

Ambulation after lower extremity amputation requires increased metabolic cost (percentage above normal):

- Symes – 15 %
- BKA, traumatic – 25 %

- BKA, vascular – 40 %
- Bilateral BKA, traumatic – 40 %
- AKA, traumatic – 60 %
- AKA, vascular – 100 %
- Bilateral AKA – 200 %

Self-selected walking speed and rate of oxygen consumption are significantly higher in patients with traumatic amputation compared to those with vascular amputation.

Complications

Postsurgical Edema

Reduction of edema promotes wound healing, minimizes postoperative pain, and shapes the residual limb for prosthetic fitting

Post-op dressings:

- Soft dressing – elastic wrap or elastic stockinet (e.g., Ace wrap)
- Semi-rigid dressing – Unna dressing, air splint
- Rigid dressing – plaster, plastic, or fiberglass; can be removable or nonremovable

Pain

Phantom limb pain: painful sensations in the portion of the amputated limb that is missing, involves both central and peripheral neural mechanisms. Treatments include desensitization and pharmacologic treatment including antidepressants (tricyclic antidepressants, noradrenergic, and serotonergic agents) and anticonvulsants.

Residual limb pain: pain in the portion of the amputated limb that is physically present. Multiple types including prosthesis related, arthrogenic (bone spurs, heterotopic ossification, osteoarthritis, osteopenia), and neurogenic (neuromas, radiculopathy).

Back pain present in up to 70 % of lower limb amputees

Joint Contractures

Prolonged sitting can lead to knee flexion, hip flexion, hip abduction, and external rotation contractures.

Ambulation is compromised by knee flexion contracture greater than 5° or hip flexion contracture greater than 15°.

Prevention: avoid knee under pillow or pillow between legs, utilize knee board in wheelchair, lay prone several times per day for 10–15 min intervals.

Skin Disorders

- Contact dermatitis: skin inflammatory reaction
- Reactive hyperemia
- Cellulitis
- Verrucous hyperplasia: wart-like lesion on end of residual limb; related to "choking" of the residual limb – prosthesis fits tightly proximally with lack of distal pressure and creates vascular congestion.

- Callus formation
- Folliculitis
- Epidermoid cyst: blocked sebaceous gland, most common in popliteal fossa and upper thigh
- Hidradenitis
- Fungal infection: nonspecific scaling erythema; tinea corporis and tinea cruris

Psychological Sequelae
Initial grief and depression common, persistent clinical depression present in 21–35 % of amputees.

Anxiety and post-traumatic stress disorder are also common. Acceptance of altered body image may be difficult.

Bibliography

1. Pasquina P, Bryant P, Huang M, Roberts T, Nelson V, Flood K. Advances in amputee care. Arch Phys Med Rehabil. 2006;87(3 Suppl 1):S34–43.
2. Pinzur M, Gottschalk F, Pinto M, Smith D. Controversies in lower-extremity amputation. J Bone Joint Surg Am. 2007;89(5):1118–27.
3. Smith D, McFarland L, Sangeorzan B, Reiber G, Czerniecki J. Postoperative dressing and management strategies for transtibial amputations: a critical review. J Rehabil Res Dev. 2003;40(3):213–24.

Amputation and Prosthetics of the Upper Extremity

Katherine Payne and Jessica Pruente

1 Amputation: Upper Extremity

Take-Home Message

- Transradial amputation allows for the highest level of functional recovery with long limb length ideal for body-powered prostheses and medium limb length ideal for externally powered prostheses.
- Voluntary opening is the most common terminal device control mechanism.
- Early prosthetic fitting is essential to promote acceptance of upper extremity prosthesis.

Definition Major amputation: any amputation performed above the level of the wrist

Etiology/Epidemiology Approximately 10,000 upper limb amputations annually in the United States

- Trauma – 77 % of acquired upper limb amputations
- Tumor
- Congenital
- Other (infection, burn, cardiovascular disease)

60 % of upper limb amputations occur in persons between ages 21 and 64 years old.
Most common major upper limb amputation is the transradial level (57 %).
Only 8 % of upper limb amputations are proximal to the finger.

K. Payne, MD (✉) • J. Pruente, MD
University of Colorado, Aurora, Colorado, USA
e-mail: katherine.payne@ucdenver.edu

C. Mauffrey, D.J. Hak (eds.), *Passport for the Orthopedic Boards and FRCS Examination*, DOI 10.1007/978-2-8178-0475-0_44

Classification: Levels of Amputation

Finger amputation – DIP, PIP, and MCP levels

Transcarpal amputation, wrist disarticulation – limited functional outcomes; preserves supination and pronation, but prosthetic fitting is difficult

Transradial amputation (below elbow) – allows for highest level of functional recovery

- Long (preserve 55–90 % of length of radius) – preferred when optimal body-powered prosthetic restoration is the goal; ideal for performing physically demanding work
- Medium (preserve 35–55 % of length of radius) – good function and cosmesis; preferred when optimal externally powered prosthetic restoration is goal
- Short (preserve 0–35 % of length of radius) – difficult suspension, limited elbow flexion and range of motion

Elbow disarticulation – poor cosmesis, unable to use externally powered elbow

Transhumeral amputation – ideal length 7–10 cm from distal humeral condyle

Treatment: Upper Limb Prostheses Early prosthetic fitting after upper limb amputation is essential, prosthetic fitting should occur within 1–4 months of amputation in order to promote greater acceptance and integration of an artificial arm

Preprosthetic Training

Fabrication and fitting can start 4–8 weeks post operatively.

Rebalancing – the amputation will cause shoulder elevation and scapular rotation; focus on correcting static posture.

Therapy – learning of single-hand techniques, retrain hand dominance, trunk and core strengthening.

Movements to control prosthesis

- Scapular abduction – provides tension for a figure of eight harness that may open terminal device.
- Humeral flexion – used to open terminal device.
- Shoulder depression, extension, and abduction – operates the internal locking elbow of transhumeral prosthesis.
- Elbow flexion/extension
- Supination/pronation
- Chest expansion
- Excursion – amount of movement achieved by the residual limb. Important for control of prosthesis. High transhumeral amputations have 40 % less excursion compared to transradial.

Pre-myoelectric testing: occupational therapist plays large role in determining electrode placement. Use biofeedback to aid motor training to increase needed muscle activity at sites to control terminal device.

Prosthetic Systems

- Passive – enhanced cosmesis and stabilization.
- Body powered – uses patient's strength and range of motion for control of terminal device motion. Benefits: durable, higher sensory feedback, and economical.
- Externally powered – uses battery power to enhance movements. Use either muscle contraction (myoelectric) or manual switch (switch control) to activate different terminal device movements.
- Co-contraction – simultaneous contraction of two muscle groups can be used to change function, e.g., hand to wrist. Benefits: more proximal function, better grip strength.
- Hybrid – combination of body powered and externally powered.

Suspension Systems

- Harness – the only option in shoulder disarticulation or short transhumeral amputation, often used in combination with other suspension systems and used with body-powered systems.
- Pin lock – often used with passive prosthetic systems, mid or long transhumeral or transradial amputations.
- Suction – often used to interface with myoelectric systems or transhumeral amputation.
- Anatomical – uses bony prominences to facilitate suspension. Can reduce harness use. Will likely decrease available ROM

Terminal Device

Categorized as passive or active
Passive: good cosmesis but less functional
Active: 2 styles

- Hook – lateral grasp, simple, lightweight, efficient grasp, and durable
- Prosthetic hand – Tripod grasp, heavier, and better cosmesis

Five Types of Grip

- Pincer (precision)
- Palmar (tripod, 3-jaw chuck)
- Lateral (key pinch)
- Hook
- Spherical

Control Mechanism

Utilize rubber bands to control the force of closing or grasp
Voluntary open: closed at rest, actively opened by patient; most common control mechanism
Voluntary close: open at rest, actively closed by patient
Specialized devices – can be custom made for variety of activities, sports, and hobbies per patient preference.

Complications Postoperative complications include edema, pain, and skin disorders as described in complications of lower limb amputation (Chapter 43 "Amputation and prosthetics lower extremity").

Common joint contractures are elbow flexion and shoulder adduction

Bibliography

1. Datta D, Selvaraja K, Davey N. Functional outcome of patients with proximal upper limb deficiency – acquired and congenital. Clin Rehabil. 2004;18(2): 172–7.
2. Smurr L, Gulick K, Ganz O. Managing the upper extremity amputee: a protocol for success. J Hand Ther. 2008;21(2):160–76.
3. Lake C, Dodson R. Progressive Upper Limb Prosthetics. Physical Medicine and Rehabilitation Clinics of North America. 2006;17(1):49–72.

Part XI
Sports Surgery

Freddie Fu, Dharmesh Vyas, and James M. Bullock

Knee

James M. Bullock, Scott Kling, Justin Arner, Joseph Labrum, Freddie Fu, and Dharmesh Vyas

1 ACL and PCL

Justin Arner

Take-Home Message

ACL

- Two functional bundles named for their insertion sites, the anteromedial (AM) bundle and the posterolateral (PL) bundle (Figs. 1 and 2).
- The natural history of the ACL-deficient knee in young and active patients may be worsening of meniscal pathology, chondral injury, and early arthritic progression.

J.M. Bullock, MD • S. Kling, MD
Sports Medicine, University of Pittsburgh Medical Center, 3200 South Water Street, Pittsburgh, PA 15203, USA
e-mail: srkling@gmail.com; jamesbullock.md@gmail.com

J. Arner, MD • J. Labrum, BS
Labrum is University of Pittsburgh Medical School, Arner is Orthopedic Residency UPMC, University of Pittsburgh Medical Center, 3200 South Water Street, Pittsburgh, PA 15203, USA
e-mail: justin.arner@gmail.com; josephlabrum@gmail.com

F. Fu
Speartment of Orthopaedics, Sports Medicine, University of Pittsburgh Medical Center, 3200 South Water Street, Pittsburgh, PA 15203, USA
e-mail: fudr@upmc.edu

D. Vyas (✉)
Department of Orthopaedic Surgery, UPMC at Oxford Drive, 600 Oxford Dr., Suite 200, Monroeville, PA 15146, USA
e-mail: vyasdr@upmc.edu

C. Mauffrey, D.J. Hak (eds.), *Passport for the Orthopedic Boards and FRCS Examination*, DOI 10.1007/978-2-8178-0475-0_45

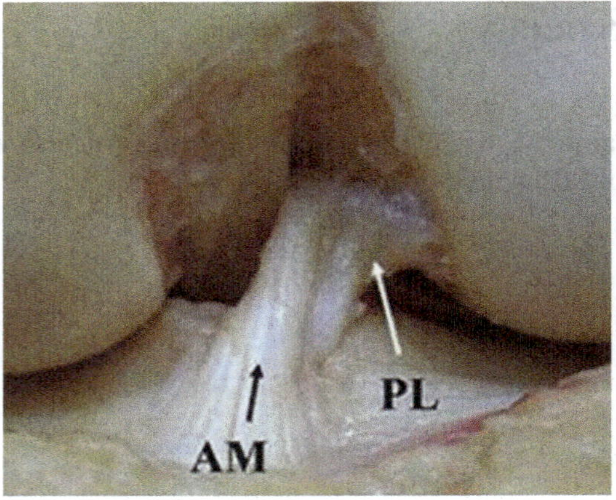

Fig. 1 Cadaveric dissection of human knee delineating the two-bundle composition of the ACL: anteromedial (*AM*) and posterolateral (*PL*) bundles (figure courtesy of Dr. Freddie Fu)

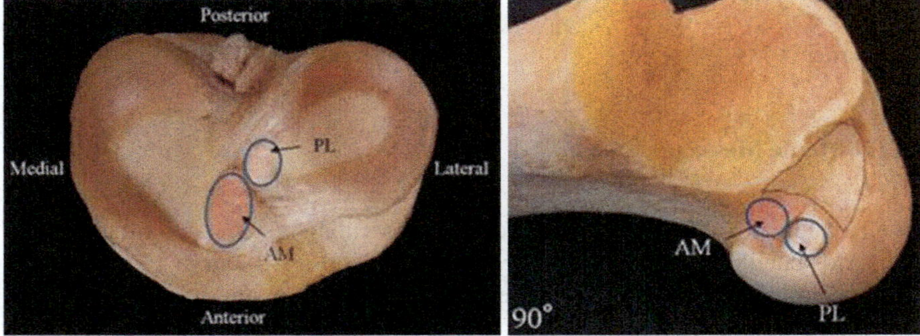

Fig. 2 Cadaveric dissection of human knee depicting the anatomic attachments of the ACL bundles on the tibia and the femur with the knee in 90° of flexion (Courtesy of Dr. Freddie Fu)

- No upper age limit exists for reconstruction, should be based on symptoms and activity.
- Females have increased risk for ACL rupture.
- The MCL and lateral meniscus are common concomitant injuries in acute ACL tears; medial meniscus injuries are seen more in chronic tears.
- Many ACL graft options exist; hamstring and bone-tendon-bone grafts both have shown good outcomes.

PCL

- Three bundles exist: anterolateral, posteromedial, and meniscofemoral ligaments.
- The PCL and PLC work synergistically.
- Evaluation of the PLC, LCL, and PCL is important.
- PCL has some healing capacity.
- Single bundle, double bundle, tibial and transtibial inlay, and PCL augmentation are all options.

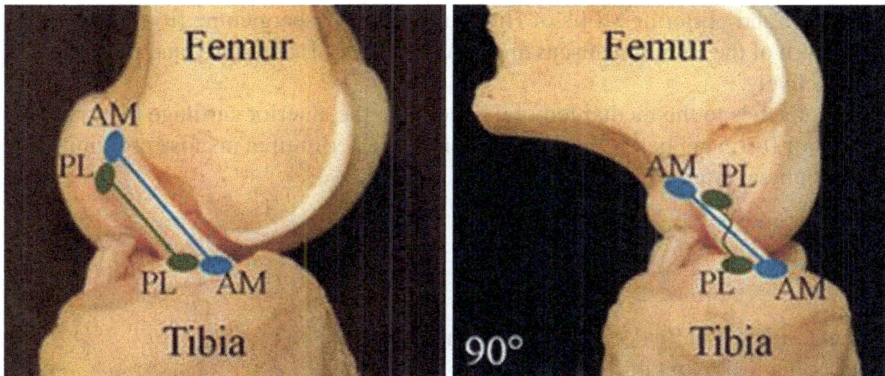

Fig. 3 Schematic showing that when the knee is in extension, the two bundles are parallel to each other. With the knee bent at 90°, the AM bundle is tight and the PL bundle is loose. This allows the knee to remain stable in the anterior direction but also concomitantly allow rotation of the tibiofemoral articulation. The two bundles work synergistically to allow for knee function (Courtesy of Dr. Freddie Fu)

Definitions Anterior cruciate ligament (ACL) and posterior cruciate ligament (PCL) are important knee stabilizers, can be injured to different degrees, and may lead to knee instability and possibly further knee injury.

Anatomy is essential; anatomic reconstruction has shown to improve outcomes.

Anatomy

ACL

- Origin on the medial wall of the lateral femoral condyle, insertion on the tibial articular surface.
- Two functional bundles named for their insertion sites, the anteromedial (AM) bundle and the posterolateral (PL) bundle (Figs. 1 and 2):
  - AM bundle is tight in flexion.
  - PL bundle is tight in extension (Fig. 3).
- 90 % type I and 10 % type III collagen.
- Innervation via the posterior articular nerve, a branch of the tibial nerve.
- Provides anteroposterior stability and is a secondary rotatory stabilizer.
- Blood supply is primarily via the middle genicular artery, a branch of the popliteal artery.

PCL

- Technically is extra-articular; synovium reflects around the PCL from the posterior capsule.
- Blood supply from the synovium plus same vascular supply (middle genicular artery) and innervation (posterior articular nerve) as the ACL.
- Made up of the larger and stronger anterolateral (AL) bundle, posteromedial (PM) bundle, and meniscofemoral ligaments (MFLs):
  - PM bundle is tight in extension.
  - AL bundle is tight in flexion.

- Anterior and posterior MFLs of Humphrey and Wrisberg come from the posterior horn of the lateral meniscus and attach to the PCL anteriorly and posteriorly, respectively.
- PCL attaches to the medial femoral condyle at the anterior cartilage margin and inserts 1.0–1.5 cm below the joint line on the posterior tibia in close proximity to the popliteal artery.

Etiology

ACL

- Acute injury usually occurs as a noncontact pivoting injury.
- Accompanied by feeling a "pop" with pain and swelling.

PCL

- More commonly injured in trauma than sports-related injuries; concomitant injuries are common, particularly to the posterior lateral corner (PLC).
- Patients rarely complain of a "pop" or instability but rather posterior knee pain with decreased knee flexion.

Pathophysiology

ACL

- Acute ACL tears are often associated with lateral meniscal tears and medial collateral ligament injury (MCL).
- Chronic ACL-deficient knees also often have meniscal tears secondary to knee instability and chondral injuries.
- More common in women compared with men (4.5:1):
  - Due to valgus leg alignment, landing biomechanics (landing more in extension, higher valgus movement), more quadriceps dominant, smaller ligaments, smaller notches, hormone levels, and genetic factors related to collagen production

PCL

- Patients more likely to be symptomatic if they have a combined ligamentous knee injury.
- After the acute effects of the knee injury resolve, patients' symptoms vary from little to severe impairment. Some only complain of instability while walking up inclines.

Radiography

ACL

- Radiographs should be done initially and usually are normal.
- Segond fracture may be seen which is pathognomonic for an ACL tear:
  - Due to an avulsion fracture of the proximal lateral tibia

- MRI should be done to further evaluate for ACL tears, meniscal tears, subchondral injury, loose bodies, and bone bruising.
- Bone bruising occurs from direct impact of the tibia and femur and classically occurs in the middle 1/3 of the lateral femoral condyle and posterior 1/3 of the lateral tibial plateau.

PCL

- X-rays should include bilateral standing anteroposterior, flexion 45° weight bearing, lateral, and merchant views.
- Evaluation of tibial subluxation is key as well as any fractures, particularly avulsion fractures.
- MRI is very sensitive in acute PCL injury but less so with chronic tears:
  - Allows evaluation of the meniscus, articular surface, and other ligamentous structures.
  - Locations of bone bruises vary.

Classification

ACL

- An effusion is usually seen and quadriceps avoidance gait is utilized where the patient does not actively extend the knee.
- Lachman's test is the most sensitive exam:
  - Grades I–III and A or B
    - Grade I is <5 mm translation.
    - Grade II is 5–10 mm translation.
    - Grade III is >10 mm translation.
    - A is when a firm end point is felt.
    - B with no endpoint.
- Anterior drawer is another option and KT-1000 testing can be used to quantify anterior laxity.
- Pivot shift is done by internally rotating the lower leg 20° and a valgus force applied while the knee is flexed:
  - Positive test when the tibial plateau reduces and a clunk can be felt at 20–30° of flexion.

PCL

- Classification is based on chronicity (acute vs. chronic), associated knee injuries, and the amount of translation of the tibia.
- Key to diagnosis is whether the injury is isolated or combined as treatment varies:
  - Isolated PCL injuries many times can be treated nonoperatively with good to excellent results.
  - Combined injuries many times have better prognosis with early surgical intervention. Commonly combined with other ligamentous injuries, fractures, vascular, and nerve injuries.

- Knee dislocation should be suspected with ACL and PCL injury or any three-ligament disruption:
  - Vascular evaluation is important.
- Chronicity is important as PLC scarring occurs if surgery is not undertaken within 3 weeks and more rotational instability may exist due to capsular stretching.
- Posterior drawer test is the most accurate test:
  - At 90° of flexion a posterior directed fore is applied on the proximal tibia. Normally, an anterior step-off of 1 cm from the medial femoral condyle to the tibial plateau exists.
- Classification is like with the ACL:
  - Grade I injury has a translation of 1–5 mm but maintains the anterior step-off.
  - Grade II translates 5–10 mm and the condyle and plateau are flush.
  - Grade III has >10 mm of translation, and the plateau is posterior to the condyle and is a complete tear.
- Posterior sag test or Godfrey's test is the evaluation of this step-off due to the weight of the tibia translating the plateau posteriorly.
- Quadriceps activation test is when the knee is held in 60° of flexion and the patient contracts the quadriceps muscle to extend their knee:
  - In grade III tears, the tibia will reduce anteriorly.
- The dial test or external rotation of the tibia is important to evaluate PLC injury as this can change the prognosis and intervention.
- Evaluation of the meniscus as well as the other ligamentous structures is also very important as outlined previously.

Treatment

ACL

- Nonoperative treatment—physical therapy and lifestyle modifications:
  - Appropriate in low demand and older individuals
- ACL repair has high failure rates and poor outcomes; therefore, reconstruction of the ACL is done in younger, more active patients.
- Proper anatomic tunnel placement is imperative to restore rotation stability.
- The tunnels should be placed anatomically within the native footprints.
- Single-bundle and double-bundle reconstruction are options:
  - Double bundle has shown to give improved rotational stability in laboratory evaluation and some clinical studies.

- Knees without ACL reconstruction many times have worsening meniscal pathology and chondral injury, and early arthritic progression may be linked:
  - Reconstruction is recommended in young, active patients.
- Graft selection is controversial.
- Options include bone patellar bone autograft, hamstring autograft, quadriceps tendon autograft, and allograft:
  - Bone patellar bone autograft allows bone healing and therefore may incorporate faster and is rigidly fixed:
    - Negatives include possible anterior knee pain from graft harvesting, patella fracture, or patella tendon rupture.
  - Hamstring autograft has a smaller incision and less anterior knee pain but fixation strength may be decreased:
    - Some concern for hamstring weakness in elite athletes and a "windshield wiper" effect because femoral fixation is further from the joint so the graft may rub in the tunnel and be impinged.
  - Quadriceps tendon autograft allows a large graft with possible bone fixation and good biomechanical properties.
  - Many different allografts can be used:
    - Take longer to incorporate and sterilization impairs its native properties and rarely disease transmission can occur.

PCL

- Nonoperative versus operative treatment of isolated PCL injuries is controversial.
- Rarer injury and therefore few larger long-term follow-up studies exist.
- Isolated acute partial PCL injuries have good outcomes with nonoperative treatment.
- A more aggressive treatment approach is suggested if the patient has persistent knee instability and pain due to the increased loading of the medial compartment in isolated complete tears.
- PCL does have healing potential so some recommend extension bracing.
- PCL avulsion fractures are less common and have more agreed upon treatment:
  - Minimally displaced fractures do well with brief immobilization.
  - Displaced fractures require operative intervention.
- Multiple graft options exist as well as fixation techniques without any clear superior option.
- Transtibial and tibial inlay procedures are arthroscopic versus open techniques, respectively, and each has their strengths and risks.
- Single- versus double-bundle reconstruction is another area of controversy:
  - Most reconstructions currently involve the AL single bundle only.

- The popliteal artery lies just posterior to the insertion of the PCL; great care must be taken during surgical intervention.
- In chronic PCL-deficient knees, high tibial osteotomy can unload the medial compartment and increase the tibial slope to eliminate varus angulation and lessen the posterior tibial sag.
- In isolated PCL and multi-ligamentous injuries, each patient must be dealt with individually as a wide array of injuries and outcomes exist.

Bibliography

1. Amis AA, et al. Anatomy of the posterior cruciate ligament and the meniscofemoral ligaments. Knee Surg Sports Traumatol Arthrosc. 2006;14(3):257–63.
2. Anderson AF, Snyder RB, Lipscomb AB Jr. Anterior cruciate ligament reconstruction. A prospective randomized study of three surgical methods. Am J Sports Med. 2001;29(3):272–9.
3. Bathala EA, et al. Radiologic case study. Segond fracture. Orthopedics. 2007;30(9):689, 797–8.
4. Boynton MD, Tietjens BR. Long-term followup of the untreated isolated posterior cruciate ligament-deficient knee. Am J Sports Med. 1996;24(3):306–10.
5. Chhabra A, et al. Anatomic, radiographic, biomechanical, and kinematic evaluation of the anterior cruciate ligament and its two functional bundles. J Bone Joint Surg Am. 2006;88(Suppl 4):2–10.
6. Ciccotti MG, et al. Non-operative treatment of ruptures of the anterior cruciate ligament in middle-aged patients. Results after long-term follow-up. J Bone Joint Surg Am. 1994;76(9):1315–21.
7. Freedman KB, et al. Arthroscopic anterior cruciate ligament reconstruction: a metaanalysis comparing patellar tendon and hamstring tendon autografts. Am J Sports Med. 2003;31(1):2–11.
8. Giffin JR, et al. Effects of increasing tibial slope on the biomechanics of the knee. Am J Sports Med. 2004;32(2):376–82.
9. Hensler D, et al. Correlation between femoral tunnel length and tunnel position in ACL reconstruction. J Bone Joint Surg Am. 2013;95(22):2029–34.
10. Honkamp NJ, Ranawat A, Harner CD. Posterior cruciate ligament injuries in the adult. In: DeLee JC, Drez D, Miller MD, editors. DeLee & Drez's orthopaedic sports medicine: principles and practice. Philadelphia: Elsevier; 2009. p. SECTION E.
11. Honkamp NJ, Shen W, Okeke N, Ferretti M, Fu FH. Anterior cruciate ligament injuries in the adult. In: DeLee JC, Drez D, Miller MD, editors. DeLee & Drez's orthopaedic sports medicine: principles and practice. Philadelphia: Elsevier; 2009. p. SECTION D.
12. Hoshino Y, et al. Quantitative evaluation of the pivot shift by image analysis using the iPad. Knee Surg Sports Traumatol Arthrosc. 2013;21(4):975–80.
13. Huston LJ, Greenfield ML, Wojtys EM. Anterior cruciate ligament injuries in the female athlete. Potential risk factors. Clin Orthop Relat Res. 2000;(372):50–63.

14. Illingworth KD, et al. Relationship between bone bruise volume and the presence of meniscal tears in acute anterior cruciate ligament rupture. Knee Surg Sports Traumatol Arthrosc. 2014;22:2181–6.
15. Kennedy JC, Weinberg HW, Wilson AS. The anatomy and function of the anterior cruciate ligament. As determined by clinical and morphological studies. J Bone Joint Surg Am. 1974;56(2):223–35.
16. Mair SD, et al. Incidence and location of bone bruises after acute posterior cruciate ligament injury. Am J Sports Med. 2004;32(7):1681–7.
17. Meyers MH. Isolated avulsion of the tibial attachment of the posterior cruciate ligament of the knee. J Bone Joint Surg Am. 1975;57(5):669–72.
18. Rabuck SJ, et al. Anatomic anterior cruciate ligament reconstruction with quadriceps tendon autograft. Clin Sports Med. 2013;32(1):155–64.
19. Race A, Amis AA. The mechanical properties of the two bundles of the human posterior cruciate ligament. J Biomech. 1994;27(1):13–24.
20. Schulz MS, et al. Epidemiology of posterior cruciate ligament injuries. Arch Orthop Trauma Surg. 2003;123(4):186–91.
21. Sekiya JK, et al. Clinical outcomes after isolated arthroscopic single-bundle posterior cruciate ligament reconstruction. Arthroscopy. 2005;21(9):1042–50.
22. Seroyer ST, Musahl V, Harner CD. Management of the acute knee dislocation: the Pittsburgh experience. Injury. 2008;39(7):710–8.
23. Shino K, et al. Conservative treatment of isolated injuries to the posterior cruciate ligament in athletes. J Bone Joint Surg Br. 1995;77(6):895–900.
24. Thompson WO, Fu FH. The meniscus in the cruciate-deficient knee. Clin Sports Med. 1993;12(4):771–96.
25. Viskontas DG, et al. Bone bruises associated with ACL rupture: correlation with injury mechanism. Am J Sports Med. 2008;36(5):927–33.
26. West RV, Harner CD. Graft selection in anterior cruciate ligament reconstruction. J Am Acad Orthop Surg. 2005;13(3):197–207.
27. Yoon KH, Yoo JH, Kim KI. Bone contusion and associated meniscal and medial collateral ligament injury in patients with anterior cruciate ligament rupture. J Bone Joint Surg Am. 2011;93(16):1510–8.

2 Collateral Ligament Injury

Justin Arner

Take-Home Message

Medial Knee

- Superficial MCL is the primary static stabilizer against valgus and external rotation stress.
- Isolated MCL injuries have valgus laxity at 30°.
- Combined MCL and ACL injuries have valgus laxity at 0°.

Lateral Knee

- Injuries occur by an excessive valgus force, external tibial rotation, or hyperextension.
- The lateral collateral ligament (LCL) is the main stabilizer, is rarely an isolated injury, but commonly is seen with posterolateral corner (PLC) injury:
  - Varus stress and dial testing helps distinguish if a combined injury exists.

Definitions Main structures include MCL and LCL.

Anatomy

Medial Knee

- Major static stabilizers: superficial MCL, deep MCL, and posterior oblique ligament.
- Dynamic stabilizers: pes anserinus, semimembranosus, medial head of the gastrocnemius, and vastus medialis.
- These structures can be divided into three layers:
  - Layer I: sartorial fascia
  - Layer II: superficial MCL
    - Superficial MCL originates at the medial femoral epicondyle and broadly inserts 5–7 cm below the joint line on the anteromedial tibial metaphysis:
      - Primary restraint to valgus stress
  - Layer III: capsule and deep MCL
    - Deep MCL is a thickening of capsule and has the same origin but inserts into the meniscus (meniscofemoral) and then runs from the meniscus to the tibia (meniscotibial).
- Layers II and III conjoin posteriorly to form the posteromedial corner.
- The posterior oblique ligament runs from the adductor tubercle of the femur to the tibia and posterior capsule.
- The MCL is supplied by the superior medial and inferior medial geniculate arteries.

Lateral Knee

- Separated in three layers:
  - Layer I—iliotibial (IT) band and the biceps femoris tendon:
    - The common peroneal nerve lies between layers I and II.

- Layer II—patellar retinaculum and patellofemoral ligament.
- Layer III includes a superficial region made up of the LCL, fabellofibular ligament, and the deep region which includes the arcuate ligament, coronary ligament, popliteus tendon, popliteofibular ligament, and the capsule:
  - Between the two subsets in layer 3 lies the inferior lateral geniculate artery.

- PLC is made up of the LCL, popliteus tendon, popliteofibular ligament, lateral capsule, arcuate ligament, and the fabellofibular ligament.
- The LCL originates on the lateral femoral condyle, proximal and posterior to the popliteus insertion, and inserts on the anterolateral fibular head:
  - Its attachment to the fibula is the most anterior structure as the popliteofibular ligament and biceps femoris attachments lay posterior to the LCL, respectively.
- The primary function of the LCL is resisting varus stress with a secondary role of resisting posterolateral rotation when the knee is in less than 50° of flexion.
- Because its axis is behind that of the knee axis, it is tight in extension and lax in flexion.
- The blood supply is via the superolateral and inferolateral geniculate arteries.

Etiology

Medial Knee

- The MCL is a valgus stabilizer.
- Commonly injured when the knee is forced into valgus and external rotation.
- Commonly seen in combined injuries with the anterior cruciate ligament (ACL) and meniscus.
- Usually a direct blow to the lateral knee leads to a more severe injury compared with a noncontact injury.
- Rupture more commonly occurs at the femoral insertion which is also the location where the MCL heals best.
- Chronic MCL deficiency can lead to calcification of the MCL femoral insertion site and is known as Pellegrini-Stieda syndrome.

Lateral Knee

- Lateral knee injuries most commonly is seen in motor vehicle accidents and athletic injuries and occurs by an excessive varus force, external tibial rotation, or hyperextension.
- The lateral collateral ligament (LCL) is the main stabilizer of the lateral knee and is rarely an isolated injury but commonly is seen with posterolateral corner (PLC) injury.

Pathophysiology

Medial Knee

- The typical history of MCL injury is hearing a "pop" and medial joint line pain with difficulty ambulating.
- On exam, patients are classically tender on the medial knee with an effusion and swelling.
- Valgus stress testing at 30° of knee flexion isolates the superficial MCL.
- If medial laxity at 0° of knee flexion as well, a posterior medial capsule or cruciate ligament injury is considered.
- It is important to evaluate the patient for other ligamentous, meniscal, and chondral lesions.
- A neurovascular exam should be performed with special attention to the saphenous nerve distribution.

Lateral Knee

- Symptoms of injury to the LCL is lateral joint line pain, swelling, difficulty ascending and descending stairs, instability with knee extension, and problems with cutting or pivoting.
- On exam, patients classically walk in hyperextension or a varus thrust gait and have lateral joint line tenderness.
- Isolated LCL injury:
  - Instability to varus stress test at 30°
- LCL combined with ACL and/or PCL injury:
  - Varus instability at both 0 and 30°.
  - If increased tibial external rotation is seen at 30°, a combined PLC and LCL injury is likely.
- Dial test—patient prone and applying external rotation stress on tibia:
  - >10° tibial external rotation asymmetry at 30°: isolated PLC injury
  - >10° external rotation asymmetry at 30° and 90°: PLC and PCL injury
- A complete neurovascular exam is critical as common peroneal nerve injuries do occur.

Radiographs

- MCL: AP and lateral X-rays and MRI to identify the location and severity of MCL injury as well as other knee structures.
- LCL: similar radiographic analysis is recommended as well as a varus stress view.

Classification

Medial Knee

- Three grades based on the amount of valgus opening:
  - Grade I: 1–5 mm
  - Grade II: 5–10 mm
  - Grade III: gross laxity with no endpoint and >10 mm of gapping

Lateral Knee

- Injuries of the LCL and PLC are graded by the amount of lateral opening on varus stress:
  - Grade I is 0–5 mm.
  - Grade II is 5–10 mm.
  - Grade 3 is >10 mm.
- Grade I and II are partial tears while grade III is a complete tear.

Treatment

Medial Knee

- Treatment is based on the grade of injury.
- Grade I injuries:
  - Rest, nonsteroidal anti-inflammatories (NSAIDs), and immediate physical therapy.
  - Return to play is usually 5–7 days.
- Isolated grade II and III injuries:
  - Rest, NSAIDS, therapy, and hinged knee bracing.
  - Return to play is typically 2–4 weeks for grade II injuries and 4–8 weeks for grade III injuries.
- Functional knee bracing for prophylactic MCL treatment has been shown to be successful in football.
- Operative intervention is utilized with combined ligamentous injuries and grade III injuries with continued instability after nonoperative treatment.
- Repairing the MCL is successful in acute avulsion injuries where suture anchors are used.
- MCL reconstruction is utilized in chronic instability or if repairing the MCL is not possible.
- Graft types include semitendinosus, hamstring autograft, tibialis anterior, or Achilles allograft.

Lateral Knee

- Nonoperative treatment is many times successful in isolated grade I or II LCL injury and includes immobilization and functional rehabilitation.
- Return to sports usually possible in 6–8 weeks.

Operative Indications

- Grade III LCL injuries.
- Rotatory instability (combined LCL and PLC).
- Posterolateral instability (combined LCL/PCL and ACL/PCL injuries).
- The proper order of repair/reconstruction of these combined knee injuries is not well defined and is a source of controversy.
- Outcomes are improved when operative intervention occurs in the acute setting.
- Avulsed LCL injuries have shown good outcomes with suture anchor fixation and direct suture repair of midsubstance injuries within 2 weeks of injury.
- When reconstruction is required in isolated LCL injury, patellar tendon autograft has shown good outcomes.
- In combined LCL and popliteofibular ligament reconstruction, the Larson technique can be used where the hamstring graft is passed through a fibular head bone tunnel and is fixed to the lateral femur to create a figure of eight.
- Another option for this same injury is a transtibial double-bundle technique:
  - Achilles tendon allograft is fixed to the femoral epicondyle and half of the tendon is fixed to the fibular head with sutures through a bone tunnel and the other half is fixed to the posterior tibia.
- Careful physical exam is critical for quick diagnosis of combined injuries which improves outcomes.

Bibliography

1. Albright JP, et al. Medial collateral ligament knee sprains in college football. Brace wear preferences and injury risk. Am J Sports Med. 1994;22(1):2–11.
2. Chen FS, Rokito AS, Pitman MI. Acute and chronic posterolateral rotatory instability of the knee. J Am Acad Orthop Surg. 2000;8(2):97–110.
3. Cooper JM, McAndrews PT, LaPrade RF. Posterolateral corner injuries of the knee: anatomy, diagnosis, and treatment. Sports Med Arthrosc. 2006;14(4):213–20.
4. Halinen J, et al. Operative and nonoperative treatments of medial collateral ligament rupture with early anterior cruciate ligament reconstruction: a prospective randomized study. Am J Sports Med. 2006;34(7):1134–40.
5. Hughston JC, et al. Classification of knee ligament instabilities. Part II. The lateral compartment. J Bone Joint Surg Am. 1976;58(2):173–9.
6. Kannus P. Long-term results of conservatively treated medial collateral ligament injuries of the knee joint. Clin Orthop Relat Res. 1988;(226):103–12.
7. Kannus P. Nonoperative treatment of grade II and III sprains of the lateral ligament compartment of the knee. Am J Sports Med. 1989;17(1):83–8.

8. LaPrade RF, et al. The posterolateral attachments of the knee: a qualitative and quantitative morphologic analysis of the fibular collateral ligament, popliteus tendon, popliteofibular ligament, and lateral gastrocnemius tendon. Am J Sports Med. 2003;31(6):854–60.
9. LaPrade RF, et al. The anatomy of the medial part of the knee. J Bone Joint Surg Am. 2007;89(9):2000–10.
10. Singhal M, PJ, Johnson D. Medial ligament injuries. In: DeLee JC, Drez D, Miller MD, editor. DeLee & Drez's orthopaedic sports medicine: principles and practice. Philadelphia: Elsevier; 2009. p. section C.

3 Chronic Exertional Compartment Syndrome

Scott Kling

Take-Home Message

- The anterior compartment is most commonly affected, followed by the lateral compartment. Posterior compartment involvement is rare and has less predictable surgical outcomes.
- Diagnostic criteria for compartment pressure measurement are the following: (1) resting pressure >15 mmHg, (2) immediate postexercise pressure >30 mmHg, and (3) continuous postexercise pressure that does not return to resting level or fall below 15 mmHg after 15 min after completing activity.
- The mainstay of treatment is surgical decompression fasciotomy of the involved compartments. This can be performed using an open or endoscopic approach with similar results.

Definition

- Exertional compartment syndrome is a relatively uncommon cause of leg pain in the athletic population.
- It is defined as reversible muscle ischemia within one of the compartments of the leg that is induced by exercise and relieved by rest.
- There are no permanent sequelae in the affected tissues.

Epidemiology

- Exertional compartment syndrome is found most commonly in male in the third decade of life.
- Athletes who perform significant amounts of running are frequently affected.

Anatomy

- There are four compartments of the leg (anterior, lateral, superficial posterior, and deep posterior):
  - The anterior compartment contains the anterior tibial artery and the deep peroneal nerve.
  - The lateral compartment contains the superficial peroneal nerve.
  - The superficial posterior compartment contains the sural nerve.
  - The deep posterior compartment contains both the posterior tibial and peroneal arteries and the posterior tibial nerve.
- The anterior compartment is most commonly affected in approximately 70 % of cases.
- The lateral compartment is involved in 10 % of cases.
- Posterior compartment involvement is rare and has less predictable surgical outcomes.

Pathophysiology

- The exact mechanism by which exertional compartment syndrome induces pain remains unknown.
- It is theorized that increasing blood perfusion, muscle hypertrophy, and increased interstitial fluid volume within a confined fascial compartment lead to significantly elevated pressures. Accordingly, there is decreased venous return, leading to impaired tissue oxygenation and ischemia. Individual muscle cells are unable to clear the metabolic waste products at a sufficient rate, and they accumulate within the cell membrane.
- Additionally, fascial hernias are suspected to be causal in some cases, with an incidence of 40 % during surgical decompression. The most common location is the intermuscular septum between the anterior and lateral compartments at the exit of the superficial peroneal nerve.

Presentation

- Patients generally present complaining of aching or burning leg pain that is induced by running. It is both predictable and reproducible in nature, often beginning 10 min or so after the onset of exercise, escalating during activity, and slowly resolving after a 30 min period of rest.
- The patient may note a recent increase in training intensity that exceeds their threshold for generating symptoms.
- There is no history of trauma.
- Bilateral involvement is common.
- Pain is localized to the involved compartment.
- Occasionally, patients will complain of distal neurologic findings in addition to pain, specifically numbness, paresthesias, or weakness in the affected nerve distribution. However, the physical exam is frequently normal.
- The diagnosis is commonly confused with medial tibial stress syndrome, colloquially referred to as “shin splints.” However, in medial tibial stress syndrome, pain is worst at the onset of exercise and tends to decrease during training.

Imaging

- Plain film radiographs, magnetic resonance imaging, and bone scan are often normal in patients with exertional compartment syndrome. However, these studies are often helpful in excluding other diagnoses such as tibial stress fracture and medial tibial stress syndrome.

Evaluation

- Exertional compartment syndrome is definitively diagnosed by measuring compartment pressures. Measuring compartment pressures during exercise proves difficult and impractical.
- Per Pedowitz criteria, three pressures must be measured for each suspected compartment: resting pressure, immediate postexercise pressure, and continuous postexercise pressure for 30 min. Diagnostic criteria are the following: (1) resting pressure >15 mmHg, (2) immediate postexercise pressure >30 mmHg, and (3) continuous postexercise pressure that does not return to resting level or fall below 15 mmHg after 15 min after completing activity.
- While the anterior and lateral compartments may be tested fairly reliably, the deep posterior compartment can be challenging.
- Alternative methods of diagnosis are being explored. Near-infrared spectroscopy will show increased deoxygenation of muscle during activity with delayed normalization after activity cessation. T2-weighted magnetic resonance imaging during exercise will demonstrate increase signal in the involved compartments when compared to normal surrounding tissue. SPECT bone scan has also demonstrated potential to localize an ischemic compartment.

Treatment

- Nonoperative treatment includes activity modification and antiinflammatory medications but often proves ineffective. Patients generally do not improve unless they completely eliminate the inciting activity.
- The mainstay of treatment is surgical decompression fasciotomy of the involved compartments, most commonly anterior and lateral. This can be performed using an open or endoscopic approach with similar results.
- The open approach involves a longitudinal incision over the anterolateral leg, identification of the intermuscular septum, and proximal and distal fascial division of both compartments. Careful attention should be paid to localize and protect the superficial peroneal nerve.
- Posterior compartments may be accessed through an extensile anterolateral dissection or a separate medial approach. The superficial compartment is easily decompressed, and the deep compartment must be reached by undermining the soleus to access the posterior tibial margin.
- Many surgeons advocate an individual release of the tibialis posterior muscle as well.
- Most patients are able to return to sports postoperatively within 4 weeks.
- Success rates are greater than 80 % when involving anterior and lateral compartments but fall to between 50 and 65 % when involving posterior compartments, particularly the deep.
- Patients note a high level of pain relief and satisfaction with the surgical result.

Complications

- The most common complication is recurrence of symptoms, which has been found in 7–17 % of operative cases. This is often attributed to incomplete fasciotomy and not specifically releasing the tibialis posterior during deep posterior decompression.
- Less frequent complications include wound infection, nerve injury (most commonly the superficial peroneal), and deep venous thrombosis.

Bibliography

1. Edwards P, Myerson MS. Exertional compartment syndrome of the leg: steps for expedient return to activity. Phys Sportsmed. 1996;24:31–46.
2. George CA, Hutchinson MR. Chronic exertional compartment syndrome. Clin Sports Med. 2012;31(2):307–19.
3. Hislop M, Batt ME. Chronic exertional compartment syndrome. Br J Sports Med. 2011;45:954–5.
4. Pedowitz RA, Hargens AR, Mubarak SJ, et al. Modified criteria for the objective diagnosis of chronic compartment syndrome of the leg. Am J Sports Med. 1990;18:35–40.

4 Extensor Mechanism Rupture

Joseph Labrum

Take-Home Message

- Quadriceps tendon rupture is generally seen in patients >40 years old, while patellar tendon disruptions tend to occur in those <40 years old.
- Patella alta or patella baja may be seen on radiographs.
- Significant swelling may mask any appreciable defect at rupture site, and misdiagnosis is very common.
- For complete tears, early surgical intervention is paramount, usually within 1 month.

Definition

- The extensor mechanism of the knee consists of the quadriceps muscle and tendon, the patella, the patellar tendon, and the tibial tubercle. Disruption of any of these components can lead to extensor mechanism failure.
- Compared with other more common injuries to the knee, such as ligamentous injury, meniscal tears, and fractures, disruptions of the extensor mechanism are relatively rare.
- Of the components of the extensor mechanism, injury to the patellar and quadriceps tendons is more commonly seen and will be highlighted here.

Epidemiology and Etiology

- Age has been observed to have considerable influence on where disruption occurs, with patellar tendon tears occurring in younger individuals and those over 40 years of age more likely to rupture the quadriceps tendon.
- Extensor mechanism rupture is more common in males, with a male to female ratio of 6:1.
- Tendon rupture most often occurs secondary to trauma, but a variety of conditions also increase the risk of spontaneous rupture, including diabetes mellitus, gout, chronic renal failure, systemic lupus erythematosus, rheumatoid arthritis, systemic steroid use, and endocrine disorders.

Patellar Tendon

Epidemiology

- Isolated rupture of the patella tendon has a peak incidence in the third and fourth decades, with 80 % of tears occurring in patients under the age of 40.

Pathophysiology

- Younger individuals—incur the injury as an end result of microtrauma from repetitive activity.
- Older patients—mechanism of tendon weakening is thought to be tendon degeneration.
- Tendon rupture most commonly occurs in the proximal portion of the tendon, close to the inferior patellar pole.
- Weakened tendon ruptures at subnormal threshold—load experienced in the patellar tendon while climbing stairs has been calculated to be 3.2 times body weight, with a force of 17.5 times body weight estimated to cause rupture in normal tendons.

Radiographs

- Plain radiographs can help confirm the diagnosis and classically show a high-riding patella or patella alta.
- Insall-Salvati ratio is defined as the length from the tibial tubercle to the inferior pole of the patella divided by the total patellar length.
- Ratio of greater than 1.2 is used to make the radiographic diagnosis of patella alta.

Classification

- Several classification schemes have been proposed to categorize patellar tendon ruptures, including those based on time since injury, pattern of tear observed at time of surgery, and level of tendon rupture, among others:
  - Classification based on chronicity of the tear before diagnosis and treatment has proven to be the most useful in determining prognosis after surgery.

Treatment

- Nonoperative treatment has a very limited role in the care of patellar tendon rupture:
  - Candidates for conservative management may include those with partial tears and maintenance of active extension and patellar height.

Quadriceps Tendon

Epidemiology

- Extensor mechanism disruption in those over age 40 is more likely to occur at the level of the quadriceps tendon, with one series reporting that 88 % of patients with quadriceps tendon tears occurred in this age group.

Etiology

- Rupture of the quadriceps tendon often occurs during a rapid, eccentric contraction of the quadriceps muscle, such as while trying to regain balance and avoid a fall.
- Other causes may include blunt trauma (especially falls), lacerations, and iatrogenic etiologies.

Pathophysiology

- The rupture site in most cases localizes to an area 1–2 cm away from the upper patellar pole, which corresponds to the avascular region of the quadriceps tendon.
- Ruptures 0–1 cm from the superior pole are also common.
- In nearly all cases, pathologic changes are degenerative in nature and commonly affect tendon blood supply.

Imaging

- Plain radiographs are generally ordered first and may show a suprapatellar mass, obliteration of the quadriceps tendon shadow, or patella baja, among other things.
- Insall-Salvati ratio less than 0.8.
- Ultrasound and MRI can also be very helpful in diagnosis, with MRI being particularly useful when the diagnosis is unclear.

Treatment

- Conservative treatment is generally indicated for partial tears, while complete tears necessitate prompt surgical intervention.

Diagnostic Considerations

- Patellar and quadriceps tendon rupture can present a diagnostic challenge. In part, this is due to their relatively uncommon occurrence, but diagnosis can be difficult even when suspected:
  - The acute phase of the injury is often accompanied by swelling and hematoma formation, and the patient may present with an inability to bear weight.
  - Unfortunately, more common injuries to the knee—such as cruciate ligament injury, meniscal tears, and collateral ligament sprains—may also present this way.
  - Additionally, the presence of significant swelling makes palpation of the suspected rupture site difficult.

- The diagnosis of extensor mechanism disruptions is often delayed as a result or even misdiagnosed entirely.
- The rate of misdiagnosis varies in the literature but has been reported as high as 67 % by some researchers.
- On physical exam, the hallmark of extensor mechanism rupture is an inability to perform active leg extension:
  - However, many patients retain the ability to perform active extension against gravity (e.g., straight leg raise) due to an intact iliotibial band or medial and lateral patellar retinaculum.
  - May therefore be preferable to examine the patient with the knee in a starting position of 90° of flexion hanging off the exam table and instructing the patient to actively extend the knee.
  - The examiner should verify that complete knee extension is achieved, as some patients with extensor mechanism disruptions will retain the ability to partially extend the knee.

Treatment

- Successful treatment of patellar or quadriceps tendon rupture hinges on early diagnosis and surgical intervention.
- Nonoperative treatment for complete tears is rarely indicated, although there is a role for nonoperative treatment in a partial tear when the patient has intact active extension and is not a high-demand athlete or laborer.
- While no consensus exists as to exact time interval of surgery, good results have been reported with early operative treatment within 1 month of injury.

Bibliography

1. Insall J, Salvati E. Patella position in the normal knee joint. Radiology. 1971;101:101–4.
2. Kaneko K, DeMouy EH, Brunet ME, Benzian J. Radiographic diagnosis of quadriceps tendon rupture: analysis of diagnostic failure. J Emerg Med. 1994;12:225–9.
3. Kuechle DK, Stuart MJ. Isolated rupture of the patellar tendon in athletes. Am J Sports Med. 1994;22:692–5.
4. Lobenhoffer P, Thermann H. Quadriceps and patellar tendon ruptures. Orthopade. 2000;29:228–343.
5. Lombardi LJ, Cleri DJ, Epstein E. Bilateral spontaneous quadriceps tendon rupture in a patient with renal failure. Orthopedics. 1995;18:187–91.
6. Matava MJ. Patellar tendon ruptures. J Am Acad Orthop Surg. 1996;4:287–96.
7. McGrory JE. Disruption of the extensor mechanism of the knee. J Emerg Med. 2003;24:163–8.
8. Ramseier LE, Werner CM, Heinzelmann M. Quadriceps and patellar tendon rupture. Injury. 2006;37(6):516–9.
9. Ramsey RH, Muller GE. Quadriceps tendon rupture: a diagnostic trap. Clin Orthop. 1970;70:161–4.
10. Rougraff BT, Reeck CC, Essenmacher J. Complete quadriceps tendon ruptures. Orthopedics. 1996;19:509–14.

11. Scuderi C. Ruptures of the quadriceps tendon; study of twenty tendon ruptures. Am J Surg. 1958;95:626–34.
12. Siwek CW, Rao JP. Ruptures of the extensor mechanism of the knee joint. J Bone Joint Surg Am. 1981;63:932–7.
13. Zanetti M, Hodler J. Ultrasonography and magnetic resonance tomography (MRI) of tendon injuries. Orthopade. 1995;24:200–8.
14. Zernicke RF, Garhammer J, Jobe FW. Human patellar-tendon rupture: a kinetic analysis. J Bone Joint Surg. 1977;59:179–83.
15. Zimmermann T, Kelm C, Heinrichs C, Herold G. Bilateral rupture of the quadriceps tendon—case report and review of the literature. Zentralbl Chir. 1993;118:368–71.

5 Meniscus and Discoid Meniscus

James M. Bullock

5.1 *Meniscus*

Take-Home Message

- Healing potential of the meniscus decreases from the periphery towards the central avascular area.
- MRI is less sensitive and specific in diagnosis of meniscus tears in the pediatric population.
- Tears in the vascular zone tend to respond well to meniscus repair surgery, with the inside-out technique considered the gold standard.
- Tears in the avascular zone have a poor prognosis after repair, and partial meniscectomy brings more predictable results.
- Discoid menisci are at increased risk of developing tears.

Definition

Anatomy and Function

- Menisci are wedge shaped and are located between the femoral condyles and tibial plateaus medially and laterally.
- Both menisci are connected anteriorly via the intermeniscal ligament and are further stabilized by attachments at the anterior and posterior horns called roots.
- Lateral meniscus posterior horn has attachments to the posterior medial femoral condyle near the PCL insertion via the meniscofemoral ligaments (Humphrey and Wrisberg).

- Medial meniscus is crescent shaped, while the lateral meniscus is more circular and also covers a larger part of the lateral tibial plateau.
- Majority of the meniscus is wet weight (72 %), and its ability to absorb water is attributed to the proteoglycan composition (aggrecan being the main one). The dry weight is predominantly composed of collagen type I. The characteristic cell found in the meniscus is the fibrochondrocyte.
- The meniscus converts axial tibiofemoral forces to horizontal hoop stresses, and also shear forces are dissipated by deformation of the meniscus radially. The menisci function in load transmission, joint stability (secondary), shock absorption, lubrication, and proprioception.

Etiology

- Injuries to the meniscus are the most common intraarticular knee injury.
- Predominantly sports related in the young patient, with a high association with ACL injury.
- Middle-aged and elderly patients predominantly have tears from long-term degeneration and are often associated with osteoarthritis.

Pathophysiology

- Ability of meniscus injuries/tears to heal is highly dependent on the zone of injury and the vascularity.
- The vascular supply changes with maturity from near-complete vascularity at birth to only the peripheral 25 % by age ten:
  - Peripheral well-vascularized area is called the red-red zone.
  - Inner avascular area is the white-white zone.
  - Watershed area between is the red-white region.
- Healing potential of the meniscus decreases from the periphery towards the central avascular area.

Presentation and Workup

- Patients present with sharp pain in the acute setting.
- May be accompanied by swelling.
- Mechanical symptoms (catching/locking).
- Locked knee if there is a displaced fragment stuck in intracondylar notch.

Physical Examination

- Joint effusion, joint line tenderness, loss of motion (with displaced/bucket handle tears), and positive McMurray test

Radiographs

- Useful to rule out bony injury or in older patients to determine if there is any associated osteoarthritis.
- MRI is advanced imaging modality of choice.
- MRI is less sensitive and specific in diagnosis of meniscus tears in the pediatric population.

Classification Tears may be classified based on

- Location (peripheral/outer versus central/inner)
- Depth (partial or full thickness)
- Types (vertical, horizontal, oblique, radial, longitudinal, complex)

Treatment

Nonsurgical Treatment

- Try for asymptomatic tears.
- Symptomatic tears that are stable and peripheral which have a good chance of healing.

Additionally, tears in the setting of significant osteoarthritis may be treated non-operatively due to possibility of ongoing knee pain from arthritis.

Surgical Treatment

- Tears in the vascular zone tend to respond well to meniscus repair surgery, with the inside-out technique considered the gold standard.
- Tears in the avascular zone have a poor prognosis after repair, and partial meniscectomy brings more predictable results.
- Meniscus repair healing rates are better when performed in conjunction with ACL reconstruction.

Complications of Meniscus Surgery *May Include*

Hemarthrosis, infection, venous thromboembolic events, neurovascular injury, repair failure, arthrofibrosis, and iatrogenic cartilage injury

5.2 Discoid Meniscus

- Most common anatomic variant of the meniscus.
- Is typically located in the lateral compartment.
- Bilateral discoid meniscus may occur in 20 % of cases.

The Watanabe classification is most commonly used with three types:

- Type I: most common. Complete discoid meniscus covering the entire tibial plateau.
- Type II: is incomplete but has normal peripheral attachments.
- Type III: least common type. Lacks normal posterior peripheral attachments, with stabilization provided by the more posterior meniscofemoral ligament (Wrisberg ligament). This variant is the most unstable.

Discoid menisci are at increased risk of developing tears:

- Becomes clinically symptomatic when peripheral attachment incompetence leads to mechanical symptoms of instability, popping, or snapping.
- Also, tears that cause peripherally stable discoid menisci to become painful or cause mechanical symptoms can be another reason for presentation.

Arthroscopic saucerization is the recommended treatment for peripherally stable (types I and II) symptomatic meniscus tears.

Saucerization with peripheral stabilization (meniscus repair) is recommended for peripherally unstable symptomatic discoid meniscus pathology (type III).

5.3 *Meniscus Transplantation*

Ideal Candidate

- Young (<50 years) patient.
- With unicompartmental activity-related knee pain in the setting of meniscal deficiency.
- Should have normal axial alignment and normal joint stability (native or post-reconstruction).
- Advanced, diffuse arthritic changes are a contraindication.

Bibliography

1. Kramer DE, Micheli LJ. Meniscal tears and discoid meniscus in children: diagnosis and treatment. J Am Acad Orthop Surg. 2009;17:698–707.
2. Makris EA, Hadidi P, Athanasiou KA. The knee meniscus: structure-function, pathophysiology, current repair techniques, and prospects for regeneration. Biomaterials. 2011;32:7411–31.
3. Noyes FR, Barber-Westin SD. Arthroscopic repair of meniscus tears extending into the avascular zone with or without anterior cruciate ligament reconstruction in patients 40 years of age and older. Arthroscopy. 2000;16:822–9.

6 Osteochondritis Dissecans and Articular Cartilage Defects

James M. Bullock

6.1 Osteochondritis Dissecans

Take-Home Message
- Etiology is unknown.
- Most commonly involved area is the lateral aspect of the medial femoral condyle.
- Most important prognostic factor is skeletal maturity.
- Evidence of fluid (high signal on T2) crossing the subchondral plate behind the lesion on MRI correlates with less successful nonoperative management.

Definition Osteochondritis dissecans (OCD) is an acquired idiopathic lesion that affects articular cartilage and/or subchondral bone.

Is seen most commonly in patients aged 10–15 years old. Males have a two-time higher incidence than females.

Etiology

- Etiology of OCD is not known.
- Theories include: genetic predisposition, hypovascularity (although osteonecrosis is not seen in fragment analysis), and traumatic or microtraumatic injury.

Presentation and Workup

- May have vague knee pain complaints, intermittent swelling, and anteromedial knee tenderness in flexion.
- May be an antalgic gait.
- If mechanical symptoms, then have a high suspicion for a loose fragment and pursue more urgent advanced imaging workup.
- Wilson sign is when there is pain with passive internal rotation and extension when ranging the knee from 90 to 0°. The pain is elicited at about 30° of flexion and should be relieved by passive external rotation which reduces the impingement of the lateral aspect of the medial femoral condyle against the medial tibial spine. This test has been shown to lack sensitivity however.
- A thorough knee exam to evaluate range of motion and ligament integrity and to determine any meniscal pathology should always be pursued.

Radiographs

Plain Radiographs

- Plain radiographs of bilateral knees should be performed to evaluate for OCD lesions. OCD may occur bilaterally in up to 30 % of cases, so workup must include bilateral knee radiographs.
- Evaluate growth plate maturity, lesion location, and stability.
- Views that should be obtained include standard weight-bearing AP, lateral views in addition to notch views. Though less common, patella involvement may occur and so merchant views should be included.
- The most commonly involved area is the lateral aspect of the medial femoral condyle.
- Larger lesions on plain film or those associated with sclerosis have been thought to have worse prognosis for nonoperative management success.

Advanced Imaging

- Classically bone scans have also been used to evaluate osteochondritis dissecans but have given way more recently to MRI.
- MRI provides useful information about cartilage integrity, as well as the subchondral bone, extent of bony edema, and presence of loose bodies.
- Evidence of fluid (high signal on T2) crossing the subchondral plate behind the lesion on MRI correlates with less successful nonoperative management results and is found in almost three quarters of all unstable lesions.

Classification Classified based on specific location, fragmentation, and/or displacement and skeletal maturity.

Patients with open physes at presentation have juvenile-onset OCD versus those that present when skeletal mature have adult OCD.

Treatment Most important prognostic factor is skeletal maturity, and this plays a role in determining appropriate treatment.

- Nonoperative management techniques include:

Activity modification that can range from cessation of sporting activity to non-weight-bearing restrictions with use of crutches and/or immobilization braces, pain medication (typically non-antiinflammatory medication), and strengthening.

- Nonoperative management is generally speaking more favorable in juvenile OCD, whereas adult forms typically do worse with nonoperative treatment:
  - Even in the juvenile OCD population, families should be counseled that the success rate might be as low as 50 %.

Surgical Treatment

- Cases that have failed nonoperative management or that have imaging findings consistent with unstable lesions are candidates for surgical treatment.

- The size, location, and stability of the lesion play a role in deciding repair versus reconstructive surgery.
- Arthroscopic findings of cartilage appearance and stability play a significant role in decision making.

Possible surgical interventions according to cartilage integrity and fragment stability are

- Stable lesions with intact cartilage → retrograde (transarticular) or antegrade (transepiphyseal avoiding the articular cartilage) drilling have good success, especially in the skeletally immature patient. The aim is to create channels for revascularization to promote healing. Success of drilling is higher in patients with open physes and is worse in cases with lesions in atypical locations, with multiple lesions, or with medical comorbidities.
- Unstable lesions with intact cartilage → open reduction and internal fixation ± compression and bone grafting are advocated. Excision has classically had poor results.
- Full-thickness cartilage defects → salvage options include osteochondral autograft, autologous chondrocyte implantation, mosaicplasty, and osteochondral allograft.
- In the adult population there may be an association with limb malalignment, and in these cases full-length lower extremity radiographs should be utilized to determine if corrective surgery for malalignment is indicated.
- Postoperative immobilization and weight-bearing restrictions are typically employed with progression over time to normal ambulation when there is comfort with course of healing.
- MRI may be employed in operative and nonoperative cases to follow the lesions and assess healing.

6.2 Articular Cartilage Defects

Articular Cartilage

- Poor intrinsic ability to heal.
- Various techniques have been developed to try and address articular cartilage injury.

The modified outerbridge system is one classification system for full-thickness articular cartilage defects:

- Grade I: softening
- Grade II: fibrillation/fissures
- Grade III: deep fissures but no exposed subchondral bone
- Grade IV: subchondral bone exposed

Bone Marrow Reparative Techniques

- Microfracture or drilling leads to development of fibrocartilage which is predominantly type I collagen, in contrast to type II collagen which predominates in hyaline cartilage.

Microfracture

- Will have best success when the lesion is contained, and the edges are prepared to stable cartilage with removal of the calcified cartilage base prior to drilling.
- Younger patients (less than 40 years old) have superior outcomes with microfracture.

Osteochondral Transplantation

- For full-thickness cartilage defects:
- May be autologous or allograft transplantation

Osteochondral Autograft Transplantations

- Better results in some series versus microfracture but is a more involved procedure with potential donor site morbidity and mismatch of cartilage thickness from donor site

Allograft Osteochondral Procedures

- No donor site morbidity but cell viability is lower, and there are risks of disease transmission versus autograft.

Autologous Chondrocyte Implantation

- Costly and involves staged procedures for harvesting, time for growth of chondrocytes, additional procedure for implantation, and potential issues with the periosteal flap used to stabilize the chondrocytes.
- Matrix-associated autologous chondrocyte implantation was created to have an appropriate implantable carrier for the chondrocytes that lacked the donor site morbidity of periosteal flaps.

Bibliography

1. Bedi A, Feeley BT, Williams RJ 3rd. Management of articular cartilage defects of the knee. J Bone Joint Surg Am. 2010;92(4):994–1009.
2. Cahill BR. Osteochondritis dissecans of the knee: treatment of juvenile and adult forms. J Am Acad Orthop Surg. 1995;3:237–47.
3. Chiroff RT, Cooke CP III. Osteochondritis dissecans: a histologic and microscopic analysis of surgically excised lesions. J Trauma. 1975;15:689–96.
4. Crawford DC, Safran MR. Osteochondritis dissecans of the knee. J Am Acad Orthop Surg. 2006;14:90–100.
5. De Smet AA, Ilahi OA, Graf BK. Untreated osteochondritis dissecans of the femoral condyles: prediction of patient outcome using radiographic and MR findings. Skeletal Radiol. 1997;26:463–7.
6. Kocher MS, Tucker R, Ganley TJ, Flynn JM. Management of osteochondritis dissecans of the knee. Current concepts review. Am J Sports Med. 2006;34(7):1181–91.
7. Kreuz PC, Erggelet C, Steinwachs MR, Krause SJ, Lahm A, Niemeyer P, Ghanem N, Uhl M, Sudkamp N. Is microfracture of chondral defects in the knee associated with different results in patients aged 40 years or younger? Arthroscopy. 2006;22(11):1180–6.

7 Osteotomies About the Knee

James M. Bullock

7.1 *Osteotomy for Knee Instability/Ligament-Deficient Knees*

High Tibial Osteotomies

- Classically been used for coronal plane malalignment correction.
- More recently indications expanded to include cruciate-ligament-deficient knees that have sagittal plane imbalance:
  - A high tibial osteotomy that is fashioned to decrease posterior tibial slope can aid the ACL-deficient knee.
  - A high tibial osteotomy fashioned to increase anterior tibial slope can be used to aid the PCL-deficient knee by causing anterior tibial translation.
- In patients with chronic posterolateral instability and varus thrust, biplanar osteotomy can be a part of treatment to address the combined PCL and posterolateral corner-deficient knee:
  - However, this may possibly only impact the static instability of the knee according to some biomechanical evaluation.

7.2 *Osteotomy for Patellofemoral Pathology*

While the majority of patient-athletes that present with anterior knee pain from patellofemoral etiology will respond to nonoperative treatment, some patients require further intervention to alleviate their symptoms.

Workup of Anterior Knee Pain

- Requires thorough history, physical exam, and appropriate imaging tests.
- Static evaluation of the Q angle may have some utility, though controversial in the literature.
- Dynamic evaluation of the patient ambulating and ranging the knee actively and passively are critical components of the exam.
- Evaluating stability of the patella with lateral translation at 30° will give important information about the status of the MPFL ligament in instability cases.
- Muscle tone evaluation of the extensor mechanism is also crucial.
- Comparison to the contralateral knee is a necessary component of the exam.
- Evaluate for generalized ligament laxity.
- Patella height and tilt must be evaluated clinically as well as radiographically.

Patella height can be evaluated by a number of ratios (Fig. 4).

- An Insall-Salvati ratio of >1.2 is considered patella alta. This method may be flawed because of variations in nonarticular portion of the inferior patella.
- Modified Insall-Salvati index addresses this potential error and has a normal mean of 1.25, and any value over 2 is considered patella alta.

Tibial Tubercle-Trochlear Groove (TT-TG) Distance

- Initially described based on CT scan.
- Greater than 20 mm is abnormal.
- Obtained by drawing a perpendicular line to a line tangential to posterior cortex to the center of the patella tendon at tibial tubercle and the center of the trochlea at its deepest point. The distance between the two points is the TT-TG distance.

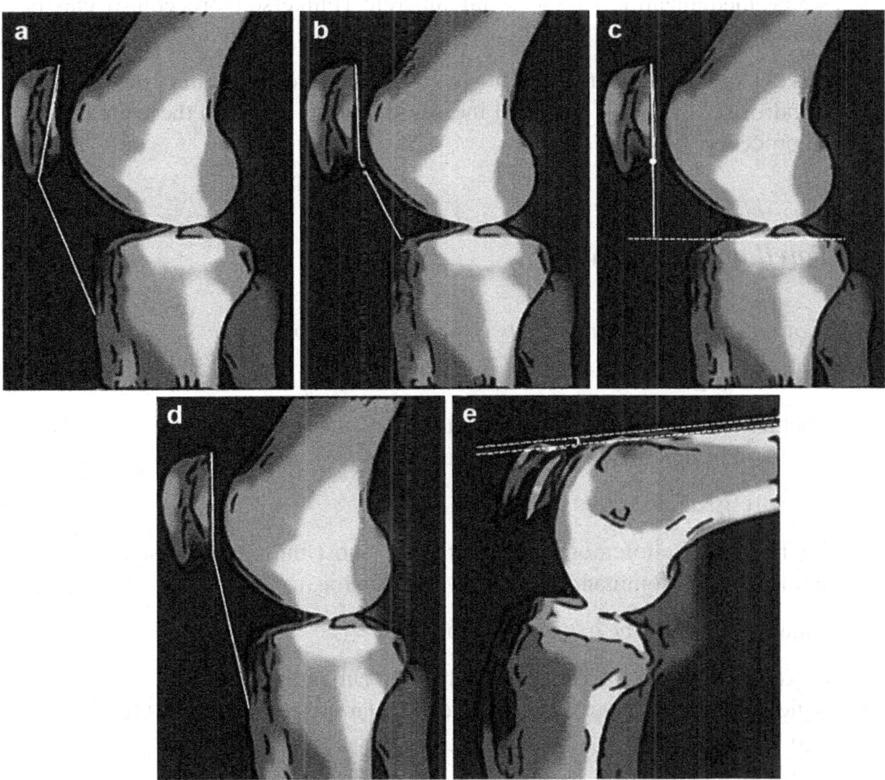

Fig. 4 Measurements of patellar height on lateral radiographs. (**a**) Insall-Salvati index. (**b**) Caton-Deschamps index. (**c**) Blackburne-Peel index. (**d**) Modified Insall-Salvati index. (**e**) Labelle-Laurin measurement (Figure adapted from Feller JA. Distal realignment (tibial tuberosity transfer). Sports Med Arthr 2012.)

- It can help understand the extent of lateralization that needs to be corrected and should be reduced to a range from 10 to 15 mm.
- MRI has been employed to measure TT-TG distance recently; however, the distance for pathologic lateralization when using MRI should be >18 mm.

7.3 Patellofemoral Osteoarthritis/Articular Cartilage Lesions

Distal realignment procedures (osteotomies of the tibial tubercle) have been described in various forms.

- Originally, straight anteriorization was described by Maquet, but this leads to unfavorable results and issues with skin necrosis.
- Currently in patients with patella alta and lateral facet or distal patella chondrosis, anteromedialization of the tibial tubercle (Fulkerson procedure) can be performed:
  - This is recommended in a patient who does not have proximal or medial facet chondrosis, because of potential increased contact forces in these areas after the procedure.

7.4 Patellar Instability

Stability of the Patellofemoral Joint Is Dependent on Appropriate

- Articular/bony geometry
  - Trochlea groove anatomy is the most important bony restraint, particularly of the lateral trochlea groove more distally.
- Passive soft tissue restraints
  - The medial patellofemoral ligament is the most important passive restraint and does so predominantly at 30° of knee flexion.
- Muscular function of the extensor mechanism
  - In extension lateral displacement with quad activation.
  - In flexion quad activation seats the patellar posteriorly into the trochlea groove.

Treatment Recommendations After Failed Nonoperative Management

If there is normal trochlea geometry, normal TT-TG distance, and normal patella height → MPFL reconstruction

In cases with normal patella height and increased TT-TG distance → medicalization

If there is increased TT-TG distance as well as patella alta → distalization and medialization of the tibial tubercle

Complications of Tibial Tubercle Transfer

- Proximal tibia fracture
- Acute compartment syndrome
- Nonunion or delayed union
- Medial compartment osteoarthritis as a result of overloading medial compartment
- Persistent patellofemoral pain
- Hardware prominence
- Patella baja

Bibliography

1. Camp CL, Stuart MJ, Krych AJ, et al. CT and MRI measurements of tibial tubercle-trochlear groove distances are not equivalent in patients with patellar instability. Am J Sports Med. 2013;41:1835–40.
2. Colvin AC, West RV. Patellar instability. J Bone Joint Surg Am. 2008;90:2751–62.
3. Feller JA. Distal realignment (tibial tuberosity transfer). Sports Med Arthrosc. 2012;20:152–61.
4. Fulkerson JP. Diagnosis and treatment of patients with patellofemoral pain. Am J Sports Med. 2002;30:447–56.
5. Giffin JR, Stabile KJ, Zantop T, Vogrin TM, Woo SL, Harner CD. Importance of tibial slope for stability of the posterior cruciate ligament-deficient knee. Am J Sports Med. 2007;35:1443–9.
6. Petrigliano FA, Suero EM, Voos JE, Pearle AD, Allen AA. The effect of proximal tibial slope on dynamic stability testing of the posterior cruciate ligament- and posterolateral corner-deficient knee. Am J Sports Med. 2012;40:1322–8.
7. Savarese E, Bisicchia S, Romeo R, Amendola A. Role of high tibial osteotomy in chronic injuries of posterior cruciate ligament and posterolateral corner. J Orthop Traumatol. 2011;12:1–17.

8 Osteotomies About the Knee for Coronal Malalignment: High Tibial Osteotomy and Distal Femoral Osteotomy

James M. Bullock

Peak forces during walking can be up to three times the body weight. In the coronal plane if there is deformity, the medial or lateral compartment may see an unequal share of the load across the knee, if there is significant varus or valgus deformity, respectively.

Osteotomies are aimed at correcting this deformity to normalize peak stress sharing across the knee and to offload a compartment that may be seeing increased forces leading to arthrosis. Oftentimes though corrective osteotomies have effects on other planes, and in high tibial osteotomies, this includes the sagittal plane typically.

Goals

- Off-load compartment that has arthritic changes.
- Delay need for total knee arthroplasty.

Workup

Thorough History and Physical (H&P). Enquire about duration of any symptoms of pain, any injury history.

Assess lower-limb alignment in all three planes (coronal, sagittal, and rotational).

Evaluate gait (look for varus thrust).

Evaluate ROM.

Radiographs should include standard knee series as well as foot-to-hip standing alignment films.

Indications

- Unicompartmental osteoarthritis
- Varus or valgus malalignment
- Osteochondral lesions/osteochondritis dissecans/osteonecrosis
- Posterolateral instability
- Correct malalignment in conjunction with chondral resurfacing procedures

Ideal candidate is young (<65 years), is active, and has isolated unicompartmental tibiofemoral degenerative joint disease, with preserved motion and stable ligamentous status.

Contraindications

- *Significant involvement of other compartment(s)*
  - *Bi- or tricompartmental DJD*
- *Advanced arthrosis of involved compartment to be off-loaded*
- *Insufficient meniscal tissue on lateral compartment*
- *Inflammatory arthritis*
- *Elderly* (>65 years; may benefit more from TKA)
- *Need for massive correction* (>20°)

8.1 Varus Malalignment

Options for valgus producing osteotomies include:

- Medial opening wedge
- Lateral closing wedge

- Dome osteotomies

The Medial Opening Wedge Osteotomy

- Is the *most common* high tibial osteotomy (HTO) performed for varus malalignment.
- Surgical goal is to typically introduce slight valgus alignment (3–6°) of a varus knee by moving the mechanical axis from falling in the medial compartment to the Fujisawa point 62 % of the width of the knee from medial to lateral.

Complications/Things to Avoid in HTO

- *Peroneal nerve palsy:*
  - With lateral closing wedge osteotomy where proximal fibula cuts are made, the nerve is most at risk. The proximal 2 cm is considered a safe zone.
- *Vascular injury:*
  - Popliteal artery at risk for posterior tibia cortical cuts. Flexion causes retraction away from the cortex and careful retractor placement and technique will help minimize risk.
- In all patients but especially in those with cruciate ligament insufficiency, there *must be particular focus on potential alteration to tibial slope*. For medial opening wedge osteotomies, if the cut for correction is centered anterior to midline, it will create increased tibial slope posteriorly. This has the effect of increasing contact area posteriorly as well as tension on the ACL. Avoid by elevating posterior portion just as much by centering elevation midline or posterior to midline.
- If tibial tubercle remains attached to distal fragment when the opening wedge is created, it can lead to *patella baja* and overload of the patella. Therefore, perform opening wedge with tibial tuberosity on proximal fragment.
- *Fracture* through cortex or into articular surface:
  - Should be addressed if recognized intraoperatively
  - Increases nonunion rates
- *Nonunion* rate is higher with medial opening wedge osteotomy than lateral closing wedge osteotomy. Risk factors are diabetes, smoking/tobacco use, and fracture of far cortex.
- *Compartment syndrome.*
- *Infection.*
- *Venous thromboembolism.*
- *Hardware failure.*

8.2 Valgus Malalignment and Distal Femoral Osteotomy

- Isolated lateral compartment DJD is less common.
- A medial closing wedge osteotomy of the proximal tibia can correct the malalignment but leaves an oblique tibiofemoral joint line:

 – Results of medial closing wedge osteotomies are not as successful as the opening wedge osteotomies for varus malalignment:
 • One of the reasons for this is that the obliquity of the joint line may remain, leading to dynamic problems of malalignment despite correcting the mechanical axis.
 – The coronal obliquity of the joint line should be ≤5°, at the end of malalignment correction. A key point in osteotomies in general for coronal malalignment is to address the deformity in the bone that sees most of the deformity.
- In deformities requiring 12° or more of correction, high tibial osteotomy for valgus malalignment should not be considered.
- As a result of the poorer success of medial closing wedge proximal tibial osteotomies, varus producing *distal femoral osteotomy is recommended.*
 – *Medial wedge closing distal femoral osteotomy is the procedure of choice.*
 – Lateral opening wedge distal femur osteotomy can also be used to correct valgus malalignment but delayed union/nonunion can be an issue.
 – This can be done with blade plate fixation or locking plates and has had higher rates of healing in studies than staples.
 – With severe valgus malalignment, the patellofemoral joint is often involved due to effects on the Q angle and lateral subluxation. There have been studies that show however that patella tracking is improved with distal femoral osteotomy and clinical results have not been adversely affected in the presence of patellofemoral arthritis.
 – *The goal is to move the mechanical axis to be centered in the medial portion of the tibial interspinous region but not over into the medial compartment.*

Bibliography

1. Amis AA. Biomechanics of high tibial osteotomy. Knee Surg Sports Traumatol Arthrosc. 2013;21:197–205.
2. Gardiner A, Richmond JC. Periarticular osteotomies for degenerative joint disease of the knee. Sports Med Arthrosc. 2013;21:38–46.
3. Rossi R, Bonasia DE, Amendola A. The role of high tibial osteotomy in the varus knee. J Am Acad Orthop Surg. 2011;19:590–9.
4. Wang JW, Hsu CC. Distal femoral varus osteotomy for osteoarthritis of the knee. J Bone Joint Surg Am. 2005;87:127–33.
5. Wang JW, Hsu CC. Distal femoral varus osteotomy for osteoarthritis of the knee. Surgical technique. J Bone Joint Surg Am. 2006;88(Suppl 1 Pt 1): 100–8.
6. Wright JM, Crockett HC, Slawski DP, Madsen MW, Windsor RE. High tibial osteotomy. J Am Acad Orthop Surg. 2005;13:279–89.

9 Patellofemoral Disorders

Scott Kling

Take-Home Message

- The MPFL is the primary restraint to lateral translation of the patella during the first 20° of knee flexion.
- There is no significant difference with regard to pain, functional level, and re-dislocation rate when comparing nonoperative and operative treatment of first-time dislocators. Recurrent dislocation is an indication for surgical intervention.
- Radiographic criterion warranting a realignment procedure is TT-TG distance greater than 20 mm.
- MPFL reconstruction is an extremely effective technique, with near 0 % re-dislocation rate.

Epidemiology

- Patellofemoral instability most commonly occurs in the second to third decades of life.
- It can be classified into two categories: acute and chronic.
- Acute instability occurs secondary to trauma and occurs with equal frequency in both genders.
- Chronic instability is far more common in women, is characterized by multiple atraumatic episodes, and is often associated with extremity malalignment.

Anatomy

- The primary restraint to lateral translation of the patella during the first 20° of knee flexion is the medial patellofemoral ligament (MPFL).
- The MPFL inserts between the medial epicondyle and the adductor tubercle of the femur:
  - The femoral side is the most common site of avulsion.
- With deeper knee flexion, additional constraint is contributed by trochlear morphology, patellar height, and patellofemoral axis alignment.
- Dynamic restraint is primarily initiated by the vastus medialis obliquus (VMO).

Pathophysiology

- The mechanism of injury is often a noncontact twisting injury with the knee fully extended.
- Immediate reduction of the dislocated patella often occurs manually after the patient contracts the quadriceps.

- Direct blows to the knee are a less common cause of dislocation.
- Multiple predisposing factors exist for patellofemoral instability and should be investigated during the evaluation. These include patella alta, lateral femoral condyle hypoplasia/trochlear dysplasia, increased Q angle/tibial tubercle-trochlear groove (TT-TG) distance, generalized ligamentous laxity, "miserable malalignment syndrome" (femoral anteversion, genu valgum, external tibial torsion), and previous patellar instability event (MPFL insufficiency).

Presentation

- Patients often recount a noncontact twisting injury to the knee and experience a "pop" sensation. They note significant anterior knee pain, often localized over the MPFL.
- Physical examination will often demonstrate a large hemarthrosis. Standing alignment and gait should be assessed. There may be quadriceps atrophy or inhibition in the presence of an effusion. A straight leg raise with inspection of extensor lag should be conducted. Patellar translation is increased when compared to the contralateral knee (often assessed via patellar quadrants). Greater than two quadrants, or when the medial patellar border can be forcibly translated to the lateral edge of the trochlear groove, is considered abnormal. Patellar apprehension is commonly found, with guarding during passive lateral translation. In cases of chronic instability, an increased Q angle may be measured. Additionally, a J sign may be observed where the patella rides laterally in extension and then abruptly reduces into the trochlear groove with increasing flexion.
- A thorough ligamentous exam of the knee must be performed to rule out confounding injuries such as cruciate ligament, collateral ligament, and meniscal tear.
- Beighton's signs of ligamentous laxity should also be tested.

Imaging

- A standard knee X-ray series should always be obtained, including flexion weight-bearing PA, lateral, and merchant views.
- The lateral view is critical in determination of patellar height, which may be assessed using any of the published methodologies such as Insall-Salvati ratio.
- The classic "crossing sign" may also be visualized on the lateral view as an indicator or trochlear dysplasia.
- The merchant view may be used to measure lateral patellar displacement, sulcus and congruence angle, and lateral patellofemoral angle.
- CT scan is helpful in determining TT-TG distance (greater than 20 mm is considered abnormal).
- MRI will consistently demonstrate the bone bruising pattern in the medial patellar facet and lateral femoral condyle. Chondral lesions with associated loose bodies are frequently visualized. Axial cuts will reliably indentify the integrity of the MPFL and its location of injury.

Nonoperative Treatment

- Nonoperative management is the mainstay of treatment for the first-time dislocator. This initially consists of brace treatment in extension 10–14 days (some advocate up to 6 weeks).
- There is a three times greater likelihood of re-dislocation with immediate mobilization.
- This is followed by rehabilitation for 3–6 weeks. This includes early mobilization with advancement of weight bearing, quadriceps strengthening sets, and patellar mobilizations. Once active and passive range of motion is restored, closed kinetic chain strength training and proprioception may be initialized (includes core and hip strengthening to improve limb positioning and balance). Finally, the patient should undertake functional and sports-specific training.
- Return to play is 16 % at 6 weeks and 69 % at 6 months.
- Multiple randomized control trials demonstrate no significant difference with regard to pain, functional level, and re-dislocation rate when comparing nonoperative and operative treatment of first-time dislocators.
- Up to 50 % of patients will progress to recurrent dislocations regardless of treatment method.
- Nonoperative management is not indicated in the treatment or recurrent dislocations, though bracing and rehabilitation may prove helpful in the short term for patient comfort.

Operative Treatment

- Indications for surgical intervention include recurrent traumatic dislocations and recurrent atraumatic dislocations that fail bracing and physical therapy, as well as concomitant osteochondral defect or loose body.
- Radiographic criterion warranting a realignment procedure is TT-TG distance greater than 20 mm.
- Surgical options for acute dislocators include medial retinacular reefing or MPFL repair/augmentation. These procedures have not proven more effective than nonoperative treatment.
- The primary indication for lateral release is patellar tilt or lateral patellar compression syndrome. It has not shown to reduce lateral subluxation and may cause iatrogenic medial subluxation, as well as increase the rate of lateral dislocation.
- There are multiple options for surgical management of chronic instability.
- The mainstay of distal realignment is the tibial tubercle osteotomy. This may be accomplished via pure medialization (Elmslie-Trillat) or anteromedialization (Fulkerson). Distalization can be incorporated to compensate for patella alta.
- Anteromedialization unloads lateral facet and distal pole of the patella, but should not exceed greater than 15 mm.
- Degenerative changes are correlated with worse clinical results, with proximal and medial chondral lesions having a particularly poor prognosis.
- Satisfactory surgical outcomes are seen in 70–90 % of patients.
- MPFL reconstruction is an extremely effective technique, with 80–96 % good to excellent results and near 0 % re-dislocation rates.

- Intraoperatively, the location of the femoral MPFL insertion may be reliably identified radiographically at Schottle point.
- Autograft or allograft may be used in the setting of preexisting ligamentous laxity.
- MPFL reconstruction may be combined successfully with a distal realignment procedure.
- Proximal realignment (VMO advancement) and trochleoplasty/trochlear osteotomy are additional, less studied surgical options.
- Postoperative rehabilitation is similar to nonoperative treatment, with expected return to sports-related activities at 3 months.

Complications

- Complications of surgical treatment include recurrent instability, excessive medial constraint, persistent pain, arthrofibrosis, tibial or patella fracture, and cutaneous nerve injury.

Bibliography

1. Alexis Chiang Colvin, West RV. Patellar instability. J Bone Joint Surg Am. 2008;90:2751–62.
2. Dejour H, Walch G, Nove-Josserand L, et al. Factors of patellar instability: an anatomic radiographic study. Knee Surg Sports Traumatol Arthrosc. 1994;(2)1:19–26.
3. Fithian DC, Paxton EW, Stone ML, Silva P, Davis DK, Elias DA, White LM. Epidemiology and natural history of acute patellar dislocation. AJSM. 2004;32:1114–21.
4. Schöttle PB, Schmeling A, Rosenstiel N, Weiler A. Radiographic landmarks for femoral tunnel placement in medial patellofemoral ligament reconstruction. Am J Sports Med. 2007;35(5):801–4. Epub 2007 Jan 31.

10 Knee Osteonecrosis

Justin Arner

Take-Home Message

- Osteonecrosis is a difficult disease to treat due to its unknown etiology, mechanism, and its lack of definitive treatment options.
- Spontaneous ON of the knee is more commonly seen in older female patients and is unilateral in the medial femoral condyle.
- Secondary ON is classically seen in younger male patients and is often bilateral with other joint involvement.
- Early diagnosis is key to prevent disease progression to debilitating arthritis, and treatment is individualized based on symptomatology and stage.

Definitions

- Osteonecrosis (ON) of the knee is a progressive disease which comes in three forms:
  - Spontaneous osteonecrosis of the knee
  - Secondary osteonecrosis
  - Postarthroscopic osteonecrosis

Etiology

Spontaneous ON

- Exact etiology is unknown:
  - One possible cause is subchondral insufficiency fracture.
- Commonly in elderly women with osteopenia.

Secondary ON

- Etiology is unknown.
- Risk factors: corticosteroid use, alcohol abuse, sickle cell disease, myeloproliferative disorders, caisson disease, and Gaucher disease.

Postarthroscopic ON

- Rare complication after arthroscopic knee surgery with unknown etiology

Pathophysiology

- Clinical diagnosis can be difficult as physical exam findings are many times nonspecific.
- Conditions such as osteochondritis dissecans, osteoarthritis, bone bruises, meniscal tears, transient osteopenia of the knee, and pes anserine bursitis can all have similar presentations.

Spontaneous ON

- Most common site: epiphysis of the medial femoral condyle, and it occurs unilaterally:
  - ~2 % of cases involve the medial tibial plateau.
  - Rarely the patella and lateral femoral condyle are involved.
- Presentation is sudden well-defined medial knee pain which is often worse at night and with weight bearing.
- More commonly unilateral and in women.

Secondary ON

- Often multifocal, involves both femoral condyles, and occurs in the epiphysis, metaphysis, and diaphysis.

- More commonly in men, patients <45 years of age, and with defined risk factors.
- Bilateral in 80 % of patients, and about 75 % of patients have other joint involvement (shoulder, hip, ankle).
- More insidious and nonspecific onset.

Postarthroscopic ON

- Most common location is on the medial femoral condyle but also occurs in the lateral femoral condyle and very rarely in the other bony regions of the knee (Table 1).

Radiographs

X-Ray

- Findings are not always evident initially.
- AP and lateral X-ray may show advanced osteonecrosis with collapse or impending collapse.
- Flattening of the weight-bearing portion of the joint is the first radiographic evidence.
- As the disease progresses, subchondral radiolucency with surrounding sclerosis can be seen which can progress to subchondral bone collapse and therefore secondary arthritis.
- As mentioned previously, the most common location differs among the two types:
  - Spontaneous ON: medial femoral condyle.
  - Secondary ON: both condyles are equally affected.

MRI

- Is the imagining modality of choice for further investigation of ON.
- It can reveal the extent of disease earlier and more completely.
- However, the finding of bone marrow edema is nonspecific:
  - Conditions such as bone bruise, microfracture, osteoarthritis, or transient osteoporosis can have a similar look on MRI.
- Serpentine lesions with a well-demarcated border are necessary to make the disease diagnosis.
- Because secondary ON is very commonly bilateral and involves other joints, screening of other joint involvement is a reasonable consideration but has not been well established.

Technetium-99 m Bone Scans

- Also can be used to evaluate ON.
- In one study, bone scans only detected 64 % of ON, while MRI detected all histologically found lesions.
- Bone scans have been shown to be more effective in diagnosing spontaneous ON than secondary ON but are only 40–70 % specific.
- Secondary ON is more difficult to diagnose because bilateral and multifocal uptake could indicate other processes such as degenerative change and malignancy.

Table 1 Osteonecrosis of the knee

	Sex	Age	Presentation	Other joint involvement	Risk factors	Anatomic location	Possible mechanisms	Treatment options
Spontaneous ON of the knee	Female	>50 years	Sudden well defined pain	Rare	Idiopathic, microtrauma, osteoporosis	Medical femoral condyle	Subchondral fracture	Conservative treatment, if no improvement in 3 months, surgical intervention
Secondary ON of the knee	Male	<45 years	Insidious onset, non specific	>80 % bilateral, >90 % other joint involvement	Trauma, caisson disease, Gaucher disease, chemotherapy, alcohol abuse, coagulopathies, corticosteriod use, smoking, systemic lupus erythematosus, organ transplant, inflammatory bowel disease	Epiphysis, metaphysis, diaphysis	Reduced blood flow	Conservative treatment has not been shown to be successful, surgical intervention suggested
Postarthroscopic ON of the knee	Any	Any	After arthoscopic knee surgery	Never	Cartilage debridement, meniscectomy, ACL reconstruction	Medical femoral condyle	Direct trauma, subchondral fracture	Conservative treatment

Current recommendations suggest initial evaluation by plain radiographs with MRI as a more specific and confirmatory test.

If malignancy is a consideration, core biopsy may be preformed.

Microscopic evaluation shows empty lacunae with a center of fatty degeneration and surrounding osseous formation with osteoblasts and fibrovascular granulation and cartilage formation.

Other possible workup to evaluate this condition includes a lipid profile, a workup of sickle cell disease, and testing for coagulopathies.

Classification

- There are four stage systems to classify ON.
- Ficat classification is commonly used.
- Stage III is always a crescent sign meaning subchondral collapse has occurred and surgical intervention is usually indicated.
- Larger lesions have been shown to predict progression.

Treatment Treatment is not well established.

Spontaneous ON

- Nonoperative treatment has produced good outcomes.
- Precollapse spontaneous ON:
  - Treatment should involve protected weight bearing, pain medications, and nonsteroidal anti-inflammatory medications.
  - Over 89 % of patients show resolution of symptoms without radiographic progression with this conservative treatment.
- Surgical intervention is reserved for patients who do not improve 3 months after onset.

Secondary ON

- Nonoperative treatment has not been proven to be as successful.
- Progression to advanced stages occurs in about 80 % of patients.
- For this reason, operative intervention is recommended.
- Pharmacologic agents, such as diphosphonates, iloprost, and anticoagulants, have not shown consistent results and lack large randomized trials and therefore are not currently recommended for ON.

Postarthroscopic ON

- Nonoperative treatment includes protected weight bearing, analgesics, and NSAIDs.
- Few studies exist evaluating treatment modalities with this rare disease.

Surgical intervention includes arthroscopic debridement, osteochondral grafts, core decompression, bone grafting, high tibial osteotomy, and knee arthroplasty.

- Arthroscopic debridement
  - Has shown inconclusive results as it is not treating the underlying cause but rather concomitant meniscal and joint pathology.
  - Arthroscopy can however give the surgeon additional information regarding the lesions and coexisting knee pathology.

Osteochondral autologous transplantation

- Beneficial in spontaneous ON as it is usually unifocal

Core decompression

- Proposed mechanism is to decompress the marrow pressure and allow for revascularization.
- Has shown success in early ON and can delay the need for total knee arthroplasty.
- Must be performed before subchondral collapse.

Bone graft

- Spontaneous ON
  - Report a significant decrease in pain without radiographic progression of disease at 2 years.
- Secondary ON
  - Shown good results in early disease
  - Provides a new scaffold to subchondral bone to help prevent its collapse

High tibial osteotomy (HTO)

- Spontaneous ON
  - Good outcomes in the right patient but is rarely utilized
- Secondary ON
  - No utilized as usually multifocal

Unicompartmental knee arthroplasty

- Used to treat advanced ON in spontaneous ON and postarthroscopic ON if the lesions are unicondylar

Total knee arthroplasty

- Has led to excellent results in secondary osteonecrosis as well as in postarthroscopic ON

Bibliography

1. Adachi N, Ochi M, Deie M, Ishikawa M, Ito Y. Osteonecrosis of the knee treated with a tissue-engineered cartilage and bone implant. A case report. J Bone Joint Surg Am. 2007;89(12):2752–7.

2. Ahlbäck S, Bauer GCH, Bohne WH. Spontaneous osteonecrosis of the knee. Arthritis Rheum. 1968;11:705–33.
3. Akamatsu Y, Mitsugi N, Hayashi T, Kobayashi H, Saito T. Low bone mineral density is associated with the onset of spontaneous osteonecrosis of the knee. Acta Orthop. 2012;83:249–55.
4. Breer S, Oheim R, Krause M, Marshall RP, Amling M, Barvencik F. Spontaneous osteonecrosis of the knee (SONK). Knee Surg Sports Traumatol Arthrosc. 2013;21(2):340–5.
5. Deie M, Ochi M, Adachi N, Nishimori M, Yokota K. Artificial bone grafting [calcium hydroxyapatite ceramic with an interconnected porous structure (IP-CHA)] and core decompression for spontaneous osteonecrosis of the femoral condyle in the knee. Knee Surg Sports Traumatol Arthrosc. 2008;16(8):753–8.
6. Duany NG, Zywiel MG, McGrath MS, Siddiqui JA, Jones LC, Bonutti PM, Mont MA. Joint-preserving surgical treatment of spontaneous osteonecrosis of the knee. Arch Orthop Trauma Surg. 2010;130(1):11–6. doi: 10.1007/s00402-009-0872-2.
7. Flynn JM, Springfield DS, Mankin HJ. Osteoarticular allografts to treat distal femoral osteonecrosis. Clin Orthop Relat Res. 1994;(303):38–43.
8. Forst J, Forst R, Heller KD, Adam G. Spontaneous osteonecrosis of the femoral condyle: causal treatment by early core decompression. Arch Orthop Trauma Surg. 1998;117(1–2):18–22.
9. Glueck CJ, Freiberg RA, Boppana S, Wang P. Thrombophilia, hypofibrinolysis, the eNOS T-786C polymorphism, and multifocal osteonecrosis. J Bone Joint Surg Am. 2008;90(10):2220–9. doi: 10.2106/JBJS.G.00616.
10. Johnson TC, Evans JA, Gilley JA, DeLee JC. Osteonecrosis of the knee after arthroscopic surgery for meniscal tears and chondral lesions. Arthroscopy. 2000;16(3):254–61.
11. Jureus J, Lindstrand A, Geijer M, Roberts D, Tägil M. Treatment of spontaneous osteonecrosis of the knee (SPONK) by a bisphosphonate. Acta Orthop. 2012;83(5):511–4.
12. Juréus J, Lindstrand A, Geijer M, Robertsson O, Tägil M. The natural course of spontaneous osteonecrosis of the knee (SPONK): a 1- to 27-year follow-up of 40 patients. Acta Orthop. 2013;84(4):410–4.
13. Koshino T. The treatment of spontaneous osteonecrosis of the knee by high tibial osteotomy with and without bone-grafting or drilling of the lesion. J Bone Joint Surg Am. 1982;64(1):47–58.
14. Koshino T, Okamoto R, Takamura K. Arthroscopy in spontaneous osteonecrosis of the knee. Orthop Clin North Am. 1979;10(3):609–18.
15. Lieberman JR, Varthi AG, Polkowski GG 2nd. Osteonecrosis of the knee – which joint preservation procedures work? J Arthroplasty. 2014;29:52–6.
16. MacDessi SJ, Brophy RH, Bullough PG, Windsor RE, Sculco TP. Subchondral fracture following arthroscopic knee surgery. A series of eight cases. J Bone Joint Surg Am. 2008;90(5):1007–12. doi: 10.2106/JBJS.G.00445. Review. PubMed PMID: 18451392.
17. Mears SC, McCarthy EF, Jones LC, Hungerford DS, Mont MA. Characterization and pathological characteristics of spontaneous osteonecrosis of the knee. Iowa Orthop J. 2009;29:38–42.

18. Meier C, Kraenzlin C, Friederich NF, Wischer T, Grize L, Meier CR, Kraenzlin ME. Effect of ibandronate on spontaneous osteonecrosis of the knee: a randomized, double-blind, placebo-controlled trial. Osteoporos Int. 2014;25:359–66.
19. Mont MA, Baumgarten KM, Rifai A, Bluemke DA, Jones LC, Hungerford DS. Atraumatic osteonecrosis of the knee. J Bone Joint Surg Am. 2000;82(9):1279–90.
20. Mont MA, Marker DR, Zywiel MG, Carrino JA. Osteonecrosis of the knee and related conditions. J Am Acad Orthop Surg. 2011;19(8):482–94.
21. Mont MA, Tomek IM, Hungerford DS. Core decompression for avascular necrosis of the distal femur: long term followup. Clin Orthop. .1997;(334):124–30.
22. Mont MA, Ulrich SD, Seyler TM, Smith JM, Marker DR, McGrath MS, Hungerford DS, Jones LC. Bone scanning of limited value for diagnosis of symptomatic oligofocal and multifocal osteonecrosis. J Rheumatol. 2008;35(8):1629–34. Epub 2008 Jun 1.
23. Motohashi M, Morii T, Koshino T. Clinical course and roentgenographic changes of osteonecrosis in the femoral condyle under conservative treatment. Clin Orthop Relat Res. 1991;(266):156–61.
24. Myers TG, Cui Q, Kuskowski M, Mihalko WM, Saleh KJ. Outcomes of total and unicompartmental knee arthroplasty for secondary and spontaneous osteonecrosis of the knee. J Bone Joint Surg Am. 2006;88(Suppl 3):76–82.
25. Parratte S, Argenson JN, Dumas J, Aubaniac JM. Unicompartmental knee arthroplasty for avascular osteonecrosis. Clin Orthop Relat Res. 2007;464:37–42.
26. Prués-Latour V, Bonvin JC, Fritschy D. Nine cases of osteonecrosis in elderly patients following arthroscopic meniscectomy. Knee Surg Sports Traumatol Arthrosc. 1998;6(3):142–7.
27. Servien E, Verdonk PC, Lustig S, Paillot JL, Kara AD, Neyret P. Medial unicompartimental knee arthroplasty for osteonecrosis or osteoarthritis. Knee Surg Sports Traumatol Arthrosc. 2008;16(11):1038–42. doi: 10.1007/s00167-008-0617-8. Epub 2008 Sep 10.
28. Son IJ, Kim MK, Kim JY, Kim JG. Osteonecrosis of the knee after arthroscopic partial meniscectomy. Knee Surg Relat Res. 2013;25(3):150–4.
29. Soucacos PN, Xenakis TH, Beris AE, Soucacos PK, Georgoulis A. Idiopathic osteonecrosis of the medial femoral condyle. Classification and treatment. Clin Orthop Relat Res. 1997;(341):82–9.
30. Tanaka Y, Mima H, Yonetani Y, Shiozaki Y, Nakamura N, Horibe S. Histological evaluation of spontaneous osteonecrosis of the medial femoral condyle and short-term clinical results of osteochondral autografting: a case series. Knee. 2009;16(2):130–5.
31. Türker M, Cetik O, Cırpar M, Durusoy S, Cömert B. Postarthroscopy osteonecrosis of the knee. Knee Surg Sports Traumatol Arthrosc. 2013.
32. Illingworth KD1, Hensler D, Casagranda B, Borrero C, van Eck CF, Fu FH. Relationship between bone bruise volume and the presence of meniscal tears in acute anterior cruciate ligament rupture. Knee Surg Sports Traumatol Arthrosc. 2014;22(9):2181–6. doi: 10.1007/s00167-013-2657-y. Epub 2013 Sep 4.
33. Yamamoto T, Bullough PG. Spontaneous osteonecrosis of the knee: the result of subchondral insufficiency fracture. J Bone Joint Surg Am. 2000;82(6):858–66.

34. Yates PJ, Calder JD, Stranks GJ, Conn KS, Peppercorn D, Thomas NP. Early MRI diagnosis and non-surgical management of spontaneous osteonecrosis of the knee. Knee. 2007;14(2):112–6.
35. Zizic TM, Marcoux C, Hungerford DS. Corticosteroid therapy associated with ischemic necrosis of bone in systemic lupus erythematosus. Am J Med. 1985;79(5):596–604.

11 Knee Arthrodesis

Scott Kling

Take-Home Message

- The most common indication for knee arthrodesis is salvage of a failed total knee arthroplasty (TKA).
- The optimal position of fusion is approximately 5–8° of valgus, 0–15° of flexion, and 0–10° of external rotation.
- Fusion rates in the literature range between 38 and 100 % depending on technique, with intramedullary nailing maintaining a significantly higher success rate.

Introduction

- For the carefully selected patient, knee arthrodesis remains an ultimate option to provide pain relief and ambulatory function in the circumstance of a knee that is not amenable to reconstruction.

Indications

- The most common indication for knee arthrodesis is salvage of a failed total knee arthroplasty (TKA), often secondary to persistent infection, massive bone or soft tissue loss, or irreparable damage to the extensor mechanism.
- Additional indications include painful arthrosis after infection or trauma, painful ankylosis, neuropathic arthropathy, and periarticular tumor resection.
- An absolute contraindication is active infection.
- Relative contraindications include ipsilateral hip arthrodesis, contralateral knee arthrodesis, contralateral leg amputation, ipsilateral hip or ankle arthrosis, and significant bone loss.
- Resection arthroplasty remains a viable option in patients with contraindications.

Preoperative Planning

- Conditions that may compromise wound healing should be optimized prior to surgical intervention, namely, diabetes mellitus, rheumatoid arthritis, chronic renal failure, peripheral vascular disease, and corticosteroid use.
- Extremity malalignment, flexion contracture, and knee range of motion should be documented.

- Radiographic assessment including long cassette weight-bearing films should be obtained.
- Consider trialing the patient in a knee immobilizer or cast preoperatively in order to demonstrate the potential difficulties of a knee arthrodesis during activities of daily living.

Position of Fusion

- The optimal position of fusion is approximately 5–8° of valgus, 0–15° of flexion, and 0–10° of external rotation.
- Slight limb shortening may be advantageous for self-care and also allows ground clearance during swing phase of gait.
- Minimal bony resection should be performed in the setting of TKA in order to maintain length.

Surgical Technique

- Soft tissue management during knee arthrodesis is critical in order to minimize postoperative wound problems. Skin flaps should not be raised more than necessary for adequate exposure in hopes of preserving cutaneous circulation.
- There are multiple surgical techniques for fixation. The use of fundamental fracture fixation principles such as bony contact, adequate blood supply, and rigid fixation will improve the likelihood of success.
- Intramedullary fusion may be accomplished by a long nail with a piriformis fossa starting point or a modular two-part nail that connects at the joint line. It is the preferred technique in the setting of extensive bone loss, demonstrating significantly higher fusion rates (95 %). Intramedullary fixation allows for fairly rapid postoperative mobilization and weight bearing.
- Compression plate osteosynthesis is another viable option.
- External fixation with compression at the fusion site may be accomplished with a uniplanar bar or a wire-ring device. These methods minimize soft tissue damage and eliminate retained hardware. Pin site infections, loss of pin fixation and fracture, and delayed weight bearing remain the disadvantages of external fixation. A lower fusion rate has been observed using external fixation techniques (approximately 60 %).
- The patella may be left alone, incorporated into the fusion, used as bone graft, or excised to remove tension on the skin.
- Intercalary allograft or autograft, such as local vascularized fibula, can be used to augment the fusion in scenarios of advanced bone loss.

Outcomes

- Fusion rates in the literature range between 38 and 100 % depending on technique, with intramedullary nailing maintaining a significantly higher success rate.
- Fusion rate after TKA is lower than in knees that have not undergone TKA. This is secondary to multiple factors including bone loss, limb shortening, persistent infection, and poor bone apposition.

- Unlike fusion of the hip, conversion of knee arthrodesis to an arthroplasty at a later date is not recommended due to an extremely high complication rate.

Complications

- The most common complication is pain resulting from nonunion. Nonunions may be either atrophic or hypertrophic and should be treated with bone grafting or more rigid fixation, respectively.
- Additional complications include infection, lumbar back pain, ipsilateral hip degenerative changes, contralateral knee degenerative changes, peroneal nerve palsy, and fracture of the supracondylar femur or proximal tibial metaphysis.
- Modular intramedullary nails inserted through the knee present a significant challenge when removal is necessitated.

Bibliography

1. Bargiotas K, Wohlrab D, Sewecke JJ, Lavinge G, Demeo PJ, Sotereanos NG. Arthrodesis of the knee with a long intramedullary nail following the failure of a total knee arthroplasty as the result of infection. J Bone Joint Surg Am. 2006;88(3):553–8.
2. Conway JD, Mont MA, Bezwada HP. Arthrodesis of the knee. J Bone Joint Surg Am. 2004;86-A(4):835–48.
3. MacDonald JH, Agarwal S, Lorei MP, Johanson NA, Freiberg AA. Knee arthrodesis. J Am Acad Orthop Surg. 2006;14(3):154–63.

Hip

Joseph Labrum, Justin Arner, Scott Kling, and James M. Bullock

1 Hip Anatomy and Blood Supply

Joseph Labrum

Take-Home Message

- The normal acetabulum is anteverted and caudally oriented.
- The iliofemoral, pubofemoral, and ischiofemoral ligaments surround the hip joint and place limitations on hip movement.
- The ascending cervical branches of the medial and lateral femoral circumflex arteries are the primary blood supply of the femoral head and neck.
- Acetabular and labral blood supply is derived mainly from the superior gluteal, inferior gluteal, and obturator arteries.

Introduction

- Prototypical ball-and-socket joint provides a wide range of motion that is surpassed only by the shoulder. The femoral head and the acetabulum comprise the osseous elements of the hip.

J. Labrum, BS (✉) • J. Arner, MD
Labrum is University of Pittsburgh Medical School,
Arner is Orthopedic Residency UPMC, University of Pittsburgh Medical Center,
3200 South Water Street, Pittsburgh, PA 15203, USA
e-mail: josephlabrum@gmail.com; justin.arner@gmail.com

S. Kling, MD • J.M. Bullock, MD
Sports Medicine, University of Pittsburgh Medical Center,
3200 South Water Street, Pittsburgh, PA 15203, USA
e-mail: srkling@gmail.com; jamesbullock.md@gmail.com

C. Mauffrey, D.J. Hak (eds.), *Passport for the Orthopedic Boards and FRCS Examination*, DOI 10.1007/978-2-8178-0475-0_46

- The femoral head closely approximates a sphere and is entirely covered by hyaline cartilage, except for a central depression termed the fovea capitis, which serves as the femoral attachment site for the ligamentum teres.
- The acetabulum is often described as horseshoe shaped and is the result of fusion between the ischium, ilium, and pubis bones. The anterior wall of the acetabulum is thin and provides only minimal support, whereas the acetabular roof and posterior wall are composed of much denser bone. The acetabulum is deficient inferiorly, giving rise to the acetabular notch—which is bridged by the transverse ligament.
- Due to the variation in wall thickness, the orientation of the acetabulum does not lie in standard anatomical planes; rather, the normal acetabulum faces forward with slight anteversion and also faces downward with caudal orientation.

Ligaments

- Three strong ligaments span the hip joint and integrate with surrounding connective tissue to help form the hip capsule.
  - Iliofemoral ligament (Y ligament of Bigelow)—Located anteriorly and prevents hyperextension at the hip
  - Pubofemoral ligament—Blends with the lower fibers of the iliofemoral ligament and limits excessive abduction
  - Ischiofemoral ligament—Lies posteriorly and also resists hyperextension
- Taken together, the restrictions placed on the hip joint by these three ligaments result in a capsule that is taught with extension and external rotation and relaxed with flexion and internal rotation.

Acetabular Labrum

- Several important intra-articular structures are present within the hip capsule, including the labrum and ligamentum teres.
- The labrum is a fibrocartilaginous structure attached to the edges of the acetabulum. Inferiorly, the labrum blends with the transverse ligament at the margins of the acetabular notch.
- The function of the labrum continues to be investigated, although it is commonly held that it serves to
  - Stabilize the hip by deepening the socket
  - Act as a seal to maintain joint fluid within the intra-articular space
  - Contain the femoral head during acetabular formation
- Evidence suggests that the labrum does not participate in direct load transmission.

Ligamentum Teres Femoris

- Originates in the fovea capitis.
- Courses along the inferior aspect of the hip joint where it attaches distally and medially to the transverse ligament and to several surrounding structures, including the central nonarticular acetabular surface.

- Forms the pulvinar, in conjunction with the small fat pad within the acetabular fossa.
- Long felt to be of no real importance in the adult hip; however, there is increasing evidence that it plays a role in hip stability.

Blood Supply of the Femoral Head and Neck

- Branches of the medial and lateral femoral circumflex arteries form the primary blood supply to the femoral head and neck. These arteries may originate as branches from either the profunda femoris or femoral arteries.
- The medial femoral circumflex artery courses posteriorly between the iliopsoas and pectineus muscles before giving rise to medial, posterior, and lateral ascending cervical branches.
- The lateral femoral circumflex artery runs anterior to the iliopsoas and gives rise to an anterior ascending cervical branch.
- Together, these four ascending branches form the extracapsular arterial ring; of the four, the lateral branch is responsible for providing most of the blood supply to the femoral head.
- The ascending cervical arteries proceed to traverse the capsule along its attachment at the base of the femoral neck. Within the capsule, they form a subsynovial anastomotic ring on the surface of the femoral neck at the margin of articular cartilage. This is known as the subsynovial intra-articular arterial ring.
- A second and much smaller source of blood to the femoral head is the artery of the ligamentum teres or foveal artery. This artery arises from the acetabular branch of the obturator artery, which itself is a branch of the external iliac artery. However, this artery is said to be often occluded in adults.

Acetabular Blood Supply

- Acetabular blood supply comes primarily from branches of the superior gluteal, inferior gluteal, and obturator arteries.
  - Superior gluteal artery—Deep branches supply the superior rim of the acetabulum
  - Inferior gluteal artery—Reaches the gluteal region by coursing through the lower part of the greater sciatic foramen. Once outside the pelvis, its branches travel inferiorly to supply the posteroinferior regions of the acetabulum
  - Obturator artery—Several branches contribute to acetabular blood supply. Of these, the acetabular branch is most significant, which emerges from the acetabular notch beneath the transverse ligament and supplies the acetabular fossa

Labral Blood Supply

- Blood supply of the acetabular labrum has received increased attention as diagnosis and treatment of labral pathology continues to evolve.
- As with the acetabular osseous tissue, the labrum derives its blood supply from branches of the superior gluteal, inferior gluteal, and obturator arteries.

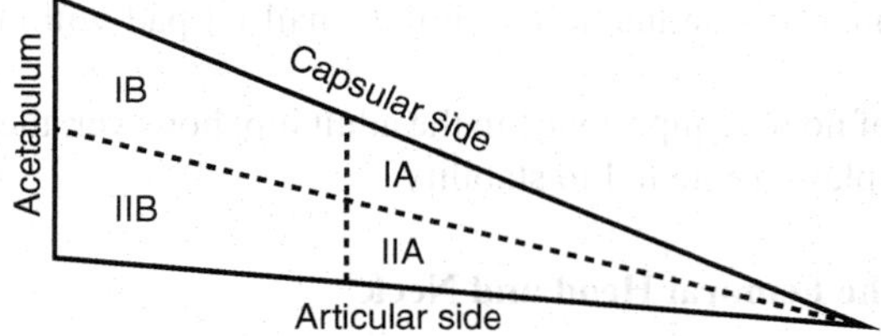

Fig. 1 Four quadrants of labral vascularity. Zones IA and IB receive a peripheral vascular contribution largely derived from the capsule, whereas zones IIA and IIB are relatively avascular (Adapted from Kelly et al. Vascularity of the hip labrum: a cadaveric investigation. Arthroscopy. 2005;21:3–11)

- Labral vascularity differs by region and can be divided into four quadrants, as demonstrated in Fig. 1.
  - Zones IA and IB receive a peripheral vascular contribution largely derived from the capsule, whereas zones IIA and IIB are relatively avascular.
- Thus, the majority of the vessels present within the labrum come from the capsular periphery and show minimal penetration into the central articular-sided region.

Bibliography

1. Bardakos NV, Villar RN. The ligamentum teres of the adult hip. J Bone Joint Surg Br. 2009;91:8–15.
2. Blankenbaker DG, De Smet AA, Keene JS, Del Rio AM. Imaging appearance of the normal and partially torn ligamentum teres on hip MR arthrography. AJR Am J Roentgenol. 2012;199(5):1093–8.
3. Chung SM. The arterial supply of the developing proximal end of the human femur. J Bone Joint Surg Am. 1976;58:961–70.
4. Ferguson SJ, Bryant JT, Ganz R, Ito K. The acetabular labrum seal: a poroelastic finite element model. Clin Biomech. 2000;15:463–8.
5. Itokazu M, Takahashi K, Matsunaga T, Hayakawa D, Emura S, Isono H, Shoumura S. A study of the arterial supply of the human acetabulum using a corrosion casting method. Clin Anat. 1997;10(2):77–81.
6. Kelly BT, Shapiro GS, Digiovanni CW, Buly RL, Potter HG, Hannafin JA. Vascularity of the hip labrum: a cadaveric investigation. Arthroscopy. 2005;21:3–11.
7. Kim Y-H. Acetabular dysplasia and osteoarthritis developed by an eversion of the acetabular labrum. Clin Orthop. 1987;215:289–93.
8. Konrath GA, Hamel AJ, Olson SA, et al. The role of the acetabular labrum and the transverse acetabular ligament in load transmission in the hip. J Bone Joint Surg Am. 1998;80:1781.
9. Rao J, Zhou YX, Villar RN. Injury to the ligamentum teres: mechanism, findings and results of treatment. Clin Sports Med. 2001;20:791–9.
10. Takechi H, Nagashima H, Ito S. Intra-articular pressure of the hip joint outside and inside the limbus. Nihon Seikeigeka Gakkai Zasshi. 1982;56(6):529–36.

2 Biomechanics of the Hip Joint

Joseph Labrum

Take-Home Message

- Analysis of biomechanics using free body diagrams is performed assuming a one-legged stance and static conditions.
- The force exerted by the abductor musculature must be approx. 2.5 times greater than that of the gravitational force to keep the pelvis level.
- In equilibrium, the joint reaction force is approx. 2.7 times body weight.
- Ways of decreasing the joint reaction force include decreasing body weight or altering the lever arms of the abductors or gravitational force.
- The joint reaction force reaches three to four times body weight while walking and seven to eight times while running in-line.

Hip Joint Characteristics

- Principal link between the axial skeleton and lower extremity, responsible for transferring weight between the two
- Central role in generation and transmission of forces
- Exceptional amount of inherent osseous stability due to anatomy of the femoro-acetabular interface
- Motion is almost entirely in rotational plane with no detectable amount of translation; predictable motion allows for simplifications necessary to analyze biomechanics

Simplifications for Analysis

- It should be noted that biomechanics of the hip are not influenced solely by local anatomy; as the trunk and lower limb are connected through the hip, remote structures in these areas can have considerable impact on hip biomechanics.
- However, it is customary to simplify the analysis by excluding the contribution of remote structures.
- Additional assumptions must also be made: although the femoral head is slightly aspherical and, therefore, does not have a single center of rotation throughout hip motion, the analysis presented here will assume a perfectly round femoral head.

Free Body Diagram

- Analysis using free body diagrams of the hip joint have traditionally been performed assuming a one-legged stance under static conditions and evaluating forces that occur in the frontal plane.
- While this scenario is somewhat artificial, it presents a powerful illustration of the impact that even subtle changes in body position or hip anatomy can have on hip biomechanics.

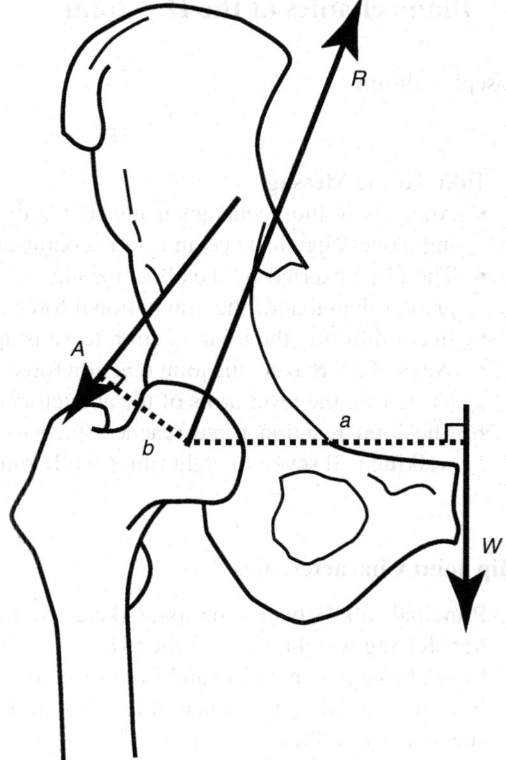

Fig. 2 Free body diagram of forces acting on the hip during a one-legged stance under static conditions. *W* gravitational force, *A* force of abductor musculature, *R* joint reaction force, *a* lever arm of gravitational force, *b* lever arm of abductor musculature

- Given the simplifications above, there are three main forces acting on the hip to consider (Fig. 2).
  - The gravitational force, *W*—calculated as the weight of the body minus the weight of the ipsilateral lower limb.
    - This gravitational force acts on a lever arm, *a*, that is the distance between the body's center of gravity and the center of the femoral head.
    - Under conditions of equilibrium, the center of gravity is situated in the midline of the trunk, just anterior to the sacrum.
  - The force exerted by the abductor musculature, *A*—acts on a lever arm, *b*, that extends from the lateral aspect of the greater trochanter to the center of the femoral head.
  - The joint reaction force, *R*—the compressive force experienced between the femoral head and the acetabulum.
- In order to hold the pelvis level during a one-legged stance, the abductor musculature must exert a moment that is equal to that of the gravitational pull. Likewise, it must exert a moment that is greater than the gravitational pull if the pelvis is to be tilted to the same side while walking.

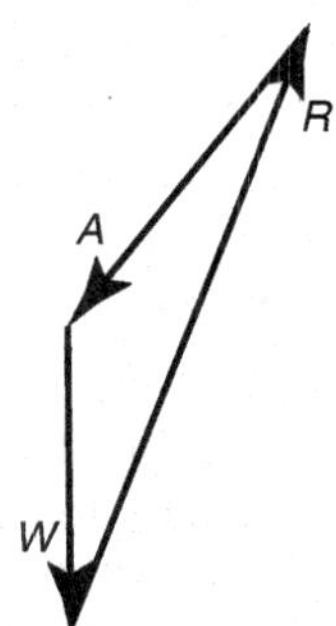

Fig. 3 Sum of force vectors acting on the hip. In order to maintain the pelvis level, the sum of vectors *A* and *W* must equal the magnitude of vector *R*

- However, since the length of the lever arms for the two forces differs, forces *W* and *A* will not be equal when the pelvis is held level; instead, force *A* must be approximately 2.5 greater than force *W* since that is the approximate ratio of lever arm *a* to lever arm *b*.

Calculation of the Joint Reaction Force

- Under static conditions, the sum of the force vectors *W*, *A*, and *R* must equal to zero in order to keep the pelvis level.
- Thus, *R* can be calculated as the sum of the vectors *W* and *A* (Fig. 3).
- In equilibrium, *R* is calculated to be 2.7 times greater than body weight and is directed 69° from the horizontal during a single leg stance.
- The joint reaction force can be determined if the abductor force is known, according to the equation

$$A = \frac{5/6 Wxa}{b}$$

- *A* is calculable if the weight and lever arms *a* and *b* are known. This equation approximates the weight of one lower limb as 1/6 total body weight.

Reduction of Joint Reaction Force

- The equation above also illustrates the potential routes of decreasing the joint reaction force:
  - Decreasing total body weight
  - Decreasing the lever arm of the gravitational force
  - Increasing the lever arm of the abductor musculature
- Any of these changes allow for a decrease in the force exerted by the abductor musculature and thus decrease the joint reaction force.
- The classic Trendelenburg lurch provides an example of this principle. During such a gait, the individual's weight is shifted over the standing leg, bringing the center of gravity closer to the center of hip rotation and thus decreasing the lever arm of the gravitational force.

  - The result is a decrease in the amount of force generated by the abductor musculature necessary to stabilize the pelvis and consequent decrease in joint reactive force.

Cane Use

- Use of a cane can also help reduce the load experienced across the hip joint.
- When used in the contralateral hand, the cane also allows for a reduction in abductor force by creating an upward directed force that helps offset the gravitational pull from the patient's weight.
- The resultant decrease in load across the hip can be substantial, with some researchers reporting up to a 42 % decrease in abductor muscle activity when near-maximal effort with a cane is used.
  - Correlates to a reduction in hip joint reaction force from 3.4 times body weight to 2.2 times body weight

Motion and Dynamic Loading

- Examining the forces about the hip under static conditions, while useful, is not entirely practical.
- The effects of motion and dynamic loading conditions are likely more relevant when considering the athlete. Researchers have calculated estimated loads across the hip joint under walking and running conditions.
  - Between three and four times body weight during walking, at various points of the gait cycle and at different speeds.
  - Approximately seven to eight times body weight are transmitted across the hip joint during running.
- However, calculations were performed for straight-line movement, and do not include potential forces encountered during cutting, pivoting, and other changes of direction.
- In vivo measurements have been made possible in recent years by implanting pressure transducers into prosthetic components.

Bibliography

1. Bergmann G, Deuretzbacher G, Heller M, et al. Hip contact forces and gait patterns from routine activities. J Biomech. 2001;34:859–71.
2. Brinckmann P, Frobin W, Leivseth G. Musculoskeletal biomechanics. New York: Thieme New York; 2002:69–84.
3. Harding L, Barbe M, Shepard K, et al. Posterior-anterior glide of the femoral head in the acetabulum: a cadaver study. J Orthop Sports Phys Ther. 2003;33:118–25.
4. Kabada MP, Ramakaishnan HK, Wooten ME, et al. Repeatability of kinematic, kinetic and electromyographic data in normal adult gait. J Orthop Res. 1989;7:849–60.
5. Neumann DA. Hip abductor muscle activity as subjects with hip prostheses walk with different methods of using a cane. Phys Ther. 1998;78:490–501.

6. Nordin M, Frankel VH. Basic biomechanics of the musculoskeletal system. 3rd ed. Baltimore: Lippincott Williams & Wilkins; 2001. p. 203–21.
7. Polkowski GG, Clohisy JC. Hip biomechanics. Sports Med Arthrosc. 2010;18:56–62.
8. Rydell N. Biomechanics of the hip-joint. Clin Orthop Relat Res. 1973;(92):6–15.

3 Hip Osteonecrosis

Justin Arner

Take-Home Message

- Osteonecrosis of the hip comes in two forms, traumatic and atraumatic.
- The most serious atraumatic risk factors including alcohol and corticosteroid use.
- Early diagnosis is imperative to try to prevent almost certain progression.
- Nonoperative treatments are limited and include bisphosphonates.
- Operative treatments with the most evidence for use include core decompression, vascularized free fibular grafting, and total hip arthroplasty.

Definitions

- Osteonecrosis of the hip is a fairly common condition which can occur atraumatically or traumatically.
- The most common complaint is deep groin pain, while knee or buttock pain also can be complaints.
- This pain is worse with weight bearing and can lead to decreased motion, internal rotation being the most problematic.
- Bilateral in 40–80 % of sufferers

Etiology

- Etiology is not well defined.
- The basis of osteonecrosis of the hip rests on the disruption of vascular supply to the femoral head.
- Decreased blood flow leads to osteocyte death which in turn creates edema and therefore increased pressure which further decreases vascular flow to the femoral head.
- This newly weakened necrotic bone cannot support the same stresses, and therefore microfractures occur in the femoral head which are unable to be repaired by the body to the pre-disease state.
- With more stresses, the femoral head will continue to collapse leading to abnormal joint congruity and joint degradation.

Traumatic Hip Osteonecrosis

- Occurs secondary to injury including include femoral neck fracture and hip dislocation

Atraumatic Hip Osteonecrosis

- Plays an important role in preventing, diagnosing, and treating the disease
- Most significant risk factors with the worst prognosis:
  - Alcohol and corticosteroids.
  - The dose to cause steroid-induced osteonecrosis is unknown, but higher doses increase the risk, and disease is almost always bilateral.
  - Alcohol-induced osteonecrosis is more common in long-term heavy consumers and those that drink over 400 mL of alcohol per week.
- Other risk factors:
  - Slipped capital femoral, epiphysis, substance abuse, coagulopathies, smoking, pregnancy, chronic renal failure, chronic pancreatitis, radiation therapy, immunosuppression, hypercortisolism, systemic lupus erythematosus, and sickle cell
- Laboratory evaluation may include coagulopathy workup, lipid testing, and sickle cell testing.
- Core biopsy and interosseous pressure measurements are options to better evaluate the process.

Pathophysiology

- No matter the risk factors or cause of osteonecrosis, the microbiology is the same.
  - Empty lacunae with dead osteocytes and bone marrow necrosis
- Osteoclasts resorb the necrotic tissue, and osteoblasts begin laying down new bone.
- Small lesions sometimes are able to be totally resorbed and replaced.
- With large lesions, bone is only able to be remodeled along the periphery leaving a center with limited vascularity and therefore risk of collapse.
- When the center collapses, a crescent sign may be seen from a fracture between the subchondral bone and the necrotic areas.
  - Best seen on a frog leg lateral radiograph
- Later, subchondral bone can collapse leading to a flattened femoral head.
- As expected, altered femoral head morphology leads to abnormal wear of the hip joint and therefore degenerative changes.
- After remodeling occurs, a sclerotic zone may develop between the living and necrotic bone.

Radiographs

X-rays should include anteroposterior and frog leg lateral views.

- Lesion size, crescent sign, and degenerative changes such as joint space narrowing, subchondral sclerosis, subchondral cysts, and osteophyte formation should be evaluated.
- Lesions are very commonly bilateral, and therefore both hips should be investigated (IMAGING).
- The role of bilateral imaging is not well defined but should be considered.

MRI

- Many times allows earlier diagnosis when clinical suspicion persists even with negative X-rays.
- MRI findings include bone marrow edema encapsulated in a ring of low intensity signal.
- Femoral head collapse can be predicted by MRI via a modified Kerboul angle.
  - This is the sum of the necrotic portion of the arc of the femoral surface measured on the midcoronal and midsagittal slices (photo).
  - In a study of 37 disease sufferers, none collapsed with angles of <190°, 50 % collapsed with angles 190–240°, and all femoral heads collapsed with an angle of >240°.
  - This evaluation may be a useful adjunct for evaluation of disease progression.

Classification

- Staging of osteonecrosis can be done with the Ficat-Arlet classification which allows better definition of the state of the disease and its risk of progression.

Treatment

Nonoperative Treatment

- Options are unfortunately limited.
- Includes activity modification/physical therapy, nonsteroidal anti-inflammatories, bisphosphonates, and hyperbaric oxygen therapy.
- The most conservative option is altered weight bearing with the thought that the femoral head will remodel and therefore become less likely to collapse.
  - Has not been proven to have satisfactory outcomes in most patients.
- Bisphosphonates
  - Thought to work by preventing the resorption of the structural boney matrix by inhibition of osteoclasts and therefore may prevent boney collapse and consequential arthritis.
  - If utilized early, bisphosphonates have been shown to improve function, decrease collapse, and delay total hip replacement surgery in level 1 studies.

- There is no clear nonoperative management for this difficult disease.
- Most nonsurgical options have not been proven to decrease disease progression and focus on symptom management.

Operative Interventions

- Include articulated hip distraction, osteotomy, core decompression, numerous grafting techniques, and total hip arthroplasty.
- Articulated hip distraction is done with the thought that remodeling may occur when the pressure over the diseased bone is relieved.
  - Studies show this may delay joint replacement temporarily but does not change long-term outcomes.
- Core decompression is thought to work by decreasing the increased intraosseous pressure.
  - This is thought to allow increased blood flow to the femoral head in early disease.
  - Good outcomes have been seen although it is important to perform this surgery before any femoral head collapse occurs.
- Bone graft can be added to the decompressed region.
  - Options include cancellous bone (iliac crest or allograft), cortical bone strut grafting (iliac crest or vascularized free fibular graft), osteochondral allograft, muscle pedicle bone graft (iliac crest with the quadratus femoris attached), growth factors (rhBMP-2), and strut grating with tantalum implants (porous metal cylinder).
  - Vascularized free fibular grafting after core decompression has been shown to provide pain relief and delay joint replacement and therefore has become popular.
- Another option includes dislocation of the hip where debridement of the necrotic bone can be accomplished before bone graft packing through a trapdoor procedure.
  - This has shown good results in advanced cases.
- Autologous bone marrow transplantation into the core decompression site has produced pain relief and decreased progression in early stages, while after hips showed collapse, poorer results were seen.
- Due to donor site morbidity, porous tantalum rod implantation was designed and has again shown better results in pre-collapse hips but not enough to recommend its use.
- None of these techniques have been definitively proven in the literature to be superior to core decompression alone.
- Proximal femoral osteotomy can be helpful in select patients where small lesion exists that can be unloaded to prevent collapse.
  - Good preoperative planning is essential to assess the osteonecrotic area which is most commonly the anterosuperior region of the head.
  - If this is the lesions' location, one can rotate the proximal femur through the trochanters to off-load the area.

- Valgus osteotomy can be done in young patients with small anterolateral lesions.
- Varus intertrochanteric osteotomy can be done when osteonecrosis occurs in the medial portion of the femoral head to off-load the affected region.
- Arthroplasty is a good option in severe osteonecrosis or in patients where other interventions have failed.
- Hemiresurfacing is one option, but increased wear on the acetabulum can lead to pain.
- Some advocate for the use of total hip resurfacing arthroplasty as some studies show that it can be as successful as total hip arthroplasty in young people and can allow them to be more active.
  - One drawback to this technique is the use of metal on metal components which may carry their own issues.
- Total hip arthroplasty is a successful option in end-state disease and in patients where other treatments failed.
- Arthrodesis is an end-stage option in low-demand patients.
  - This is the current standard in advanced disease.

Bibliography

1. Amanatullah DF, Strauss EJ, Di Cesare PE. Current management options for osteonecrosis of the femoral head part 1, diagnosis and nonoperative management. Am J Orthop (Belle Mead NJ). 2011a;40(9):E186–92.
2. Amanatullah DF, Strauss EJ, Di Cesare PE. Current management options for osteonecrosis of the femoral head: part II, operative management. Am J Orthop (Belle Mead NJ). 2011b;40(10):E216–25.
3. Ficat RP. Idiopathic bone necrosis of the femoral head. Early diagnosis and treatment. J Bone Joint Surg Br. 1985;67(1):3–9.
4. Ha YC, et al. Prediction of collapse in femoral head osteonecrosis: a modified Kerboul method with use of magnetic resonance images. J Bone Joint Surg Am. 2006;88(Suppl 3):35–40.
5. Korompilias AV, et al. Femoral head osteonecrosis: why choose free vascularized fibula grafting. Microsurgery. 2011;31(3):223–8.
6. Lai KA, et al. The use of alendronate to prevent early collapse of the femoral head in patients with nontraumatic osteonecrosis. A randomized clinical study. J Bone Joint Surg Am. 2005;87(10):2155–9.
7. Lavernia CJ, Sierra RJ, Grieco FR. Osteonecrosis of the femoral head. J Am Acad Orthop Surg. 1999;7(4):250–61.
8. Mont MA, Carbone JJ, Fairbank AC. Core decompression versus nonoperative management for osteonecrosis of the hip. Clin Orthop Relat Res. 1996;(324):169–78.
9. Mont MA, et al. The trapdoor procedure using autogenous cortical and cancellous bone grafts for osteonecrosis of the femoral head. J Bone Joint Surg Br. 1998;80(1):56–62.
10. Mont MA, et al. The natural history of untreated asymptomatic osteonecrosis of the femoral head: a systematic literature review. J Bone Joint Surg Am. 2010;92(12):2165–70.

11. Nadeau M, et al. Short term clinical outcome of a porous tantalum implant for the treatment of advanced osteonecrosis of the femoral head. Mcgill J Med. 2007;10(1):4–10.
12. Rajagopal M, Balch Samora J, Ellis TJ. Efficacy of core decompression as treatment for osteonecrosis of the hip: a systematic review. Hip Int. 2012;22(5):489–93.
13. Rajpura A, Wright AC, Board TN. Medical management of osteonecrosis of the hip: a review. Hip Int. 2011;21(4):385–92.
14. Scher DL, Belmont PJ Jr., Owens BD. Case report: osteonecrosis of the femoral head after hip arthroscopy. Clin Orthop Relat Res. 2010;468(11):3121–5.
15. Stiehl JB, et al. Bone morphogenetic proteins in total hip arthroplasty, osteonecrosis and trauma surgery. Expert Rev Med Devices. 2008;5(2):231–8.
16. Urbaniak JR, Harvey EJ. Revascularization of the femoral head in osteonecrosis. J Am Acad Orthop Surg. 1998;6(1):44–54.

4 Transient Osteoporosis

Scott Kling

Take-Home Message

- ITOH is a self-limiting disease. Treatment remains nonoperative and is directed at minimizing clinical symptoms.
- ITOH is found in two distinct populations: (1) middle-aged men (40–55 years) and (2) pregnant women in their third trimester.
- The discrepancy between the physical exam findings and history is a characteristic finding of ITOH.

Definition

- Idiopathic transient osteoporosis of the hip (ITOH), also known as bone marrow edema syndrome

Epidemiology

- ITOH affects men three times more frequently than women.
- It is found in two distinct populations: (1) middle-aged men (40–55 years) and (2) pregnant women in their third trimester.
- It has also been observed in the immediate postpartum period.
- It is extremely rare in patients of Asian descent.

Pathophysiology

- The pathogenesis of ITOH remains poorly understood.
- One theory hypothesizes that local hyperemia and impaired venous return with marrow edema and increased intramedullary pressure within the proximal femur are responsible.
- Transient ischemia to proximal nerve roots and resulting temporary denervation has also been proposed as a cause.
- Some authors have proposed ITOH to be an abortive form of avascular necrosis (AVN) or a type of reflex sympathetic dystrophy syndrome.
- Bone biopsy reveals irregularly woven bone, osteoid seams, and lining osteoblast cells indicative of periarticular osseous demineralization.
- Synovial biopsy shows minimal synovial inflammation despite an increase in synovial fluid volume.

Presentation

- ITOH is most commonly unilateral in nature.
- Patients generally present complaining gradual onset hip and groin pain without any history of inciting trauma. The pain is progressive and worsens over several weeks.
- Physical exam may demonstrate focal tenderness about the proximal femur and reduced range of motion of the hip joint at the extremes. Grossly limited range of motion and crepitus are not observed. Often patients will refuse to bear weight on the involved extremity and describe fairly severe disability. Rarely, patients will complain of other lower extremity joint involvement.
- The discrepancy between the physical exam findings and history is a characteristic finding of ITOH.

Imaging

- Diagnostic workup should begin with plain film radiographs of the pelvis and hip. The joint space itself is always preserved in ITOH. There will be diffuse osteopenia of the femoral head and neck, with subchondral cortical bone loss. The "phantom appearance" is a well-described phenomenon in the later stages of ITOH with complete loss of the osseous architecture of the femoral head with preservation of the trochanters and acetabulum.
- The radiographic findings often lag behind the clinical symptoms by 4–6 weeks. This is opposed to the findings of AVN, most notably a localized sclerosis in early stages that progresses to the classic crescent sign and ultimately collapses.
- Bone scan may be useful in the early diagnosis of ITOH because increased homogenous radionuclide uptake occurs only days after onset of symptoms and well prior to radiographic findings.

- Magnetic resonance imaging is the modality of choice for making a definitive diagnosis of ITOH. T1-weighted sequences show decreased signal with loss of fatty marrow, while T2 sequences show diffuse high-signal marrow edema and often a reactive joint effusion. AVN will yield subchondral focal changes most commonly in the anterosuperior quadrant of the femoral head with decreased signal intensity on both T1 and T2 sequences.

Evaluation

- ITOH remains a diagnosis of exclusion. Femoral neck fracture, osteomyelitis, avascular necrosis, inflammatory arthritis, and malignancy must be ruled out prior to making a diagnosis.
- A history of trauma, acute onset of pain, systemic symptoms such as fever or weight loss, and chronic alcohol or steroid use should warn the physician of an alternative diagnosis.
- Laboratory tests do not aid in making the diagnosis, but certainly should be performed to rule out aggressive metastatic or metabolic bone disease with long-term sequelae. Early differentiation from other such conditions in the differential diagnosis is critical to prevent unnecessary treatment.
- Nonspecific markers of bone turnover such as alkaline phosphatase have normal serum levels in patients with ITOH.
- Histology is generally not performed unless other entities are suspected.

Treatment

- ITOH is a self-limiting disease. Thus, treatment remains nonoperative and is directed at minimizing clinical symptoms. This includes nonsteroidal anti-inflammatory drugs (NSAIDs), as well as protected weight bearing to limit pain and avoid propagation of a stress fracture.
- ITOH typically resolves within 6–8 months, but may infrequently recur.
- After the bone marrow edema has resolved, significant trabecular bone loss remains. Treatments aimed at increasing bone mineral density, such as calcium, vitamin D, and bisphosphonates, are indicated. Accordingly, DEXA scan may play a role in the management of ITOH.

Bibliography

1. Guerra JJ, Steinberg ME. Distinguishing transient osteoporosis from avascular necrosis of the hip. J Bone Joint Surg Am. 1995;77:616–24.
2. Korompilias AV, Karantanas AH, Lykissas MG, Beris AE. Transient osteoporosis. J Am Acad Orthop Surg. 2008;16:480–9.
3. Takatori Y, Kokubo T, Ninomiya S, Nakamura T, Okutsu I, Kamogawa M. Transient osteoporosis of the hip. Magnetic resonance imaging. Clin Orthop Relat Res. 1991;(271):190–4.

5 Hip Arthrodesis

Scott Kling

Take-Home Message

- The classic indication for hip arthrodesis is a young, active laborer with painful isolated unilateral arthrosis after infection or trauma.
- The optimal position of fusion is approximately 20–30° of flexion, 0–5° of adduction, and 5–10° of external rotation.
- Long-term hip arthrodesis may cause degenerative changes in the lumbar spine, ipsilateral knee, and contralateral hip. The constellation of these findings is an indication for conversion THA.

Introduction

- The management of young adults with severe osteoarthritis of the hip is a difficult problem due to high failure rates of total hip arthroplasty (THA) necessitating multiple revision surgeries.
- Hip arthrodesis remains a viable option in this population. However, it is perceived as having inferior outcomes to THA despite the high failure rate of arthroplasty in this population (revision rate of 33–45 %).
- Cementless fixation and alternate bearings have not been studied long term in this population.
- When performed correctly, arthrodesis provides pain relief, allows for an active lifestyle, and may be converted to a later THA with minimal morbidity.

Indications

- The classic indication is a young, active laborer with painful isolated unilateral arthrosis after infection or trauma. This is often in the setting of failed previous pelvic or hip surgery. THA will fail at an unacceptable rate in this patient, and thus arthrodesis is a reasonable choice.
- Salvage of failed THA is a second common indication.
- Other indications are neuropathic arthropathy and tumor resection about the proximal femur and acetabulum.
- An absolute contraindication is active infection. Relative contraindications include contralateral hip, ipsilateral knee, and lumbar spine degenerative disease, bilateral developmental hip dysplasia, as well as severe osteoporosis.
- Preexisting contralateral THA is controversial, but known to have a failure rate of approximately 40 %. Advocates support the use of an anterior approach to minimize dislocation risk.

Position of Fusion

- The optimal position of fusion is approximately 20–30° of flexion, 0–5° of adduction, and 5–10° of external rotation.
- Limb length discrepancy should be less than 2 cm.
- Abduction induces pelvic obliquity and may result in lumbar back pain.
- Occupation (sitting versus standing) of the patient should influence flexion position.

Surgical Technique

- The surgeon must be constantly aware of future conversion to THA with respect to femoral bone loss, limb length discrepancy, and active infection.
- The most important determining factor for success is proper positioning of the extremity in all three planes.
- The classic cobra head plating technique (a tension band construct) requires stripping of the abductor musculature from the iliac wing in combination with a pelvic osteotomy and placement of a lateral plate. A trochanteric osteotomy modification should be considered if future conversion to THA is expected.
- The anterior plating technique spares abductor musculature, allows for easier hip positioning intraoperatively, and may be beneficial for patients with decreased bone stock. The extended Smith-Peterson approach is utilized to bridge the internal iliac fossa, anterior acetabular rim, and intertrochanteric region of the proximal femur.
- The double plating technique may prove effective in multiple revision situations, avascularity, unreduced dislocations, and poor patient compliance.
- With significant leg length discrepancies greater than 4 cm, a two-stage approach should be utilized.

Outcomes

- When proper patient selection is utilized, a fusion rate of greater than 80 % is expected with maximal preservation of bone stock.
- Surgical technique is paramount with adequate position of fusion and negligible limb length discrepancy.
- Most patients note adequate pain relief and are able to return to an active lifestyle, including manual labor.
- Biomechanically, hip arthrodesis necessitates a 30 % increase in energy expenditure for ambulation. Gait undergoes a shortened stance phase with a prolonged swing phase and a resultant decreased velocity.
- If indicated, conversion THA results in decreased pain in adjacent joints, marked correction of limb length discrepancy, and improved hip mobility (range of motion is slightly decreased when compared to primary THA).
- Survivorship of conversion THA is comparable to primary THA in a patient older than 50 years.
- Preservation of hip abductor function is critical to the success of conversion THA in reference to gait. Abductor function can be assessed with preoperative electromyogram and nerve conduction studies.

- More than half of conversion THA patients require the use of an assistive device for ambulation.
- Full recovery may require up to 2 years and necessitate prolonged physical therapy.

Complications

- A predictable cascade of joint degeneration often ensues due to a transfer of forces, notably in the lumbar spine, ipsilateral knee, and contralateral hip (in order of decreasing frequency). This process can be delayed approximately 20 years with proper fusion position. However, the constellation of these three findings is an indication for conversion to THA.
- There is a significantly higher complication rate of conversion THA as compared to primary THA, including infection, component loosening, and recurrent dislocation.
- Less common complaints of hip arthrodesis patients include sexual dysfunction and self-urination due to excessive adduction.

Bibliography

1. Beaulé PE, Matta JM, Mast JW. Hip arthrodesis: current indications and techniques. J Am Acad Orthop Surg. 2002;10(4):249–58.
2. Callaghan JJ, Brand RA, Pedersen DR. Hip arthrodesis. A long-term follow-up. J Bone Joint Surg Am. 1985;67(9):1328–35.
3. Panagiotopoulos KP, Robbins GM, Masri BA, Duncan CP. Conversion of hip arthrodesis to total hip arthroplasty. Instr Course Lect. 2001;50:297–305.
4. Richards CJ, Duncan CP. Conversion of hip arthrodesis to total hip arthroplasty: survivorship and clinical outcome. J Arthroplasty. 2011;26(3):409–13. doi:10.1016/j.arth.2010.02.005. Epub 2010 Mar 26.
5. Stover MD, Beaulé PE, Matta JM, Mast JW. Hip arthrodesis: a procedure for the new millennium? Clin Orthop Relat Res. 2004;(418):126–33.

6 Hip Arthroscopy

James M. Bullock

Take-Home Message

- MRI arthrogram can be used to better assess labral anatomy.
- Patients who have arthritic changes noted at arthroscopy have poorer outcomes after arthroscopic hip surgery.
- Cam-type impingement is femoroacetabular impingement (FAI) on the femoral side with abnormality of the femoral head-neck junction.
- Pincer-type impingement is when there is FAI on the acetabular side with ossification of the labrum.
- Thorough history and physical exam will help to determine if there is true intra-articular pathology associated with the patient's "hip" pain.

Hip arthroscopy allows minimally invasive access to intra-articular as well as extra-articular hip pathologies of various kinds.

Indications

- Symptomatic labral tears
- Chondral lesions of the femoral head or acetabulum
- Femoroacetabular impingement (FAI)
- Ligamentum teres injuries
- Synovial chondromatosis
- Hip instability
- Snapping hip
- Loose bodies
- Septic hip
- Adhesive capsulitis
- Osteonecrosis (limited role, mostly diagnostic)
- Degenerative joint disease (low success rates)

Contraindications

- Severe medical comorbidities
- Poor bone quality (unable to withstand traction forces)
- Ankylosis of hip joint

Clinical Workup

Thorough history and physical with layered approach to possible etiologies of hip pain/pathology.

Plain radiographs: AP pelvis and modified Dunn lateral radiograph to evaluate femoral head-neck junction.

CT scan can be helpful to evaluate bony morphology. 3D reconstructions can be helpful.

MRI can be utilized to better assess soft tissue structures about the hip as well as cartilage status. Labral tears can be better appreciated with MRI with intra-articular gadolinium contrast arthrography (MR arthrogram).

Outcomes

Patients who have arthritic changes noted at arthroscopy have poorer outcomes after arthroscopic hip surgery.

Complications

From recent studies the major complication rate is less than 1 %, and the minor complication rate is approximately 8 %. Experienced hip arthroscopists have lower complication rates.

- Iatrogenic chondrolabral injury
  - Most common complication

- Temporary neuropraxia from traction
- Direct injury to nerves from portal placement
  - Anterolateral portal—superior gluteal nerve at risk
  - Anterior portal—lateral femoral cutaneous nerve at risk
  - Posterolateral portal—sciatic nerve at risk. Risk decreased with internal rotation of the hip
- Perineal skin injury
- Conversion to THA
  - Higher rate in patients with joint space narrowing who are over 50 years old
- Iatrogenic instability
- Intra-abdominal or intrathoracic fluid extravasation and associated compartment syndrome
- Thromboembolic phenomena
- Femoral neck fracture
- Avascular necrosis
  - Secondary to injury of lateral epiphyseal artery branches of medial femoral circumflex artery
- Death

6.1 *Femoroacetabular Impingement*

Cam-Type Impingement

- Femoral head-neck junction overgrowth deformity
  - Alpha angle >50°
  - Femoral head-neck offset <8 mm
- Leads to abutment against anterosuperior acetabular rim during internal rotation and flexion
- Compressive and shearing force at labro-chondral junction and at subchondral tidemark

Pincer-Type Impingement

- Excessive acetabular coverage causes increased compression of superolateral acetabular labrum and subsequent ossification of labrum.
  - Lateral center edge angle >39° on AP

Mixed-type impingement can occur with findings of both cam- and pincer-type impingement.

6.2 Labral Tears

Labral tears with no coexisting bony dysmorphism can also benefit from arthroscopic treatment.

Labral debridement may remove painful tissue but based on basic science studies may be concerning for subsequent progression to osteoarthritis due to possible effect on fluid seal and control of fluid flow between central and peripheral compartments of the hip which affects articular surface friction.

Labral repair when possible helps to improve chance of healing of unstable labral tears, by preserving tissue that may be vascularized on the acetabular bony side of the labrum-acetabulum complex.

Bibliography

1. Bedi A, Chen N, Robertson W, Kelly BT. The management of labral tears and femoroacetabular impingement of the hip in the young, active patient. Arthroscopy. 2008;24:1135–45.
2. Bedi A, Kelly BT, Khanduja V. Arthroscopic hip preservation surgery: current concepts and perspective. Bone Joint J. 2013;95-B:10–19.
3. Byrd JW. Hip arthroscopy. J Am Acad Orthop Surg. 2006;14:433–44.
4. Byrd JW, Jones KS. Prospective analysis of hip arthroscopy with 10-year followup. Clin Orthop Relat Res. 2010;468:741–6.
5. Field RE, Rajakulendran K. The labro-acetabular complex. J Bone Joint Surg Am. 2011;93(Suppl 2):22–7.
6. Harris JD, McCormick FM, Abrams GD, et al. Complications and reoperations during and after hip arthroscopy: a systematic review of 92 studies and more than 6,000 patients. Arthroscopy. 2013;29:589–95.
7. Haviv B, O'Donnell J. Arthroscopic treatment for acetabular labral tears of the hip without bony dysmorphism. Am J Sports Med. 2011;39(Suppl):79S–84S.
8. Safran MR. The acetabular labrum: anatomic and functional characteristics and rationale for surgical intervention. J Am Acad Orthop Surg. 2010;18:338–45.
9. Stevens MS, Legay DA, Glazebrook MA, Amirault D. The evidence for hip arthroscopy: grading the current indications. Arthroscopy. 2010;26:1370–83.
10. Tannast M, Siebenrock KA, Anderson SE. Femoroacetabular impingement: radiographic diagnosis–what the radiologist should know. AJR Am J Roentgenol. 2007;188:1540–52.

Part XII
Orthopedic Pathology

Frank J. Frassica, Renee Genoa, and Gregory Osgood

1.1 Introduction

One must be able to separate non-oncologic processes from oncologic ones. The corollary of this is that the surgeon needs to know which lesions can be safely observed and which require referral to an orthopedic oncologist.

There are several processes that the surgeon must be able to do. These include the following:

1. Evaluate an adult patient with a destructive bone lesion and decide whether to initiate treatment or refer the patient to an orthopedic oncologist.
2. Evaluate a young patient with a destructive bone lesion and decide whether to initiate treatment or refer the patient to an orthopedic oncologist.
3. Evaluate a patient with a soft tissue mass and decide on the next step in treatment: (1) observation, (2) incisional or needle biopsy, or (3) excisional biopsy.
4. Know ten characteristic radiographic appearances (non-ossifying fibroma, osteochondroma, enchondroma, stress fracture, Paget's disease, fibrous dysplasia, bone infarct, bone island, heterotopic ossification, and osteoid osteoma).

Part XII
Orthopedic Pathology

Frank J. Frassica, Renee Genos, and Gregory Osgood

1.1 Introduction

One must be able to separate non-oncologic processes from oncologic ones. The corollary of this is that the surgeon needs to know which lesions can be safely observed and which require referral to an orthopedic oncologist.

There are several processes that the surgeon must be able to do. These include the following:

1. Evaluate an adult patient with a destructive bone lesion and decide whether to initiate treatment or refer the patient to an orthopedic oncologist.
2. Evaluate a young patient with a destructive bone lesion and decide whether to initiate treatment or refer the patient to an orthopedic oncologist.
3. Evaluate a patient with a soft tissue mass and decide on the next step in treatment: (1) observation, (2) incisional or needle biopsy, or (3) excisional biopsy.
4. Know ten characteristic radiographic appearances (non-ossifying fibroma, osteochondroma, enchondroma, stress fracture, Paget's disease, fibrous dysplasia, bone infarct, bone island, heterotopic ossification, and osteoid osteoma).

Adult Patient with a Destructive Bone Lesion (Ages 40–80+ Year)

Frank J. Frassica, Renee Genoa, and Gregory Osgood

Take-Home Message

- All patients who undergone surgery for metastatic bone disease are also treated with external beam irradiation and bisphosphonates.
- Prior to surgery for metastatic bone disease in a patient with a single bone lesion, an evaluation (which might include a biopsy) must be done.
- The treatment of myeloma of bone is chemotherapy and bisphosphonates. Surgery is reserved for fractures or impending fractures.
- The treatment of lymphoma of bone is chemotherapy. There is no role for resection.
- Chondrosarcomas are treated with wide resection without chemotherapy or radiation.

As adults age, the patient may develop a destructive lesion in their bone (Table 1). The most common cause of a destructive lesion is a bone metastasis. Other common causes include multiple myeloma, lymphoma, chondrosarcoma, and malignant fibrous histiocytoma.

Very few benign lesions cause symptoms in adults. Paget's disease occasionally causes symptoms. Patients with bone destruction secondary to hyperparathyroidism may also have symptoms. In general enchondromas and bone infarcts do not cause pain.

F.J. Frassica, MD (✉) • G. Osgood, MD
Department of Orthopaedic Surgery, Johns Hopkins University, Baltimore, MD, USA
e-mail: fjfrassica@aol.com

R. Genoa, MD
Department of Orthopaedics, Johns Hopkins University, Baltimore, MD, USA

C. Mauffrey, D.J. Hak (eds.), *Passport for the Orthopedic Boards and FRCS Examination*, DOI 10.1007/978-2-8178-0475-0_47

Table 1 Differential diagnosis of a destructive lesion in the adult patients (ages 40–80+ years)

Benign lesions	Malignant lesions
Enchondroma	Metastatic bone disease
Bone islands	Multiple myeloma
Paget's disease	Lymphoma
Hyperparathyroidism	Chondrosarcoma
	Malignant fibrous histiocytoma (undifferentiated sarcoma)

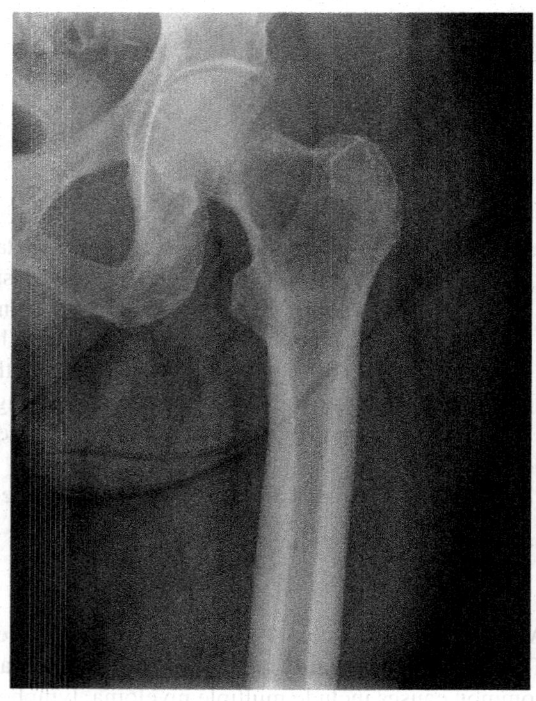

Fig. 1 Anteroposterior radiograph showing a destructive lesion in the proximal femur. The differential diagnosis of this lesion includes metastatic bone disease, multiple myeloma, lymphoma, chondrosarcoma, and malignant fibrous histiocytoma

When a patient presents with a destructive bone lesion (Fig. 1), the clinician does an evaluation to try to find the cause of the destructive lesion. The evaluation scheme is quite simple:

- Computerized tomography scan of the chest, abdomen, and pelvis: This test is rapid (generally less than 3 min) and can be done without contrast. This test is very sensitive for:
  - Lung cancer
  - Kidney cancer
  - Pulmonary metastases
  - Liver metastases
  - Lymph node enlargement

- Technetium bone scan: This test is very sensitive for detecting bone metastases. If there is more than one destructive lesion present (increased uptake on the technetium bone scan and correlation with a radiograph), the differential diagnosis narrows as one can exclude monostotic processes (such as chondrosarcoma or malignant fibrous histiocytoma).
- Laboratory tests
  - Complete blood count
    - Hemoglobin level – low levels of hemoglobin are often indicative of replacement of the bone marrow by a malignancy. Hemoglobin levels of less than 12 mg/dl are a presenting finding in two thirds of patients with muliple myleoma. Patients who have a hemoglobin less than 12 mg/dl and a sedimentation rate greater than 50 mm/h often have multiple myeloma.
    - White blood cell count – high white blood cell counts can occur in patients with hematologic malignancies.
  - Erythrocyte sedimentation rate – elevations of this serum level are found in inflammatory states. Two thirds of patients who present with multiple myeloma have an elevated sedimentation rate (rate greater than 50 mm/h.)
  - Serum calcium and phosphate – high serum calcium level and a low serum phosphorus level suggest hyperparathyroidism as the cause for multiple bone lesions. Certain cancers which are metastatic to the bone such as lung cancer, breast cancer, and lymphomas may have an elevated calcium level and a normal phosphate level.

Decision-making – using this evaluation scheme, there is an 80–90 % chance of finding a cause of a destructive bone lesion. When a cause is not found, a biopsy must be done to determine the nature of the lesion. A biopsy needs to be done as the treatment for the different diagnoses is different.

Depending on the diagnosis, a number of different treatment options are available for each patient. The diagnosis determines what treatment should be offered to the patient:

- Metastatic bone disease – once the malignant cells have spread to the bone, the treatment is palliative for the patient – controlling pain and preventing or treating fracture.
  - Long bone lesions without fracture – the radiation oncologists and the medical oncologist often will ask the surgeon whether there is a risk of fracture (impending fracture). It can be very difficult to predict the risk, but there are several helpful factors to consider.
    - Amount of cortical bone destruction—when there is greater than 50 % cortical bone destruction, there is a greater risk of fracture
    - Localization of the lesion in the bone – when a lesion is eccentric in the bone, there is a much greater risk of fracture than a concentric lesion.
    - Purely lytic bone destruction – when there is no reaction from the bone and a lesion is purely lytic, there is a greater risk of fracture.

    - Location of the lesion in the bone –lesions that involve the diaphysis has a greater risk of fracture than ones in the metaphysis or epiphysis.
    - Hip lesions – lesions in the proximal femur are subject to very high bending and torsional loads. Lesions in this location are very prone to fracture especially when weight-bearing pain is present.

      If the lesion meets the criteria of impending fracture, surgery should be done to prevent fracture. In contrast, if one does not believe the criteria for impending fracture have been met, then nonoperative treatment is chosen.
  - Long bone lesion with fracture – in this scenario, the surgeon must decide whether rigid internal fixation can be accomplished. If rigid fixation is not feasible, then arthroplasty may be the best choice for the patient. If the joint surfaces have been destroyed, then arthroplasty is probably the best method of treatment.
  - Adjuvant treatment – all patients following surgery for metastatic disease need postoperative radiation and bisphosphonate therapy. The external beam irradiation is used to kill the tumor which prevents progression and improves pain scores.

- Multiple myeloma – multiple myeloma is a condition in which a single line of plasma cells (hence monoclonal) becomes a neoplasm with unregulated growth.
  - The treatment of myeloma is chemotherapy and bisphosphonates. The chemotherapy kills the tumors cells, and the bisphosphonates halt the bone destruction.
  - The orthopedic surgeon has three roles
    - At times it is necessary to evaluate the patient and help make the diagnosis with the described evaluation regimen.
    - To evaluate the patient for impending fracture (the same criteria as metastatic disease).
    - To treat fractures with the same criteria that one uses for metastatic bone disease.

- Lymphoma – lymphoma can occur in a single bone or as a manifestation of a patient with widespread disease. Patients with lymphoma of bone present with pain. The pain may start at a very low level such that the pain waxes and wanes in intensity. The symptoms may mimic arthritis, a sports injury, or tendinitis.
  - The role of the orthopedic surgeon is primarily in the diagnosis. When a patient presents with pain suggestive of a tumor and the radiographs are normal, an MRI is necessary to evaluate the bone marrow. If the bone marrow is abnormal, a biopsy must be done to determine the nature of the lesion.
  - The treatment of lymphoma is chemotherapy (referral to a medical oncologist).

- Chondrosarcoma – this is the most common sarcoma in the adult patient. Patients present with pain and sometimes a soft tissue mass. When the clinician does the evaluation scheme, the workup reveals a monostotic lesion.
  - Imaging – the radiographs often show a very characteristic appearing lesion. Intramedullary chondrosarcomas are lesions which often mineralize – show characteristic rings, arcs, and stipples. There are also large erosions, thickening of the cortex, and lysis in the cortex. These findings are so characteristic that the clinician should be able to place chondrosarcoma high on the differential list.
  - Treatment – wide excision of the lesion which involves removal of the entire tumor with a margin of normal tissue. There is no role for chemotherapy or irradiation.
- Malignant fibrous histiocytoma (undifferentiated sarcoma) – this sarcoma can arise in the bone spontaneously or within a preexisting lesion such as a bone infarct, following irradiation, or Paget's disease.
  - Imaging – this high-grade malignant tumor is very nonspecific in its appearance. Usually the lesion is both large and very destructive.
  - Treatment – wide excision of the tumor with a cuff of normal tissue and most patients also receive chemotherapy.

Evaluation of Patients Between 10 and 40 Years of Age (Young Patient)

Frank J. Frassica, Renee Genoa, and Gregory Osgood

Take-Home Message

- The most common sites of metastasis in osteosarcoma are the lungs and bone. A computerized tomography scan and technetium bone scan are used to detect these potential metastases.
- Ewing's tumor may present with bone destruction, fever, and an elevated white blood cell count mimicking osteomyelitis.
- The treatment of osteosarcoma and Ewing's tumor is multi-agent chemotherapy and wide resection.
- Solitary eosinophilic granuloma of bone is treated with aspiration and a cortisone injection.
- Cultures may be negative in osteomyelitis but often will show *Staphylococcus aureus*.

In contrast to the adult patient, the differential diagnosis in the young patient is completely different. In young patients, osteosarcoma and Ewing's tumor are the most common malignancies, while osteomyelitis and eosinophilic granuloma are common benign causes of a destructive lesion. Occasionally, leukemia and lymphoma can be causes of a destructive lesion. In contrast to the adult patient where the evaluation usually precedes biopsy, in the young patient biopsy is often done after the radiographs, and magnetic resonance imaging has been performed. The treatment is often different for the different lesions.

F.J. Frassica, MD (✉) • G. Osgood, MD
Department of Orthopaedic Surgery, Johns Hopkins University, Baltimore, MD, USA
e-mail: fjfrassica@aol.com

R. Genoa, MD
Department of Orthopaedics, Johns Hopkins University,
Baltimore, MD, USA

C. Mauffrey, D.J. Hak (eds.), *Passport for the Orthopedic Boards and FRCS Examination*, DOI 10.1007/978-2-8178-0475-0_48

- Osteosarcoma – this is the most common bone sarcoma in the young patient. Patients present with pain and there is often a soft tissue mass.
  - Imaging – the radiographs often show a destructive lesion in the metaphysis, and there is often evidence of new bone formation either in the medullary cavity or in the soft tissues (Fig. 1).
  - Staging evaluation – a magnetic resonance imaging of the lesion determines the size of the lesion and the absence or presence of discontinuous tumor (skip metastases). A computerized tomography scan of the chest is used to look for pulmonary metastases (appears as one or more nodules), and a technetium bone scan is used to search for bone metastases.
  - Treatment – the preoperative chemotherapy is followed by wide resection of the tumor and reconstruction. Most patients receive postoperative chemotherapy for 6–12 months. Patients who present with localized disease (Stage II) have a 60–70 % long-term survival, while patients who present with pulmonary nodules (Stage IV disease) have a survival of approximately 25 %.

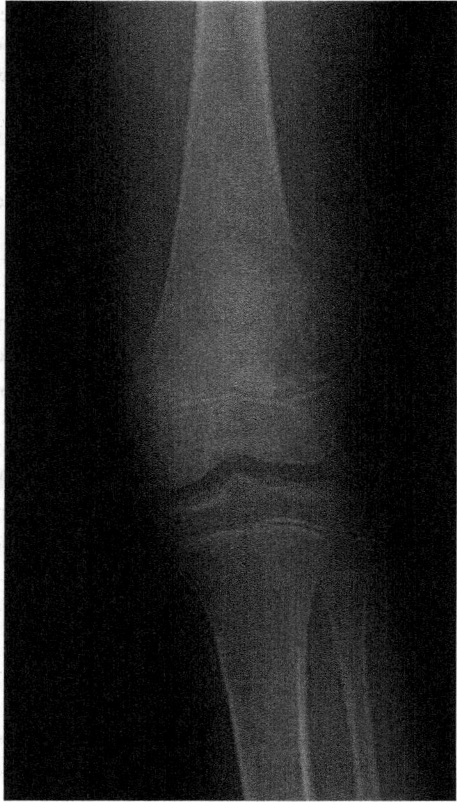

Fig. 1 Anteroposterior radiograph of the distal femur showing a destructive lesion in the lateral aspect of the metaphysis. Note the bone destruction and periosteal reaction. This appearance is very typical of osteosarcoma

- Ewing's tumor – this is the second most common cause of a malignant bone sarcoma in the young patient. In addition to presenting with pain and a soft tissue mass, patients may also have constitutional symptoms such as fever and fatigue. The erythrocyte sedimentation rate and white blood cell count may be elevated. When the radiographs and the systemic manifestations are considered, osteomyelitis is often considered higher in the differential diagnosis than Ewing's tumor.
  - Imaging – the radiographs often show a destructive lesion (Fig. 2). The magnetic resonance imaging scan often shows a large soft tissue mass, and there may be a high level of periosteal reaction.
  - Staging evaluation – in addition to the computerized tomography scan and technetium bone scan, sampling of the iliac crest is often performed to look for bone marrow involvement. This sampling is most commonly done with bilateral iliac crest biopsies. In some centers, magnetic resonance imaging or positive emission tomography may be utilized.

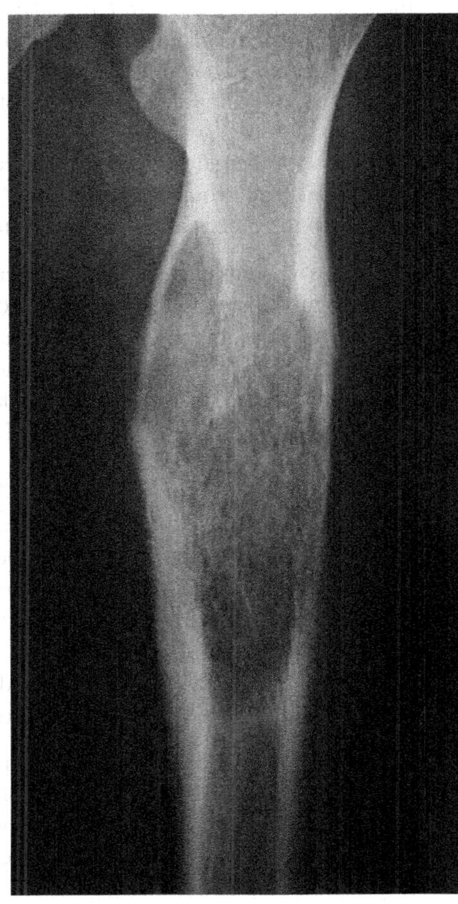

Fig. 2 Anteroposterior radiograph of the proximal femur showing a very destructive lesion, which is lytic with marked periosteal reaction. The differential diagnosis of this lesion can include osteosarcoma, Ewing's tumor, osteomyelitis, and eosinophilic granuloma

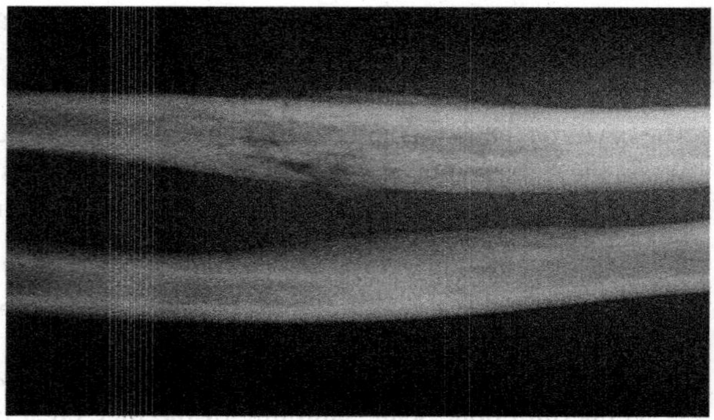

Fig. 3 Lateral radiograph showing a destructive lesion in the mid-shaft with lytic bone destruction and periosteal reaction

- Treatment – preoperative chemotherapy and wide resection are performed. Chemotherapy is also given postoperatively. Ewing's tumor is very sensitive to external beam irradiation so that patients may choose radiation as an alternative to surgery. Local failure is higher following radiation than surgery and there is of pathologic fracture following radiation. The risk of second sarcoma occurring in the irradiated bone is probably as high is five percent in the Ewing's patient. The prognosis for patients with localized disease is 60–70 %, while patients who prevent with metastases, it is less than 25 %.

- Osteomyelitis – hematogenous osteomyelitis is most commonly seen in the young patient (age group 10–40 years). Although, hematogenous osteomyelitis may occur in the older patient, the incidence is very low.
  - Imaging – radiographs show a destructive lesion, and it is often not possible to distinguish osteomyelitis from osteosarcoma, Ewing's tumor, and eosinophilic granuloma based on the radiographs alone. There is often a destructive lesion present with lytic bone formation and reactive new bone (Fig. 3). Periosteal reaction and cortical bone destruction are often present. The MRI scan will usually show low signal on T1 and high signal on T2. There is usually a large amount of edema (high signal on T2-weighted images) present.
  - Evaluation – in active disease the erythrocyte sedimentation rate and C-reactive protein are often elevated (but not always). There may be an elevation in the white blood cell count (or be completely normal).
  - Treatment – debridement of all the non-vascularized bone and antibiotics are usually necessary.

- Eosinophilic granuloma – this self-limited process often occurs in a single bone and can cause diagnostic confusion with other processes.
  - Imaging – although this lesion can mimic the appearance of many destructive processes, a punched out lesion in a long bone is the most common finding.
  - Evaluation – this lesion originates in the bone marrow so that evaluation with a skeletal survey or technetium bone scan can be used to evaluate for polyostotic lesions.
  - Treatment – injection with cortisone is a very common method of treatment.

Evaluation of Patients with a Soft Tissue Mass

Frank J. Frassica, Renee Genoa, and Gregory Osgood

Take-Home Message

- The most common MRI appearance of a sarcoma is a centripetal appearing mass that is low on T1-weighted images and high on T2.
- The most common sarcoma to mineralize is synovial sarcoma.
- Excisional biopsy should never be performed on an indeterminate mass.
- Lipomas are determinate masses and always completely suppress on fat suppression MRI techniques.
- The most common adult soft tissue sarcoma is malignant fibrous histiocytoma (also called undifferentiated sarcoma), and the thigh is the most common location.

The evaluation of a patient with a soft tissue mass is a very common problem that orthopedic surgeons will face. There are very features that help the clinician decide whether the mass is malignant or benign, so a very careful evaluation is necessary. The orthopedic surgeon has three choices as he or she plans treatment: (1) observation, (2) incisional or needle biopsy, and (3) excisional biopsy. Excisional biopsy is a very dangerous procedure to perform – the surgeon must be sure that the lesion is benign.

The first step is a radiograph to see if the underlying bone is involved or whether there is any mineralization in the mass. If there is mineralization in the mass, the differential diagnosis is often narrowed (Table 1).

F.J. Frassica, MD (✉) • G. Osgood, MD
Department of Orthopaedic Surgery, Johns Hopkins University, Baltimore, MD, USA
e-mail: fjfrassica@aol.com

R. Genoa, MD
Department of Orthopaedics, Johns Hopkins University, Baltimore, MD, USA

C. Mauffrey, D.J. Hak (eds.), *Passport for the Orthopedic Boards and FRCS Examination*, DOI 10.1007/978-2-8178-0475-0_49

Table 1 Mineralization in a soft tissue mass

Phleboliths	Round bodies with a lucent center	Hemangioma
Globular amorphous	Centered on a joint	Tumoral calcinosis
Zonal pattern	Mineralized at the periphery and lucent in the center	Heterotopic calcification
Scattered	Calcification or mineralization	Synovial sarcoma

Table 2 Determinate soft tissue masses

Lipoma
Ganglions
Heterotopic ossification
Soft tissue hemangioma
Schwannomas

A magnetic resonance imaging scan is often necessary to fully evaluate most lesions. The clinician and radiologist then study the imaging studies to determine if they can precisely identify the nature of the soft tissue mass. If they can determine the nature of the mass (determinate lesion), then treatment can proceed without obtaining a biopsy (Table 2). If, in contrast, the clinician and radiologist cannot determine the nature of the mass, then the soft tissue mass is indeterminate (Fig. 1). All indeterminate masses must be biopsied before treatment is initiated.

A typical lipoma is a determinate mass. The lipoma is the same high signal on T1-weighted images that subcutaneous fat is. With fat suppression, the lipoma completely loses its entire fat signal and is completely low signal. Lipomas can be removed with an excisional biopsy, and the margin can be intralesional or marginal.

Ganglions are also determinate masses. A ganglion is very low signal on T1-weighted images and very high signal on T2-weighted images. To be sure that the ganglion is a fluid-filled structure, contrast is added to the MRI study. The contrast will show the rim enhancement, which is seen in virtually all ganglions. The contrast accumulates around the thin capsule (hence the rim enhancement) and does not enhance in the center where there is avascular fluid. A ganglion can be removed with an intralesional or a marginal margin.

Heterotopic ossification is also a determinate lesion with very characteristic radiographic and MRI features. Radiographic or a computerized tomography scan shows mineralization at the periphery and lucency in the center.

Schwannomas and neurofibromas are benign nerve sheath tumors. Nerve sheath tumors sometimes show a very characteristic target sign on T2-weighted images. On T1-weighted images the lesion is low signal, while on T2-weighted images one will see high signal at the periphery and low signal in the center (target sign).

In contrast to determinate lesions which are always benign, all the sarcomas are indeterminate. One might guess that one is present, but it is impossible to predict the

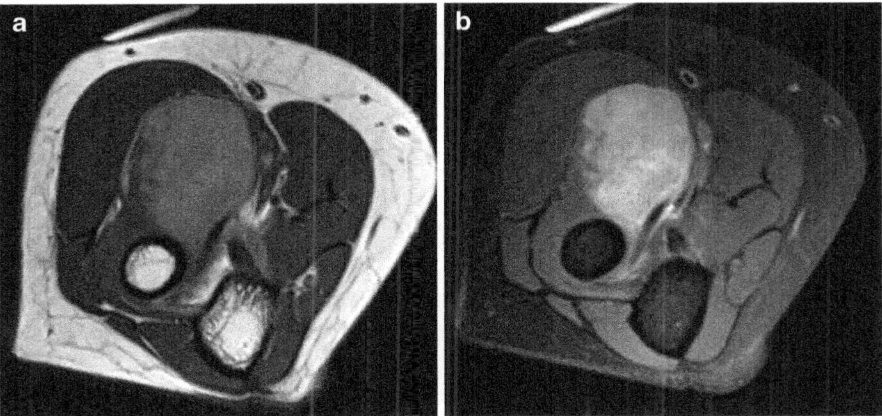

Fig. 1 (**a**) T1-weighted image showing a low signal mass in the proximal forearm. Notice the centripetal nature of the mass. This mass is indeterminate. (**b**) T2-weighted image with fat suppression showing a large centripetal mass in the proximal forearm. This mass is indeterminate in nature

Table 3 Common soft tissues sarcomas

Synovial sarcoma	1. 90 % not in a joint BUT 5–10 % intra-articular
	2. Most common soft tissue sarcoma of the foot and ankle
Epithelioid sarcoma	1. Most common soft tissue sarcoma in the hand
	2. Often presents as small soft tissue masses
Liposarcoma	1. Most common location is the thigh
	2. Usually the older patient
Malignant fibrous histiocytoma (also called undifferentiated sarcoma)	1. Most common location is the thigh

diagnosis with any certainty. In addition, many benign lesions also have an indeterminate appearance. This appearance is low signal on T1-weighted images and high signal on T2-weighted sequences. The only way to make a definitive diagnosis is for a biopsy to be done.

Certain sarcomas do occur more commonly in certain age groups and locations (Table 3). Soft tissue sarcomas are treated the same regardless of the different histologic diagnoses. Resection if the tumor with a cuff of normal tissue (wide margin) and irradiation are the mainstays of treatment. Many patients are also treated with chemotherapy. Children with rhabdomyosarcomas, soft tissue Ewing's tumor, and synovial sarcoma are always treated with chemotherapy. For adults, lesions that are below the fascia and greater than 8 cm in diameter are often treated with chemotherapy.

Characteristic Radiographic Appearances

Frank J. Frassica, Renee Genoa, and Gregory Osgood

Take-Home Message

- NOF have a characteristic radiographic appearance – metaphyseal, eccentric, a sclerotic rim, and involve the cortex. These lesions should be treated with observation if the lesion is asymptomatic.
- Enchondromas do not alter the cortex and should be treated by observation.
- Stress fractures have discordant radiographic findings – almost normal on T1 images and very high signal on T2.
- The radiographic appearance of Paget's disease is cortical thickening and coarsening of the bone trabeculae.
- Heterotopic ossification shows mineralization at the periphery and lucency in the center.

On the recertification examination, there are virtually no histology slides to interpret, but one does need to be able to interpret imaging studies. Certain lesions have a very characteristic appearance. These lesions include: non-ossifying fibroma, osteochondroma, enchondroma, stress fracture, Paget's disease, fibrous dysplasia, bone infarct, bone island, heterotopic ossification, unicameral bone cyst, and osteoid osteoma.

F.J. Frassica, MD (✉) • G. Osgood, MD
Department of Orthopaedic Surgery, Johns Hopkins University, Baltimore, MD, USA
e-mail: fjfrassica@aol.com

R. Genoa, MD
Department of Orthopaedics, Johns Hopkins University, Baltimore, MD, USA

C. Mauffrey, D.J. Hak (eds.), *Passport for the Orthopedic Boards and FRCS Examination*, DOI 10.1007/978-2-8178-0475-0_50

- Non-ossifying fibroma – this is a very common developmental abnormality that completely disappears as we age. These lesions are usually discovered incidentally when a child sustains trauma to the extremity. The vast majority of non-ossifying fibromas are asymptomatic, and treatment is simply observation.
  - Imaging appearance – most common locations are the distal femur, proximal tibia, or distal tibia (Fig. 1).
    - Metaphyseal.
    - Eccentric.
    - Sclerotic border.
    - Overlying cortex is thinned but intact.
- Osteochondroma – this is a very common developmental abnormality that occurs when a portion of the growth plate becomes entrapped in the surface of the bone. Solitary osteochondromas very seldom progress on to malignancy. If an osteochondroma is asymptomatic, the patient is treated by observation. If the patient has symptoms, then simple removal is necessary (intralesional or marginal margin).
  - Imaging appearance – most common locations are the distal femur, proximal tibia, distal tibia, proximal femur, and proximal humerus (Fig. 2).

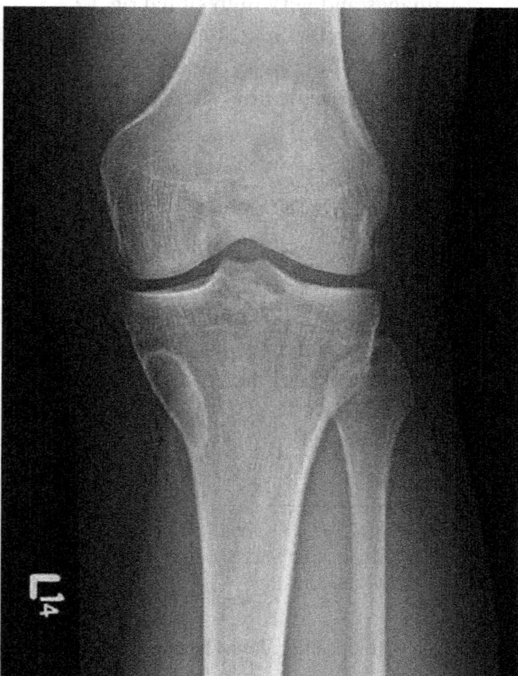

Fig. 1 Anteroposterior radiograph of the knee. Notice the lesion in the medial proximal tibia. This is a non-ossifying fibroma. The lesion is metaphyseal, eccentric, and has a sharply defined sclerotic rim, and thinning of the overlying cortex

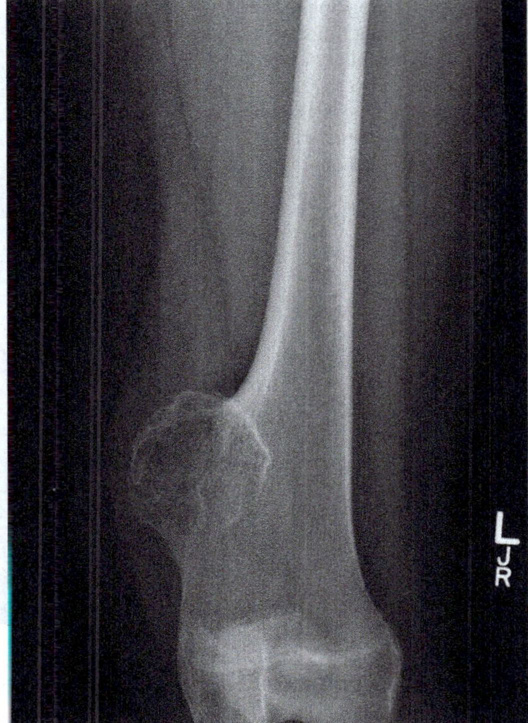

Fig. 2 Anteroposterior radiograph of the distal femur. Note the continuity of the medullary cavity and this lesion. There is also widening of the metaphysis. This is the typical appearance of an osteochondroma

- Metaphyseal or metaphyseal-diaphyseal
- Medullary cavity flows into the lesion
- Shares the cortex with the host bone
- Eccentric

- Enchondroma – this is a very common mineralized, intramedullary lesion in the adult. This lesion does not cause pain and is often discovered incidentally. Enchondromas of the long bones are always treated by careful observation.
  - Imaging appearance – common locations include the proximal humerus, distal femur, proximal tibia, and proximal tibia (Fig. 3).
    - Metaphyseal
    - Mineralized – rings, arcs, commas, stipples
    - No or very minor cortical changes
    - No cortical thickening, greater than 50 % endosteal erosions, soft tissue extension, cortical lysis
  - MRI appearance – this lesion sits in the medullary cavity with no suggestions of active growth
    - T1-weighted images – low signal
    - T2-weighted images – high signal

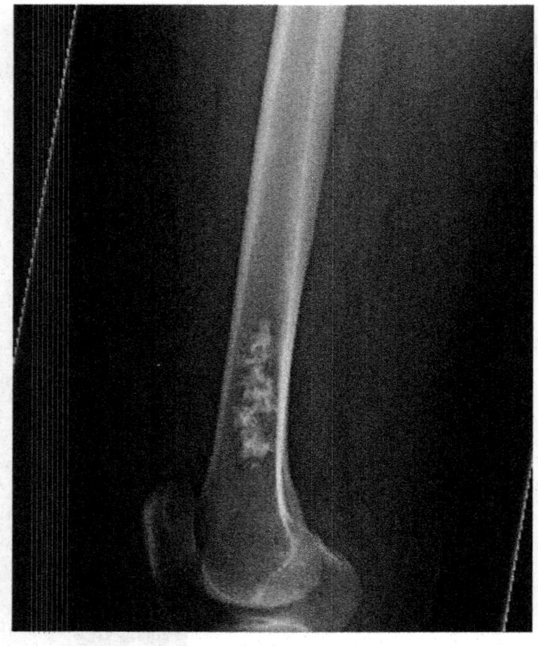

Fig. 3 Lateral radiograph of the distal femur showing rings, arcs, and commas in the medullary cavity. Notice that the cortices are not involved (no erosions, thickening, or lysis). This is the characteristic appearance of an enchondroma)

    - No peri-tumoral edema
    - No periosteal reaction

- Stress fracture – these injuries caused by repetitive stress occur in two age groups – young athletes (Fig. 4) and the geriatric patient (usually on bisphosphonates). For young athletes, the presentation is pain and difficulty ambulating. There is almost always a history of increased physical activity or mileage. In the older patient, there may or may not be a history of a fall or other injury. Patients who have been on long-term bisphosphonates are especially at risk.
  - Imaging – the radiographs are not very sensitive. If positive one can often see periosteal reaction or lysis within the cortex (gray cortex).
    - MRI is very sensitive for stress fractures, often described as discordant – minimal findings on T1-weighted images and very high signal on T2-weighted images.
      - T1-weighted images – low density streaking in the normal marrow
      - T2-weighted images – very high signal

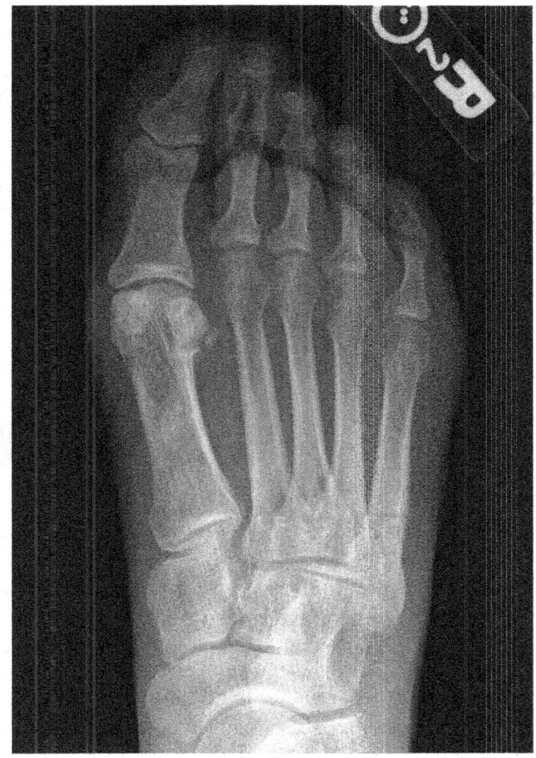

Fig. 4 Anteroposterior radiograph of the foot. Notice the transverse fracture of the shaft of the fifth metatarsal with periosteal reaction. This is a stress fracture

- Treatment
  - Young athletes – almost always nonoperative with reduced weight bearing. One major exception is the tension side of the femoral neck (pin fixation is necessary).
  - Geriatric patient – lesions in the femur do not reliably heal with nonoperative treatment necessitating internal fixation to prevent progression to a complete fracture and to allow healing.

- Paget's disease – this is a remodeling disease with a multifactorial etiology including viral, geographic, and genetic factors, There is resorption of the bone followed by bone formation. The bone is thickened and weakened to the point that multiple stress fractures and curvature of the bone occur.
  - Imaging – radiographs are often diagnostic (Fig. 5)

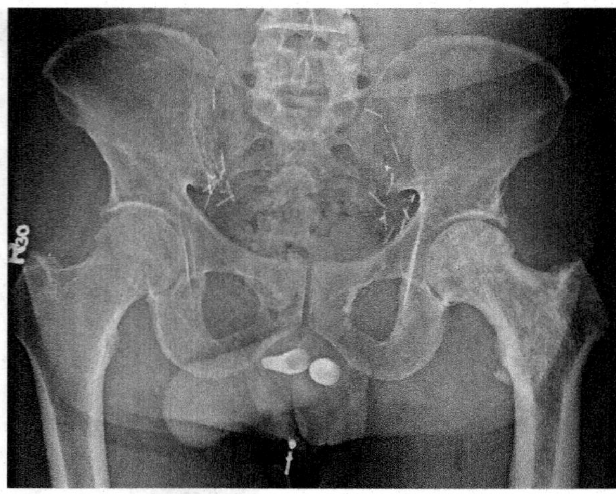

Fig. 5 Anteroposterior radiograph of the pelvis showing marked cortical thickening of the cortices of the right proximal femur. There is also coarsening of the bone trabeculae. This is the very characteristic appearance of Paget's disease

    - Coarsening of the bone trabeculae.
    - Cortical thickening.
    - Loss of definition between the cortex and medullary cavity.
    - Enlargement and bowing of the bone.
    - The cortex may be thickened but is always intact.
  - Three-dimensional imaging – computerized tomography or magnetic resonance imaging scans can be used to exclude degeneration into a sarcoma by detecting cortical bone destruction and a soft tissue mass. Conversion into a sarcoma occurs in about one percent of patients.
  - Treatment – therapy with a bisphosphonate is the main therapy. Patients with severe arthritis are treated with arthroplasty. Patients who have no symptoms are generally not treated.

- Fibrous dysplasia – this is a condition where a mutation occurs so that individuals lose the ability to form lamellar bone. This often involves a single bone but may affect all the bones on one side of the body.
  - Imaging – this lesion occurs in the medullary cavity and may expand the bone. The most characteristic appearance is the "ground glass" lesion (Fig. 6).
    - Intramedullary lesions with a "ground glass" appearance
    - Sclerotic rim around the lesion
    - May have deformity in the bone
  - Treatment – symptomatic treatment usually involves a corrective osteotomy or internal fixation of a stress fracture. Patients with no symptoms are treated by observation.

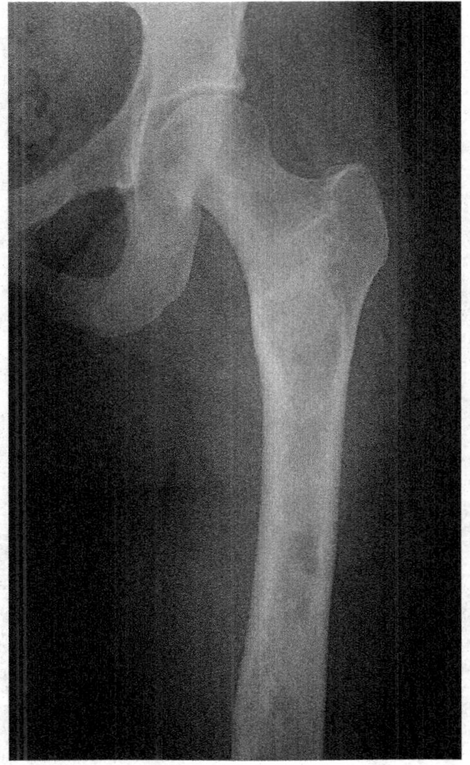

Fig. 6 Anteroposterior radiograph of the proximal femur with a ground glass intramedullary appearance. This is the typical appearance of fibrous dysplasia. This is a long lesion in a long bone

- Bone infarcts – there may be a number of etiologies including steroid use, alcohol, trauma, chemotherapy, and others.
  - Imaging – the most characteristic appearance is an intramedullary lesion with sclerotic rims and a lucent center. There is usually no involvement of the cortex or periosteal reaction (Fig. 7).
  - Treatment – these lesions that do not involve a joint surface do not require treatment.
- Bone island – this lesion is also called an enostosis. This is a developmental abnormality which never causes symptoms. The most common locations are the pelvis and proximal femur.
  - Imaging – well-demarcated sclerotic lesion often with speculated edges (Fig. 8).
  - Treatment – none is necessary.

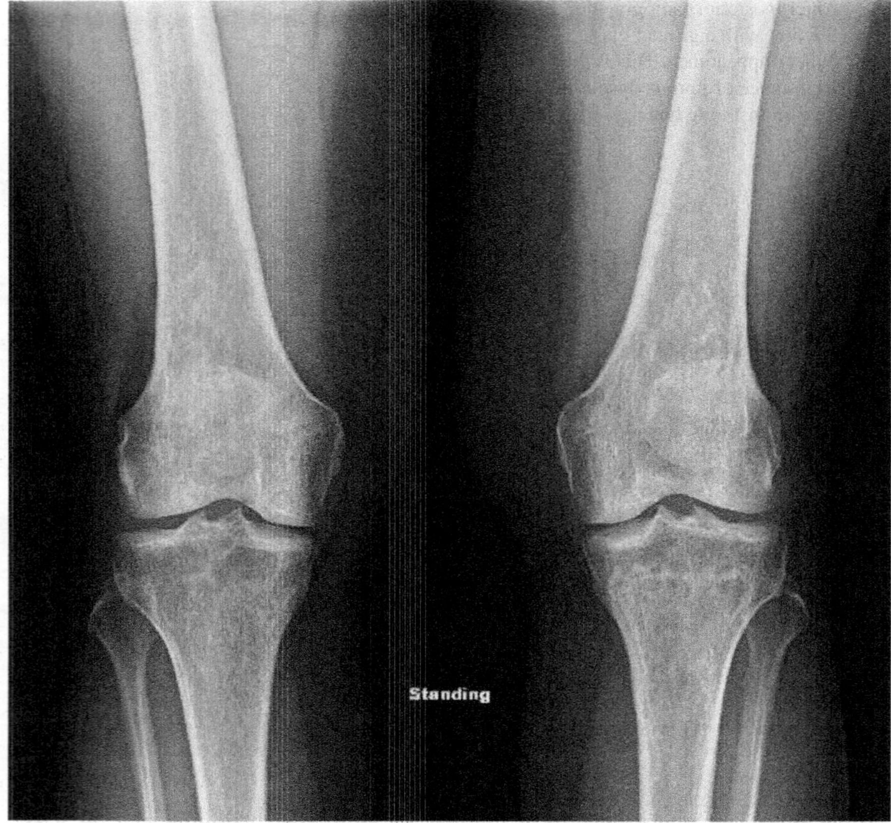

Fig. 7 Anteroposterior radiograph of the left and right knees. There are intramedullary lesions with sclerotic rims. Notice that the cortices are intact. This is the typical appearance of bone infarcts

- Heterotopic ossification – this lesion occurs in the muscle bellies of the quadriceps and brachialis muscles most commonly and always is secondary to a traumatic episode.
  - Imaging – mineralized at the periphery and lucent in the center
    - MRI
      - T1 – marked swelling of the involved muscle
      - T2 – high signal throughout the abnormal area
    - CT
      - Mineralized at the periphery
      - Lucent in the center

Fig. 8 Computerized tomography scan of the pelvis showing a densely sclerotic lesion in the ischium. This is a bone island

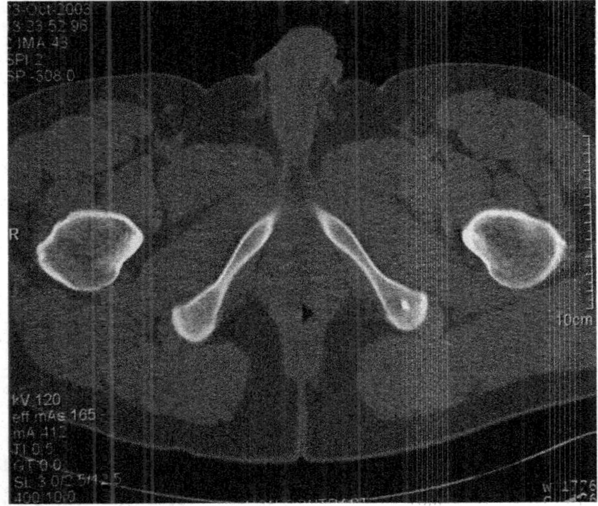

- Unicameral bone cyst – this lesion is most common in the proximal humerus and is found following minor trauma. There are usually no antecedent symptoms. The fracture heals quickly and is seldom displaced.
  - Imaging (Fig. 9)
    - Concentric thinning of all the cortices
    - Expansion equals that of the phases
    - Almost always open physes
    - Usually purely lucent
  - Treatment – when this lesion occurs in the proximal humerus, aspiration and cortisone injection are usually employed. When the lesion occurs in the proximal femur, curettage, bone grafting, and internal fixation are necessary.
- Osteoid osteoma – this lesion occurs in patients less than 45 years old and is associated with severe, constant pain. The pain is completely relieved by aspirin or nonsteroidal anti-inflammatory medication.
  - Imaging – a small round or oval lucent area is seen on the radiograph or CT scan (Fig. 10).
    - 5–15 mm lucent nidus
    - Surrounding sclerosis
    - Central ossification of the lesion
  - Treatment – percutaneous radiofrequency ablation

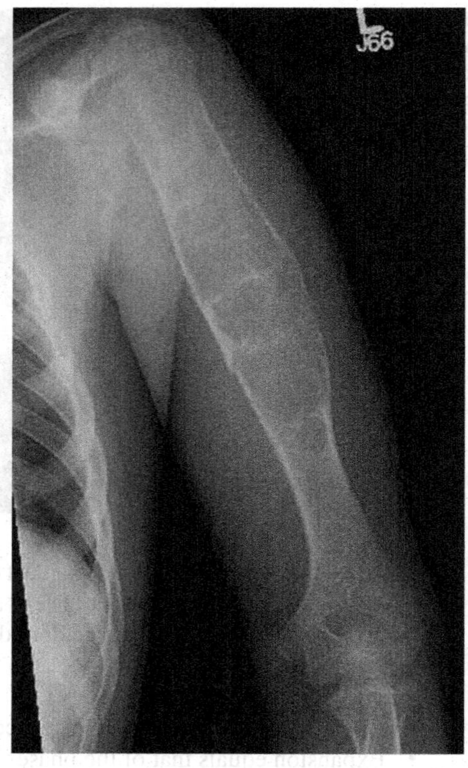

Fig. 9 Anteroposterior view of the humerus in an adolescent. Notice that all the cortices are thinned and there is mild symmetric expansion. This is the typical appearance of unicameral bone cyst

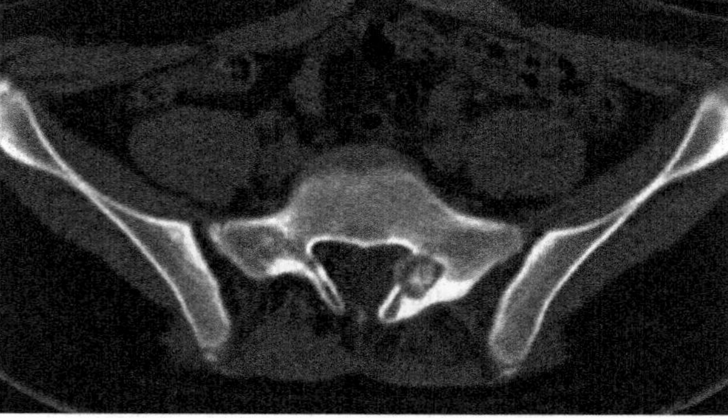

Fig. 10 Computerized tomography scan of the pelvis with a round to oval nidus in the posterior elements. Note the central mineralization and surrounding sclerosis. This is an osteoid osteoma

Bibliography

1. Fayad LM, Kamel IR, Kawamoto S, Bluemke DA, Frassica FJ, Fishman EK. Distinguishing stress fractures from pathologic fractures: a multimodality approach. Skeletal Radiol. 2005;34(5):245–59.
2. Frassica FJ, Frassica DA, McCarthy EF, Riley LH, III. Metastatic bone disease: evaluation, clinicopathologic features, biopsy, fracture risk, nonsurgical treatment, and supportive management. Instr Course Lect. 2000;49:453–9.
3. Frassica FJ, Khanna JA, McCarthy EF. The role of MR imaging in soft tissue tumor evaluation: perspective of the orthopedic oncologist and musculoskeletal pathologist. Magn Reson Imaging Clin North Am. 2000;8(4):915–27.
4. Frassica FJ, McCarthy EF, Bluemke DA. Soft-tissue masses: when and how to biopsy. Instr Course Lect. 2000;49:437–42.
5. Frassica FJ, Thompson RC, Jr. Evaluation, diagnosis, and classification of benign soft-tissue tumors. Instr Course Lect. 1996;45:447–60.
6. Ma LD, McCarthy EF, Bluemke DA, Frassica FJ. Differentiation of benign from malignant musculoskeletal lesions using MR imaging: pitfalls in MR evaluation of lesions with a cystic appearance. AJR Am J Roentgenol. 1998;170(5):1251–8.
7. Papp DF, Khanna AJ, McCarthy EF, Carrino JA, Farber AJ, Frassica FJ. Magnetic resonance imaging of soft-tissue tumors: determinate and indeterminate lesions. J Bone Joint Surg Am. 2007;89(Suppl 3):103–15.
8. Rougraff BT, Frassica FJ. Presentation and staging of metastatic bone disease. Clin Orthop Relat Res. 2003;415S:S129–S131.
9. Weber KL, Peabody T, Frassica FJ, Mott MP, Parsons TW 3rd. Tumors for the general orthopedist: how to save your patients and practice. Instr Course Lect. 2010;59:579–91.

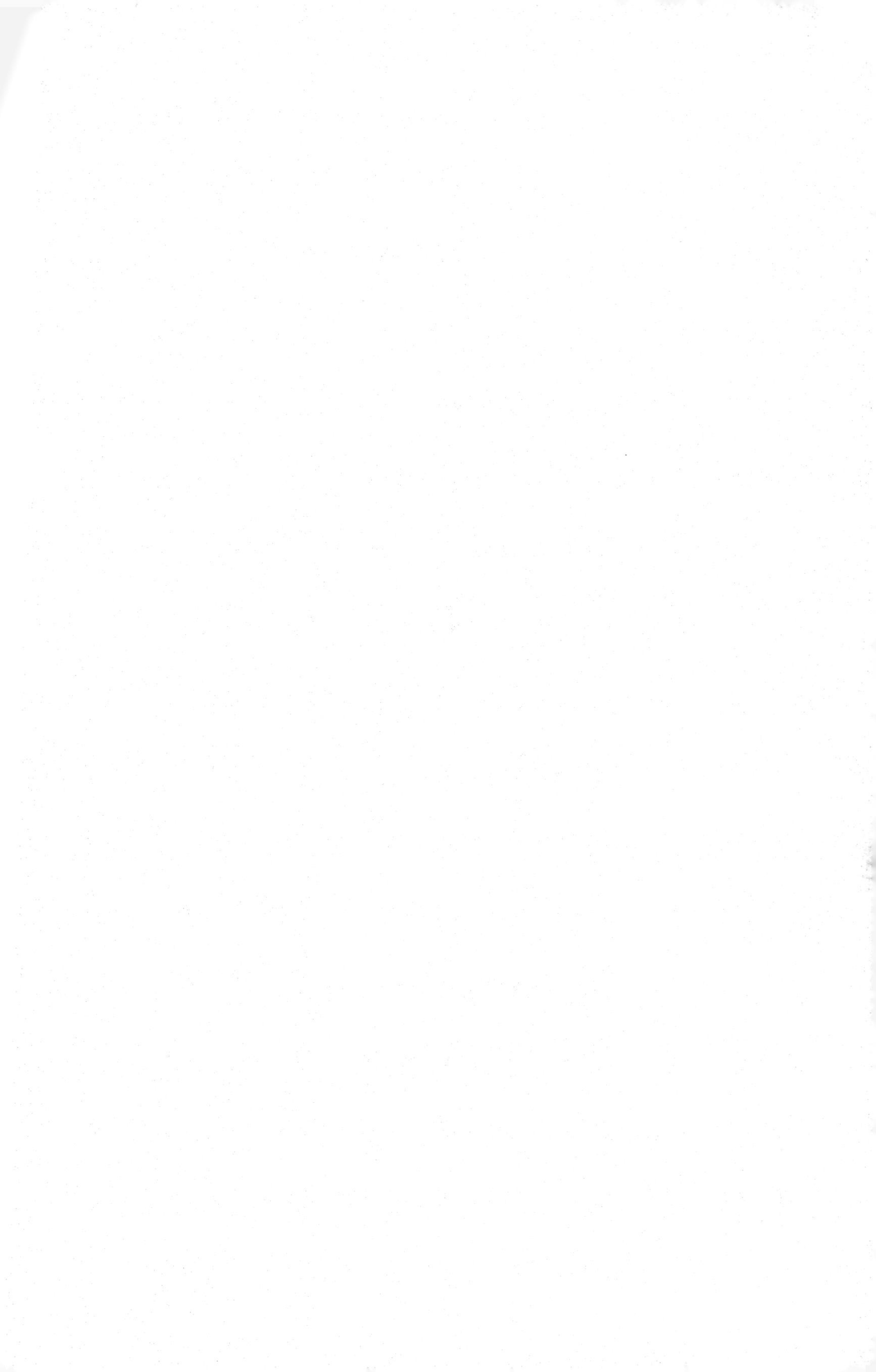

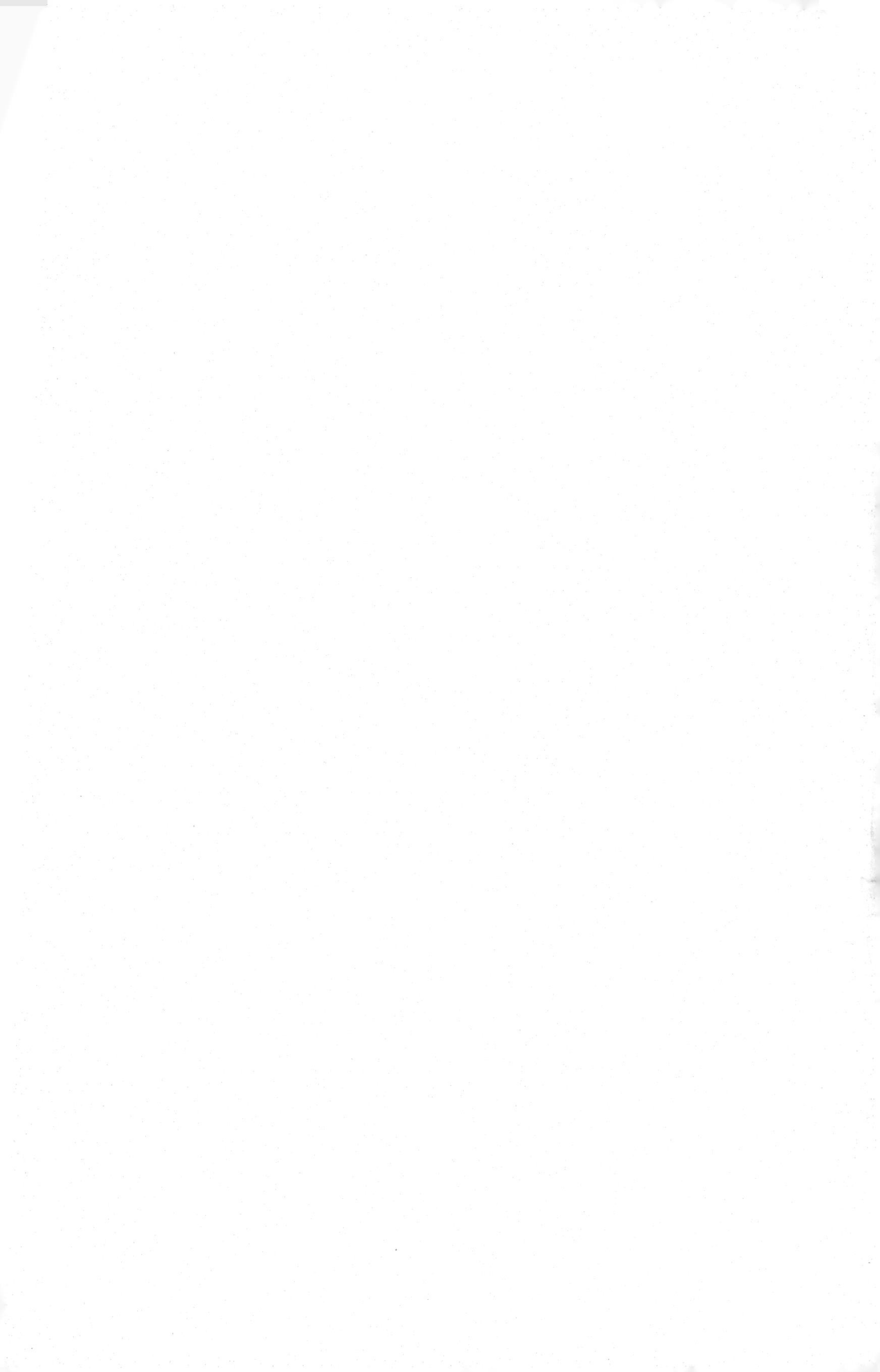

Printed by Printforce, United Kingdom